Metastatic Progression and Tumour Heterogeneity

Metastatic Progression and Tumour Heterogeneity

Special Issue Editors

Frédéric Hollande
Delphine Merino

MDPI • Basel • Beijing • Wuhan • Barcelona • Belgrade • Manchester • Tokyo • Cluj • Tianjin

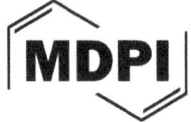

Special Issue Editors
Frédéric Hollande
University of Melbourne
Australia

Delphine Merino
Olivia Newton-John Cancer Research Institute
Australia

Editorial Office
MDPI
St. Alban-Anlage 66
4052 Basel, Switzerland

This is a reprint of articles from the Special Issue published online in the open access journal *Cancers* (ISSN 2072-6694) (available at: https://www.mdpi.com/journal/cancers/special_issues/tumour_heterogeneity).

For citation purposes, cite each article independently as indicated on the article page online and as indicated below:

LastName, A.A.; LastName, B.B.; LastName, C.C. Article Title. *Journal Name* **Year**, *Article Number*, Page Range.

ISBN 978-3-03928-853-3 (Hbk)
ISBN 978-3-03928-854-0 (PDF)

Cover image courtesy of Carolyn Shembrey.

© 2020 by the authors. Articles in this book are Open Access and distributed under the Creative Commons Attribution (CC BY) license, which allows users to download, copy and build upon published articles, as long as the author and publisher are properly credited, which ensures maximum dissemination and a wider impact of our publications.

The book as a whole is distributed by MDPI under the terms and conditions of the Creative Commons license CC BY-NC-ND.

Contents

About the Special Issue Editors vii

Preface to "Metastatic Progression and Tumour Heterogeneity" ix

Beatriz P. San Juan, Maria J. Garcia-Leon, Laura Rangel, Jacky G. Goetz and
Christine L. Chaffer
The Complexities of Metastasis
Reprinted from: *Cancers* **2019**, *11*, 1575, doi:10.3390/cancers11101575 1

Miriam Teeuwssen and Riccardo Fodde
Cell Heterogeneity and Phenotypic Plasticity in Metastasis Formation: The Case of
Colon Cancer
Reprinted from: *Cancers* **2019**, *11*, 1368, doi:10.3390/cancers11091368 23

Alexandr Samocha, Hanna Doh, Kai Kessenbrock and Jeroen P. Roose
Unraveling Heterogeneity in Epithelial Cell Fates of the Mammary Gland and Breast Cancer
Reprinted from: *Cancers* **2019**, *11*, 1423, doi:10.3390/cancers11101423 43

James H. Monkman, Erik W. Thompson and Shivashankar H. Nagaraj
Targeting Epithelial Mesenchymal Plasticity in Pancreatic Cancer: A Compendium of
Preclinical Discovery in a Heterogeneous Disease
Reprinted from: *Cancers* **2019**, *11*, 1745, doi:10.3390/cancers11111745 63

Nako Maishi, Dorcas A. Annan, Hiroshi Kikuchi, Yasuhiro Hida and Kyoko Hida
Tumor Endothelial Heterogeneity in Cancer Progression
Reprinted from: *Cancers* **2019**, *11*, 1511, doi:10.3390/cancers11101511355 95

Jamie R. Kutasovic, Amy E. McCart Reed, Anna Sokolova, Sunil R. Lakhani and
Peter T. Simpson
Morphologic and Genomic Heterogeneity in the Evolution and Progression of Breast Cancer
Reprinted from: *Cancers* **2020**, *12*, 848, doi:10.3390/cancers12040848 111

Su Bin Lim, Chwee Teck Lim and Wan-Teck Lim
Single-Cell Analysis of Circulating Tumor Cells: Why Heterogeneity Matters
Reprinted from: *Cancers* **2019**, *11*, 1595, doi:10.3390/cancers11101595 133

Carolyn Shembrey, Nicholas D. Huntington and Frédéric Hollande
Impact of Tumor and Immunological Heterogeneity on the Anti-Cancer Immune Response
Reprinted from: *Cancers* **2019**, *11*, 1217, doi:10.3390/cancers11091217 155

Helen Tower, Meagan Ruppert and Kara Britt
The Immune Microenvironment of Breast Cancer Progression
Reprinted from: *Cancers* **2019**, *11*, 1375, doi:10.3390/cancers11091375 179

Susanna Leskela, Belen Pérez-Mies, Juan Manuel Rosa-Rosa, Eva Cristobal,
Michele Biscuola, María L. Palacios-Berraquero, SuFey Ong, Xavier Matias-Guiu Guia and
José Palacios
Molecular Basis of Tumor Heterogeneity in Endometrial Carcinosarcoma
Reprinted from: *Cancers* **2019**, *11*, 964, doi:10.3390/cancers11070964 195

Lehang Lin and De-Chen Lin
Biological Significance of Tumor Heterogeneity in Esophageal Squamous Cell Carcinoma
Reprinted from: *Cancers* **2019**, *11*, 1156, doi:10.3390/cancers11081156 217

Estíbaliz López-Fernández and José I. López
The Impact of Tumor Eco-Evolution in Renal Cell Carcinoma Sampling
Reprinted from: *Cancers* **2018**, *10*, 485, doi:10.3390/cancers10120485 231

Clément Bailly, Caroline Bodet-Milin, Mickaël Bourgeois, Sébastien Gouard, Catherine Ansquer, Matthieu Barbaud, Jean-Charles Sébille, Michel Chérel, Françoise Kraeber-Bodéré and Thomas Carlier
Exploring Tumor Heterogeneity Using PET Imaging: The Big Picture
Reprinted from: *Cancers* **2019**, *11*, 1282, doi:10.3390/cancers11091282 241

Camille Evrard, Gaëlle Tachon, Violaine Randrian, Lucie Karayan-Tapon and David Tougeron
Microsatellite Instability: Diagnosis, Heterogeneity, Discordance, and Clinical Impact in Colorectal Cancer
Reprinted from: *Cancers* **2019**, *11*, 1567, doi:10.3390/cancers11101567 5 259

David E. Korenchan and Robert R. Flavell
Spatiotemporal pH Heterogeneity as a Promoter of Cancer Progression and Therapeutic Resistance
Reprinted from: *Cancers* **2019**, *11*, 1026, doi:10.3390/cancers11071026 285

About the Special Issue Editors

Frédéric Hollande obtained his PhD in 1994 from the University of Montpellier, France. He worked as a Research Fellow for CNRS (France) from 1996 to 2012, studying molecular mechanisms that underlie the progression of colon cancer. In parallel with his academic work, he co-founded in 2007 a small biotech company developing therapeutic monoclonal antibodies. He was the joint-scientific director of this company and designed its Intellectual Property portfolio until 2011. Fred also headed the Oncology Research Department at the Institute of Functional Genomics of Montpellier in 2011–2012. Fred moved to Melbourne in September 2012 to take up a position at the Department of Pathology at the University of Melbourne. He currently is the Deputy Head of Department @ Dept of Clinical Pathology. He leads a research group and a tumour organoid platform at the University of Melbourne Centre for Cancer Research, located within the Victorian Comprehensive Cancer Centre. His research interests include the analysis of cancer stem cell regulation by their surrounding environment, as well as the study of the impact of inter and intra-tumour heterogeneity on metastatic progression and treatment response. His work focuses on cancers with poor clinical outcomes, such as advanced/metastatic colorectal cancer and, more recently, pancreatic cancer.

Delphine Merino is a faculty member and laboratory head at the Olivia Newton-John Cancer Research Institute, in Melbourne, Australia. Her current research interests are focussed on understanding the cellular and molecular events regulating breast cancer progression and drug resistance. Her team uses patient samples and patient-derived xenografts to dissect the journey of human metastases and to study tumour heterogeneity. A major focus of Dr Merino's research is on identifying the survival pathways responsible for the spread of cancer cells to different metastatic sites. Understanding how cancer cells survive in their microenvironment and resist current treatments will ultimately lead to the identification of new therapies for the treatment of advanced breast cancer.

Preface to "Metastatic Progression and Tumour Heterogeneity"

Tumor heterogeneity is one of the biggest current challenges for cancer therapy. Exciting developments in single-cell -omics, cellular tracking, and imaging, alongside the expansion of new tools to study patient samples enable a deeper understanding of the molecular mechanisms that drive tumor progression. These approaches have recently highlighted the broad inter- and intra-tumoral heterogeneity that exists amongst patient cohorts and across tumor streams, while longitudinal studies indicate that the diversity of malignant cell populations that make up primary tumors and metastases can evolve in space and time.

Furthermore, the cellular and molecular features of the tumor microenvironment, including immune cells, have to be taken into consideration for the understanding of tumor progression. Targeting both tumor cells and tumor microenvironment is also an exciting area of investigation, with new approaches such as immunotherapy now emerging as powerful treatment alternatives.

Thus, comprehensive analyses of tumor heterogeneity are essential to both improve the overall treatment of patients with cancer and further progress towards precision medicine. This Special Issue highlights some of the state-of-the-art technologies aiming to dissect the heterogeneity of malignant cells and their microenvironment and will cover some of the promising discoveries that are likely to improve cancer patients' outcome.

Frédéric Hollande, Delphine Merino
Special Issue Editors

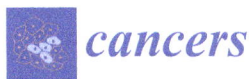

Review

The Complexities of Metastasis

Beatriz P. San Juan [1,2,†], Maria J. Garcia-Leon [3,4,5,†], Laura Rangel [1,2], Jacky G. Goetz [3,4,5,*,‡] and Christine L. Chaffer [1,2,*,‡]

1. The Kinghorn Cancer Centre, Garvan Institute of Medical Research, Darlinghurst 2010, Australia; b.perez@garvan.org.au (B.P.S.J.); l.rangel@garvan.org.au (L.R.)
2. St Vincent's Clinical School, University of New South Wales Medicine, University of New South Wales, Darlinghurst 2010, Australia
3. INSERM UMR_S1109, Tumor Biomechanics, 67000 Strasbourg, France; m.garcia@inserm.fr
4. Université de Strasbourg, 67000 Strasbourg, France
5. Fédération de Médecine Translationnelle de Strasbourg (FMTS), 67000 Strasbourg, France
* Correspondence: jacky.goetz@inserm.fr (J.G.G.); c.chaffer@garvan.org.au (C.L.C.)
† These authors contributed equally to this manuscript.
‡ Co-senior authors.

Received: 13 September 2019; Accepted: 11 October 2019; Published: 16 October 2019

Abstract: Therapies that prevent metastatic dissemination and tumor growth in secondary organs are severely lacking. A better understanding of the mechanisms that drive metastasis will lead to improved therapies that increase patient survival. Within a tumor, cancer cells are equipped with different phenotypic and functional capacities that can impact their ability to complete the metastatic cascade. That phenotypic heterogeneity can be derived from a combination of factors, in which the genetic make-up, interaction with the environment, and ability of cells to adapt to evolving microenvironments and mechanical forces play a major role. In this review, we discuss the specific properties of those cancer cell subgroups and the mechanisms that confer or restrict their capacity to metastasize.

Keywords: metastasis; heterogeneity; plasticity; epithelial-to-mesenchymal transition; biomechanics; circulating tumor cells (CTCs); extracellular vesicles; metastatic niche; epigenetics; CTC-clusters

---

1. Cancer Cell Heterogeneity: A Hierarchical Matter?

1.1. Cancer Origin and Evolution

A normal cell transforms into a cancer cell by accrual of multiple genetic mutations over time, which ultimately lead to uncontrolled cellular proliferation. Genetic drift may arise from a combination of germline or spontaneous mutations, exposure to environmental carcinogens, genome rearrangements, and/or increased genome instability [1]. Those genetic changes can subsequently impact a cancer cell's epigenetic landscape by changing chromatin regulatory machinery or by aberrant expression of transcription factors that normally drive cellular differentiation and specify cellular fate [2]. To add to that complexity, the genomic/epigenomic drivers of a cancer can change over time. Standard-of-care treatment for most solid tumors comprises a series of aggressive chemotherapies that, in combination with aberrant cancer cell divisions and fluctuating microenvironmental landscapes, create opportunity for cancer cells to further mutate, adapt, and evolve, often toward a more aggressive phenotype. In this way, genetic and epigenetic modifications create phenotypic and functional heterogeneity [3] that fuel tumor progression and, consequently, represent a major therapeutic obstacle [4].

1.2. A Cancer Cell Hierarchy

Notwithstanding the genetic component to cancer development and progression, it is also well established that epigenetic mechanisms can create functional heterogeneity in genetically identical cancer cells, which is fundamentally important to tumor growth and metastasis. That notion is solidified in the idea that genetically identical cancer cells can be hierarchically organized according to phenotype, in this case, tumor-initiating potential [5–9]. At the top of the hierarchy sit the aggressive cancer stem cells (CSCs, or tumor-initiating cells), which, in a manner akin to stem cell divisions in normal tissues, self-renew to maintain the tumor-initiating cell pool or divide asymmetrically to produce non-tumor-initiating cell progeny (Figure 1). The balance between self-renewal and differentiation is determined by a combination of cell-intrinsic and environmental factors, which can dynamically impact cellular heterogeneity observed within a tumor. Generally, a higher percentage of tumor-initiating cells is associated with more aggressive and metastatic tumors [10,11]. With the unique capacity to fuel tumor growth, to metastasize, and to resist therapeutic treatment, attempts to better identify and functionally characterize those aggressive cells are of great interest.

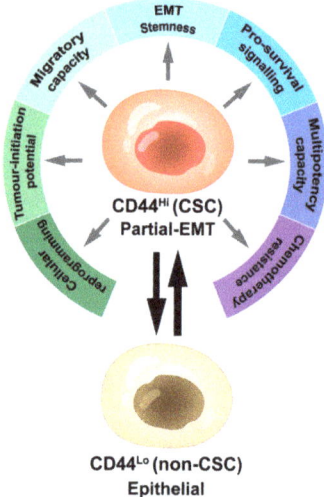

Figure 1. Schematic overview of cancer cell phenotypic heterogeneity. Cancer cells with an identical genetic background can be hierarchically organized according to cell phenotype. CD44^{Hi} cancer stem cells (CSC) are an aggressive cell type that have likely undergone a partial-epithelial-to-mesenchymal transition (partial-EMT) to acquire multiple biological traits that enhance their tumorigenic and metastatic potential. Cells residing in a CD44^{Hi} CSC state sit at the top of the hierarchy, where they can self-renew to maintain the aggressive CSC pool or, alternatively, undergo asymmetric divisions to form more differentiated CD44^{Lo} (non-CSC) progeny. In some cancer types, CD44^{Lo} epithelial cells have the potential to ascend the hierarchy and enter into the aggressive CD44^{Hi} state.

The origins of tumor-initiating cells are not yet clearly defined; however, it has been hypothesized that they may arise via oncogenic transformation of normal tissue stem or progenitor cells [12–14]. Alternatively, tumor-initiating cells may also arise via reversion of non-tumor-initiating cancer cells into a tumor-initiating cell state [7,10,15]. That idea is conceptually important as it implies that tumor-initiating cells can be continually replenished throughout tumorigenesis. Moreover, it provides a mechanism for non-aggressive tumors to transition toward more aggressive and metastatic disease. Accordingly, the characterization of signaling mechanisms that generate and maintain highly tumorigenic, metastatic, and chemotherapy-resistant tumor-initiating cells should provide novel avenues for therapeutic design. In that regard, the development of new technologies, such as single-cell sequencing [16,17] and barcoding-based functional assays [9,18–20], applied to clinically relevant models, should be able to address these issues in the near future.

1.3. CD44: Defining Aggressive Cancer Cells

The use of membrane-anchored protein markers to distinguish subpopulations of aggressive cancer cells has proven a useful tool in cancer research [21–25]. In a wide variety of solid tumors, including those of breast [6], gastric [26], pancreas [27], ovary and colon [28–30], and also in blood malignancies [31], residence in, or transition into the aggressive tumor-initiating cell state can be monitored by high expression of the cancer stem cell marker CD44—where the nomenclature CD44^{Hi} represents cells enriched for that aggressive cancer cell phenotype [32–36]. The CD44 molecule can exist in a variety of splice isoforms that are functionally important. Recent findings link the expression of different CD44 isoform variants with cancer progression and specific tumor cell features, including pro-survival signaling [37], cellular reprogramming [38], acquisition of migratory capacity [39], and tumor initiation [40–42]. CD44 can also facilitate the arrest of circulating tumor cells prior to extravasation [43]. Together, these findings emphasize the cellular and molecular heterogeneity that exists within cancer cell populations, which belie the power of bulk population analyses to define putative therapeutic options.

1.3.1. CD44^{Lo} versus CD44^{Hi} Cells: Epithelial versus Mesenchymal Cell States

Compared to the bulk tumor mass, the aggressive CD44^{Hi} cancer stem cell subpopulation is often associated with loss of epithelial characteristics and gain of mesenchymal traits [10,15]. Consistent with those findings, activation of the epithelial-to-mesenchymal transition (EMT) program is one means by which poorly aggressive CD44^{Lo} epithelial cancer cells gain entrance into a more aggressive CD44^{Hi} cancer stem-like state [44–46]. The EMT transcription factors SNAI1 (snail family transcriptional repressor 1), SNAI2, ZEB1 (zinc finger E-box binding homeobox 1), among others, are key mediators of that process [47]. Indeed, ZEB1 also drives splicing of CD44 in a manner that promotes tumorigenicity, recurrence, and drug-resistance [48,49]. Along with the acquisition of cancer stem-like traits, the EMT also increases a cancer cell's ability to invade and migrate, promotes cancer cell spread away from the primary tumor, entrance into the circulation, and extravasation at a secondary site [50]. In line with those findings, single-cell expression analysis of disseminated tumor cells isolated from breast cancer patient-derived xenograft (PDX) models at early stages of metastatic disease display gene expression profiles consistent with the EMT [17]. Additional studies in preclinical models also establish a correlation between existence of mesenchymal CSC populations and metastatic burden, and that inhibiting EMT-transcription factor expression abolishes tumor-initiation and metastatic potential of aggressive cancer cells [51,52]. Moreover, loss of an epithelial phenotype and gain of mesenchymal features correlates with poor clinical outcome in some tumor types [53–58].

1.3.2. Novel Markers to Define Metastatic Cells

The search for additional markers to refine the aggressive cancer stem cell population has revealed that the CD44^{Hi} cancer cell compartment is heterogeneous and encompasses a variety of phenotypic cell states [6,59,60]. For example, expression of the marker CD24 has been used to distinguish between different cancer cell phenotypes, where enhanced tumor-initiating potential correlates with residence in a CD44^{Hi}CD24^{Lo} state and the CD44^{Hi}CD24^{Hi} cell state is further associated with tolerance to chemotherapy [61]. In addition, a recent study showed a novel role for integrin β4 (CD104) in the regulation of cell transitions across the epithelial–mesenchymal spectrum, where CD44^{Hi}CD104$^+$ cells reside in a more epithelial state than their CD44^{Hi}CD104$^-$ counterparts [60]. That study characterized a CD104 expression 'sweet spot' for tumor-initiating potential that defined a CD44^{Hi}CD104$^+$ intermediate epithelial–mesenchymal state [60]. Furthermore, a follow-up study demonstrated that non-canonical WNT signaling drives CD44^{Hi} cells through the CD104$^+$ to CD104$^-$ transition with a concomitant shift from a partial-EMT state to a mesenchymal state. That phenotypic change is indeed associated with a significant decrease in tumor-initiating potential, suggesting that retention of certain epithelial characteristics, i.e., a partial-EMT state, provides optimal tumorigenicity [54,62–66].

2. Cancer Cell Plasticity: Shaping Metastatic Fitness

We and others have shown that CD44^{Lo} cell populations are not locked in their epithelial state, rather they can transition into the aggressive CD44^{Hi} state via activation of components of the EMT program [15,33,35,44]. Those findings suggest that poorly tumorigenic CD44^{Lo} cells may also have the intrinsic potential to seed metastases by transitioning into a CD44^{Hi} state, albeit with far more biological effort than pre-existing CD44^{Hi} cells. If true, CD44^{Lo} cells may also be present at very early stages of metastatic dissemination. Accordingly, while pre-existing CD44^{Hi} cells are highly enriched for metastatic potential, defining a tumor's CD44^{Hi} content at one specific time point may not adequately capture the tumor's true metastatic potential. Additionally, and although yet to be clarified, it has been suggested that certain tumor cells are more suited to sense, compute, and respond to signals from their microenvironment that initiate the EMT program [44]. Indeed, we have previously identified that tumor cells maintaining the ZEB1 promoter in a bivalent chromatin configuration are highly conducive to activating the EMT program, or part thereof. In contrast, tumor cells that maintain the ZEB1 promoter in a repressed state are less likely to undergo the EMT [44]. Together, these studies suggest that strategies designed to prevent cellular plasticity combined with strategies to eradicate existing CD44^{Hi} cells will be required to treat cancer effectively.

3. The Seed, the Journey, and the Soil: The Metastatic Cascade

Metastasis is initiated when cells migrate away from the primary tumor and invade into neighboring tissue toward blood or lymphatic vessels. After vessel wall barrier transmigration (intravasation), the invasive cells, now referred to as circulating tumor cells (CTCs), are exposed to a variety of arduous conditions, including a novel microenvironment, exposure to new cell types and signals, anchorage-independent growth, and shear forces from the blood flow. As such, survival in the circulation poses an extremely harsh selection process that very few CTCs can withstand. While CTCs are indeed detected in the majority of patients with carcinoma [67,68], it has been suggested that as few as 1–4% of CTCs successfully complete the metastatic cascade and successfully form metastatic foci [67–70]. That inefficiency suggests that CTC intrinsic features likely co-operate with surrounding tumor stroma and vascular environments to determine overall metastatic success [71,72]. CTCs thus represent a minority subpopulation of a patient's tumor, where the role of hemodynamic forces, endothelial fitness, and blood cells are capital for tuning CTC metastatic potential. CD44^{Hi} tumor-initiating cells and the EMT program endow cancer cells with the very ability to survive these arduous conditions. Indeed, studies analyzing CTCs in human patients are enriched for an EMT phenotype [73,74].

3.1. Entering the Circulation, Off They Go

Tumor cells invade into their surrounding tissues toward the lymphatic and/or vascular circulation as single mesenchymal or amoeboid cell types, or collectively as epithelial sheets or clumps [75,76]. A common way for tumor cells to gain access to the circulation is via disruption of tumor vasculature integrity that enables transendothelial migration. That process is enhanced in the setting of tumor-induced chronic inflammation [77], where endothelial cell integrity and selective permeability are lost [78]. Endothelial disruption is predominantly caused by tumor infiltrating leukocytes, such as neutrophils [79,80] and macrophages [81], that communicate with tumor cells to promote intravasation by facilitating angiogenesis together with the breakdown and remodeling of the extracellular matrix [82]. In fact, macrophage depletion in mice completely abrogates breast cancer metastasis. Endothelial integrity disruption also exposes extracellular matrix proteins such as von Willebrand factor (vWF), collagen, or fibronectin, which in turn, recruit and activate platelets that act in concert to further tune tumor cell intravasation [83,84] (Figure 2). Interestingly, and together with cytokines and growth factors secreted by the tumor stroma, activated platelets at tumor vessel disruption sites can directly contribute to the initial invasive phenotype of tumor cells by the release of transforming growth factor beta TGFβ [85,86]. Indeed, platelet-derived TGFβ can induce the EMT in tumor cells entering the circulation [85,87].

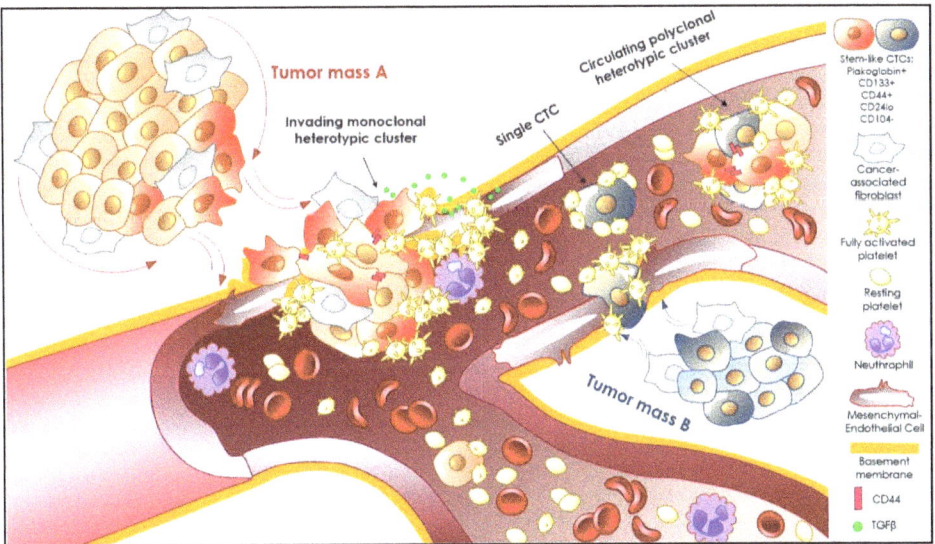

Figure 2. From invasion into the circulation. Tumor cells can reach the vasculature and enter the circulation as single circulating tumor cells (CTCs) or CTC clusters. The latter may show a variable degree of complexity according to cell heterogeneity within the primary tumor (tumor mass A) and/or the cells encountered during the process of intravasation and in the circulation, such as blood cells (e.g., platelets, neutrophils) or due to encounters with tumor cells from a different primary site (tumor mass B). Cancer cells within the primary tumor can reside in diverse stages of differentiation along an epithelial-to-mesenchymal spectrum. Cells that display mesenchymal features may have enhanced survival, proliferation, and invasiveness and express cancer stem-like markers, including the adhesion molecules CD44 or plakoglobin. Homotypic interactions between tumor cells, mediated by CD44 among others, may lead to the formation of a CTC cluster. At the moment of intravasation, disruption of endothelial integrity by invasive tumor cells exposes extracellular matrix proteins (yellow line) including von Willebrand factor (vWF), collagen, or fibronectin, which recruit and activate blood platelets. In turn, platelets secrete transforming growth factor beta TGFβ, among many other angiogenic and pro-inflammatory factors that can induce tumor cells to undergo the EMT and induce a mesenchymal phenotype in endothelial cells, thereby increasing endothelial permeability and the expression of Notch ligands. Activation of Notch signaling in tumor cells supports survival and proliferation, mostly on CSC populations. Once tumor cells have entered the circulation, activated or resting platelets (unpublished observation) can bind to single CTCs or CTC clusters and support survival by protecting them from shear stress as well as enhancing cell adhesion at distant sites of arrest.

Besides platelets, CTCs may also tune intravasation themselves and take advantage of the endothelial microenvironment. For example, human breast cancer cells induce mesenchymal characteristics in endothelial cells, as evidenced by upregulation of smooth muscle actin (ACTA2) and fibroblast specific protein 1 (FSP1), a phenotype also detectable in human neoplastic breast biopsies. Subsequently, the altered endothelial cells display enhanced survival, migratory, and angiogenic properties and are in turn capable of improving tumor cell survival and invasiveness via the TGFβ and Notch–Jagged1 signaling pathways [88]. Indeed, Notch ligands are frequently present on tumor-associated endothelial cells [89–92], and, independently of their roles in angiogenesis [93], they can also activate Notch signaling in tumor cells, thus enhancing aggressiveness, survival, and metastasis in diverse cancers [94–96]. Those advantages were precisely observed in CD44^{Hi}CD24$^{Lo/-}$ CTCs [97]. Similarly, a CD133$^+$ cancer-stem cell phenotype is induced by Notch signaling in colon cancer [98]. Together, these observations indicate that the stem-like CTC phenotype may be enhanced by endothelial cell crosstalk.

3.2. In Transit: Better Together

3.2.1. CTC Clustering

The phenotypic, morphological, and functional properties of heterogeneous tumor cell populations at the primary tumor site, may lead to differential mechanisms of tumor cell shedding into circulation. In this sense, single CTCs and/or collectively migrating clusters—ranging from two to 50 cells—are both detected within the circulation of patients with metastatic solid cancers [99–102]. Some CTC clusters have been characterized as polyclonal tumor cell groupings suggesting that 1) they may arise from different tumor masses or metastatic foci [103,104] or 2) clustering does not necessarily occur prior to departure from the primary site, but during intravasation [105,106], transit in the circulation [103,104], or at the secondary arrest site [107] (Figure 3). Recent data derived from pre-clinical murine models demonstrate that CTC clusters show a 23–50-fold increased metastatic potential over single CTCs and are known to increase in number during disease recurrence and the development of chemotherapy resistance [74,103].

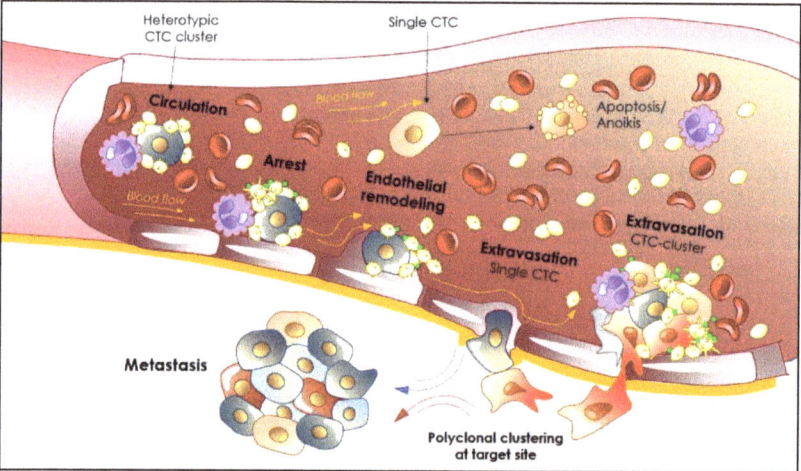

Figure 3. From the circulation to extravasation. CTCs that survive the harsh conditions of the blood microenvironment will eventually come into contact with, and arrest, on the endothelial cells lining the blood vessels at the metastatic site. Adhesion to the endothelial cells depends on the adhesion receptor repertoire of the tumor cells and in the case of heterotypic clusters, on the adhesion receptor repertoire of accompanying cells, for example, neutrophils and platelets. In addition to their role in adhesion, neutrophils and platelets can further enhance extravasation by increasing endothelial permeability via TGFβ and vascular endothelial growth factor A (VEGF secretion. Endothelial arrest predominantly takes place at sites where blow flow is low enough to allow stable adhesion to the vasculature. After this point, higher flow profiles are needed to induce endothelial remodeling around the arrested CTC, an essential process for successful extravasation. Clustering of polyclonal CTCs can occur at the site of arrest and/or extravasation, together with blood cells.

The mechanisms behind a CTC cluster's enhanced metastatic fitness are currently under investigation. One hypothesis suggests that differential expression of cell junction proteins may play a relevant role, as cell–cell junctions are important regulators of cell phenotype and function. Indeed, preserving cell–cell contacts protects clusters from anoikis [74] and enhances their survival and colony-forming potential [103,106]. For example, knockdown of the cell junction protein plakoglobin in mouse models abrogates CTC cluster formation and drastically inhibits lung metastasis [103]. Additionally, recent findings demonstrate that CTC clusters are enriched for cells with cancer stem cell-like features [74,105], whereby intercellular homotypic interactions between the cancer stem cell marker CD44 molecules enhance cluster formation [104]. Hence, intercellular cell–cell contacts within the cluster, in addition to paracrine signals, may be key to the maintenance of that aggressive stem-like cancer cell state. Furthermore, during development, loss of cell–cell junctions is an initiating step in the EMT, while maintenance of cell–cell junctions is required to preserve the embryonic stem cell state and to reprogram somatic cells into induced-pluripotent stem cells [108–110]. Consistent with those findings, it has recently been shown that classic binding sites for pluripotency and proliferation-associated transcription factors such as POU class 5 homeobox 1 (POU5F1/OCT4), SRY-box transcription factor 2 (SOX2), and Nanog homeobox (NANOG, are specifically hypomethylated in clustered CTCs [111] and that pharmacological dissociation of CTC clusters reverts their methylation profile and suppresses metastasis. Those findings suggest that the distinct differentiation states between single CTCs and CTC clusters, driven in part by pluripotency factors, may account for differences in their metastatic potential. The hypothesis that hypomethylation of pluripotency sites may account for the differential metastatic potential of CTC clusters versus single CTCs is supported by data demonstrating that the DNA methylation profile of CTC clusters is detected in primary breast tumors with poor prognosis [111]. However, the specific role of EMT in CTC cluster formation and the resultant enhanced metastatic fitness remains unclear. For example, it has been shown that CTC clusters encapsulated by tumor-induced blood vessels are highly metastatic by a Slug/Snail-independent mechanism [112]. Furthermore, another report by using quantitative 3D histology at the cancer–host interface revealed that collective migration is the predominant mechanism of cancer cell invasion, positioning single cell migration as an extremely rare event [113]. These findings suggest that CTC-extrinsic mechanisms, such as vascular patterning during tumor progression, can influence CTC clustering and shedding without a compulsory phenotypic change toward the mesenchymal fate. As evidenced by a recent longitudinal analysis of patient-derived single and clustered CTCs, the number and size of CTC clusters add additional prognostic value to single CTCs' enumeration alone [114]. Nevertheless, the mechanisms involved in the generation of a certain number and/or size of CTC clusters are yet to be studied. Interestingly, recent findings in this direction point to CTC plasticity as a key regulator of CTC-cluster size. Indeed, the prevention of a full EMT transition and thus a hybrid epithelial/mesenchymal phenotype, regulates the formation of large CTC clusters, suggesting that the balance between intermediate epithelial/mesenchymal phenotypes improved the metastatic fitness of CTC clusters [115].

3.2.2. Interactions That Matter: Heterotypic Clustering

The metastatic fitness of CTCs may be regulated by their physical and functional interactions with cell types other than cancer cells established at the primary tumor site or during their transit through the circulation, thus creating not only polyclonal but also heterotypic clusters (Figure 2). These heterotypic CTC clusters can include neutrophils [79,116], dendritic cells [117], or cancer-associated fibroblasts derived from the primary tumor stroma [118] that accompany CTCs to their secondary site [119]. Those companions are likely to modify the phenotype and intravascular behavior of CTCs by diverse means, including enhanced resistance to shear stress, EMT/MET induction, adhesion, survival, or proliferation. Moreover, the variety of cytokines and growth factors arising from those heterotypic CTC clusters may play a fundamental role in remodeling the distant niche during and after extravasation, thereby facilitating colonization [119,120]. One well-studied heterotypic interaction is that of CTCs and blood platelets (Figure 3). The implication of blood platelets in cancer is a rather old song [121,122]; however, their role in metastasis is not yet completely understood.

In general terms, platelets have shown a pro-metastatic role in several mouse models [86,123–125], and their number, size, and thrombotic properties have been linked to poor prognosis in human cancers [83,84,126]. The most compelling evidence for pro-metastatic platelets is the inhibition of metastasis by platelet depletion in experimental murine lung metastasis models [122,127,128]. Additionally, it is generally accepted that CTCs are able to bind, activate, and aggregate platelets in a process called tumor cell-induced platelet aggregation (TCIPA) [129]. TCIPA has been shown to correlate with the metastatic potential of CTCs [130,131] and to protect CTCs from shear stress and/or immune system cytotoxicity by forming a physical shield or by releasing immunosuppressive molecules [86,132]. The mechanism(s) involved in TCIPA-metastatic potential correlation are not yet clear, as not all metastatic cells aggregate platelets [129,133–135]. In that sense, TCIPA involvement in metastatic potential may have historically suffered from a lack of consensus about what TCIPA actually is: The induction of homotypic clumps of activated platelets, or the formation of platelet–tumor cell heterotypic clusters? In the later scenario, resting or low-activated platelets could bind and shield cells without classic TCIPA occurrence (unpublished observation). Additionally, and contrary to their well-established pro-metastatic role, specific platelets receptors have been shown to mediate anti-metastatic effects [136,137], questioning their precise contribution to metastasis and suggesting a spatiotemporal role of platelets in the metastatic cascade [138]. Nonetheless, heterotypic interactions are likely to prove a key component of metastatic success and may be refined in the future to include platelet binding to specific CTC populations where adhesive capacity is enhanced, and platelet-dependent tuning of CTC–endothelial adhesion/extravasation.

Whether the effects of platelets on metastasis involve physical and continuous CTC–platelet interactions whilst in the circulation and/or during extravasation remains an open question. Steric interference of CTC–platelet interactions directed at the alpha2beta3 integrin expressed on platelets does inhibit metastatic burden [139–141]. On the CTC side, the adhesion protein CD97 that is expressed in several primary and metastatic cancers [142] has been shown to directly interact and activate platelets. In turn, the lysophosphatidic acid (LPA) released by the platelets promotes experimental metastasis [143,144] by a mechanism involving CD97–LPAR (LPA receptor) dimerization at the CTC plasma membrane. LPA binding to CD97–LPAR heterodimer may also induce a pre-EMT invasive phenotype via a RHO family GTPase signaling-dependent mechanism [145,146]. Other cell surface antigens expressed on tumor cells can serve as adhesive receptors for platelets, including podoplanin: CLEC2 [147], the HMGB1: TLR4 [148], and the CD24: P-selectin interactions [149]. Interestingly, CD24 knockdown decreases metastatic burden in vivo, whether this is due to changes in platelet interactions remains to be determined [150,151]. Platelets may also support CTC survival and subsequent metastasis by inhibiting anoikis in a Yes associated protein 1 (YAP1)-dependent manner [152]. They can also tune endothelial fitness and favor adhesion to the vessel wall by activating the purigenic receptor, $P2Y_2$ [153,154] or by their natural ability to link to endothelial selectin P ligand (PSGL-1) [155,156], highlighting the important spatiotemporal role of platelets during the metastatic cascade.

3.2.3. Going with the Flow: Biomechanics of CTCs Extravasation

In order to reach secondary sites, circulating tumor cells (CTCs) have to avoid the hostile blood or lymphatic flow forces to arrest and stably adhere to the endothelium of the target organ [157,158]. CTC-extrinsic mechanisms such hemodynamic forces have been proven to be key in CTC endothelial arrest and extravasation [43,159]. We have recently identified a threshold of hemodynamic forces that allow stable arrest of CTCs in low-flow venous-like vascular regions, and active endothelial remodeling in higher-flow regions. Endothelial remodeling is an essential event for successful CTC extravasation (Figure 3). In this sense, endothelial fitness and crosstalk with CTCs at the extravasation site may define the final metastatic outcome. Indeed, we have observed that only flow-activated endothelium shows plasma membrane protrusions and accomplishes endothelial remodeling in vitro [159]. Others have additionally demonstrated that flow forces are able to regulate endothelial cell barrier function via non-canonical Notch signaling [160], making endothelial cells more permeable to CTCs, and inducing vascular cell adhesion molecule 1 (VCAM1) expression, leading to increased neutrophil infiltration and metastasis [161]. Interestingly, the areas with endothelial remodeling show deposition of fibrillar material and platelet recruitment [162,163], supporting a role for platelets in CTC flow-dependent adhesion and/or extravasation processes. Whether CTC clusters equally extravasate by endothelial remodeling in flow-permissive regions remains to be further elucidated. A recent study conducted in the zebrafish embryo, that requires further validation, demonstrates that clusters of CTCs mostly extravasate upon endothelium remodeling [164]. It has become evident that clustering increases CTC resistance to shear stress and protects from immune cell clearance [103,165]. Furthermore, the trajectories traveled by CTC clusters in the circulation are different to the paths of single CTCs, in large part due to size and shape. Compact clusters flow closer to the endothelial barrier than linear clusters or single CTCs and, thus, slowly [166,167], which increases their ability of adhering to the endothelium [168]. Interestingly, the intrinsic differentiation state of a CTC cluster may also influence its flow-dependent adhesive and biomechanical properties. It has been demonstrated that breast cancer cells showing the stem-like $CD44^+/CD24^-/ALDH1^+$ phenotype were significantly more deformable than non-CSCs. In addition, more-deformable cells were found to roll with shear-independent velocities in vitro [169]. Those findings have provided motivation to consider mechanical properties as a possible biomarker for cancer cell stemness. Indeed, we have recently shown that CD44 plays a key role in early endothelial arrest, as CD44 mediates the early weak-magnitude adhesion forces required for CTC arrest at the endothelial wall [43]. Hence, the increased metastatic potential of CTC clusters could be explained in part by a higher propensity to arrest on endothelial cells and to extravasate, which might be directly linked to the cell deformability index of CTC clusters.

4. Secondary Organ Colonization: Shedders or Seeders?

Not all CTCs that reach a secondary site have the capacity to colonize it [170]. In an elegant study utilizing barcoding clonal analysis of patient-derived xenografts, Merino et al. recently demonstrated that the extent of clonal diversity at metastatic sites is highly dependent on continual shedding of CTCs from the primary tumor. Hence, once the primary tumor is removed, clonal heterogeneity in secondary organs is dramatically reduced [18]. It is thus possible that while a variety of heterogeneous cancer cells may continually enter the circulation via active or passive processes at the primary tumor site, only CTCs with tumor-initiating potential have the ability to efficiently seed metastases. This idea is in line with the observation that cancer cells with high tumor-initiating/metastatic potential, for example $CD44^{Hi}$ cells, are observed at low frequency in patient primary tumors (~15% of the cancer cell population [6]).

There are likely other mechanisms by which poorly metastatic cells overcome their own metastatic inefficiency, including that of subclonal co-operation. It has recently been shown that minor subclones expressing interleukin 11 (IL11) and vascular endothelial growth factor D (VEGFD) within the primary tumor can modulate the immune system in a manner that enhances polyclonal metastatic growth of otherwise non-metastatic clones [171]. Those findings demonstrate how intra-tumor heterogeneity can mechanistically progress disease to advanced stages [172] and highlight the complex and co-operative interactions that contribute to metastatic success.

Metastatic Niche: A Driving Force or a Barrier?

Irrespective of whether cancer cells arrive at the secondary tumor site as single, clusters, or polyclonal clusters of cells, there are still multiple extrinsic stresses that must be overcome in order to generate a robustly growing metastasis (Figure 4). In 1889, Steven Paget proposed that the ability of tumor cells to initiate secondary tumor growth largely depends on crosstalk between metastatic tumor cells—the seeds—and the host microenvironment—the soil [173]. For a cancer cell entering a secondary tissue, it is likely that the growth-supportive signals from the local stroma and interactions with other cancer cells are quite different to those formerly present at the primary tumor site. Consequently, even a metastasis-competent disseminated cancer cell may be forced into a state of senescence, apoptosis, or latency if it is not able to rapidly adapt to its new environment. The fate of a disseminated cancer cell at the secondary site can be markedly influenced by location, where proximity to the microvasculature niche is related to dormancy, an effect mediated by tissue specific mechanisms. For example, cancer cell quiescence in the lung is mediated by thrombospondin 1 (TSP1) and bone morphogenetic protein 4 (BMP4), whereas in the bone marrow, TSP1, BMP7, transforming growth factor β2 (TGFβ2), and growth arrest-specific 6 (GAS6) induce and maintain quiescence [174,175].

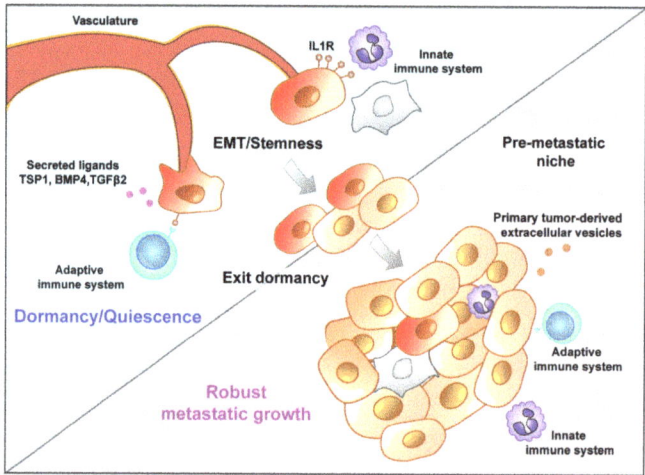

Figure 4. Metastatic colonization. Cancer cells with the intrinsic potential (e.g., CSCs) to initiate a secondary tumor must overcome multiple extrinsic stresses to establish a robustly growing metastasis. Signaling in the secondary tumor environment (initiated by the innate/adaptive immune system, stromal cells, or vasculature) can induce cells into a state of quiescence or dormancy. A permissive pre-metastatic niche may be created by signals arising from the primary tumor (via primary tumor-derived extracellular vesicles or polarization of the adaptive and/or innate immune systems) that enables cancer cells to avoid or exit dormancy and subsequently proliferate to establish a metastatic colony.

Metastatic colonization can also be restricted by the immune system. In melanoma, disseminated tumor cells enter into an immuno-induced dormant state following arrival at a secondary site [176]. Upon depletion of cytotoxic CD8$^+$ T cells however, metastatic growth reactivates, indicating an active role of the immune system in inhibiting tumor cell proliferation after dissemination. Similarly, in breast and lung carcinomas, interaction between tumor cells and natural killer (NK) cells suppress NK cell-activating ligands, a process that appears to be coupled with entrance into a quiescent state [177]. Our recent work demonstrated that the immune system can restrict metastatic growth by modulating a cancer cell's phenotype. In models of breast cancer, the primary tumor activated the innate immune system such that macrophages at sites of metastasis inhibit metastatic outgrowth by locking cancer cells in a stem-like state [178]. In that setting, interleukin 1 beta IL1B released by macrophages signals via the interleukin 1 receptor type 1 (IL1R1) on the cancer cells to maintain high expression of ZEB1. Implicit here is the notion that preventing CD44^{Hi} cells from undergoing asymmetric divisions to produce their highly proliferative epithelial CD44^{Lo} progeny significantly inhibits metastatic growth. Conversely, forcing cells to undergo a complete mesenchymal-to-epithelial transition (MET) at the metastatic site can deplete the tumor of the tumor-initiating cells that sustain secondary tumor growth [179]. Together those studies highlight the intricate balance between epithelial and mesenchymal cancer cell states and their impact on tumorigenicity.

In other instances, including the example of co-operative growth leading to robust metastasis [171], the immune system can act in a manner that enhances secondary tumor growth. In that setting, a hypoxic primary tumor microenvironment creates a pre-metastatic niche comprising $CD11b^+/Ly6C^{med}/Ly6G^+$ immune suppressor cells that compromise NK cell cytotoxicity, thereby diminishing a key mechanism for disseminated tumor cell elimination [180]. Additionally, recruitment of monocytes/macrophages and neutrophils can promote tumor cell survival, colonization, and pre-metastatic niche establishment in mice [181–183]. Neutrophils have been shown to enhance metastasis by grouping CTCs in circulation through the formation of neutrophil traps (NETs)—nets of extracellular neutrophil DNA fibers. In addition, neutrophil-derived leukotrienes were shown to be responsible for colonization at sites of metastasis by selectively expanding a subpopulation of cancer cells that retain high tumorigenic potential. Neutrophils can also remodel the host extracellular matrix to promote metastatic growth and direct signaling that maintains aggressive metastasis-initiating phenotypes [171,182–184].

The EMT itself is another mechanism that can impart several advantages on disseminated tumor cells during early stages of colonization. Tumor cells are subjected to high levels of oxidative stress due to hypoxic conditions at the primary tumor site, in the circulation, and at secondary sites of colonization [185]. Expression of EMT transcription factors can protect from the damaging cytotoxic effects induced by oxygen radicals and DNA damage [186]. Furthermore, oxidative stress has been linked with activation of the EMT [187], setting up a positive feedback loop that may enhance metastatic cell survival under stressful conditions. The EMT also plays a key role in enabling disseminated tumor cells to evade immune surveillance [188]. Accordingly, epithelial cells have been shown to express high major histocompatibility (MHC) class I and low CD274 (PD-L1) levels, while more mesenchymal carcinoma cell lines exhibiting EMT markers expressed low levels of MHC-I, high levels of PD-L1 [189]. Indeed, ZEB1 can directly regulate PD-L1 levels [190,191]. Consequently, epithelial tumors can be more susceptible to elimination by immunotherapy than corresponding mesenchymal tumors [189]. Mechanisms of immune evasion attributable to the EMT may also include downregulation of immunoproteasome subunits and consequently, downregulation of MHC class I -bound peptides [192].

Another important determinant of metastatic success is the preparation of a favorable pre-metastatic niche via primary tumor cell-derived extracellular vesicles (EV) [193]. A recent study by Hoshino et al. showed that uptake of tumor-derived integrin exosomes by resident cells at secondary sites determines organotropic metastasis. Exosomal expression of $\alpha6\beta4$ and $\alpha6\beta1$ is associated with lung metastasis, while exosomal integrin $\alpha v\beta5$ was linked to liver metastasis. Reduction of those distinct integrin complexes decreased exosome uptake and subsequently metastasis, via inhibition of Src signaling and activation of pro-inflammatory signals in resident cells [194]. Additionally, our recent work has shown that patrolling monocytes and endothelial cells are key cellular types in charge of tumor EV uptake [195] and may therefore be early activators of the metastatic niche. Indeed, uptake of metastatic tumor cell-derived molecules reprograms the resident normal tissue cells in a manner that aids metastatic growth [196]. Clearly, interactions between the seed and soil are intricately linked to metastatic success. Determining the mechanisms that define those interactions may form the basis of future therapeutic strategies to inhibit metastasis.

5. Conclusions

Metastasis is not a linear process, rather, it is a highly dynamic interplay of intrinsic cellular properties and extrinsic host factors that are constantly evolving throughout the course of tumorigenesis to positively or negatively influence the metastatic process. We have discussed phenotypic traits that promote a cancer cell's ability to complete specific stages of the metastatic cascade, encompassing the notion that there is not a single phenotypic state that equates with metastatic success. Instead, it is likely that metastatic success lies in tumor cell's ability to adapt its phenotype, at each step of the cascade, to survive the variety of challenges encountered along its journey; including constant turnover of transitional cellular states, interactions with host components and between different clonal populations. The extent to which a given cell/clone completes the metastatic cascade likely depends upon its epigenetic, transcriptomic, and proteomic landscape, and whether it travels alone or with companions. Those properties, in turn, determine how that cell processes and responds to incoming signals. In some tumor types, it is likely that specialized cancer cells are equipped with most, if not all of the biological traits required for metastasis. In less adept cancer cell populations, a favorable metastatic niche environment, traveling with a support team, or a permissive environment created by the primary tumor may be the prime determinants of metastatic success. Elucidating the prominent mechanisms at play in different tumor types and subtypes will lead to more effective means to therapeutically target and inhibit metastatic growth.

Funding: B.P.S.J. is supported by the Rebecca Wilson Fellowship in Breast Cancer Research, Nelune Foundation. C.L.C. is supported by a Cancer Institute New South Wales Fellowship. This work has been funded by the National Breast Cancer Foundation Australia (C.L.C.), the French National Cancer Institute (INCa) and by institutional funds from INSERM and University of Strasbourg to J.G. M.J.G.L. is supported by INCa (National Cancer institute) and University of Strasbourg (Idex).

Conflicts of Interest: The authors declare no conflict of interest.

References

1. Weinstein, B.T.; Lavrentovich, M.O.; Möbius, W.; Murray, A.W.; Nelson, D.R. Genetic drift and selection in many-allele range expansions. *PLoS Comput. Biol.* **2017**, *13*, e1005866. [CrossRef]
2. Feinberg, A.P.; Koldobskiy, M.A.; Göndör, A. Epigenetic modulators, modifiers and mediators in cancer aetiology and progression. *Nat. Rev. Genet.* **2016**, *17*, 284–299. [CrossRef]
3. Rubin, H.; Rubin, A.L. Phenotypic selection as the biological mode of epigenetic conversion and reversion in cell transformation. *Proc. Natl. Acad. Sci. USA* **2018**, *115*, E725–E732. [CrossRef] [PubMed]
4. Rybinski, B.; Yun, K. Addressing intra-tumoral heterogeneity and therapy resistance. *Oncotarget* **2016**, *7*, 72322–72342. [CrossRef] [PubMed]
5. Bonnet, D.; Dick, J.E. Human acute myeloid leukemia is organized as a hierarchy that originates from a primitive hematopoietic cell. *Nat. Med.* **1997**, *3*, 730–737. [CrossRef] [PubMed]
6. Al-Hajj, M.; Wicha, M.S.; Benito-Hernandez, A.; Morrison, S.J.; Clarke, M.F. Prospective identification of tumorigenic breast cancer cells. *Proc. Natl. Acad. Sci. USA* **2003**, *100*, 3983–3988. [CrossRef]
7. Choi, Y.-J.; Ingram, P.N.; Yang, K.; Coffman, L.; Iyengar, M.; Bai, S.; Thomas, D.G.; Yoon, E.; Buckanovich, R.J. Identifying an ovarian cancer cell hierarchy regulated by bone morphogenetic protein 2. *Proc. Natl. Acad. Sci. USA* **2015**, *112*, E6882–E6888. [CrossRef]
8. Driessens, G.; Beck, B.; Caauwe, A.; Simons, B.D.; Blanpain, C. Defining the mode of tumour growth by clonal analysis. *Nature* **2012**, *488*, 527–530. [CrossRef]
9. Lan, X.; Jörg, D.J.; Cavalli, F.M.G.; Richards, L.M.; Nguyen, L.V.; Vanner, R.J.; Guilhamon, P.; Lee, L.; Kushida, M.M.; Pellacani, D.; et al. Fate mapping of human glioblastoma reveals an invariant stem cell hierarchy. *Nature* **2017**, *549*, 227–232. [CrossRef]
10. Mani, S.A.; Guo, W.; Liao, M.J.; Eaton, E.N.; Ayyanan, A.; Zhou, A.Y.; Brooks, M.; Reinhard, F.; Zhang, C.C.; Shipitsin, M.; et al. The epithelial-mesenchymal transition generates cells with properties of stem cells. *Cell* **2008**, *133*, 704–715. [CrossRef]
11. McAllister, S.S.; Weinberg, R.A. The tumour-induced systemic environment as a critical regulator of cancer progression and metastasis. *Nat. Cell Biol.* **2014**, *16*, 717–727. [CrossRef] [PubMed]
12. Goldstein, A.S.; Huang, J.; Guo, C.; Garraway, I.P.; Witte, O.N. Identification of a cell of origin for human prostate cancer. *Science* **2010**, *329*, 568–571. [CrossRef] [PubMed]
13. Vanharanta, S.; Massagué, J. Origins of Metastatic Traits. *Cancer Cell* **2013**, *24*, 410–421. [CrossRef] [PubMed]
14. Li, L.; Neaves, W.B. Normal Stem Cells and Cancer Stem Cells: The Niche Matters: Figure 1. *Cancer Res.* **2006**, *66*, 4553–4557. [CrossRef]
15. Chaffer, C.L.; Brueckmann, I.; Scheel, C.; Kaestli, A.J.; Wiggins, P.A.; Rodrigues, L.O.; Brooks, M.; Reinhardt, F.; Su, Y.; Polyak, K.; et al. Normal and neoplastic nonstem cells can spontaneously convert to a stem-like state. *Proc. Natl. Acad. Sci. USA* **2011**, *108*, 7950–7955. [CrossRef]

16. Koboldt, D.C.; Fulton, R.S.; McLellan, M.D.; Schmidt, H.; Kalicki-Veizer, J.; McMichael, J.F.; Fulton, L.L.; Dooling, D.J.; Ding, L.; Mardis, E.R.; et al. Comprehensive molecular portraits of human breast tumours. *Nature* **2012**, *490*, 61–70.
17. Lawson, D.A.; Bhakta, N.R.; Kessenbrock, K.; Prummel, K.D.; Yu, Y.; Takai, K.; Zhou, A.; Eyob, H.; Balakrishnan, S.; Wang, C.Y.; et al. Single-cell analysis reveals a stem-cell program in human metastatic breast cancer cells. *Nature* **2015**, *526*, 131–135. [CrossRef]
18. Merino, D.; Weber, T.S.; Serrano, A.; Vaillant, F.; Liu, K.; Pal, B.; Di Stefano, L.; Schreuder, J.; Lin, D.; Chen, Y.; et al. Barcoding reveals complex clonal behavior in patient-derived xenografts of metastatic triple negative breast cancer. *Nat. Commun.* **2019**, *10*, 766. [CrossRef]
19. Wagenblast, E.; Soto, M.; Gutiérrez-Ángel, S.; Hartl, C.A.; Gable, A.L.; Maceli, A.R.; Erard, N.; Williams, A.M.; Kim, S.Y.; Dickopf, S.; et al. A model of breast cancer heterogeneity reveals vascular mimicry as a driver of metastasis. *Nature* **2015**, *520*, 358–362. [CrossRef]
20. Nguyen, L.V.; Cox, C.L.; Eirew, P.; Knapp, D.J.H.F.; Pellacani, D.; Kannan, N.; Carles, A.; Moksa, M.; Balani, S.; Shah, S.; et al. DNA barcoding reveals diverse growth kinetics of human breast tumour subclones in serially passaged xenografts. *Nat. Commun.* **2014**, *5*, 5871. [CrossRef]
21. Maleki, M.; Ghanbarvand, F.; Behvarz, M.R.; Ejtemaei, M.; Ghadirkhomi, E. Comparison of Mesenchymal Stem Cell Markers in Multiple Human Adult Stem Cells. *Int. J. Stem Cells* **2014**, *7*, 118–126. [CrossRef] [PubMed]
22. Kryczek, I.; Liu, S.; Roh, M.; Vatan, L.; Szeliga, W.; Wei, S.; Banerjee, M.; Mao, Y.; Kotarski, J.; Wicha, M.S.; et al. Expression of aldehyde dehydrogenase and CD133 defines ovarian cancer stem cells. *Int. J. Cancer* **2012**, *130*, 29–39. [CrossRef] [PubMed]
23. Curley, M.D.; Therrien, V.A.; Cummings, C.L.; Sergent, P.A.; Koulouris, C.R.; Friel, A.M.; Roberts, D.J.; Seiden, M.V.; Scadden, D.T.; Rueda, B.R.; et al. CD133 expression defines a tumor initiating cell population in primary human ovarian cancer. *Stem Cells* **2009**, *27*, 2875–2883. [CrossRef] [PubMed]
24. Singh, S.K.; Hawkins, C.; Clarke, I.D.; Squire, J.A.; Bayani, J.; Hide, T.; Henkelman, R.M.; Cusimano, M.D.; Dirks, P.B. Identification of human brain tumour initiating cells. *Nature* **2004**, *432*, 396–401. [CrossRef]
25. Boiko, A.D.; Razorenova, O.V.; van de Rijn, M.; Swetter, S.M.; Johnson, D.L.; Ly, D.P.; Butler, P.D.; Yang, G.P.; Joshua, B.; Kaplan, M.J.; et al. Human melanoma-initiating cells express neural crest nerve growth factor receptor CD271. *Nature* **2010**, *466*, 133–137. [CrossRef]
26. Takaishi, S.; Okumura, T.; Tu, S.; Wang, S.S.W.; Shibata, W.; Vigneshwaran, R.; Gordon, S.A.K.; Shimada, Y.; Wang, T.C. Identification of gastric cancer stem cells using the cell surface marker CD44. *Stem Cells* **2009**, *27*, 1006–1020. [CrossRef]
27. Li, C.; Heidt, D.G.; Dalerba, P.; Burant, C.F.; Zhang, L.; Adsay, V.; Wicha, M.; Clarke, M.F.; Simeone, D.M. Identification of pancreatic cancer stem cells. *Cancer Res.* **2007**, *67*, 1030–1037. [CrossRef]
28. Lin, J.; Ding, D. The prognostic role of the cancer stem cell marker CD44 in ovarian cancer: A meta-analysis. *Cancer Cell Int.* **2017**, *17*, 8. [CrossRef]
29. O'Brien, C.A.; Pollett, A.; Gallinger, S.; Dick, J.E. A human colon cancer cell capable of initiating tumour growth in immunodeficient mice. *Nature* **2007**, *445*, 106–110. [CrossRef]
30. Dobbin, Z.C.; Katre, A.A.; Steg, A.D.; Erickson, B.K.; Shah, M.M.; Alvarez, R.D.; Conner, M.G.; Schneider, D.; Chen, D.; Landen, C.N. Using heterogeneity of the patient-derived xenograft model to identify the chemoresistant population in ovarian cancer. *Oncotarget* **2014**, *5*, 8750–8764. [CrossRef]
31. Garcia-Peydro, M.; Fuentes, P.; Mosquera, M.; Garcia-Leon, M.J.; Alcain, J.; Rodriguez, A.; Garcia de Miguel, P.; Menendez, P.; Weijer, K.; Spits, H.; et al. The NOTCH1/CD44 axis drives pathogenesis in a T cell acute lymphoblastic leukemia model. *J. Clin. Investig.* **2018**, *128*, 2802–2818. [CrossRef] [PubMed]
32. Senbanjo, L.T.; Chellaiah, M.A. CD44: A Multifunctional Cell Surface Adhesion Receptor Is a Regulator of Progression and Metastasis of Cancer Cells. *Front. Cell Dev. Biol.* **2017**, *5*, 18. [CrossRef] [PubMed]
33. Anido, J.; Sáez-Borderías, A.; Gonzàlez-Juncà, A.; Rodón, L.; Folch, G.; Carmona, M.A.; Prieto-Sánchez, R.M.; Barba, I.; Martínez-Sáez, E.; Prudkin, L.; et al. TGF-β Receptor Inhibitors Target the CD44high/Id1high Glioma-Initiating Cell Population in Human Glioblastoma. *Cancer Cell* **2010**, *18*, 655–668. [CrossRef] [PubMed]
34. Liu, J.; Xiao, Z.; Wong, S.K.-M.; Tin, V.P.-C.; Ho, K.-Y.; Wang, J.; Sham, M.-H.; Wong, M.P. Lung cancer tumorigenicity and drug resistance are maintained through ALDH(hi)CD44(hi) tumor initiating cells. *Oncotarget* **2013**, *4*, 1698–1711. [CrossRef]

35. Bansal, N.; Davis, S.; Tereshchenko, I.; Budak-Alpdogan, T.; Zhong, H.; Stein, M.N.; Kim, I.Y.; DiPaola, R.S.; Bertino, J.R.; Sabaawy, H.E. Enrichment of human prostate cancer cells with tumor initiating properties in mouse and zebrafish xenografts by differential adhesion. *Prostate* **2014**, *74*, 187–200. [CrossRef]
36. Shen, S.; Yang, W.; Wang, Z.; Lei, X.; Xu, L.; Wang, Y.; Wang, L.; Huang, L.; Yu, Z.; Zhang, X.; et al. Tumor-Initiating Cells Are Enriched in CD44hi Population in Murine Salivary Gland Tumor. *PLoS ONE* **2011**, *6*, e23282. [CrossRef]
37. Chen, C.; Zhao, S.; Karnad, A.; Freeman, J.W. The biology and role of CD44 in cancer progression: Therapeutic implications. *J. Hematol. Oncol.* **2018**, *11*, 64.
38. Todaro, M.; Gaggianesi, M.; Catalano, V.; Benfante, A.; Iovino, F.; Biffoni, M.; Apuzzo, T.; Sperduti, I.; Volpe, S.; Cocorullo, G.; et al. CD44v6 Is a Marker of Constitutive and Reprogrammed Cancer Stem Cells Driving Colon Cancer Metastasis. *Cell Stem Cell* **2014**, *14*, 342–356. [CrossRef]
39. Bourguignon, L.Y.W.; Gunja-Smith, Z.; Iida, N.; Zhu, H.B.; Young, L.J.T.; Muller, W.J.; Cardiff, R.D. CD44v3,8-10 is involved in cytoskeleton-mediated tumor cell migration and matrix metalloproteinase (MMP-9) association in metastatic breast cancer cells. *J. Cell Physiol.* **1998**, *176*, 206–215. [CrossRef]
40. Zeilstra, J.; Joosten, S.P.J.; van Andel, H.; Tolg, C.; Berns, A.; Snoek, M.; van de Wetering, M.; Spaargaren, M.; Clevers, H.; Pals, S.T. Stem cell CD44v isoforms promote intestinal cancer formation in Apc(min) mice downstream of Wnt signaling. *Oncogene* **2014**, *33*, 665–670. [CrossRef]
41. Li, Z.; Chen, K.; Jiang, P.; Zhang, X.; Li, X.; Li, Z. CD44v/CD44s expression patterns are associated with the survival of pancreatic carcinoma patients. *Diagn. Pathol.* **2014**, *9*, 79. [CrossRef] [PubMed]
42. Xu, Y.-Y.; Guo, M.; Yang, L.-Q.; Zhou, F.; Yu, C.; Wang, A.; Pang, T.-H.; Wu, H.-Y.; Zou, X.-P.; Zhang, W.-J.; et al. Regulation of CD44v6 expression in gastric carcinoma by the IL-6/STAT3 signaling pathway and its clinical significance. *Oncotarget* **2017**, *8*, 45848–45861. [CrossRef] [PubMed]
43. Osmani, N.; Follain, G.; Garcia Leon, M.J.; Lefebvre, O.; Busnelli, I.; Larnicol, A.; Harlepp, S.; Goetz, J.G. Metastatic Tumor Cells Exploit Their Adhesion Repertoire to Counteract Shear Forces during Intravascular Arrest. *Cell Rep.* **2019**, *28*, 2491–2500 e2495. [CrossRef] [PubMed]
44. Chaffer, C.L.; Marjanovic, N.D.; Lee, T.; Bell, G.; Kleer, C.G.; Reinhardt, F.; D'Alessio, A.C.; Young, R.A.; Weinberg, R.A. Poised chromatin at the ZEB1 promoter enables breast cancer cell plasticity and enhances tumorigenicity. *Cell* **2013**, *154*, 61–74. [CrossRef]
45. Guo, W.; Keckesova, Z.; Donaher, J.L.; Shibue, T.; Tischler, V.; Reinhardt, F.; Itzkovitz, S.; Noske, A.; Zürrer-Härdi, U.; Bell, G.; et al. Slug and Sox9 cooperatively determine the mammary stem cell state. *Cell* **2012**, *148*, 1015–1028. [CrossRef]
46. Larsen, J.E.; Nathan, V.; Osborne, J.K.; Farrow, R.K.; Deb, D.; Sullivan, J.P.; Dospoy, P.D.; Augustyn, A.; Hight, S.K.; Sato, M.; et al. ZEB1 drives epithelial-to-mesenchymal transition in lung cancer. *J. Clin. Investig.* **2016**, *126*, 3219–3235. [CrossRef]
47. Nieto, M.A.; Huang, R.Y.; Jackson, R.A.; Thiery, J.P. EMT: 2016. *Cell* **2016**, *166*, 21–45. [CrossRef]
48. Preca, B.T.; Bajdak, K.; Mock, K.; Sundararajan, V.; Pfannstiel, J.; Maurer, J.; Wellner, U.; Hopt, U.T.; Brummer, T.; Brabletz, S.; et al. A self-enforcing CD44s/ZEB1 feedback loop maintains EMT and stemness properties in cancer cells. *Int. J. Cancer.* **2015**, *137*, 2566–2577. [CrossRef]
49. Jolly, M.K.; Preca, B.T.; Tripathi, S.C.; Jia, D.; George, J.T.; Hanash, S.M.; Brabletz, T.; Stemmler, M.P.; Maurer, J.; Levine, H. Interconnected feedback loops among ESRP1, HAS2, and CD44 regulate epithelial-mesenchymal plasticity in cancer. *APL Bioeng.* **2018**, *2*, 031908. [CrossRef]
50. Ye, X.; Weinberg, R.A. Epithelial-Mesenchymal Plasticity: A Central Regulator of Cancer Progression. *Trends Cell Biol.* **2015**, *25*, 675–686. [CrossRef]
51. Shen, M.; Xu, Z.; Xu, W.; Jiang, K.; Zhang, F.; Ding, Q.; Xu, Z.; Chen, Y. Inhibition of ATM reverses EMT and decreases metastatic potential of cisplatin-resistant lung cancer cells through JAK/STAT3/PD-L1 pathway. *J. Exp. Clin. Cancer Res.* **2019**, *38*, 149.
52. Ponnusamy, L.; Mahalingaiah, P.K.S.; Chang, Y.-W.; Singh, K.P. Role of cellular reprogramming and epigenetic dysregulation in acquired chemoresistance in breast cancer. *Cancer Drug Resist.* **2019**. [CrossRef]
53. Chen, X.; Liao, R.; Li, D.; Sun, J. Induced cancer stem cells generated by radiochemotherapy and their therapeutic implications. *Oncotarget* **2017**, *8*, 17301–17312. [CrossRef] [PubMed]
54. Grosse-Wilde, A.; Fouquier d'Herouel, A.; McIntosh, E.; Ertaylan, G.; Skupin, A.; Kuestner, R.E.; del Sol, A.; Walters, K.A.; Huang, S. Stemness of the hybrid Epithelial/Mesenchymal State in Breast Cancer and Its Association with Poor Survival. *PLoS ONE* **2015**, *10*, e0126522. [CrossRef] [PubMed]

55. Ginestier, C.; Hur, M.H.; Charafe-Jauffret, E.; Monville, F.; Dutcher, J.; Brown, M.; Jacquemier, J.; Viens, P.; Kleer, C.G.; Liu, S.; et al. ALDH1 is a marker of normal and malignant human mammary stem cells and a predictor of poor clinical outcome. *Cell Stem Cell* **2007**, *1*, 555–567. [CrossRef] [PubMed]
56. Gjerdrum, C.; Tiron, C.; Hoiby, T.; Stefansson, I.; Haugen, H.; Sandal, T.; Collett, K.; Li, S.; McCormack, E.; Gjertsen, B.T.; et al. Axl is an essential epithelial-to-mesenchymal transition-induced regulator of breast cancer metastasis and patient survival. *Proc. Natl. Acad. Sci. USA* **2010**, *107*, 1124–1129. [CrossRef]
57. Soundararajan, R.; Paranjape, A.N.; Barsan, V.; Chang, J.T.; Mani, S.A. A novel embryonic plasticity gene signature that predicts metastatic competence and clinical outcome. *Sci. Rep.* **2015**, *5*, 11766. [CrossRef]
58. Kim, J.; Hong, S.J.; Park, J.Y.; Park, J.H.; Yu, Y.S.; Park, S.Y.; Lim, E.K.; Choi, K.Y.; Lee, E.K.; Paik, S.S.; et al. Epithelial-mesenchymal transition gene signature to predict clinical outcome of hepatocellular carcinoma. *Cancer Sci.* **2010**, *101*, 1521–1528. [CrossRef]
59. Collins, A.T.; Berry, P.A.; Hyde, C.; Stower, M.J.; Maitland, N.J. Prospective identification of tumorigenic prostate cancer stem cells. *Cancer Res.* **2005**, *65*, 10946–10951. [CrossRef]
60. Bierie, B.; Pierce, S.E.; Kroeger, C.; Stover, D.G.; Pattabiraman, D.R.; Thiru, P.; Liu Donaher, J.; Reinhardt, F.; Chaffer, C.L.; Keckesova, Z.; et al. Integrin-beta4 identifies cancer stem cell-enriched populations of partially mesenchymal carcinoma cells. *Proc. Natl. Acad. Sci. USA* **2017**, *114*, E2337–E2346. [CrossRef]
61. Goldman, A.; Majumder, B.; Dhawan, A.; Ravi, S.; Goldman, D.; Kohandel, M.; Majumder, P.K.; Sengupta, S. Temporally sequenced anticancer drugs overcome adaptive resistance by targeting a vulnerable chemotherapy-induced phenotypic transition. *Nat. Commun.* **2015**, *6*, 6139. [CrossRef] [PubMed]
62. Kroger, C.; Afeyan, A.; Mraz, J.; Eaton, E.N.; Reinhardt, F.; Khodor, Y.L.; Thiru, P.; Bierie, B.; Ye, X.; Burge, C.B.; et al. Acquisition of a hybrid E/M state is essential for tumorigenicity of basal breast cancer cells. *Proc. Natl. Acad. Sci. USA* **2019**, *116*, 7353–7362. [CrossRef] [PubMed]
63. Cooper, J.; Giancotti, F.G. Integrin Signaling in Cancer: Mechanotransduction, Stemness, Epithelial Plasticity, and Therapeutic Resistance. *Cancer Cell* **2019**, *35*, 347–367. [CrossRef] [PubMed]
64. Jolly, M.K.; Huang, B.; Lu, M.; Mani, S.A.; Levine, H.; Ben-Jacob, E. Towards elucidating the connection between epithelial-mesenchymal transitions and stemness. *J. R. Soc. Interface* **2014**, *11*, 20140962. [CrossRef] [PubMed]
65. Pastushenko, I.; Brisebarre, A.; Sifrim, A.; Fioramonti, M.; Revenco, T.; Boumahdi, S.; Van Keymeulen, A.; Brown, D.; Moers, V.; Lemaire, S.; et al. Identification of the tumour transition states occurring during EMT. *Nature* **2018**, *556*, 463–468. [CrossRef]
66. Jolly, M.K.; Somarelli, J.A.; Sheth, M.; Biddle, A.; Tripathi, S.C.; Armstrong, A.J.; Hanash, S.M.; Bapat, S.A.; Rangarajan, A.; Levine, H. Hybrid epithelial/mesenchymal phenotypes promote metastasis and therapy resistance across carcinomas. *Pharmacol. Ther.* **2019**, *194*. [CrossRef]
67. Yu, M.; Stott, S.; Toner, M.; Maheswaran, S.; Haber, D.A. Circulating tumor cells: Approaches to isolation and characterization. *J. Cell Biol.* **2011**, *192*, 373–382. [CrossRef]
68. Alix-Panabieres, C.; Pantel, K. Circulating tumor cells: Liquid biopsy of cancer. *Clin. Chem.* **2013**, *59*, 110–118.
69. Luzzi, K.J.; MacDonald, I.C.; Schmidt, E.E.; Kerkvliet, N.; Morris, V.L.; Chambers, A.F.; Groom, A.C. Multistep nature of metastatic inefficiency: Dormancy of solitary cells after successful extravasation and limited survival of early micrometastases. *Am. J. Pathol.* **1998**, *153*, 865–873. [CrossRef]
70. Weiss, L. Metastatic inefficiency. *Adv. Cancer Res.* **1990**, *54*, 159–211.
71. Blazejczyk, A.; Papiernik, D.; Porshneva, K.; Sadowska, J.; Wietrzyk, J. Endothelium and cancer metastasis: Perspectives for antimetastatic therapy. *Pharmacol. Rep.* **2015**, *67*, 711–718. [CrossRef] [PubMed]
72. Nguyen-Ngoc, K.V.; Cheung, K.J.; Brenot, A.; Shamir, E.R.; Gray, R.S.; Hines, W.C.; Yaswen, P.; Werb, Z.; Ewald, A.J. ECM microenvironment regulates collective migration and local dissemination in normal and malignant mammary epithelium. *Proc. Natl. Acad. Sci. USA* **2012**, *109*, E2595–E2604. [CrossRef] [PubMed]
73. Sullivan, J.P.; Nahed, B.V.; Madden, M.W.; Oliveira, S.M.; Springer, S.; Bhere, D.; Chi, A.S.; Wakimoto, H.; Rothenberg, S.M.; Sequist, L.V.; et al. Brain tumor cells in circulation are enriched for mesenchymal gene expression. *Cancer Discov.* **2014**, *4*, 1299–1309. [CrossRef] [PubMed]
74. Yu, M.; Bardia, A.; Wittner, B.S.; Stott, S.L.; Smas, M.E.; Ting, D.T.; Isakoff, S.J.; Ciciliano, J.C.; Wells, M.N.; Shah, A.M.; et al. Circulating breast tumor cells exhibit dynamic changes in epithelial and mesenchymal composition. *Science* **2013**, *339*, 580–584. [CrossRef]
75. Friedl, P.; Wolf, K. Tumour-cell invasion and migration: Diversity and escape mechanisms. *Nat. Rev. Cancer* **2003**, *3*, 362–374. [CrossRef]

76. Van Zijl, F.; Krupitza, G.; Mikulits, W. Initial steps of metastasis: Cell invasion and endothelial transmigration. *Mutat. Res.* **2011**, *728*, 23–34. [CrossRef]
77. Yang, L.; Lin, P.C. Mechanisms that drive inflammatory tumor microenvironment, tumor heterogeneity, and metastatic progression. *Semin. Cancer Biol.* **2017**, *47*, 185–195. [CrossRef]
78. Zervantonakis, I.K.; Hughes-Alford, S.K.; Charest, J.L.; Condeelis, J.S.; Gertler, F.B.; Kamm, R.D. Three-dimensional microfluidic model for tumor cell intravasation and endothelial barrier function. *Proc. Natl. Acad. Sci. USA* **2012**, *109*, 13515–13520. [CrossRef]
79. Spicer, J.D.; McDonald, B.; Cools-Lartigue, J.J.; Chow, S.C.; Giannias, B.; Kubes, P.; Ferri, L.E. Neutrophils promote liver metastasis via Mac-1-mediated interactions with circulating tumor cells. *Cancer Res.* **2012**, *72*, 3919–3927. [CrossRef]
80. Gros, A.; Syvannarath, V.; Lamrani, L.; Ollivier, V.; Loyau, S.; Goerge, T.; Nieswandt, B.; Jandrot-Perrus, M.; Ho-Tin-Noe, B. Single platelets seal neutrophil-induced vascular breaches via GPVI during immune-complex-mediated inflammation in mice. *Blood* **2015**, *126*, 1017–1026. [CrossRef]
81. Wyckoff, J.B.; Wang, Y.; Lin, E.Y.; Li, J.F.; Goswami, S.; Stanley, E.R.; Segall, J.E.; Pollard, J.W.; Condeelis, J. Direct visualization of macrophage-assisted tumor cell intravasation in mammary tumors. *Cancer Res.* **2007**, *67*, 2649–2656. [CrossRef] [PubMed]
82. Condeelis, J.; Pollard, J.W. Macrophages: Obligate partners for tumor cell migration, invasion, and metastasis. *Cell* **2006**, *124*, 263–266. [CrossRef] [PubMed]
83. Prandoni, P. Venous thromboembolism risk and management in women with cancer and thrombophilia. *Gend. Med.* **2005**, *2* (Suppl. A), S28–S34. [CrossRef]
84. Varki, A. Trousseau's syndrome: Multiple definitions and multiple mechanisms. *Blood* **2007**, *110*, 1723–1729. [CrossRef]
85. Miyashita, T.; Tajima, H.; Makino, I.; Nakagawara, H.; Kitagawa, H.; Fushida, S.; Harmon, J.W.; Ohta, T. Metastasis-promoting role of extravasated platelet activation in tumor. *J. Surg. Res.* **2015**, *193*, 289–294. [CrossRef]
86. Labelle, M.; Begum, S.; Hynes, R.O. Platelets guide the formation of early metastatic niches. *Proc. Natl. Acad. Sci. USA* **2014**, *111*, E3053–E3061. [CrossRef] [PubMed]
87. Labelle, M.; Begum, S.; Hynes, R.O. Direct signaling between platelets and cancer cells induces an epithelial-mesenchymal-like transition and promotes metastasis. *Cancer Cell* **2011**, *20*, 576–590. [CrossRef] [PubMed]
88. Ghiabi, P.; Jiang, J.; Pasquier, J.; Maleki, M.; Abu-Kaoud, N.; Halabi, N.; Guerrouahen, B.S.; Rafii, S.; Rafii, A. Breast cancer cells promote a notch-dependent mesenchymal phenotype in endothelial cells participating to a pro-tumoral niche. *J. Transl. Med.* **2015**, *13*, 27. [CrossRef]
89. Kontomanolis, E.; Panteliadou, M.; Giatromanolaki, A.; Pouliliou, S.; Efremidou, E.; Limberis, V.; Galazios, G.; Sivridis, E.; Koukourakis, M.I. Delta-like ligand 4 (DLL4) in the plasma and neoplastic tissues from breast cancer patients: Correlation with metastasis. *Med. Oncol.* **2014**, *31*, 945. [CrossRef]
90. Mailhos, C.; Modlich, U.; Lewis, J.; Harris, A.; Bicknell, R.; Ish-Horowicz, D. Delta4, an endothelial specific notch ligand expressed at sites of physiological and tumor angiogenesis. *Differentiation* **2001**, *69*, 135–144. [CrossRef]
91. Patel, N.S.; Li, J.L.; Generali, D.; Poulsom, R.; Cranston, D.W.; Harris, A.L. Up-regulation of delta-like 4 ligand in human tumor vasculature and the role of basal expression in endothelial cell function. *Cancer Res.* **2005**, *65*, 8690–8697. [CrossRef] [PubMed]
92. Reedijk, M.; Odorcic, S.; Chang, L.; Zhang, H.; Miller, N.; McCready, D.R.; Lockwood, G.; Egan, S.E. High-level coexpression of JAG1 and NOTCH1 is observed in human breast cancer and is associated with poor overall survival. *Cancer Res.* **2005**, *65*, 8530–8537. [CrossRef] [PubMed]
93. Potente, M.; Gerhardt, H.; Carmeliet, P. Basic and therapeutic aspects of angiogenesis. *Cell* **2011**, *146*, 873–887. [CrossRef] [PubMed]
94. Cao, Z.; Ding, B.S.; Guo, P.; Lee, S.B.; Butler, J.M.; Casey, S.C.; Simons, M.; Tam, W.; Felsher, D.W.; Shido, K.; et al. Angiocrine factors deployed by tumor vascular niche induce B cell lymphoma invasiveness and chemoresistance. *Cancer Cell* **2014**, *25*, 350–365. [CrossRef] [PubMed]

95. Zhu, T.S.; Costello, M.A.; Talsma, C.E.; Flack, C.G.; Crowley, J.G.; Hamm, L.L.; He, X.; Hervey-Jumper, S.L.; Heth, J.A.; Muraszko, K.M.; et al. Endothelial cells create a stem cell niche in glioblastoma by providing NOTCH ligands that nurture self-renewal of cancer stem-like cells. *Cancer Res.* **2011**, *71*, 6061–6072. [CrossRef] [PubMed]
96. Sonoshita, M.; Aoki, M.; Fuwa, H.; Aoki, K.; Hosogi, H.; Sakai, Y.; Hashida, H.; Takabayashi, A.; Sasaki, M.; Robine, S.; et al. Suppression of colon cancer metastasis by Aes through inhibition of Notch signaling. *Cancer Cell* **2011**, *19*, 125–137. [CrossRef] [PubMed]
97. Ghiabi, P.; Jiang, J.; Pasquier, J.; Maleki, M.; Abu-Kaoud, N.; Rafii, S.; Rafii, A. Endothelial cells provide a notch-dependent pro-tumoral niche for enhancing breast cancer survival, stemness and pro-metastatic properties. *PLoS ONE* **2014**, *9*, e112424. [CrossRef]
98. Lu, J.; Ye, X.; Fan, F.; Xia, L.; Bhattacharya, R.; Bellister, S.; Tozzi, F.; Sceusi, E.; Zhou, Y.; Tachibana, I.; et al. Endothelial cells promote the colorectal cancer stem cell phenotype through a soluble form of Jagged-1. *Cancer Cell* **2013**, *23*, 171–185. [CrossRef]
99. Fidler, I.J. The relationship of embolic homogeneity, number, size and viability to the incidence of experimental metastasis. *Eur. J. Cancer* **1973**, *9*, 223–227. [CrossRef]
100. Liotta, L.A.; Saidel, M.G.; Kleinerman, J. The significance of hematogenous tumor cell clumps in the metastatic process. *Cancer Res.* **1976**, *36*, 889–894.
101. Molnar, B.; Ladanyi, A.; Tanko, L.; Sreter, L.; Tulassay, Z. Circulating tumor cell clusters in the peripheral blood of colorectal cancer patients. *Clin. Cancer Res.* **2001**, *7*, 4080–4085. [PubMed]
102. Cho, E.H.; Wendel, M.; Luttgen, M.; Yoshioka, C.; Marrinucci, D.; Lazar, D.; Schram, E.; Nieva, J.; Bazhenova, L.; Morgan, A.; et al. Characterization of circulating tumor cell aggregates identified in patients with epithelial tumors. *Phys. Biol.* **2012**, *9*, 016001. [CrossRef] [PubMed]
103. Aceto, N.; Bardia, A.; Miyamoto, D.T.; Donaldson, M.C.; Wittner, B.S.; Spencer, J.A.; Yu, M.; Pely, A.; Engstrom, A.; Zhu, H.; et al. Circulating tumor cell clusters are oligoclonal precursors of breast cancer metastasis. *Cell* **2014**, *158*, 1110–1122. [CrossRef] [PubMed]
104. Liu, X.; Taftaf, R.; Kawaguchi, M.; Chang, Y.F.; Chen, W.; Entenberg, D.; Zhang, Y.; Gerratana, L.; Huang, S.; Patel, D.B.; et al. Homophilic CD44 Interactions Mediate Tumor Cell Aggregation and Polyclonal Metastasis in Patient-Derived Breast Cancer Models. *Cancer Discov.* **2019**, *9*, 96–113. [CrossRef]
105. Cheung, K.J.; Gabrielson, E.; Werb, Z.; Ewald, A.J. Collective invasion in breast cancer requires a conserved basal epithelial program. *Cell* **2013**, *155*, 1639–1651. [CrossRef]
106. Cheung, K.J.; Padmanaban, V.; Silvestri, V.; Schipper, K.; Cohen, J.D.; Fairchild, A.N.; Gorin, M.A.; Verdone, J.E.; Pienta, K.J.; Bader, J.S.; et al. Polyclonal breast cancer metastases arise from collective dissemination of keratin 14-expressing tumor cell clusters. *Proc. Natl. Acad. Sci. USA* **2016**, *113*, E854–E863. [CrossRef]
107. Entenberg, D.; Voiculescu, S.; Guo, P.; Borriello, L.; Wang, Y.; Karagiannis, G.S.; Jones, J.; Baccay, F.; Oktay, M.; Condeelis, J. A permanent window for the murine lung enables high-resolution imaging of cancer metastasis. *Nat. Methods* **2018**, *15*, 73–80. [CrossRef]
108. Li, D.; Zhou, J.; Wang, L.; Shin, M.E.; Su, P.; Lei, X.; Kuang, H.; Guo, W.; Yang, H.; Cheng, L.; et al. Integrated biochemical and mechanical signals regulate multifaceted human embryonic stem cell functions. *J. Cell Biol.* **2010**, *191*, 631–644. [CrossRef]
109. Li, L.; Bennett, S.A.; Wang, L. Role of E-cadherin and other cell adhesion molecules in survival and differentiation of human pluripotent stem cells. *Cell Adh. Migr.* **2012**, *6*, 59–70. [CrossRef]
110. Pieters, T.; van Roy, F. Role of cell-cell adhesion complexes in embryonic stem cell biology. *J. Cell Sci.* **2014**, *127*, 2603–2613. [CrossRef]
111. Gkountela, S.; Castro-Giner, F.; Szczerba, B.M.; Vetter, M.; Landin, J.; Scherrer, R.; Krol, I.; Scheidmann, M.C.; Beisel, C.; Stirnimann, C.U.; et al. Circulating Tumor Cell Clustering Shapes DNA Methylation to Enable Metastasis Seeding. *Cell* **2019**, *176*, 98–112 e114. [CrossRef] [PubMed]
112. Fang, J.H.; Zhou, H.C.; Zhang, C.; Shang, L.R.; Zhang, L.; Xu, J.; Zheng, L.; Yuan, Y.; Guo, R.P.; Jia, W.H.; et al. A novel vascular pattern promotes metastasis of hepatocellular carcinoma in an epithelial-mesenchymal transition-independent manner. *Hepatology* **2015**, *62*, 452–465. [CrossRef] [PubMed]
113. Bronsert, P.; Enderle-Ammour, K.; Bader, M.; Timme, S.; Kuehs, M.; Csanadi, A.; Kayser, G.; Kohler, I.; Bausch, D.; Hoeppner, J.; et al. Cancer cell invasion and EMT marker expression: A three-dimensional study of the human cancer-host interface. *J. Pathol.* **2014**, *234*, 410–422. [CrossRef] [PubMed]

114. Wang, C.; Mu, Z.; Chervoneva, I.; Austin, L.; Ye, Z.; Rossi, G.; Palazzo, J.P.; Sun, C.; Abu-Khalaf, M.; Myers, R.E.; et al. Longitudinally collected CTCs and CTC-clusters and clinical outcomes of metastatic breast cancer. *Breast Cancer Res. Treat.* **2017**, *161*, 83–94. [CrossRef]
115. Bocci, F.; Kumar Jolly, M.; Onuchic, J.N. A biophysical model uncovers the size distribution of migrating cell clusters across cancer types. *Cancer Res.* **2019**. [CrossRef]
116. Szczerba, B.M.; Castro-Giner, F.; Vetter, M.; Krol, I.; Gkountela, S.; Landin, J.; Scheidmann, M.C.; Donato, C.; Scherrer, R.; Singer, J.; et al. Neutrophils escort circulating tumour cells to enable cell cycle progression. *Nature* **2019**, *566*, 553–557. [CrossRef]
117. Wei, D.; Zeng, X.; Yang, Z.; Zhou, Q.; Weng, X.; He, H.; Gu, Z.; Wei, X. Visualizing Interactions of Circulating Tumor Cell and Dendritic Cell in the Blood Circulation Using In Vivo Imaging Flow Cytometry. *IEEE Trans. Biomed. Eng.* **2019**. [CrossRef]
118. Gao, Q.; Yang, Z.; Xu, S.; Li, X.; Yang, X.; Jin, P.; Liu, Y.; Zhou, X.; Zhang, T.; Gong, C.; et al. Heterotypic CAF-tumor spheroids promote early peritoneal metastatsis of ovarian cancer. *J. Exp. Med.* **2019**, *216*, 688–703. [CrossRef]
119. Duda, D.G.; Duyverman, A.M.; Kohno, M.; Snuderl, M.; Steller, E.J.; Fukumura, D.; Jain, R.K. Malignant cells facilitate lung metastasis by bringing their own soil. *Proc. Natl. Acad. Sci. USA* **2010**, *107*, 21677–21682. [CrossRef]
120. Baeriswyl, V.; Christofori, G. The angiogenic switch in carcinogenesis. *Semin. Cancer Biol.* **2009**, *19*, 329–337. [CrossRef]
121. Erpenbeck, L.; Schon, M.P. Deadly allies: The fatal interplay between platelets and metastasizing cancer cells. *Blood* **2010**, *115*, 3427–3436. [CrossRef] [PubMed]
122. Gasic, G.J.; Gasic, T.B.; Stewart, C.C. Antimetastatic effects associated with platelet reduction. *Proc. Natl. Acad. Sci. USA* **1968**, *61*, 46–52. [CrossRef] [PubMed]
123. Labelle, M.; Hynes, R.O. The initial hours of metastasis: The importance of cooperative host-tumor cell interactions during hematogenous dissemination. *Cancer Discov.* **2012**, *2*, 1091–1099. [CrossRef] [PubMed]
124. Mammadova-Bach, E.; Mangin, P.; Lanza, F.; Gachet, C. Platelets in cancer. From basic research to therapeutic implications. *Hamostaseologie* **2015**, *35*, 325–336. [CrossRef]
125. Cheung, K.J.; Ewald, A.J. A collective route to metastasis: Seeding by tumor cell clusters. *Science* **2016**, *352*, 167–169. [CrossRef]
126. Chew, H.K.; Wun, T.; Harvey, D.J.; Zhou, H.; White, R.H. Incidence of venous thromboembolism and the impact on survival in breast cancer patients. *J. Clin. Oncol.* **2007**, *25*, 70–76. [CrossRef]
127. Jain, S.; Zuka, M.; Liu, J.; Russell, S.; Dent, J.; Guerrero, J.A.; Forsyth, J.; Maruszak, B.; Gartner, T.K.; Felding-Habermann, B.; et al. Platelet glycoprotein Ib alpha supports experimental lung metastasis. *Proc. Natl. Acad. Sci. USA* **2007**, *104*, 9024–9028. [CrossRef]
128. Jain, S.; Russell, S.; Ware, J. Platelet glycoprotein VI facilitates experimental lung metastasis in syngenic mouse models. *J. Thromb Haemost.* **2009**, *7*, 1713–1717. [CrossRef]
129. Jurasz, P.; Alonso-Escolano, D.; Radomski, M.W. Platelet–cancer interactions: Mechanisms and pharmacology of tumour cell-induced platelet aggregation. *Br. J. Pharmacol.* **2004**, *143*, 819–826. [CrossRef]
130. Karpatkin, S.; Ambrogio, C.; Pearlstein, E. The role of tumor-induced platelet aggregation, platelet adhesion and adhesive proteins in tumor metastasis. *Prog. Clin. Biol. Res.* **1988**, *283*, 585–606.
131. Karpatkin, S.; Pearlstein, E.; Ambrogio, C.; Coller, B.S. Role of adhesive proteins in platelet tumor interaction in vitro and metastasis formation in vivo. *J. Clin. Investig.* **1988**, *81*, 1012–1019. [CrossRef] [PubMed]
132. Nieswandt, B.; Hafner, M.; Echtenacher, B.; Mannel, D.N. Lysis of tumor cells by natural killer cells in mice is impeded by platelets. *Cancer Res.* **1999**, *59*, 1295–1300. [PubMed]
133. Katagiri, Y.; Hayashi, Y.; Baba, I.; Suzuki, H.; Tanoue, K.; Yamazaki, H. Characterization of platelet aggregation induced by the human melanoma cell line HMV-I: Roles of heparin, plasma adhesive proteins, and tumor cell membrane proteins. *Cancer Res.* **1991**, *51*, 1286–1293. [PubMed]
134. Alonso-Escolano, D.; Strongin, A.Y.; Chung, A.W.; Deryugina, E.I.; Radomski, M.W. Membrane type-1 matrix metalloproteinase stimulates tumour cell-induced platelet aggregation: Role of receptor glycoproteins. *Br. J. Pharmacol.* **2004**, *141*, 241–252. [CrossRef] [PubMed]
135. Pantel, K.; Brakenhoff, R.H. Dissecting the metastatic cascade. *Nat. Rev. Cancer* **2004**, *4*, 448–456. [CrossRef]

136. Echtler, K.; Konrad, I.; Lorenz, M.; Schneider, S.; Hofmaier, S.; Plenagl, F.; Stark, K.; Czermak, T.; Tirniceriu, A.; Eichhorn, M.; et al. Platelet GPIIb supports initial pulmonary retention but inhibits subsequent proliferation of melanoma cells during hematogenic metastasis. *PLoS ONE* **2017**, *12*, e0172788. [CrossRef]
137. Erpenbeck, L.; Nieswandt, B.; Schon, M.; Pozgajova, M.; Schon, M.P. Inhibition of platelet GPIb alpha and promotion of melanoma metastasis. *J. Investig. Dermatol.* **2010**, *130*, 576–586. [CrossRef]
138. Gay, L.J.; Felding-Habermann, B. Contribution of platelets to tumour metastasis. *Nat. Rev. Cancer* **2011**, *11*, 123–134. [CrossRef]
139. Papa, A.L.; Jiang, A.; Korin, N.; Chen, M.B.; Langan, E.T.; Waterhouse, A.; Nash, E.; Caroff, J.; Graveline, A.; Vernet, A.; et al. Platelet decoys inhibit thrombosis and prevent metastatic tumor formation in preclinical models. *Sci. Transl. Med.* **2019**, *11*. [CrossRef]
140. Amirkhosravi, A.; Mousa, S.A.; Amaya, M.; Blaydes, S.; Desai, H.; Meyer, T.; Francis, J.L. Inhibition of tumor cell-induced platelet aggregation and lung metastasis by the oral GpIIb/IIIa antagonist XV454. *Thromb Haemost.* **2003**, *90*, 549–554.
141. Millard, M.; Odde, S.; Neamati, N. Integrin targeted therapeutics. *Theranostics* **2011**, *1*, 154–188. [CrossRef] [PubMed]
142. Safaee, M.; Clark, A.J.; Ivan, M.E.; Oh, M.C.; Bloch, O.; Sun, M.Z.; Oh, T.; Parsa, A.T. CD97 is a multifunctional leukocyte receptor with distinct roles in human cancers (Review). *Int. J. Oncol.* **2013**, *43*, 1343–1350. [CrossRef] [PubMed]
143. Boucharaba, A.; Serre, C.M.; Gres, S.; Saulnier-Blache, J.S.; Bordet, J.C.; Guglielmi, J.; Clezardin, P.; Peyruchaud, O. Platelet-derived lysophosphatidic acid supports the progression of osteolytic bone metastases in breast cancer. *J. Clin. Investig.* **2004**, *114*, 1714–1725. [CrossRef] [PubMed]
144. Leblanc, R.; Lee, S.C.; David, M.; Bordet, J.C.; Norman, D.D.; Patil, R.; Miller, D.; Sahay, D.; Ribeiro, J.; Clezardin, P.; et al. Interaction of platelet-derived autotaxin with tumor integrin alphaVbeta3 controls metastasis of breast cancer cells to bone. *Blood* **2014**, *124*, 3141–3150. [CrossRef] [PubMed]
145. Ward, Y.; Lake, R.; Yin, J.J.; Heger, C.D.; Raffeld, M.; Goldsmith, P.K.; Merino, M.; Kelly, K. LPA receptor heterodimerizes with CD97 to amplify LPA-initiated RHO-dependent signaling and invasion in prostate cancer cells. *Cancer Res.* **2011**, *71*, 7301–7311. [CrossRef]
146. Ward, Y.; Lake, R.; Faraji, F.; Sperger, J.; Martin, P.; Gilliard, C.; Ku, K.P.; Rodems, T.; Niles, D.; Tillman, H.; et al. Platelets Promote Metastasis via Binding Tumor CD97 Leading to Bidirectional Signaling that Coordinates Transendothelial Migration. *Cell Rep.* **2018**, *23*, 808–822. [CrossRef]
147. Kato, Y.; Kaneko, M.K.; Kunita, A.; Ito, H.; Kameyama, A.; Ogasawara, S.; Matsuura, N.; Hasegawa, Y.; Suzuki-Inoue, K.; Inoue, O.; et al. Molecular analysis of the pathophysiological binding of the platelet aggregation-inducing factor podoplanin to the C-type lectin-like receptor CLEC-2. *Cancer Sci.* **2008**, *99*, 54–61. [CrossRef]
148. Yu, L.X.; Yan, L.; Yang, W.; Wu, F.Q.; Ling, Y.; Chen, S.Z.; Tang, L.; Tan, Y.X.; Cao, D.; Wu, M.C.; et al. Platelets promote tumour metastasis via interaction between TLR4 and tumour cell-released high-mobility group box1 protein. *Nat. Commun.* **2014**, *5*, 5256. [CrossRef]
149. Aigner, S.; Sthoeger, Z.M.; Fogel, M.; Weber, E.; Zarn, J.; Ruppert, M.; Zeller, Y.; Vestweber, D.; Stahel, R.; Sammar, M.; et al. CD24, a mucin-type glycoprotein, is a ligand for P-selectin on human tumor cells. *Blood* **1997**, *89*, 3385–3395. [CrossRef]
150. Kristiansen, G.; Sammar, M.; Altevogt, P. Tumour biological aspects of CD24, a mucin-like adhesion molecule. *J. Mol. Histol.* **2004**, *35*, 255–262. [CrossRef]
151. Yao, X.; Labelle, M.; Lamb, C.R.; Dugan, J.M.; Williamson, C.A.; Spencer, D.R.; Christ, K.R.; Keating, R.O.; Lee, W.D.; Paradis, G.A.; et al. Determination of 35 cell surface antigen levels in malignant pleural effusions identifies CD24 as a marker of disseminated tumor cells. *Int. J. Cancer* **2013**, *133*, 2925–2933. [CrossRef] [PubMed]
152. Haemmerle, M.; Taylor, M.L.; Gutschner, T.; Pradeep, S.; Cho, M.S.; Sheng, J.; Lyons, Y.M.; Nagaraja, A.S.; Dood, R.L.; Wen, Y.; et al. Platelets reduce anoikis and promote metastasis by activating YAP1 signaling. *Nat. Commun.* **2017**, *8*, 310. [CrossRef] [PubMed]
153. Schumacher, D.; Strilic, B.; Sivaraj, K.K.; Wettschureck, N.; Offermanns, S. Platelet-derived nucleotides promote tumor-cell transendothelial migration and metastasis via P2Y2 receptor. *Cancer Cell* **2013**, *24*, 130–137. [CrossRef] [PubMed]

154. Pilch, J.; Habermann, R.; Felding-Habermann, B. Unique ability of integrin alpha(v)beta 3 to support tumor cell arrest under dynamic flow conditions. *J. Biol. Chem.* **2002**, *277*, 21930–21938. [CrossRef]
155. Frenette, P.S.; Johnson, R.C.; Hynes, R.O.; Wagner, D.D. Platelets roll on stimulated endothelium in vivo: An interaction mediated by endothelial P-selectin. *Proc. Natl. Acad. Sci. USA* **1995**, *92*, 7450–7454. [CrossRef]
156. Reymond, N.; d'Agua, B.B.; Ridley, A.J. Crossing the endothelial barrier during metastasis. *Nat. Rev. Cancer* **2013**, *13*, 858–870. [CrossRef]
157. Fung, Y.C. *Biomechanics: Circulation*; Springer: New York, NY, USA, 1997.
158. Regmi, S.; Fu, A.; Luo, K.Q. High Shear Stresses under Exercise Condition Destroy Circulating Tumor Cells in a Microfluidic System. *Sci. Rep.* **2017**, *7*, 39975. [CrossRef]
159. Follain, G.; Osmani, N.; Azevedo, S.; Allio, G.; Mercier, L.; Karreman, M.A.; Solecki, G.; Garcia-Leon, M.J.; Fekonja, N.; Chabannes, V.; et al. Hemodynamic forces tune the arrest, adhesion and extravasation of circulating tumor cells. *Dev. Cell* **2018**, *45*, 33–52. [CrossRef]
160. Polacheck, W.J.; Kutys, M.L.; Yang, J.; Eyckmans, J.; Wu, Y.; Vasavada, H.; Hirschi, K.K.; Chen, C.S. A non-canonical Notch complex regulates adherens junctions and vascular barrier function. *Nature* **2017**, *552*, 258–262. [CrossRef]
161. Wieland, E.; Rodriguez-Vita, J.; Liebler, S.S.; Mogler, C.; Moll, I.; Herberich, S.E.; Espinet, E.; Herpel, E.; Menuchin, A.; Chang-Claude, J.; et al. Endothelial Notch1 Activity Facilitates Metastasis. *Cancer Cell* **2017**, *31*, 355–367. [CrossRef]
162. Karreman, M.A.; Mercier, L.; Schieber, N.L.; Solecki, G.; Allio, G.; Winkler, F.; Ruthensteiner, B.; Goetz, J.G.; Schwab, Y. Fast and precise targeting of single tumor cells in vivo by multimodal correlative microscopy. *J. Cell Sci.* **2016**, *129*, 444–456. [CrossRef] [PubMed]
163. Im, J.H.; Fu, W.; Wang, H.; Bhatia, S.K.; Hammer, D.A.; Kowalska, M.A.; Muschel, R.J. Coagulation facilitates tumor cell spreading in the pulmonary vasculature during early metastatic colony formation. *Cancer Res.* **2004**, *64*, 8613–8619. [CrossRef] [PubMed]
164. Allen, T.A.; Asad, D.; Amu, E.; Hensley, M.T.; Cores, J.; Vandergriff, A.; Tang, J.; Dinh, P.U.; Shen, D.; Qiao, L.; et al. Circulating tumor cells exit circulation while maintaining multicellularity, augmenting metastatic potential. *J. Cell Sci.* **2019**, *132*. [CrossRef] [PubMed]
165. Zhuang, X.; Long, E.O. CD28 Homolog Is a Strong Activator of Natural Killer Cells for Lysis of B7H7(+) Tumor Cells. *Cancer Immunol. Res.* **2019**, *7*, 939–951. [CrossRef] [PubMed]
166. Rejniak, K.A. Circulating Tumor Cells: When a Solid Tumor Meets a Fluid Microenvironment. *Adv. Exp. Med. Biol.* **2016**, *936*, 93–106. [PubMed]
167. Anderson, K.J.; de Guillebon, A.; Hughes, A.D.; Wang, W.; King, M.R. Effect of circulating tumor cell aggregate configuration on hemodynamic transport and wall contact. *Math Biosci.* **2017**, *294*, 181–194. [CrossRef] [PubMed]
168. Hong, Y.; Fang, F.; Zhang, Q. Circulating tumor cell clusters: What we know and what we expect (Review). *Int. J. Oncol.* **2016**, *49*, 2206–2216. [CrossRef]
169. Mohammadalipour, A.; Burdick, M.M.; Tees, D.F.J. Deformability of breast cancer cells in correlation with surface markers and cell rolling. *FASEB J.* **2018**, *32*, 1806–1817. [CrossRef]
170. Celia-Terrassa, T.; Kang, Y. Distinctive properties of metastasis-initiating cells. *Genes Dev.* **2016**, *30*, 892–908. [CrossRef]
171. Janiszewska, M.; Tabassum, D.P.; Castano, Z.; Cristea, S.; Yamamoto, K.N.; Kingston, N.L.; Murphy, K.C.; Shu, S.; Harper, N.W.; Del Alcazar, C.G.; et al. Subclonal cooperation drives metastasis by modulating local and systemic immune microenvironments. *Nat. Cell Biol.* **2019**, *21*, 879–888. [CrossRef]
172. Burrell, R.A.; Swanton, C. Re-Evaluating Clonal Dominance in Cancer Evolution. *Trends Cancer* **2016**, *2*, 263–276. [CrossRef] [PubMed]
173. Paget, S. The distribution of secondary growths in cancer of the breast. 1889. *Cancer Metastasis Rev.* **1989**, *8*, 98–101. [PubMed]
174. Ghajar, C.M.; Peinado, H.; Mori, H.; Matei, I.R.; Evason, K.J.; Brazier, H.; Almeida, D.; Koller, A.; Hajjar, K.A.; Stainier, D.Y.R.; et al. The perivascular niche regulates breast tumor dormancy. *Nat. Cell Biol.* **2013**, *15*, 807. [CrossRef] [PubMed]
175. Ghajar, C.M. Metastasis prevention by targeting the dormant niche. *Nat. Rev. Cancer* **2015**, *15*, 238–247. [CrossRef] [PubMed]

176. Eyles, J.; Puaux, A.-L.; Wang, X.; Toh, B.; Prakash, C.; Hong, M.; Tan, T.G.; Zheng, L.; Ong, L.C.; Jin, Y.; et al. Tumor cells disseminate early, but immunosurveillance limits metastatic outgrowth, in a mouse model of melanoma. *J. Clin. Investig.* **2010**, *120*, 2030–2039. [CrossRef]
177. Malladi, S.; Macalinao, D.G.; Jin, X.; He, L.; Basnet, H.; Zou, Y.; de Stanchina, E.; Massagué, J. Metastatic Latency and Immune Evasion through Autocrine Inhibition of WNT. *Cell* **2016**, *165*, 45–60. [CrossRef]
178. Castaño, Z.; San Juan, B.P.; Spiegel, A.; Pant, A.; DeCristo, M.J.; Laszewski, T.; Ubellacker, J.M.; Janssen, S.R.; Dongre, A.; Reinhardt, F.; et al. IL-1β inflammatory response driven by primary breast cancer prevents metastasis-initiating cell colonization. *Nat. Cell Biol.* **2018**, *20*, 1084–1097. [CrossRef]
179. Pattabiraman, D.R.; Bierie, B.; Kober, K.I.; Thiru, P.; Krall, J.A.; Zill, C.; Reinhardt, F.; Tam, W.L.; Weinberg, R.A. Activation of PKA leads to mesenchymal-to-epithelial transition and loss of tumor-initiating ability. *Science* **2016**, *351*, aad3680. [CrossRef]
180. Sceneay, J.; Chow, M.T.; Chen, A.; Halse, H.M.; Wong, C.S.F.; Andrews, D.M.; Sloan, E.K.; Parker, B.S.; Bowtell, D.D.; Smyth, M.J.; et al. Primary Tumor Hypoxia Recruits CD11b$^+$/Ly6C^{med}/Ly6G$^+$ Immune Suppressor Cells and Compromises NK Cell Cytotoxicity in the Premetastatic Niche. *Cancer Res.* **2012**, *72*, 3906–3911. [CrossRef]
181. Gil-Bernabe, A.M.; Ferjancic, S.; Tlalka, M.; Zhao, L.; Allen, P.D.; Im, J.H.; Watson, K.; Hill, S.A.; Amirkhosravi, A.; Francis, J.L.; et al. Recruitment of monocytes/macrophages by tissue factor-mediated coagulation is essential for metastatic cell survival and premetastatic niche establishment in mice. *Blood* **2012**, *119*, 3164–3175. [CrossRef]
182. Wculek, S.K.; Malanchi, I. Neutrophils support lung colonization of metastasis-initiating breast cancer cells. *Nature* **2015**, *528*, 413–417. [CrossRef] [PubMed]
183. Najmeh, S.; Cools-Lartigue, J.; Rayes, R.F.; Gowing, S.; Vourtzoumis, P.; Bourdeau, F.; Giannias, B.; Berube, J.; Rousseau, S.; Ferri, L.E.; et al. Neutrophil extracellular traps sequester circulating tumor cells via β1-integrin mediated interactions. *Int. J. Cancer* **2017**, *140*, 2321–2330. [CrossRef] [PubMed]
184. Albrengues, J.; Shields, M.A.; Ng, D.; Park, C.G.; Ambrico, A.; Poindexter, M.E.; Upadhyay, P.; Uyeminami, D.L.; Pommier, A.; Küttner, V.; et al. Neutrophil extracellular traps produced during inflammation awaken dormant cancer cells in mice. *Science* **2018**, *361*, eaao4227. [CrossRef] [PubMed]
185. Piskounova, E.; Agathocleous, M.; Murphy, M.M.; Hu, Z.; Huddlestun, S.E.; Zhao, Z.; Leitch, A.M.; Johnson, T.M.; DeBerardinis, R.J.; Morrison, S.J. Oxidative stress inhibits distant metastasis by human melanoma cells. *Nature* **2015**, *527*, 186–191. [CrossRef]
186. Morel, A.-P.; Ginestier, C.; Pommier, R.M.; Cabaud, O.; Ruiz, E.; Wicinski, J.; Devouassoux-Shisheboran, M.; Combaret, V.; Finetti, P.; Chassot, C.; et al. A stemness-related ZEB1–MSRB3 axis governs cellular pliancy and breast cancer genome stability. *Nat. Med.* **2017**, *23*, 568–578. [CrossRef]
187. Liu, Z.; Tu, K.; Wang, Y.; Yao, B.; Li, Q.; Wang, L.; Dou, C.; Liu, Q.; Zheng, X. Hypoxia Accelerates Aggressiveness of Hepatocellular Carcinoma Cells Involving Oxidative Stress, Epithelial-Mesenchymal Transition and Non-Canonical Hedgehog Signaling. *Cell. Physiol. Biochem.* **2017**, *44*, 1856–1868. [CrossRef]
188. Ricciardi, M.; Zanotto, M.; Malpeli, G.; Bassi, G.; Perbellini, O.; Chilosi, M.; Bifari, F.; Krampera, M. Epithelial-to-mesenchymal transition (EMT) induced by inflammatory priming elicits mesenchymal stromal cell-like immune-modulatory properties in cancer cells. *Br. J. Cancer* **2015**, *112*, 1067–1075. [CrossRef]
189. Dongre, A.; Rashidian, M.; Reinhardt, F.; Bagnato, A.; Keckesova, Z.; Ploegh, H.L.; Weinberg, R.A. Epithelial-to-Mesenchymal Transition Contributes to Immunosuppression in Breast Carcinomas. *Cancer Res.* **2017**, *77*, 3982–3989. [CrossRef]
190. Chen, L.; Gibbons, D.L.; Goswami, S.; Cortez, M.A.; Ahn, Y.H.; Byers, L.A.; Zhang, X.; Yi, X.; Dwyer, D.; Lin, W.; et al. Metastasis is regulated via microRNA-200/ZEB1 axis control of tumour cell PD-L1 expression and intratumoral immunosuppression. *Nat. Commun.* **2014**, *5*, 5241. [CrossRef]
191. Noman, M.Z.; Janji, B.; Abdou, A.; Hasmim, M.; Terry, S.; Tan, T.Z.; Mami-Chouaib, F.; Thiery, J.P.; Chouaib, S. The immune checkpoint ligand PD-L1 is upregulated in EMT-activated human breast cancer cells by a mechanism involving ZEB-1 and miR-200. *Oncoimmunology* **2017**, *6*, e1263412. [CrossRef]
192. Tripathi, S.C.; Peters, H.L.; Taguchi, A.; Katayama, H.; Wang, H.; Momin, A.; Jolly, M.K.; Celiktas, M.; Rodriguez-Canales, J.; Liu, H.; et al. Immunoproteasome deficiency is a feature of non-small cell lung cancer with a mesenchymal phenotype and is associated with a poor outcome. *Proc. Natl. Acad. Sci. USA* **2016**, *113*, E1555–E1564. [CrossRef] [PubMed]

193. Peinado, H.; Zhang, H.; Matei, I.R.; Costa-Silva, B.; Hoshino, A.; Rodrigues, G.; Psaila, B.; Kaplan, R.N.; Bromberg, J.F.; Kang, Y.; et al. Pre-metastatic niches: Organ-specific homes for metastases. *Nat. Rev. Cancer* **2017**, *17*, 302–317. [CrossRef] [PubMed]
194. Hoshino, A.; Costa-Silva, B.; Shen, T.L.; Rodrigues, G.; Hashimoto, A.; Tesic Mark, M.; Molina, H.; Kohsaka, S.; Di Giannatale, A.; Ceder, S.; et al. Tumour exosome integrins determine organotropic metastasis. *Nature* **2015**, *527*, 329–335. [CrossRef] [PubMed]
195. Hyenne, V.; Ghoroghi, S.; Collot, M.; Bons, J.; Follain, G.; Harlepp, S.; Mary, B.; Bauer, J.; Mercier, L.; Busnelli, I.; et al. Studying the Fate of Tumor Extracellular Vesicles at High Spatiotemporal Resolution Using the Zebrafish Embryo. *Dev. Cell.* **2019**, *48*, 554–572 e557. [CrossRef] [PubMed]
196. Ombrato, L.; Nolan, E.; Kurelac, I.; Mavousian, A.; Bridgeman, V.L.; Heinze, I.; Chakravarty, P.; Horswell, S.; Gonzalez-Gualda, E.; Matacchione, G.; et al. Metastatic-niche labelling reveals parenchymal cells with stem features. *Nature* **2019**, *572*, 603–608. [CrossRef]

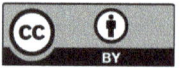

© 2019 by the authors. Licensee MDPI, Basel, Switzerland. This article is an open access article distributed under the terms and conditions of the Creative Commons Attribution (CC BY) license (http://creativecommons.org/licenses/by/4.0/).

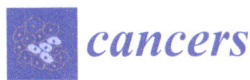

Review

Cell Heterogeneity and Phenotypic Plasticity in Metastasis Formation: The Case of Colon Cancer

Miriam Teeuwssen and Riccardo Fodde *

Department of Pathology, Erasmus MC Cancer Institute, Erasmus University Medical Center, 3015 GD Rotterdam, The Netherlands; m.teeuwssen@erasmusmc.nl
* Correspondence: r.fodde@erasmusmc.nl; Tel.: +31-010-7043896

Received: 25 July 2019; Accepted: 11 September 2019; Published: 14 September 2019

Abstract: The adenoma-to-carcinoma progression in colon cancer is driven by a sequential accumulation of genetic alterations at specific tumor suppressors and oncogenes. In contrast, the multistage route from the primary site to metastasis formation is underlined by phenotypic plasticity, i.e., the capacity of disseminated tumor cells to undergo transiently and reversible transformations in order to adapt to the ever-changing environmental contexts. Notwithstanding the considerable body of evidence in support of the role played by epithelial-to-mesenchymal transition (EMT)/mesenchymal-to-epithelial transition (MET) in metastasis, its rate-limiting function, the detailed underlying cellular and molecular mechanisms, and the extension of the necessary morphologic and epigenetic changes are still a matter of debate. Rather than leading to a complete epithelial or mesenchymal state, the EMT/MET-program generates migrating cancer cells displaying intermediate phenotypes featuring both epithelial and mesenchymal characteristics. In this review, we will address the role of colon cancer heterogeneity and phenotypic plasticity in metastasis formation and the contribution of EMT to these processes. The alleged role of hybrid epithelial/mesenchymal (E/M) in collective and/or single-cell migration during local dissemination at the primary site and more systemic spreading will also be highlighted.

Keywords: colon cancer; Wnt signaling; tumor heterogeneity; phenotypic plasticity; EMT; hybrid E/M; collective and single-cell migration; beta-catenin paradox

---

1. Introduction—Tumor Heterogeneity in Colon Cancer

Colon cancer is the third most commonly diagnosed malignancy and the second leading cause of cancer-related death worldwide. It is predicted that its mortality burden will increase by 75% by 2040 [1]. Apart from its clinical impact, colon cancer also represents a unique study model to elucidate the cellular and molecular mechanisms underlying tumor onset, progression towards malignancy, and metastasis formation at distant organ sites [2].

It is generally accepted that primary colon carcinomas are heterotypic, i.e., they feature a heterogeneous composition of epithelial cancer cells intermingled with lymphocytes, stromal fibroblasts, endothelial, and other cell types from the micro- and macro-environment [3]. This heterogeneity is matched by the diversity of parenchymal cancer cells encompassing a broad spectrum of morphologies, gene expression profiles, and functional characteristics [4–6]. Likewise, heterogeneity within the stromal compartment, i.e., the tumor microenvironment, has also been demonstrated [5,7].

Intrinsic, i.e., (epi)genetic, as well as extrinsic factors, such as spatial location within the tumor (e.g., at the invasive front vs. tumor center), inflammation, and treatment history underlie the observed intra-tumor heterogeneity. Consequently, different cellular subpopulations within the primary tumor mass and its metastatic lesions are observed [8,9]. Next to 'spatial' heterogeneity, 'temporal' heterogeneity has also been demonstrated relative to changes in the (epi)genetic landscape of colon cancer within individual tumors over time [10]. Of note, tumor heterogeneity is thought to underlie the disappointing results of many currently employed anti-cancer therapies as it not only supports tumor progression and metastatic dissemination but it also lies at the basis of the development of therapy resistance and of overall poor clinical prognosis [11].

Metastasis formation is a process encompassing multiple steps: (1) Local tumor invasion across the basement membrane into the surrounding stroma, (2) intravasation into the vasculature, (3) survival in the circulatory system, (4) extravasation into the parenchyma of the distant organ, (5) colonization into a distal organ, and (6) re-initiation of proliferation to form macroscopic metastases [12]. In order to successfully complete this challenging series of events, the most important feature of the metastasizing cancer cell is the capacity to adapt to the ever-changing environmental contexts by undergoing reversible changes in its cellular identity. This 'Dr. Jekyll and Mr. Hide' feature of migrating cancer cells is often referred to as phenotypic plasticity [13] and is controlled by epigenetic mechanisms which regulate, among other processes, epithelial-to-mesenchymal transition (EMT) and the reverse mesenchymal-to-epithelial transition (MET) [14].

A variety of chromatin remodeling complexes such as Polycomb and NuRD, play a central role in the transcriptional regulation of EMT-related transcription factors (EMT-TFs) and micro RNAs (miRs) by determining the accessibility of regulatory DNA elements and positioning of nucleosomes [15,16]. In addition, post-translational histone modifications which modulate chromatin folding and influence recruitment of regulatory proteins and control gene expression [17]. Accordingly, contextual EMT-promoting signals epigenetically modify the repression of epithelial genes and consequently drive the transition of cells into more mesenchymal-like states. These are epigenetically sustained unless the presence of EMT-promoting signals is discontinued leading to the reversion to more epithelial phenotypes [15].

Notwithstanding the considerable body of evidence in support of the role played by EMT/MET in metastasis, its rate-limiting function, and the detailed underlying cellular and molecular mechanisms, and the extension of the necessary morphologic and epigenetic changes are still a matter of debate [14,18,19]. Rather than leading to a complete epithelial or mesenchymal state, the EMT/MET programs generate migrating cancer cells displaying intermediate phenotypes featuring both epithelial and mesenchymal characteristics. These hybrid E/M cancer cells have been the focus of much attention in the most recent scientific literature as they are likely to be metastable and as such very efficient in causing metastasis [20].

Here, we will address the role of tumor cell heterogeneity and phenotypic plasticity in colon cancer metastasis formation and the contribution of EMT to these processes. The alleged role of hybrid E/M in collective and/or single-cell migration during local dissemination at the primary site and more systemic spreading will be highlighted.

2. The Adenoma-Carcinoma Sequence in Colon Cancer: The β-Catenin Paradox

Colon cancer arises and progresses through a well-defined series of histologic stages along which normal colonic epithelial cells transform in stepwise fashion into precursor lesions which eventually evolve to increasingly more invasive and malignant stages. This sequence, often referred to as 'the adenoma-carcinoma sequence', features a gradual accumulation of genetic alterations in specific tumor suppressors and oncogenes generally regarded as the main underlying and driving forces in the progression of colonic adenomas towards malignancy [21].

The initiating and rate-limiting event in the vast majority of sporadic colon cancer cases is represented by the constitutive activation of canonical Wnt signaling through loss of function mutations at the *APC* (adenomatous polyposis coli) tumor suppressor gene. Alternatively, gain of function or 'activating' mutations in Wnt agonists such as the β-catenin (*CTNNB1*) oncogene have functionally equivalent consequences, i.e., the ligand-independent and constitutive signaling activation of the pathway [2]. The reason for the pivotal role of the Wnt/β-catenin signal transduction pathway in colon cancer onset mainly resides in its functional role in the intestinal crypt of Lieberkühn where it regulates the homeostatic equilibrium between stemness, proliferation, and differentiation [22]. In the bottom third of the crypt, where stem cells reside, Wnt signaling is particularly active due to signals from the surrounding stromal environment. Moving along the crypt-villus axis however, Wnt is progressively less active in a decreasing gradient inversely proportional to the grade of differentiation of the epithelial lining [23]. Here, in the absence of canonical Wnt ligands such as Wnt3a, intracellular β-catenin levels are controlled by the formation of a multiprotein "destruction complex" encompassing protein phosphatase 2A (PP2a), glycogen synthase kinase 3 (GSK3β) and casein kinase 1α (CK1α), and the scaffold proteins adenomatous polyposis coli (APC), and Axin1/2. This complex binds and phosphorylates β-catenin at specific serine and threonine residues, thereby targeting it for ubiquitination and proteolytic degradation by the proteasome [23] (Figure 1a). In the presence of Wnt ligands instead, i.e., in the stem cell compartment, co-activation of the Frizzled and LRP5/6 (low-density lipoprotein receptor-related proteins) receptors prevents the formation of the destruction complex thus resulting in the stabilization and consequent translocation of β-catenin from the cytoplasm to the nucleus. Here, β-catenin interacts with members of the TCF/LEF family of transcription factors and modulates the expression of a broad spectrum of Wnt downstream target genes with cellular functions ranging from stemness to proliferation [23] (Figure 1a). Consequently, loss- and gain-of-function genetic alterations in *APC* and β-catenin respectively, result in the constitutive signaling of β-catenin to the nucleus [2].

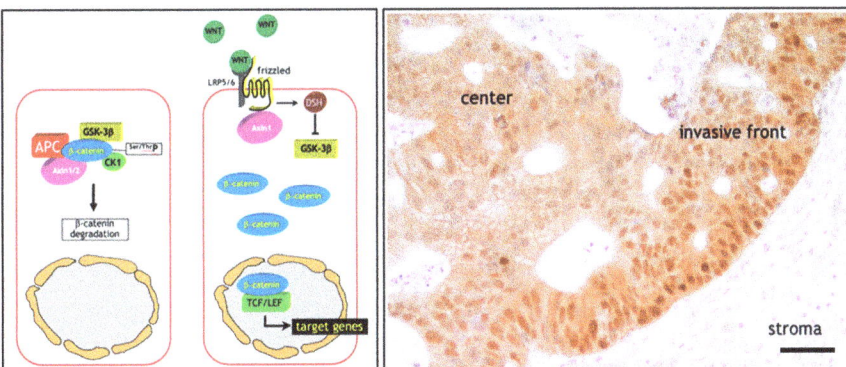

Figure 1. The (**a**) Wnt/β-catenin signal transduction pathway and the (**b**) β-catenin paradox in colon cancer. (**a**) Illustration of the canonical Wnt signaling in homeostasis. Left panel: In the absence of Wnt ligands, intracellular β-catenin levels are controlled by a destruction complex encompassing protein phosphatase 2A (PP2a), glycogen synthase kinase 3 (GSK3β) and casein kinase 1α (CK1α), adenomatous polyposis coli (APC), and Axin1/2. This complex binds and phosphorylates β-catenin at serine and threonine residues, thereby targeting it for ubiquitination and proteolytic degradation by the proteasome. Right panel: In presence of Wnt, co-activation of the Frizzled and LRP5/6 (low-density lipoprotein receptor-related proteins) receptors prevents the formation of the destruction complex leading to the stabilization and consequent translocation of β-catenin from the cytoplasm to the nucleus. Here, β-catenin interacts with members of the TCF/LEF family of transcription factors and modulates the expression of a broad spectrum of Wnt downstream target genes. Adapted from [24]. (**b**) The β-catenin paradox in colon cancer. β-catenin IHC analysis of the invasive front of a colon carcinoma show marked nuclear β-catenin accumulation in the proximity of the stromal microenvironment. In contrast, the majority of tumor cells localized inside the tumor mass are characterized by membrane-bound and cytoplasmic β-catenin staining. Scale bar: 50 µm.

This genetic model predicts that the vast majority of colon cancers, initiated by the constitutive activation of Wnt signaling, should feature nuclear β-catenin localization throughout the entire tumor mass. However, extensive immunohistochemical analysis of sporadic colon cancers has contradicted this prediction. In fact, only a minority of colon cancer cells, non-randomly distributed along the invasive front of the primary mass and of quasi-mesenchymal morphology, show nuclear β-catenin accumulation. In contrast, the majority of more differentiated (epithelial-like) tumor cells localized inside the tumor mass are characterized by an apparently normal (membrane-bound) subcellular distribution of β-catenin together with increased cytoplasmic staining [25] (Figure 1b). This "β-catenin paradox" is generally explained by the fact that the *APC* and β-catenin mutations are necessary for the constitutive activation of the pathway though insufficient for nuclear β-catenin accumulation and full-blown Wnt signaling [24] (Figure 1b). The latter is only achieved in colon cancer cells located at the invasive front where they are exposed to stromal cues capable of further promoting the nuclear translocation of β-catenin from the cytoplasm [26].

Of note, the same heterogeneous β-catenin distribution, with nuclear staining in less differentiated cells located in closer proximity to the microenvironment and membranous staining in more differentiated cells in the center of the lesion, has also been observed in colon cancer metastases [27]. The reacquisition of epithelial features at the metastatic sites is required for cancer cell proliferation, as mesenchymal-like cells are generally hindered in their proliferative activity and are therefore not able to underlie the expansion of the metastasis.

Hence, different levels of Wnt signaling activity between the tumor center and the invasive front are likely to account for the 'spatial' intra-tumor heterogeneity and to underlie distinct Wnt downstream cellular effectors such as proliferation and EMT leading to tumor growth and invasion, respectively [28]. These observations have led to the hypothesis according to which, apart from its role in colon cancer initiation, Wnt signaling and the consequent downstream EMT activation, also underlies the onset of migrating cancer stem cells (mCSC) at the invasive front of the primary lesion which locally invade the tumor microenvironment and eventually form distant metastases [29].

This paracrine—and presumably epigenetic—control of local invasion and metastasis also offers an explanation to the so-called "progression puzzle" [30], i.e., the lack of main genetic and expression differences between matched primary tumors and metastases as reported in colon cancer and other tumor types [31–33]. This suggests that although the adenoma-carcinoma progression at the primary site is clearly driven by the sequential accumulation of genetic mutations at key genes, the multistage route from dissemination into the tumor microenvironment to metastasis formation is underlined by phenotypic plasticity, i.e., the capacity of circulating tumor cells (CTCs) to undergo transient phenotypic changes to adapt to the ever-changing cellular contexts en route to distant organ sites. As previously and eloquently proposed by Thomas Brabletz and collaborators, EMT and its reverse program MET play pivotal roles in regulating phenotypic plasticity of CTCs [29].

In the next section, we will discuss the current understanding of the role of EMT in local invasion and metastasis.

3. Epithelial to Mesenchymal Transition in Local Invasion and Metastasis

As pointed out in the previous section, tumor cells within primary and metastatic tumor masses, as well as CTCs, display substantial phenotypic heterogeneity representing various intermediate stages of the EMT program [34,35]. EMT is a developmental program exploited by carcinoma cells to switch from their epithelial state, featuring cell–cell contacts and apical–basal polarity, to more motile and invasive quasi-mesenchymal phenotypes with spindle-like morphology and front-back-end polarity. During cancer invasion, EMT provides cells with the ability to produce, interact with, and digest the surrounding extracellular matrix (ECM), detach from the primary tumor, and invade into the surrounding tissue [14]. In addition to promoting cellular migration and invasion, the transient phenotypic changes associated with formation of the mesenchymal state during EMT have been associated with the acquisition of stem-like properties, resistance to therapy, and immune suppression [36–39]. The epigenetic, and as such reversible nature of EMT is crucial as the reverse mesenchymal-to-epithelial (MET) process allows migrating cancer (stem-like) cells to regain proliferative and epithelial characteristics to colonize distant organ sites [14]. The initiation and execution of EMT are orchestrated by a set of transcription factors (i.e., *ZEB1/2*, *SNAIL1/SLUG*, and *TWIST1/2*) and miRNAs (e.g., the miR200 family) [40]. Hallmarks of EMT include the silenced expression of integral members of epithelial cell adhesion structures such as adherens- and tight-junctions, and desmosomes, and/or proteins involved in cytoskeleton (re)organization and in cell-matrix adhesion. Next, EMT-TFs can also activate the expression of mesenchymal cell markers resulting in changes in cell morphology, enhanced migratory properties, and ECM remodeling. EMT is induced by cytokines and growth factors secreted from the tumor microenvironment in response to metabolic changes, hypoxia, innate and adaptive immune responses, and treatment by cytotoxic drugs [40]. In addition, the mechanical composition and properties of the ECM also play an important role in EMT regulation. Both shear stress of cancer cells and increasing matrix stiffness in the microenvironment activate EMT, tumor invasion and metastasis [41–43]. In turn, as noted before, EMT also stimulates the composition and mechanics of the ECM, thereby forming a tightly controlled feedback loop that is often dysregulated in cancer.

As mentioned above, colon carcinomas display nuclear β-catenin accumulation at the invasive front simultaneously with the acquisition of mesenchymal-like morphologic features [24]. In this respect, it has been shown that EMT can be activated downstream of canonical Wnt/β-catenin signaling as GSK3β kinase activity inhibition stabilizes SLUG, thereby initiating EMT [44]. Alternatively, active Wnt signaling also inhibits SNAIL1 phosphorylation, leading to increased protein levels of this transcriptional repressor of E-cadherin, EMT initiation, and local invasion [45]. In colon cancer, overexpression of the Wnt ligand Wnt3a is associated with EMT and cancer progression. Accordingly, Wnt3a overexpression in both in vitro and in vivo models was shown to induce *SNAIL* expression thus promoting EMT, an effect that is abrogated by the Wnt antagonist Dickkopf1 (Dkk1) [28].

More recently, the intestinal microbiome has also been shown to contribute to EMT. A variety of enterotoxins secreted by microbes, including *Bacteriodes fragilis*, *Fusobacterium nucleatum*, and *Enterococcus faecalis* have been demonstrated to alter normal cell–cell adhesion by interfering with E-cadherin function [46–48]. *F. nucleatum* adheres through FadA (*Fusobacterium adhesion A*), an adhesion protein, to E-cadherin in colon cancer cells. The FadA/E-cadherin interaction leads to activation of β-catenin signaling and of oncogenic and inflammatory responses [48]. Interestingly, *Fusobacterium* and its associated microbiome (including *Bacteroides*, *Selenomonas*, and *Prevotella*) are sustained in distal metastases and mouse xenografts of primary colorectal tumors. Treating tumor-bearing mice with the antibiotic metronidazole reduced the amount *Fusobacterium* and abrogated cancer cell proliferation and growth [49].

3.1. Role of EMT in Metastasis under Debate

EMT is often defined by the respective down- and up-regulation of epithelial (e.g., E-cadherin, catenins, and cytokeratins) and mesenchymal markers (e.g., vimentin, fibronectin, and N-cadherin) by the above-mentioned *ZEB1/2*, *SNAIL1/SLUG*, and *TWIST1/2* transcription factors (EMT-TFs). However, no single transcription factor (TF) or downstream target can universally define EMT throughout different cancer types and cellular contexts. Distinct EMT-TFs are likely to act in a tumor- and dosage-specific manner and as such differentially repress or enhance the transcription of specific downstream target genes. From this perspective, the recent debate on whether EMT is an essential requirement for metastasis to occur [14,50] reflects the complexity of the network of transcription factors and their downstream targets in the activation of the EMT program. Two provocative studies, in particular, have raised questions on the relative importance of the role played by EMT along the multistep sequence of events leading to metastasis. Fischer et al. (2015) employed in vivo mesenchymal GFP reporters to study EMT onset in the MMTV-PyMT mammary cancer model. Notwithstanding the observed mesenchymal expression within the primary lesions, albeit in low proportion, and its enrichment in CTCs, GFP-positive tumor cells did not contribute to distant metastases [18]. Moreover, *Zeb1/2* inhibition by miR-200 overexpression did not reduce lung metastasis incidence. In a second study by Zheng et al. (2015) it was shown, by taking advantage of a pancreatic ductal carcinoma mouse model, that genetic ablation of *Snail1* or *Twist1* did not affect dissemination and lung metastasis development [19]. The latter is in contrast with a later study by Krebs et al. (2017), showing that *Zeb1* downregulation in the same pancreatic cancer models negatively affects the formation of precursor lesions, tumor grading, invasion, and metastasis [51]. Additionally, other studies using different cancer mouse models point to a key role of *Snail1*- and *Twist1*-driven EMT in metastatic colonization [52–54].

Although compelling, the Fischer et al. (2015) and Zheng et al. (2015) studies are mainly based on the analysis of individual transcription factors and downstream targets in specific tumor models [39,40] and cannot as such be used to discard EMT's role in metastasis against an overwhelming body of experimental evidence from the scientific literature. Several TFs are known to cooperate in eliciting EMT and in controlling the extension of the execution of the trans-differentiation program. Also, EMT-TFs are known to act in a cooperative and context-dependent fashion, and loss of individual factors in specific organ sites may well not suffice to initiate EMT and facilitate metastasis formation. The same is true for the employed mesenchymal markers the expression of which cannot be employed as universal readouts of EMT activation [14,50].

3.2. Hybrid E/M Phenotypes and Partial EMT: Many Shades of Gray

As mentioned above, the transient and reversible nature of EMT represents an essential feature for a metastatic lesion to develop [52,54,55]. Recent experimental evidence indicates that EMT, rather than acting as a binary switch where cells transit between fully epithelial and mesenchymal states, generates a broad spectrum of intermediate E/M stages where cells co-express both types of markers [14] (Figure 2). These partial EMT states are metastable and as such confer to the cancer cell enhanced phenotypic plasticity, an essential hallmark of the migrating/metastatic cancer (stem) cell [14].

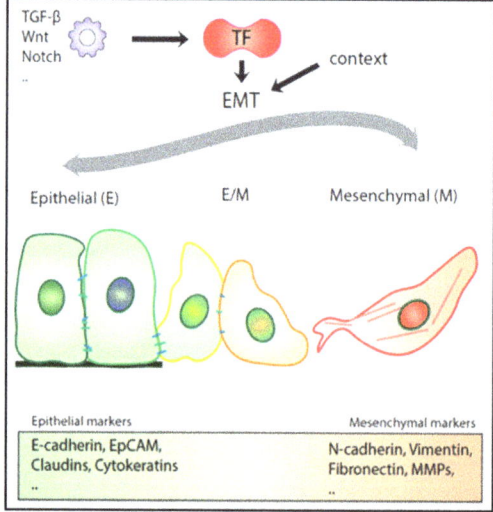

Figure 2. Epithelial to mesenchymal transition (EMT). Schematic overview of epithelial (E) cells transitioning to mesenchymal (M) phenotypes through an intermediate E/M state, and vice versa. EMT can be induced by various stimuli and is dependent on the environmental context.

Two recent studies, in particular, have highlighted the relevance of partial EMT in metastasis. In a mouse model of pancreatic ductal adenocarcinoma (PDAC), Aiello et al. (2018) sorted primary tumor cells according to their membranous expression of E-cadherin (*Cdh1*). Additional RNAseq and protein analysis of *Cdh1*-negative cancer cells revealed the presence of two distinct groups of tumors: while the first resulted from the transcriptional downregulation of E-cadherin (and of other epithelial markers), the second and major group showed E-cadherin expression both at the mRNA and protein levels. However, rather than being presented at the membrane, E-cadherin was internalized in recycling endosomes [34]. These two distinct E-cadherin negative and EMT-competent subpopulations of tumor cells were also earmarked by different invasive and metastatic behavior. Whereas cancer cells featuring a complete EMT (i.e., E-cadherin downregulated at the transcriptional level) invaded the tumor microenvironment mostly as single cells, cells with internalized E-cadherin in a partial EMT state (E/M) migrate collectively as multicellular clusters which are also found in the blood of the pancreatic cancer mouse model [34]. Of note, it has also been shown that the different degrees of epithelial-mesenchymal plasticity affect the tumor cells' metastatic organotropism, i.e., their capacity to metastasize a spectrum of different organ sites [56].

In a second study, Pastushenko et al. (2018) employed a mouse model of squamous cell carcinoma (SCC) and, by taking advantage of the different expression levels of the CD106, CD61, and CD51 cell-surface markers, identified six distinct EpCAM-negative tumor cell subpopulations, each characterized by a different degree of EMT. The different SCC subpopulations, encompassing both fully mesenchymal (complete EMT) and hybrid E/M subtypes (partial EMT), were characterized by distinct chromatin landscapes and gene expression profiles. Similar EMT-heterogeneity was also found in mouse models for metaplastic and luminal breast cancer [35]. Although the tumor-propagating capacity of hybrid E/M EpCAM-negative SCC cells was found to be comparable with that of their fully mesenchymal equivalents, those with a partial EMT phenotype showed increased CTC multiplicities and metastasis formation at distant organs [35]. Overall, partial EMT seems to confer increased phenotypic plasticity to the cancer cells especially when it comes to regaining epithelial characteristic (by MET), an essential requirement for metastasis formation at specific organ sites [14]. Of note, HNSCC (head and neck squamous cell carcinoma) cells with partial EMT are preferentially localized at the invasive front of the primary tumors in close proximity to CAFs (cancer-associated fibroblasts) [57], reminiscent of the "β-catenin paradox" in colon cancer [24].

The elucidation of the molecular mechanisms underlying partial EMT is still in its early days. Nonetheless, the different intermediate E/M phenotypes are likely to be driven by specific epigenetic and transcriptional modifications. Kröger et al. (2019) isolated subpopulation tumor cells stably residing in a hybrid E/M state from both in vitro and in vivo models using a human immortalized and transformed mammary epithelial cell line. These E/M tumor cells were characterized by upregulation of the SNAIL EMT-TF and of canonical Wnt-signaling. Ectopic *ZEB1* expression resulted in a fully mesenchymal transformation of the E/M cells accompanied by a reduction of their tumorigenic potential and a switch from canonical to non-canonical Wnt signaling [58].

Apart from SNAIL, other transcription factors including NUMB, GRLH2, and OVOL have been proposed to act as *'phenotypic stability factors'* which promote, control, and stabilize the hybrid E/M state, possibly by interfering with the core EMT decision-making circuit [59,60].

As mentioned above, the cancer cell's ability to revert back from EMT-induced phenotypes is critical for metastasis formation in distant organs and full mesenchymal transformation may result in the irreversible loss of MET capacity [58,61,62]. For example, activation of TGF-β signaling triggers EMT in carcinoma cells in a dosage-dependent fashion. Upon short-term treatment, the induced EMT is reversible. However, prolonged exposure of cancer cells to TGF-β result in more stable and irreversible transitions even upon ligand withdrawal [62].

Next to the specific expression signatures of EMT-related transcription factors and their downstream signaling pathways driving hybrid E/M and fully mesenchymal states in cancer cells, the existence of other alternative EMT-programs with distinct outcomes has been proposed [34,56].

Overall, it is still unclear whether hybrid E/M cells represent a metastable population or are just captured in a time frame transitioning from the epithelial to mesenchymal phenotype. Also, it remains uncertain which context-dependent environmental factors and downstream signaling paths are responsible for driving heterogeneous phenotypic fates during tumor progression. Nonetheless, as mentioned earlier, ample experimental evidence clearly indicates that the hybrid E/M cells state is involved in the collective invasion, migration, and dissemination of tumor cells en route to form distant metastases. In the next sections, we will portray the role of EMT in collective cell invasion into the local tumor stroma and dissemination as CTC-clusters, when compared with single migrating cancer cells that complete the full EMT-program.

4. Single versus Collective Cell Migration

The initial detachment of the cancer cell from the primary mass and its invasion in the surrounding stromal microenvironment represent critical and rate-limiting steps in the metastatic cascade responsible for 90% of deaths in patients with malignancies [12,63]. In order to invade, cancer cells employ distinct invasion modalities: single (amoeboid or mesenchymal invasion) and collective cell migration. Of note, cancer cells can switch between these invasion modes, an important feature when it comes to the development of anti-invasive and anti-metastatic therapies [64].

4.1. Single Cell Migration

Cancer cells lacking interactions with neighboring tumor cells can detach from the primary mass and migrate individually into the microenvironment. There are two different mechanisms of single-cell invasion, namely amoeboid and mesenchymal migration [64]. The involvement of one of these two modes is dependent on the rigidity of the cell-matrix adhesions, the tumor cell's capacity to remodel the extracellular matrix, and the contractility of the cytoskeleton [65]. In amoeboid invasion, an EMT-independent mechanism, cancer cells have a characteristic rounded cell shape. Here, migration relies on the contractility of cortical actomyosin, promoted by the Rho/ROCK signaling pathway [66]. The proteolysis-independent actomyosin contractility results in membrane blebbing, i.e., the formation of membrane protrusions that enable cancer cells to squeeze through gaps within the ECM [66,67]. In contrast, during mesenchymal single-cell invasion, cells adopt an elongated spindle-like phenotype with front-back polarity as a result of EMT [68,69]. Additionally, cells that engage the mesenchymal mode are dependent on the activity of enzymes such as matrix metalloproteinases (MMPs) and serine protease seprase that degrade the ECM and, as tumor cells invade, progressively create channels which can be used for the cells lagging behind the leading ones [70]. Interestingly, inhibition of ECM remodeling leads to amoeboid migration with cancer cells squeezing through pre-existing pores by actomyosin contractility [67]. Of note, MMPs are generally regarded as integral members of the EMT program. In hepatocellular carcinoma (HCC), upregulation of the EMT-TF Snail not only repressed E-cadherin transcription but also increased expression of MMP-1, MMP-2, MMP-7, and MT1-MMP leading to accelerated invasion [71,72]. Alternatively, several ECM components and even MMPs can, in some cases, act as EMT initiators [73,74]. Induction of MMP-3, also known as stromelysin-1 (SL-1), in the mammary epithelium resulted in cleavage of E-cadherin leading to removal of E-cadherin and catenins from adherens junctions, downregulation of cytokeratins, upregulation of vimentin and of endogenous MMPs [73].

Although single-cell invasion is linked to tumor cells undergoing the full EMT-program leading to suppression of E-cadherin and induction of vimentin [68,69], there is evidence that partial EMT, i.e., the retention of epithelial features, can also feature single-cell migration [75,76]. Additionally, cancer cells can switch between amoeboid and mesenchymal states spontaneously or through changes in ECM composition [67].

4.2. Collective Cell Migration and the Role of EMT

In collective cell migration, cancer cells retain intact cell–cell adhesions while invading the tumor microenvironment, the vasculature, and distant organ sites [77]. A variety of migration modalities feature collective cell migration, ranging from narrow linear connected cell strands to broad sheets or compact cluster/budding of cells [77]. Unlike single-cell migration resulting from fully mesenchymal cells, the role of EMT in collective migration is subtler. Recently, using a *Drosophila melanogaster* model of colon cancer, it was shown that the Snail homolog *Sna* can activate partial EMT in tumor cells leading to their collective invasion through the basement membrane and muscle fibers [78]. Additional evidence pointing at the correlation between hybrid E/M and collective cell migration lies in the onset of 'leader' cells at the invasive margin that are selected to guide other 'following' cancer cells [79]. These leader cells show a bi-phenotypic state with mesenchymal features as altered polarity and development of protrusions at their front. Yet, they also maintain attachments to their follower cells at their rear end. The follower cells, on the other hand, retain apical–basal polarity and migrate taking advantage of the pulling force generated by leader cells [80]. Knockdown of the epithelial marker cytokeratin 14 in leader cells is sufficient to block collective migration suggesting that the hybrid E/M state is mandatory for establishment of the leader cells [79]. The onset, activity, and maintenance of leader cells are coordinated by environmental stimuli, i.e., the local increase of compression [81], soluble factors, and chemokines [82], but is also controlled within the collective tumor group by autocrine or juxtacrine fashion. Of note, also in this case several MMPs are expressed at the leading edge to facilitate ECM degradation and to create a migration path for the cell clusters [83].

Notably, non-cancer cells can also contribute to collective cell migration. The movement of cancer cells can be conducted by migratory stromal cells such as fibroblasts [84,85]) or macrophages [86,87]. Labernadie et al. (2017) demonstrated that cancer-associated fibroblasts (CAFs) exert a physical force on cancer cells that leads to their collective migration. This intercellular force transduction is achieved by the formation of heterophilic adhesion complexes between N-cadherin on the CAF membrane and E-cadherin on the cancer cell membrane [85]. Moreover, CAFs are also a source of ECM-degrading proteases such as MMPs thereby creating micro tracks used by cancer cells to migrate through [84]. In addition to degrading the ECM, CAFs also secrete growth factors and chemokines that generate chemotactic gradients to direct cell migration [88]. Last, cancer cells can ingest exosomes secreted by CAFs thereby activating intracellular pathways known to trigger EMT [89]. In colon cancer, CAFs release exosomes containing miR-92a-3p and promote invasion and chemotherapy resistance. miR-92a-3p directly binds to FBXW7 and MOAP1 thereby activating Wnt-induced EMT and mitochondrial apoptosis [89].

Overall, single and collective cell migration share some of the underlying mechanisms (e.g., cell–cell and cell-matrix communication, and the establishment of a migratory polarity). Moreover, during invasion tumor cells can switch between different modes of migration depending on intrinsic (cell adhesion) and extrinsic cues (ECM composition and density). In general terms, a complete EMT is associated with single-cell migration, whereas collective cell migration seems to result from partial EMT. Nonetheless, the mechanisms underlying the role of EMT in determining the invasion modalities, the intercellular communication among invading cells, and the tumor microenvironmental cues leading to collective migration are yet poorly defined. This is further complicated by the fact that invasion modalities are likely to be cell type-, tissue-, and time-dependent. The plasticity of cancer cells to switch between different invasion modes is a key feature and a putative target for the development of novel therapeutic strategies [90].

5. Circulating Tumor Cells

Circulating tumor cells (CTCs) are defined as those cancer cells disseminated from the primary tumor mass and intravasated into blood vessels which are thought to underlie metastasis at distant organ sites [91]. CTCs have been identified at different multiplicities in many carcinomas including colon, breast, prostate, lung, bladder, and gastric cancer, while they are extremely rare in healthy individuals or in patients with non-malignant disease [91]. However, even in cancer patients, CTCs are extremely rare and, accordingly, their prospective isolation and characterization have proven to be a challenge [91]. Heterogeneity also exists among CTCs, possibly reflecting the above discussed intra-tumor heterogeneity. Likewise, the existence of both single CTCs, as well as CTC clusters comprising multiple (from few to hundreds) cells, has been well established in the scientific literature [92,93]. Of note, CTC clusters are not exclusively composed of epithelial cancer cells but are often intermingled with immune cells, cancer-associated fibroblasts, tumor stroma, and platelets [94–98].

In addition to this heterogeneity, CTCs and CTC clusters have been captured that express both epithelial and mesenchymal features [93,99–101].

5.1. Single CTCs versus CTC Clusters

Single CTCs disseminate into distant organs upon EMT [14]. However, the discovery of CTC clusters has raised questions on the relative role of EMT in local invasion and systemic dissemination from the primary tumor mass. CTC clusters are defined as a group of 2–3 or more tumor cells that travel as a group through the bloodstream [91]. In 1954, Watanabe showed that, by injecting bronchogenic carcinoma cells in the jugular vein of recipient mice, tumor clumps, in contrast to single cells, were able to form metastasis [102]. Accordingly, aggregated colon cancer cells also showed increased metastatic efficiency in the liver when compared with single cells after intra-portal injection in rat [103]. These initial observations, however, did not explain how and where CTC clusters are formed. More recently, it has been demonstrated that CTC clusters do not derive from the intravascular aggregation of single CTCs or from proliferating single CTCs, but rather from clumps of primary tumor cells that collectively detach from the primary mass and enter the vasculature as CTC clusters [104–106]. Moreover, it was also shown that the metastatic capacity of CTC clusters was up to fifty-fold higher when compared with single CTCs [104]. Genome-wide single-cell DNA methylation analysis demonstrated distinct methylomes between CTC clusters and single CTCs in human breast cancer patients. CTC clusters were shown to be hypo-methylated at stemness- and proliferation-associated transcription regulators including OCT4, NANOG, SOX2, and SIN3A, and hyper-methylated at Polycomb target genes [107]. Lastly, the presence of circulating tumor micro emboli in peripheral blood of patients with cancer arising from colon, breast, and lung was predictive of poor survival [104,108,109].

5.2. CTC Cluster Heterogeneity

The heterogeneous composition of CTC clusters encompassing parenchymal cancer cells together with immune cells, cancer-associated fibroblasts, tumor stroma, and platelets, seems to reflect the heterogeneity of the primary tumors they originate from [94–98]. The presence of non-malignant cells within CTC clusters contributes to their improved survival and metastatic capacity. Normal epithelial cells undergo cell anoikis upon the detachment from the extracellular matrix (ECM), which establishes an important defense mechanism to prevent abnormal growth in inappropriate places. However, EMT can circumvent anoikis in individual cells during dissemination and metastasis [110]. The transition of single CTCs to a mesenchymal phenotype results in the expression of adherence-independent survival signals that compensate for the loss of attachment to the ECM [111]. Alternatively, CTC clusters may prevent tumor cell anoikis by retaining epithelial cell–cell interactions and thus contributing to the activation of survival stimuli [104,105]. Next, the non-malignant cell microenvironment can protect CTC cells from immune cells [112,113], shield cells from mechanical stress, and promotes adhesion to the endothelium [114,115]. It also has been shown that platelets can induce EMT in CTCs via TGF-β and NF-κB signaling while enhancing their metastatic potential [97]. Thus, secretion of growth factors and cytokines by the non-cancer cells may represent an additional survival advantage for the CTC clusters in the vasculature. Last, yet another advantage of the CTC clusters when compared to single CTCs is the capacity of remodeling the microenvironment at the metastatic site, thereby facilitating colonization [95].

5.3. EMT in CTC Clusters

Next to the heterogeneity of CTC clusters in terms of cell lineage composition, the degree of EMT activation among the parenchymal cancer cells within CTCs can also vary considerably. CTC clusters display epithelial cell–cell interactions as shown by the retention of expression of several epithelial-specific genes such as K5, K8, K14, E-cadherin, P-cadherin, and plakoglobin in metastatic breast CTC clusters [116]. Accordingly, knockdown of plakoglobin, a member of the catenin protein family and homologous to β-catenin, led to disaggregation of the CTC clusters, thereby compromising metastasis formation [104]. Also, disruption of K14 expression negatively affected the expression of key downstream effectors in metastatic niche remodeling and metastasis survival, leading to compromised efficiency in metastasis formation [105]. However, CTC clusters with predominant hybrid E/M or fully mesenchymal features have been observed in human colon, prostate, lung, and breast cancer patients [93,99–101]. At least one-third of cancer cells from within CTC clusters derived from colon cancer patients were negative for cytokeratin expression [100]. In breast cancer, CTC clusters show shifts in their EMT status according to treatment modalities with predominant mesenchymal expression patterns during cancer progression and/or in refractory disease [93] (Figure 3). This dynamic EMT profile allows for cellular plasticity and adaptation to the diverse cellular contexts encountered by CTCs during dissemination and metastasis formation, and to different treatments regimes. The latter is also of relevance for the use of prognostic epithelial markers of CTCs likely to fail to detect cancer cells that have undergone EMT. Additional mesenchymal CTCs markers are needed for more accurate prognostic studies [117].

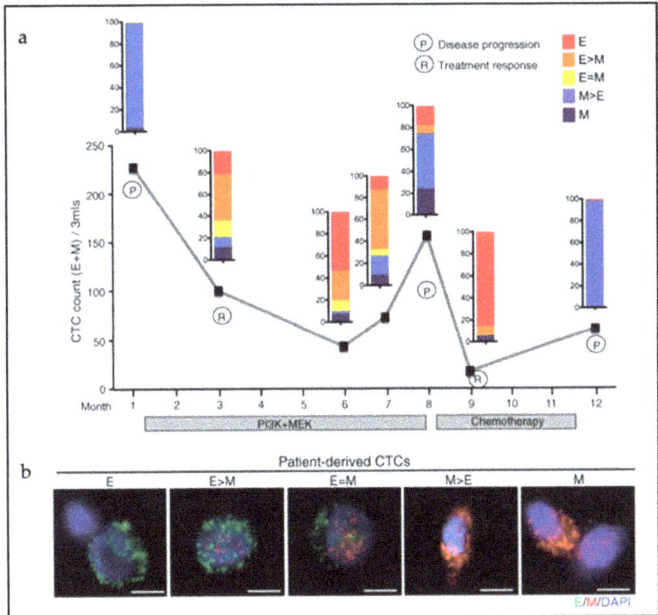

Figure 3. EMT features in single circulating tumor cells (CTCs) and CTC clusters from a metastatic breast cancer patient. (**a**) Longitudinal monitoring of EMT features in CTCs. The Y-axis indicates the number of CTCs per 3 mL of blood. The patient was monitored over time (X-axis) during treatment with inhibitors targeting the PI3K and MEK pathways (months 1–8), followed by chemotherapy with Adriamycin (8–12). The color-coded quantification bars indicate the EMT status of the CTCs based on RNA-ISH (in situ hybridization) analysis at each indicated time point. P = disease progression; R = tumor response. (**b**) RNA-ISH analysis of EMT markers in CTCs derived from patients with metastatic breast cancer. Green dots represent epithelial (E) and red marks mesenchymal (M) markers. Scale bar: 5 µm. Adapted from [93].

As mentioned above, alternative EMT-programs accounts for different CTC phenotypes. Aiello et al. (2018) suggested that single CTCs arise from cancer cells that have completed a full EMT-program, whereas tumor cells characterized by partial EMT tend to present as clusters resulting from collective migration [34]. However, it has been demonstrated that, next to those mainly composed by CTCs, cell clusters have been isolated from colon cancer patients which consist of endothelial cells without any genetic aberrations found in their matched primary tumor of origin. These cell clusters were positive for both epithelial and mesenchymal markers and are thought to result from the direct release of clusters from the tumor vasculature due to impaired neo-angiogenesis [118].

6. Partial EMT, Collective Cell Migration, and Metastasis: Therapeutic strategies

Metastasis formation involves the successful completion of a sequential series of challenging steps. Phenotypic plasticity refers to the key feature of the metastasizing cancer cell to adapt to the environment where it resides through reversible changes of its cellular identity [13]. This '*Dr. Jekyll and Mr. Hide*' feature of migrating cancer cells is controlled by epigenetic mechanisms which regulate E-to-M and M-to-E transitions (EMT and MET) [14]. However, EMT cannot be regarded as a binary process as it generates hybrid E/M cancer cells encompassing a range of intermediate stages. Partial EMT has been correlated with collective cell migration and with the presence of CTC clusters with enhanced metastatic potential in the peripheral blood of cancer patients [119]. Moreover, the unaffected CTC clusters multiplicity upon chemotherapy is indicative of treatment failure in colorectal cancer [120]. From this perspective, the elucidation of the underlying intrinsic and extrinsic mechanisms is bound to lead to the development of novel therapeutic and even preventive strategies based on the targeting of cell–cell and/or cell-matrix interactions and the disruption of CTC clusters. Gkountela et al. (2019) tested a library of approximately 2500 FDA-approved compounds and identified Na^+/K^+ ATPase inhibitors able to disaggregate derived CTC clusters derived from breast cancer patients into single cells. Mechanistically, Na^+/K^+ ATPase inhibition in tumor cells leads to an increase of intercellular Ca^{2+} concentration and to the consequent inhibition of formation of cell–cell junctions. In an in vivo xenograft model using NSG mice injected with patient-derived breast cancer cells in their fat pad, treatment with the Na^+/K^+ ATPase inhibitor ouabain resulted in a marked reduction of CTC cluster formation together with the increase of single CTC multiplicity. Although the size of the primary tumor was unaffected upon ouabain treatment, the overall number of metastatic lesions, corresponding to the number of CTC clusters, was reduced [107].

An alternative approach towards the development of therapeutic strategies based on CTC clusters may be represented by inhibition of platelet function. Platelets make integral part of CTC clusters where they are thought to protect the cancer cells from shear stress and immune attacks [121]. Acetylsalicylic acid (i.e., aspirin) inhibits platelet function by acetylation of cyclooxygenase (COX) thereby preventing arachidonic acid (and prostaglandin) production and consequently resulting in irreversible inhibition of platelet-dependent thromboxane formation. Based on this, aspirin has been employed as an anticoagulant for the prevention of thrombosis [122]. In experimental cancer models and clinical trials, inhibiting the interaction between cancer cells and platelets have been shown to hamper tumor cell survival, growth and metastasis formation [123,124].

Notwithstanding the above promising and innovative therapeutic strategies based on CTC clusters, their allegedly high degree of plasticity—as a mechanism to escape targeted treatment—is also likely to result in therapy resistance. Nonetheless, future research towards the identification of novel therapeutic targets to lower the risk of CTC cluster formation is expected to improve the efficacy of cancer treatment in the long run.

7. Final Remarks and Conclusions

EMT contributes to a considerable degree of cellular heterogeneity in both primary tumors and metastatic lesions as it affects a broad spectrum of cellular functions beyond the transitions between epithelial and mesenchymal states associated with enhanced invasive and metastatic abilities. Changes in stem cell behavior, escape from apoptosis and senescence, ECM and tumor-microenvironment remodeling, and resistance to cytotoxic treatments are only a few among the broad spectrum of downstream EMT effectors which contribute to intra-tumor cell heterogeneity with profound implications for cancer therapeutics, especially in the decade of personalized treatments [11].

In fact, EMT is thought to play key roles in each and every step of the metastatic cascade including intra- and extravasation [125], and the colonization of distant organ sites [126,127]. For the sake of brevity, these latter aspects are not discussed in this review. The observed broad spectrum of EMT effectors may well reflect the pleiotropic functional roles of the EMT-TFs such as ZEB1 [128] that go well beyond the E to M (and vice versa) trans-differentiation, and include angiogenesis, remodeling of the tumor microenvironment, immune escape, mechanotransduction, and possibly many more.

The identification and elucidation of the complex network of intrinsic and extrinsic mechanisms driving EMT at "just-right" (E/M) levels to trigger collective migration, generate CTC clusters and successfully metastasize distant organ sites represent the major future research challenge in the translation of our fundamental understanding of metastasis into therapy. From this perspective, single-cell epigenetic and transcriptomic analysis will provide powerful approaches to address this challenge. These high-resolution techniques will be key to elucidate the heterogeneous composition of malignancies including the identification of distinct and rare cell types arising transiently in time and at specific locations within tumors. Moreover, single-cell profiles will help to investigate the variability among individuals, disease states, microenvironments, and treatment history.

Overall, the realization of the importance of epigenetics and the elucidation of the mechanisms underlying transient changes in the cellular identity of individual circulating and metastasizing tumor cells will lay the basis for the development of novel treatment modalities. These will complement the current 'personalized cancer medicine' mainly directed at somatic gene mutations arisen at the primary site and unlikely to be rate-limiting in the clinical management of a more advanced malignant disease.

Funding: This research was funded by the Dutch Cancer Society (KWF), grant number EMCR 2015-7588.

Acknowledgments: The authors would like to thank Mathijs Verhagen for his assistance with the artwork.

Conflicts of Interest: The authors declare no conflict of interest.

References

1. Ferlay, J.; Ervik, M.; Lam, F.; Colombet, M.; Mery, L.; Piñeros, M.; Znaor, A.; Soerjomataram, I.; Bray, F. Global Cancer Observatory: Cancer Tomorrow. Available online: https://gco.iarc.fr/tomorrow (accessed on 2 May 2019).
2. Fodde, R.; Smits, R.; Clevers, H. APC, signal transduction and genetic instability in colorectal cancer. *Nat. Rev. Cancer* **2001**, *1*, 55–67. [CrossRef] [PubMed]
3. Hanahan, D.; Weinberg, R.A. Hallmarks of cancer: The next generation. *Cell* **2011**, *144*, 646–674. [CrossRef] [PubMed]
4. Dalerba, P.; Kalisky, T.; Sahoo, D.; Rajendran, P.S.; Rothenberg, M.E.; Leyrat, A.A.; Sim, S.; Okamoto, J.; Johnston, D.M.; Qian, D.; et al. Single-cell dissection of transcriptional heterogeneity in human colon tumors. *Nat. Biotechnol.* **2011**, *29*, 1120–1127. [CrossRef] [PubMed]
5. Li, H.; Courtois, E.T.; Sengupta, D.; Tan, Y.; Chen, K.H.; Goh, J.J.L.; Kong, S.L.; Chua, C.; Hon, L.K.; Tan, W.S.; et al. Reference component analysis of single-cell transcriptomes elucidates cellular heterogeneity in human colorectal tumors. *Nat. Genet.* **2017**, *49*, 708–718. [CrossRef] [PubMed]
6. Roerink, S.F.; Sasaki, N.; Lee-Six, H.; Young, M.D.; Alexandrov, L.B.; Behjati, S.; Mitchell, T.J.; Grossmann, S.; Lightfoot, H.; Egan, D.A.; et al. Intra-tumour diversification in colorectal cancer at the single-cell level. *Nature* **2018**, *556*, 457–462. [CrossRef] [PubMed]
7. Fiori, M.E.; Di Franco, S.; Villanova, L.; Bianca, P.; Stassi, G.; De Maria, R. Cancer-associated fibroblasts as abettors of tumor progression at the crossroads of EMT and therapy resistance. *Mol. Cancer* **2019**, *18*, 70. [CrossRef] [PubMed]
8. Lamprecht, S.; Schmidt, E.M.; Blaj, C.; Hermeking, H.; Jung, A.; Kirchner, T.; Horst, D. Multicolor lineage tracing reveals clonal architecture and dynamics in colon cancer. *Nat. Commun.* **2017**, *8*, 1406. [CrossRef] [PubMed]
9. van der Heijden, M.; Miedema, D.M.; Waclaw, B.; Veenstra, V.L.; Lecca, M.C.; Nijman, L.E.; van Dijk, E.; van Neerven, S.M.; Lodestijn, S.C.; Lenos, K.J.; et al. Spatiotemporal regulation of clonogenicity in colorectal cancer xenografts. *Proc. Natl. Acad. Sci. USA* **2019**, *116*, 6140–6145. [CrossRef]

10. Saito, T.; Niida, A.; Uchi, R.; Hirata, H.; Komatsu, H.; Sakimura, S.; Hayashi, S.; Nambara, S.; Kuroda, Y.; Ito, S.; et al. A temporal shift of the evolutionary principle shaping intratumor heterogeneity in colorectal cancer. *Nat. Commun.* **2018**, *9*, 2884. [CrossRef]
11. Fisher, R.; Pusztai, L.; Swanton, C. Cancer heterogeneity: Implications for targeted therapeutics. *Br. J. Cancer* **2013**, *108*, 479–485. [CrossRef]
12. Fidler, I.J. The pathogenesis of cancer metastasis: The 'seed and soil' hypothesis revisited. *Nat. Rev. Cancer* **2003**, *3*, 453–458. [CrossRef] [PubMed]
13. Varga, J.; Greten, F.R. Cell plasticity in epithelial homeostasis and tumorigenesis. *Nat. Cell Biol.* **2017**, *19*, 1133–1141. [CrossRef] [PubMed]
14. Nieto, M.A.; Huang, R.Y.; Jackson, R.A.; Thiery, J.P. Emt: 2016. *Cell* **2016**, *166*, 21–45. [CrossRef] [PubMed]
15. Tam, W.L.; Weinberg, R.A. The epigenetics of epithelial-mesenchymal plasticity in cancer. *Nat. Med.* **2013**, *19*, 1438–1449. [CrossRef] [PubMed]
16. Mohd-Sarip, A.; Teeuwssen, M.; Bot, A.G.; De Herdt, M.J.; Willems, S.M.; Baatenburg de Jong, R.J.; Looijenga, L.H.J.; Zatreanu, D.; Bezstarosti, K.; van Riet, J.; et al. DOC1-Dependent Recruitment of NURD Reveals Antagonism with SWI/SNF during Epithelial-Mesenchymal Transition in Oral Cancer Cells. *Cell Rep.* **2017**, *20*, 61–75. [CrossRef] [PubMed]
17. Zentner, G.E.; Henikoff, S. Regulation of nucleosome dynamics by histone modifications. *Nat. Struct Mol. Biol.* **2013**, *20*, 259–266. [CrossRef] [PubMed]
18. Fischer, K.R.; Durrans, A.; Lee, S.; Sheng, J.; Li, F.; Wong, S.T.; Choi, H.; El Rayes, T.; Ryu, S.; Troeger, J.; et al. Epithelial-to-mesenchymal transition is not required for lung metastasis but contributes to chemoresistance. *Nature* **2015**, *527*, 472–476. [CrossRef]
19. Zheng, X.; Carstens, J.L.; Kim, J.; Scheible, M.; Kaye, J.; Sugimoto, H.; Wu, C.C.; LeBleu, V.S.; Kalluri, R. Epithelial-to-mesenchymal transition is dispensable for metastasis but induces chemoresistance in pancreatic cancer. *Nature* **2015**, *527*, 525–530. [CrossRef] [PubMed]
20. Pastushenko, I.; Blanpain, C. EMT Transition States during Tumor Progression and Metastasis. *Trends Cell Biol.* **2019**, *29*, 212–226. [CrossRef] [PubMed]
21. Fearon, E.R.; Vogelstein, B. A genetic model for colorectal tumorigenesis. *Cell* **1990**, *61*, 759–767. [CrossRef]
22. Reya, T.; Clevers, H. Wnt signalling in stem cells and cancer. *Nature* **2005**, *434*, 843–850. [CrossRef] [PubMed]
23. Gregorieff, A.; Clevers, H. Wnt signaling in the intestinal epithelium: From endoderm to cancer. *Genes Dev.* **2005**, *19*, 877–890. [CrossRef] [PubMed]
24. Fodde, R.; Brabletz, T. Wnt/beta-catenin signaling in cancer stemness and malignant behavior. *Curr. Opin. Cell Biol.* **2007**, *19*, 150–158. [CrossRef] [PubMed]
25. Brabletz, T.; Jung, A.; Hermann, K.; Gunther, K.; Hohenberger, W.; Kirchner, T. Nuclear overexpression of the oncoprotein beta-catenin in colorectal cancer is localized predominantly at the invasion front. *Pathol. Res. Pract.* **1998**, *194*, 701–704. [CrossRef]
26. Le, N.H.; Franken, P.; Fodde, R. Tumour-stroma interactions in colorectal cancer: Converging on beta-catenin activation and cancer stemness. *Br. J. Cancer* **2008**, *98*, 1886–1893. [CrossRef]
27. Brabletz, T.; Jung, A.; Reu, S.; Porzner, M.; Hlubek, F.; Kunz-Schughart, L.A.; Knuechel, R.; Kirchner, T. Variable beta-catenin expression in colorectal cancers indicates tumor progression driven by the tumor environment. *Proc. Natl. Acad. Sci. USA* **2001**, *98*, 10356–10361. [CrossRef]
28. Qi, L.; Sun, B.; Liu, Z.; Cheng, R.; Li, Y.; Zhao, X. Wnt3a expression is associated with epithelial-mesenchymal transition and promotes colon cancer progression. *J. Exp. Clin. Cancer Res.* **2014**, *33*, 107. [CrossRef]
29. Brabletz, T.; Jung, A.; Spaderna, S.; Hlubek, F.; Kirchner, T. Opinion: Migrating cancer stem cells-an integrated concept of malignant tumour progression. *Nat. Rev. Cancer* **2005**, *5*, 744–749. [CrossRef]
30. Bernards, R.; Weinberg, R.A. A progression puzzle. *Nature* **2002**, *418*, 823. [CrossRef]
31. Reiter, J.G.; Makohon-Moore, A.P.; Gerold, J.M.; Heyde, A.; Attiyeh, M.A.; Kohutek, Z.A.; Tokheim, C.J.; Brown, A.; DeBlasio, R.M.; Niyazov, J.; et al. Minimal functional driver gene heterogeneity among untreated metastases. *Science* **2018**, *361*, 1033–1037. [CrossRef]
32. Goswami, R.S.; Patel, K.P.; Singh, R.R.; Meric-Bernstam, F.; Kopetz, E.S.; Subbiah, V.; Alvarez, R.H.; Davies, M.A.; Jabbar, K.J.; Roy-Chowdhuri, S.; et al. Hotspot mutation panel testing reveals clonal evolution in a study of 265 paired primary and metastatic tumors. *Clin. Cancer Res.* **2015**, *21*, 2644–2651. [CrossRef] [PubMed]

33. Brannon, A.R.; Vakiani, E.; Sylvester, B.E.; Scott, S.N.; McDermott, G.; Shah, R.H.; Kania, K.; Viale, A.; Oschwald, D.M.; Vacic, V.; et al. Comparative sequencing analysis reveals high genomic concordance between matched primary and metastatic colorectal cancer lesions. *Genome Biol.* **2014**, *15*, 454. [CrossRef] [PubMed]
34. Aiello, N.M.; Maddipati, R.; Norgard, R.J.; Balli, D.; Li, J.; Yuan, S.; Yamazoe, T.; Black, T.; Sahmoud, A.; Furth, E.E.; et al. EMT Subtype Influences Epithelial Plasticity and Mode of Cell Migration. *Dev. Cell* **2018**, *45*, 681–695.e4. [CrossRef] [PubMed]
35. Pastushenko, I.; Brisebarre, A.; Sifrim, A.; Fioramonti, M.; Revenco, T.; Boumahdi, S.; Van Keymeulen, A.; Brown, D.; Moers, V.; Lemaire, S.; et al. Identification of the tumour transition states occurring during EMT. *Nature* **2018**, *556*, 463–468. [CrossRef] [PubMed]
36. Dongre, A.; Rashidian, M.; Reinhardt, F.; Bagnato, A.; Keckesova, Z.; Ploegh, H.L.; Weinberg, R.A. Epithelial-to-Mesenchymal Transition Contributes to Immunosuppression in Breast Carcinomas. *Cancer Res.* **2017**, *77*, 3982–3989. [CrossRef] [PubMed]
37. Morel, A.P.; Lievre, M.; Thomas, C.; Hinkal, G.; Ansieau, S.; Puisieux, A. Generation of breast cancer stem cells through epithelial-mesenchymal transition. *PLoS ONE* **2008**, *3*, e2888. [CrossRef] [PubMed]
38. Mani, S.A.; Guo, W.; Liao, M.J.; Eaton, E.N.; Ayyanan, A.; Zhou, A.Y.; Brooks, M.; Reinhard, F.; Zhang, C.C.; Shipitsin, M.; et al. The epithelial-mesenchymal transition generates cells with properties of stem cells. *Cell* **2008**, *133*, 704–715. [CrossRef] [PubMed]
39. Smith, B.N.; Bhowmick, N.A. Role of EMT in Metastasis and Therapy Resistance. *J. Clin. Med.* **2016**, *5*, 17. [CrossRef]
40. Puisieux, A.; Brabletz, T.; Caramel, J. Oncogenic roles of EMT-inducing transcription factors. *Nat. Cell Biol.* **2014**, *16*, 488–494. [CrossRef]
41. Lee, H.J.; Diaz, M.F.; Price, K.M.; Ozuna, J.A.; Zhang, S.; Sevick-Muraca, E.M.; Hagan, J.P.; Wenzel, P.L. Fluid shear stress activates YAP1 to promote cancer cell motility. *Nat. Commun.* **2017**, *8*, 14122. [CrossRef]
42. Wei, S.C.; Fattet, L.; Tsai, J.H.; Guo, Y.; Pai, V.H.; Majeski, H.E.; Chen, A.C.; Sah, R.L.; Taylor, S.S.; Engler, A.J.; et al. Matrix stiffness drives epithelial-mesenchymal transition and tumour metastasis through a TWIST1-G3BP2 mechanotransduction pathway. *Nat. Cell Biol.* **2015**, *17*, 678–688. [CrossRef] [PubMed]
43. Rice, A.J.; Cortes, E.; Lachowski, D.; Cheung, B.C.H.; Karim, S.A.; Morton, J.P.; Del Rio Hernandez, A. Matrix stiffness induces epithelial-mesenchymal transition and promotes chemoresistance in pancreatic cancer cells. *Oncogenesis* **2017**, *6*, e352. [CrossRef] [PubMed]
44. Wu, Z.Q.; Li, X.Y.; Hu, C.Y.; Ford, M.; Kleer, C.G.; Weiss, S.J. Canonical Wnt signaling regulates Slug activity and links epithelial-mesenchymal transition with epigenetic Breast Cancer 1, Early Onset (BRCA1) repression. *Proc. Natl. Acad. Sci. USA* **2012**, *109*, 16654–16659. [CrossRef] [PubMed]
45. Yook, J.I.; Li, X.Y.; Ota, I.; Fearon, E.R.; Weiss, S.J. Wnt-dependent regulation of the E-cadherin repressor snail. *J. Biol. Chem.* **2005**, *280*, 11740–11748. [CrossRef] [PubMed]
46. Yang, Y.; Wang, X.; Huycke, T.; Moore, D.R.; Lightfoot, S.A.; Huycke, M.M. Colon Macrophages Polarized by Commensal Bacteria Cause Colitis and Cancer through the Bystander Effect. *Transl. Oncol.* **2013**, *6*, 596–606. [CrossRef] [PubMed]
47. Wu, S.; Lim, K.C.; Huang, J.; Saidi, R.F.; Sears, C.L. Bacteroides fragilis enterotoxin cleaves the zonula adherens protein, E-cadherin. *Proc. Natl. Acad. Sci. USA* **1998**, *95*, 14979–14984. [CrossRef] [PubMed]
48. Rubinstein, M.R.; Wang, X.; Liu, W.; Hao, Y.; Cai, G.; Han, Y.W. Fusobacterium nucleatum promotes colorectal carcinogenesis by modulating E-cadherin/beta-catenin signaling via its FadA adhesin. *Cell Host Microbe* **2013**, *14*, 195–206. [CrossRef]
49. Bullman, S.; Pedamallu, C.S.; Sicinska, E.; Clancy, T.E.; Zhang, X.; Cai, D.; Neuberg, D.; Huang, K.; Guevara, F.; Nelson, T.; et al. Analysis of Fusobacterium persistence and antibiotic response in colorectal cancer. *Science* **2017**, *358*, 1443–1448. [CrossRef]
50. Maheswaran, S.; Haber, D.A. Cell fate: Transition loses its invasive edge. *Nature* **2015**, *527*, 452–453. [CrossRef]
51. Krebs, A.M.; Mitschke, J.; Lasierra Losada, M.; Schmalhofer, O.; Boerries, M.; Busch, H.; Boettcher, M.; Mougiakakos, D.; Reichardt, W.; Bronsert, P.; et al. The EMT-activator Zeb1 is a key factor for cell plasticity and promotes metastasis in pancreatic cancer. *Nat. Cell Biol.* **2017**, *19*, 518–529. [CrossRef]
52. Tran, H.D.; Luitel, K.; Kim, M.; Zhang, K.; Longmore, G.D.; Tran, D.D. Transient SNAIL1 expression is necessary for metastatic competence in breast cancer. *Cancer Res.* **2014**, *74*, 6330–6340. [CrossRef] [PubMed]

53. Xu, Y.; Lee, D.K.; Feng, Z.; Xu, Y.; Bu, W.; Li, Y.; Liao, L.; Xu, J. Breast tumor cell-specific knockout of Twist1 inhibits cancer cell plasticity, dissemination, and lung metastasis in mice. *Proc. Natl. Acad. Sci. USA* **2017**, *114*, 11494–11499. [CrossRef] [PubMed]
54. Tsai, J.H.; Donaher, J.L.; Murphy, D.A.; Chau, S.; Yang, J. Spatiotemporal regulation of epithelial-mesenchymal transition is essential for squamous cell carcinoma metastasis. *Cancer Cell* **2012**, *22*, 725–736. [CrossRef] [PubMed]
55. Schmidt, J.M.; Panzilius, E.; Bartsch, H.S.; Irmler, M.; Beckers, J.; Kari, V.; Linnemann, J.R.; Dragoi, D.; Hirschi, B.; Kloos, U.J.; et al. Stem-cell-like properties and epithelial plasticity arise as stable traits after transient Twist1 activation. *Cell Rep.* **2015**, *10*, 131–139. [CrossRef] [PubMed]
56. Reichert, M.; Bakir, B.; Moreira, L.; Pitarresi, J.R.; Feldmann, K.; Simon, L.; Suzuki, K.; Maddipati, R.; Rhim, A.D.; Schlitter, A.M.; et al. Regulation of Epithelial Plasticity Determines Metastatic Organotropism in Pancreatic Cancer. *Dev. Cell* **2018**, *45*, 696–711.e8. [CrossRef]
57. Puram, S.V.; Tirosh, I.; Parikh, A.S.; Patel, A.P.; Yizhak, K.; Gillespie, S.; Rodman, C.; Luo, C.L.; Mroz, E.A.; Emerick, K.S.; et al. Single-Cell Transcriptomic Analysis of Primary and Metastatic Tumor Ecosystems in Head and Neck Cancer. *Cell* **2017**, *171*, 1611–1624.e24. [CrossRef]
58. Kroger, C.; Afeyan, A.; Mraz, J.; Eaton, E.N.; Reinhardt, F.; Khodor, Y.L.; Thiru, P.; Bierie, B.; Ye, X.; Burge, C.B.; et al. Acquisition of a hybrid E/M state is essential for tumorigenicity of basal breast cancer cells. *Proc. Natl. Acad. Sci. USA* **2019**, *116*, 7353–7362. [CrossRef]
59. Bocci, F.; Jolly, M.K.; Tripathi, S.C.; Aguilar, M.; Hanash, S.M.; Levine, H.; Onuchic, J.N. Numb prevents a complete epithelial-mesenchymal transition by modulating Notch signalling. *J. R. Soc. Interface* **2017**, *14*. [CrossRef]
60. Jolly, M.K.; Tripathi, S.C.; Jia, D.; Mooney, S.M.; Celiktas, M.; Hanash, S.M.; Mani, S.A.; Pienta, K.J.; Ben-Jacob, E.; Levine, H. Stability of the hybrid epithelial/mesenchymal phenotype. *Oncotarget* **2016**, *7*, 27067–27084. [CrossRef]
61. Biddle, A.; Gammon, L.; Liang, X.; Costea, D.E.; Mackenzie, I.C. Phenotypic Plasticity Determines Cancer Stem Cell Therapeutic Resistance in Oral Squamous Cell Carcinoma. *EBioMedicine* **2016**, *4*, 138–145. [CrossRef]
62. Katsuno, Y.; Meyer, D.S.; Zhang, Z.; Shokat, K.M.; Akhurst, R.J.; Miyazono, K.; Derynck, R. Chronic TGF-beta exposure drives stabilized EMT, tumor stemness, and cancer drug resistance with vulnerability to bitopic mTOR inhibition. *Sci. Signal.* **2019**, *12*. [CrossRef] [PubMed]
63. Mehlen, P.; Puisieux, A. Metastasis: A question of life or death. *Nat. Rev. Cancer* **2006**, *6*, 449–458. [CrossRef] [PubMed]
64. Friedl, P.; Wolf, K. Tumour-cell invasion and migration: Diversity and escape mechanisms. *Nat. Rev. Cancer* **2003**, *3*, 362–374. [CrossRef] [PubMed]
65. Ridley, A.J.; Schwartz, M.A.; Burridge, K.; Firtel, R.A.; Ginsberg, M.H.; Borisy, G.; Parsons, J.T.; Horwitz, A.R. Cell migration: Integrating signals from front to back. *Science* **2003**, *302*, 1704–1709. [CrossRef] [PubMed]
66. Sahai, E.; Marshall, C.J. Differing modes of tumour cell invasion have distinct requirements for Rho/ROCK signalling and extracellular proteolysis. *Nat. Cell Biol.* **2003**, *5*, 711–719. [CrossRef] [PubMed]
67. Wolf, K.; Mazo, I.; Leung, H.; Engelke, K.; von Andrian, U.H.; Deryugina, E.I.; Strongin, A.Y.; Brocker, E.B.; Friedl, P. Compensation mechanism in tumor cell migration: Mesenchymal-amoeboid transition after blocking of pericellular proteolysis. *J. Cell Biol.* **2003**, *160*, 267–277. [CrossRef] [PubMed]
68. Beerling, E.; Seinstra, D.; de Wit, E.; Kester, L.; van der Velden, D.; Maynard, C.; Schafer, R.; van Diest, P.; Voest, E.; van Oudenaarden, A.; et al. Plasticity between Epithelial and Mesenchymal States Unlinks EMT from Metastasis-Enhancing Stem Cell Capacity. *Cell Rep.* **2016**, *14*, 2281–2288. [CrossRef]
69. Zhao, Z.; Zhu, X.; Cui, K.; Mancuso, J.; Federley, R.; Fischer, K.; Teng, G.; Mittal, V.; Gao, D.; Zhao, H.; et al. In Vivo Visualization and Characterization of Epithelial-Mesenchymal Transition in Breast Tumors. *Cancer Res.* **2016**, *76*, 2094–2104. [CrossRef]
70. Friedl, P.; Wolf, K. Proteolytic interstitial cell migration: A five-step process. *Cancer Metastasis Rev.* **2009**, *28*, 129–135. [CrossRef]
71. Miyoshi, A.; Kitajima, Y.; Kido, S.; Shimonishi, T.; Matsuyama, S.; Kitahara, K.; Miyazaki, K. Snail accelerates cancer invasion by upregulating MMP expression and is associated with poor prognosis of hepatocellular carcinoma. *Br. J. Cancer* **2005**, *92*, 252–258. [CrossRef]

72. Miyoshi, A.; Kitajima, Y.; Sumi, K.; Sato, K.; Hagiwara, A.; Koga, Y.; Miyazaki, K. Snail and SIP1 increase cancer invasion by upregulating MMP family in hepatocellular carcinoma cells. *Br. J. Cancer* **2004**, *90*, 1265–1273. [CrossRef] [PubMed]
73. Lochter, A.; Galosy, S.; Muschler, J.; Freedman, N.; Werb, Z.; Bissell, M.J. Matrix metalloproteinase stromelysin-1 triggers a cascade of molecular alterations that leads to stable epithelial-to-mesenchymal conversion and a premalignant phenotype in mammary epithelial cells. *J. Cell Biol* **1997**, *139*, 1861–1872. [CrossRef] [PubMed]
74. Shintani, Y.; Wheelock, M.J.; Johnson, K.R. Phosphoinositide-3 kinase-Rac1-c-Jun NH2-terminal kinase signaling mediates collagen I-induced cell scattering and up-regulation of N-cadherin expression in mouse mammary epithelial cells. *Mol. Biol. Cell* **2006**, *17*, 2963–2975. [CrossRef] [PubMed]
75. Ilina, O.; Campanello, L.; Gritsenko, P.G.; Vullings, M.; Wang, C.; Bult, P.; Losert, W.; Friedl, P. Intravital microscopy of collective invasion plasticity in breast cancer. *Dis. Model. Mech.* **2018**, *11*. [CrossRef] [PubMed]
76. Shamir, E.R.; Pappalardo, E.; Jorgens, D.M.; Coutinho, K.; Tsai, W.T., Aziz, K.; Auer, M.; Tran, P.T.; Bader, J.S.; Ewald, A.J. Twist1-induced dissemination preserves epithelial identity and requires E-cadherin. *J. Cell Biol.* **2014**, *204*, 839–856. [CrossRef]
77. Friedl, P.; Locker, J.; Sahai, E.; Segall, J.E. Classifying collective cancer cell invasion. *Nat. Cell Biol.* **2012**, *14*, 777–783. [CrossRef] [PubMed]
78. Campbell, K.; Rossi, F.; Adams, J.; Pitsidianaki, I.; Barriga, F.M.; Garcia-Gerique, L.; Batlle, E.; Casanova, J.; Casali, A. Collective cell migration and metastases induced by an epithelial-to-mesenchymal transition in Drosophila intestinal tumors. *Nat. Commun.* **2019**, *10*, 2311. [CrossRef]
79. Cheung, K.J.; Gabrielson, E.; Werb, Z.; Ewald, A.J. Collective invasion in breast cancer requires a conserved basal epithelial program. *Cell* **2013**, *155*, 1639–1651. [CrossRef]
80. Friedl, P.; Mayor, R. Tuning Collective Cell Migration by Cell-Cell Junction Regulation. *Cold Spring Harb. Perspect. Biol.* **2017**, *9*. [CrossRef]
81. Tse, J.M.; Cheng, G.; Tyrrell, J.A.; Wilcox-Adelman, S.A.; Boucher, Y.; Jain, R.K.; Munn, L.L. Mechanical compression drives cancer cells toward invasive phenotype. *Proc. Natl. Acad. Sci. USA* **2012**, *109*, 911–916. [CrossRef]
82. Scarpa, E.; Mayor, R. Collective cell migration in development. *J. Cell Biol.* **2016**, *212*, 143–155. [CrossRef] [PubMed]
83. Wolf, K.; Wu, Y.I.; Liu, Y.; Geiger, J.; Tam, E.; Overall, C.; Stack, M.S.; Friedl, P. Multi-step pericellular proteolysis controls the transition from individual to collective cancer cell invasion. *Nat. Cell Biol.* **2007**, *9*, 893–904. [CrossRef] [PubMed]
84. Gaggioli, C.; Hooper, S.; Hidalgo-Carcedo, C.; Grosse, R.; Marshall, J.F.; Harrington, K.; Sahai, E. Fibroblast-led collective invasion of carcinoma cells with differing roles for RhoGTPases in leading and following cells. *Nat. Cell Biol.* **2007**, *9*, 1392–1400. [CrossRef] [PubMed]
85. Labernadie, A.; Kato, T.; Brugues, A.; Serra-Picamal, X.; Derzsi, S.; Arwert, E.; Weston, A.; Gonzalez-Tarrago, V.; Elosegui-Artola, A.; Albertazzi, L.; et al. A mechanically active heterotypic E-cadherin/N-cadherin adhesion enables fibroblasts to drive cancer cell invasion. *Nat. Cell Biol.* **2017**, *19*, 224–237. [CrossRef] [PubMed]
86. Condeelis, J.; Pollard, J.W. Macrophages: Obligate partners for tumor cell migration, invasion, and metastasis. *Cell* **2006**, *124*, 263–266. [CrossRef] [PubMed]
87. DeNardo, D.G.; Barreto, J.B.; Andreu, P.; Vasquez, L.; Tawfik, D.; Kolhatkar, N.; Coussens, L.M. CD4(+) T cells regulate pulmonary metastasis of mammary carcinomas by enhancing protumor properties of macrophages. *Cancer Cell* **2009**, *16*, 91–102. [CrossRef] [PubMed]
88. Roussos, E.T.; Condeelis, J.S.; Patsialou, A. Chemotaxis in cancer. *Nat. Rev. Cancer* **2011**, *11*, 573–587. [CrossRef]
89. Hu, J.L.; Wang, W.; Lan, X.L.; Zeng, Z.C.; Liang, Y.S.; Yan, Y.R.; Song, F.Y.; Wang, F.F.; Zhu, X.H.; Liao, W.J.; et al. CAFs secreted exosomes promote metastasis and chemotherapy resistance by enhancing cell stemness and epithelial-mesenchymal transition in colorectal cancer. *Mol. Cancer* **2019**, *18*, 91. [CrossRef]
90. Gandalovicova, A.; Rosel, D.; Fernandes, M.; Vesely, P.; Heneberg, P.; Cermak, V.; Petruzelka, L.; Kumar, S.; Sanz-Moreno, V.; Brabek, J. Migrastatics-Anti-metastatic and Anti-invasion Drugs: Promises and Challenges. *Trends Cancer* **2017**, *3*, 391–406. [CrossRef]
91. Aceto, N.; Toner, M.; Maheswaran, S.; Haber, D.A. En Route to Metastasis: Circulating Tumor Cell Clusters and Epithelial-to-Mesenchymal Transition. *Trends Cancer* **2015**, *1*, 44–52. [CrossRef]

92. Finkel, G.C.; Tishkoff, G.H. Malignant cells in a peripheral blood smear: Report of a case. *N. Engl. J. Med.* **1960**, *262*, 187–188. [CrossRef] [PubMed]
93. Yu, M.; Bardia, A.; Wittner, B.S.; Stott, S.L.; Smas, M.E.; Ting, D.T.; Isakoff, S.J.; Ciciliano, J.C.; Wells, M.N.; Shah, A.M.; et al. Circulating breast tumor cells exhibit dynamic changes in epithelial and mesenchymal composition. *Science* **2013**, *339*, 580–584. [CrossRef] [PubMed]
94. Ao, Z.; Shah, S.H.; Machlin, L.M.; Parajuli, R.; Miller, P.C.; Rawal, S.; Williams, A.J.; Cote, R.J.; Lippman, M.E.; Datar, R.H.; et al. Identification of Cancer-Associated Fibroblasts in Circulating Blood from Patients with Metastatic Breast Cancer. *Cancer Res.* **2015**, *75*, 4681–4687. [CrossRef] [PubMed]
95. Duda, D.G.; Duyverman, A.M.; Kohno, M.; Snuderl, M.; Steller, E.J.; Fukumura, D.; Jain, R.K. Malignant cells facilitate lung metastasis by bringing their own soil. *Proc. Natl. Acad. Sci. USA* **2010**, *107*, 21677–21682. [CrossRef] [PubMed]
96. Gasic, G.J.; Gasic, T.B.; Galanti, N.; Johnson, T.; Murphy, S. Platelet-tumor-cell interactions in mice. The role of platelets in the spread of malignant disease. *Int. J. Cancer* **1973**, *11*, 704–718. [CrossRef] [PubMed]
97. Labelle, M.; Begum, S.; Hynes, R.O. Direct signaling between platelets and cancer cells induces an epithelial-mesenchymal-like transition and promotes metastasis. *Cancer Cell* **2011**, *20*, 576–590. [CrossRef] [PubMed]
98. Szczerba, B.M.; Castro-Giner, F.; Vetter, M.; Krol, I.; Gkountela, S.; Landin, J.; Scheidmann, M.C.; Donato, C.; Scherrer, R.; Singer, J.; et al. Neutrophils escort circulating tumour cells to enable cell cycle progression. *Nature* **2019**, *566*, 553–557. [CrossRef] [PubMed]
99. Lecharpentier, A.; Vielh, P.; Perez-Moreno, P.; Planchard, D.; Soria, J.C.; Farace, F. Detection of circulating tumour cells with a hybrid (epithelial/mesenchymal) phenotype in patients with metastatic non-small cell lung cancer. *Br. J. Cancer* **2011**, *105*, 1338–1341. [CrossRef] [PubMed]
100. Molnar, B.; Ladanyi, A.; Tanko, L.; Sreter, L.; Tulassay, Z. Circulating tumor cell clusters in the peripheral blood of colorectal cancer patients. *Clin. Cancer Res.* **2001**, *7*, 4080–4085. [PubMed]
101. Yadavalli, S.; Jayaram, S.; Manda, S.S.; Madugundu, A.K.; Nayakanti, D.S.; Tan, T.Z.; Bhat, R.; Rangarajan, A.; Chatterjee, A.; Gowda, H.; et al. Data-Driven Discovery of Extravasation Pathway in Circulating Tumor Cells. *Sci. Rep.* **2017**, *7*, 43710. [CrossRef]
102. Watanabe, S. The metastasizability of tumor cells. *Cancer* **1954**, *7*, 215–223. [CrossRef]
103. Topal, B.; Roskams, T.; Fevery, J.; Penninckx, F. Aggregated colon cancer cells have a higher metastatic efficiency in the liver compared with nonaggregated cells: An experimental study. *J. Surg. Res.* **2003**, *112*, 31–37. [CrossRef]
104. Aceto, N.; Bardia, A.; Miyamoto, D.T.; Donaldson, M.C.; Wittner, B.S.; Spencer, J.A.; Yu, M.; Pely, A.; Engstrom, A.; Zhu, H.; et al. Circulating tumor cell clusters are oligoclonal precursors of breast cancer metastasis. *Cell* **2014**, *158*, 1110–1122. [CrossRef] [PubMed]
105. Cheung, K.J.; Padmanaban, V.; Silvestri, V.; Schipper, K.; Cohen, J.D.; Fairchild, A.N.; Gorin, M.A.; Verdone, J.E.; Pienta, K.J.; Bader, J.S.; et al. Polyclonal breast cancer metastases arise from collective dissemination of keratin 14-expressing tumor cell clusters. *Proc. Natl. Acad. Sci. USA* **2016**, *113*, E854–E863. [CrossRef] [PubMed]
106. Maddipati, R.; Stanger, B.Z. Pancreatic Cancer Metastases Harbor Evidence of Polyclonality. *Cancer Discov.* **2015**, *5*, 1086–1097. [CrossRef] [PubMed]
107. Gkountela, S.; Castro-Giner, F.; Szczerba, B.M.; Vetter, M.; Landin, J.; Scherrer, R.; Krol, I.; Scheidmann, M.C.; Beisel, C.; Stirnimann, C.U.; et al. Circulating Tumor Cell Clustering Shapes DNA Methylation to Enable Metastasis Seeding. *Cell* **2019**, *176*, 98–112.e14. [CrossRef] [PubMed]
108. Hou, J.M.; Krebs, M.G.; Lancashire, L.; Sloane, R.; Backen, A.; Swain, R.K.; Priest, L.J.; Greystoke, A.; Zhou, C.; Morris, K.; et al. Clinical significance and molecular characteristics of circulating tumor cells and circulating tumor microemboli in patients with small-cell lung cancer. *J. Clin. Oncol.* **2012**, *30*, 525–532. [CrossRef] [PubMed]
109. Zhang, D.; Zhao, L.; Zhou, P.; Ma, H.; Huang, F.; Jin, M.; Dai, X.; Zheng, X.; Huang, S.; Zhang, T. Circulating tumor microemboli (CTM) and vimentin+ circulating tumor cells (CTCs) detected by a size-based platform predict worse prognosis in advanced colorectal cancer patients during chemotherapy. *Cancer Cell Int.* **2017**, *17*, 6. [CrossRef] [PubMed]
110. Frisch, S.M.; Schaller, M.; Cieply, B. Mechanisms that link the oncogenic epithelial-mesenchymal transition to suppression of anoikis. *J. Cell Sci.* **2013**, *126*, 21–29. [CrossRef]

111. Mahauad-Fernandez, W.D.; Naushad, W.; Panzner, T.D.; Bashir, A.; Lal, G.; Okeoma, C.M. BST-2 promotes survival in circulation and pulmonary metastatic seeding of breast cancer cells. *Sci. Rep.* **2018**, *8*, 17608. [CrossRef]
112. Nieswandt, B.; Hafner, M.; Echtenacher, B.; Mannel, D.N. Lysis of tumor cells by natural killer cells in mice is impeded by platelets. *Cancer Res.* **1999**, *59*, 1295–1300. [PubMed]
113. Palumbo, J.S.; Talmage, K.E.; Massari, J.V.; La Jeunesse, C.M.; Flick, M.J.; Kombrinck, K.W.; Jirouskova, M.; Degen, J.L. Platelets and fibrin(ogen) increase metastatic potential by impeding natural killer cell-mediated elimination of tumor cells. *Blood* **2005**, *105*, 178–185. [CrossRef] [PubMed]
114. Borsig, L.; Wong, R.; Hynes, R.O.; Varki, N.M.; Varki, A. Synergistic effects of L- and P-selectin in facilitating tumor metastasis can involve non-mucin ligands and implicate leukocytes as enhancers of metastasis. *Proc. Natl. Acad. Sci. USA* **2002**, *99*, 2193–2198. [CrossRef] [PubMed]
115. Leblanc, R.; Peyruchaud, O. Metastasis: New functional implications of platelets and megakaryocytes. *Blood* **2016**, *128*, 24–31. [CrossRef] [PubMed]
116. Cheung, K.J.; Ewald, A.J. A collective route to metastasis: Seeding by tumor cell clusters. *Science* **2016**, *352*, 167–169. [CrossRef] [PubMed]
117. Gorges, T.M.; Tinhofer, I.; Drosch, M.; Rose, L.; Zollner, T.M.; Krahn, T.; von Ahsen, O. Circulating tumour cells escape from EpCAM-based detection due to epithelial-to-mesenchymal transition. *BMC Cancer* **2012**, *12*, 178. [CrossRef] [PubMed]
118. Cima, I.; Kong, S.L.; Sengupta, D.; Tan, I.B.; Phyo, W.M.; Lee, D.; Hu, M.; Iliescu, C.; Alexander, I.; Goh, W.L.; et al. Tumor-derived circulating endothelial cell clusters in colorectal cancer. *Sci. Transl. Med.* **2016**, *8*, 345ra389. [CrossRef]
119. Mu, Z.; Wang, C.; Ye, Z.; Austin, L.; Civan, J.; Hyslop, T.; Palazzo, J.P.; Jaslow, R.; Li, B.; Myers, R.E.; et al. Prospective assessment of the prognostic value of circulating tumor cells and their clusters in patients with advanced-stage breast cancer. *Breast Cancer Res. Treat.* **2015**, *154*, 563–571. [CrossRef]
120. Molnar, B.; Floro, L.; Sipos, F.; Toth, B.; Sreter, L.; Tulassay, Z. Elevation in peripheral blood circulating tumor cell number correlates with macroscopic progression in UICC stage IV colorectal cancer patients. *Dis. Markers* **2008**, *24*, 141–150. [CrossRef]
121. Sharma, D.; Brummel-Ziedins, K.E.; Bouchard, B.A.; Holmes, C.E. Platelets in tumor progression: A host factor that offers multiple potential targets in the treatment of cancer. *J. Cell Physiol.* **2014**, *229*, 1005–1015. [CrossRef]
122. Schror, K. Aspirin and platelets: The antiplatelet action of aspirin and its role in thrombosis treatment and prophylaxis. *Semin. Thromb. Hemost.* **1997**, *23*, 349–356. [CrossRef]
123. Kanikarla-Marie, P.; Lam, M.; Sorokin, A.V.; Overman, M.J.; Kopetz, S.; Menter, D.G. Platelet Metabolism and Other Targeted Drugs; Potential Impact on Immunotherapy. *Front. Oncol.* **2018**, *8*, 107. [CrossRef]
124. Guillem-Llobat, P.; Dovizio, M.; Bruno, A.; Ricciotti, E.; Cufino, V.; Sacco, A.; Grande, R.; Alberti, S.; Arena, V.; Cirillo, M.; et al. Aspirin prevents colorectal cancer metastasis in mice by splitting the crosstalk between platelets and tumor cells. *Oncotarget* **2016**, *7*, 32462–32477. [CrossRef]
125. Frose, J.; Chen, M.B.; Hebron, K.E.; Reinhardt, F.; Hajal, C.; Zijlstra, A.; Kamm, R.D.; Weinberg, R.A. Epithelial-Mesenchymal Transition Induces Podocalyxin to Promote Extravasation via Ezrin Signaling. *Cell Rep.* **2018**, *24*, 962–972. [CrossRef]
126. Stankic, M.; Pavlovic, S.; Chin, Y.; Brogi, E.; Padua, D.; Norton, L.; Massague, J.; Benezra, R. TGF-beta-Id1 signaling opposes Twist1 and promotes metastatic colonization via a mesenchymal-to-epithelial transition. *Cell Rep.* **2013**, *5*, 1228–1242. [CrossRef]
127. Ocana, O.H.; Corcoles, R.; Fabra, A.; Moreno-Bueno, G.; Acloque, H.; Vega, S.; Barrallo-Gimeno, A.; Cano, A.; Nieto, M.A. Metastatic colonization requires the repression of the epithelial-mesenchymal transition inducer Prrx1. *Cancer Cell* **2012**, *22*, 709–724. [CrossRef]
128. Sanchez-Tillo, E.; Siles, L.; de Barrios, O.; Cuatrecasas, M.; Vaquero, E.C.; Castells, A.; Postigo, A. Expanding roles of ZEB factors in tumorigenesis and tumor progression. *Am. J. Cancer Res.* **2011**, *1*, 897–912.

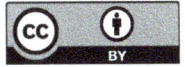

© 2019 by the authors. Licensee MDPI, Basel, Switzerland. This article is an open access article distributed under the terms and conditions of the Creative Commons Attribution (CC BY) license (http://creativecommons.org/licenses/by/4.0/).

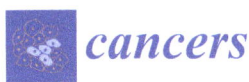

Review

Unraveling Heterogeneity in Epithelial Cell Fates of the Mammary Gland and Breast Cancer

Alexandr Samocha [1,†], Hanna Doh [1], Kai Kessenbrock [2] and Jeroen P. Roose [1,*]

[1] Department of Anatomy, University of California, San Francisco, CA 94143, USA; ajsamocha@gmail.com (A.S.); hanna.doh@ucsf.edu (H.D.)
[2] Department of Biological Chemistry, University of California, Irvine, CA 92697, USA; kai.kessenbrock@uci.edu
[*] Correspondence: Jeroen.Roose@ucsf.edu; Tel.: +1-415-476-3977
[†] Current address: Wild Type, Inc. 953 Indiana Street, San Francisco, CA 94107, USA.

Received: 21 August 2019; Accepted: 22 September 2019; Published: 24 September 2019

Abstract: Fluidity in cell fate or heterogeneity in cell identity is an interesting cell biological phenomenon, which at the same time poses a significant obstacle for cancer therapy. The mammary gland seems a relatively straightforward organ with stromal cells and basal- and luminal- epithelial cell types. In reality, the epithelial cell fates are much more complex and heterogeneous, which is the topic of this review. Part of the complexity comes from the dynamic nature of this organ: the primitive epithelial tree undergoes extensively remodeling and expansion during puberty, pregnancy, and lactation and, unlike most other organs, the bulk of mammary gland development occurs late, during puberty. An active cell biological debate has focused on lineage commitment to basal- and luminal- epithelial cell fates by epithelial progenitor and stem cells; processes that are also relevant to cancer biology. In this review, we discuss the current understanding of heterogeneity in mammary gland and recent insights obtained through lineage tracing, signaling assays, and organoid cultures. Lastly, we relate these insights to cancer and ongoing efforts to resolve heterogeneity in breast cancer with single-cell RNAseq approaches.

Keywords: mammary gland; breast cancer; cell fate; heterogeneity; 3D cultures; organoids; signaling; single-cell RNAseq

---

1. Introduction into Mammary Gland Structure, Function and Early Development

The mammary gland is comprised of many different interacting cell types. Epithelial cells form a primitive structure early during embryonic development, which later form the nipple and a ductal network that expands into the fat pad. These epithelial ducts are surrounded by fat cells, and become innervated with a variety of stromal cells including endothelial cells, immune cells, and fibroblasts [1]. Maturation of the gland is regulated at first by mesenchymal interactions, and later by hormone and growth factor receptor signaling during puberty and pregnancy. Mammary epithelial cells assemble into their normal morphology between E16-E18 (embryonic day), forming a bilayered duct with an inner lumen [2]. Together, the mammary epithelial subtypes interact to carry out the organ's functions. After pregnancy, mature epithelial cells can later differentiate into alveolar cells and subsequently produce milk proteins.

Mammary epithelial cells (MECs) typically form a bilayered epithelium and can be broadly separated into two distinct compartments: an inner layer of luminal and outer layer of basal MECs. However, additional heterogeneity exists within both luminal and basal MECs. Luminal populations are often sub classified based on hormone and growth factor receptor status. The basal epithelium contains a subset of so-called myoepithelial cells that lie along the outside of the ductal epithelial tree and assist in the motility of milk protein along the lumen. The MEC system also contains subsets of basal and luminal stem and progenitor cells, which will be covered in greater detail later. For example, within the luminal compartment a population of luminal progenitor cells can go on to form ductal or alveolar cells. In addition, basal cells contain a subset of mammary stem cells (MaSCs) forming a small, heterogeneous, and to date poorly defined population that drive development, repair and organ reconstitution when transplanted into epithelium-cleared fat pads of recipient mice [3].

Puberty is the most dynamic and striking period during the development of the mammary gland. The rudimentary duct undergoes significant expansion, resulting in the formation of bulbous multilayered structures called terminal end buds (TEBs) [4] (Figure 1). TEBs are the proliferative centers that drive elongation, bifurcation, and branching until the entirety of the mammary fat pad is filled, thereby creating the mature epithelial tree [5]. The TEB contains cap cells, a rapidly growing and dividing progenitor cell population that later goes on to form the tree's outer myoepithelial layer [6].

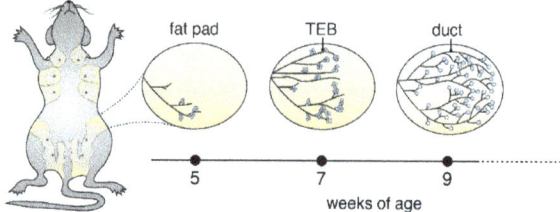

Figure 1. Schematic of mouse mammary gland development during puberty. During puberty, the rudimentary duct undergoes significant expansion, resulting in the formation of bulbous multilayered structures called terminal end buds (TEBs). These TEBs are the proliferative centers that drive elongation, bifurcation, and branching of ducts until the entirety of the mammary fat pad is filled, thereby creating the mature epithelial tree.

2. Luminal Cells and Luminal-Specific Progenitors

The luminal compartment contains different mature, differentiated cell populations with specified functions as well as progenitor-cell populations that are each distinguished by specific gene and extracellular ligand profiles.

Several classifications of luminal cells exist within the mammary gland. Luminal cells are segregated based on functional, morphological, and expression profiling evidence. Histologically, luminal cells can be broadly separated into two types: ductal and alveolar. Mature ductal cells can be either estrogen receptor (ER) positive or negative, and feature the following marker expression profile: $CD49f^{lo}CD29^{lo}CD24^{+}CD14^{-}EpCAM^{hi}c\text{-}kit^{-}Sca1^{+}CD61^{-}CD49b^{-}$ [7], in which the CD numbers and other markers represent different gene products. Mature alveolar cells are always estrogen receptor (ER) negative and can be more precisely characterized through a $CD49f^{lo}CD29^{lo}CD24^{+}CD14^{-}EpCAM^{hi}Sca1^{lo}CD61^{-}$ expression pattern. Alveolar cells can be distinguished by their secretory morphology and histologically by the accumulation of milk proteins within.

Transcription factors have been demonstrated to drive luminal cell fate commitment throughout development. The Elf5 (E74-like factor 5) transcription factor is one of the major drivers of luminal cell specification and differentiation. Elf5 is able to directly repress Slug (Zinc Finger Protein SNAI2) transcription, thereby blocking basal cell determination and promoting luminal cell fate [8,9]. Progesterone acts on mature, progesterone receptor-positive cells and induces expression and secretion of the chemokine RANKL (Receptor activator of nuclear factor kappa-B ligand) that subsequently, in a paracrine manner, induces progenitor cells to express Elf5 [10]. The transcription factor Gata-3 (GATA binding protein 3) is another key regulator of luminal cell identity. Gata-3 expression is important for the maturation of luminal progenitor cells into mature ductal and alveolar cells [11]. Stat5a (Signal Transducer and Activator of Transcription 5A), a transcription factor activated by activated by ligands including prolactin, growth hormone, and EGF (Epidermal Growth Factor) drives the expansion of luminal progenitors and subsequent differentiation into alveolar cells [12].

Luminal progenitor populations can be distinguished using many of the above extracellular markers. For example, ductal progenitors are CD61$^+$, CD49b$^+$, CD14$^+$, and c-kit$^+$ whereas their mature counterparts are negative for the surface expression of these proteins [13–15]. Sca-1 (Spinocerebellar ataxia type 1) expression can be used to separate ductal progenitors from alveolar progenitors since alveolar progenitor cells lack membrane expression of the protein. It should be noted that expression of these extracellular receptors is not ubiquitous between mouse model lines. Neither c-kit nor CD61 are expressed in mammary epithelial cells derived from C57BL/6 mice, while they are both found in MECs from FVB/N mice [16]. The fate and biology of these luminal progenitor cell populations has been further characterized by lineage tracing experiments, which we will discuss in Section 4.

3. Basal Cells and Progenitors

Unlike luminal cells, the factors that control and label different basal cell populations are less clear. Both stem cells and bipotent progenitor cells have been identified within the broader basal cell lineage. The use of extracellular markers to distinguish these discrete populations, however, has not yet yielded clear profiles. Mature myoepithelial basal cells are typically CD29^{hi}CD49f^{hi}CD24$^+$EpCAM$^{lo/med}$ [7]. The undifferentiated population that is enriched for MaSCs is believed to be CD49f^{hi}CD29^{hi}CD24^{hi}EpCAM$^{lo/med}$Sca1$^-$. Markers that are specific for a restricted basal cell progenitor have not been identified and neither have specific markers for a restricted myoepithelial cell progenitors. Luminal progenitors are thought to arise from an early basal cell population.

Several epithelial-mesenchymal transition (EMT) factors have been identified as molecular regulators of the basal/MaSC population. The transcription factor Slug is a key for the basal/MaSC lineage as it suppresses luminal cell fate. Slug-deficient mice have delayed ductal morphogenesis and aberrantly express luminal signature genes in basal cell populations [17,18]. The transcription factor Sox9 cooperates with Slug to suppress luminal fate and exogenous expression of these two factors can convert differentiated luminal cells into MaSCs with long-term mammary gland-reconstituting ability [18]. Tumor protein TP63 loss blocks the formation of the primitive epithelial duct [19]. Perhaps one of the strongest drivers of basal cell identity, p63 overexpression in luminal cells leads to an identity shift from luminal to a basal phenotype [20]. Notch1/3 signaling has been reported to down-regulate TP63 expression as basal progenitors restrict to a luminal cell fate [21]. The transcription factor p53, on the other hand, restricts basal/MaSC renewal and drives differentiation [22].

4. Lineage Tracing to Identify Restricted and Bipotent Progenitor Cells

Lineage tracing is a powerful tool to observe and track the function of adult-, stem- and progenitor-cells during normal homeostasis, and various studies have utilized this approach to shed light on the lineage hierarchies of the MECs. K8-creER targeted cells exclusively differentiate into luminal cells when observed in vitro [23]. MECs marked with this label are maintained in small numbers following several rounds of growth and differentiation. Elf5, a well-studied luminal progenitor cell gene, was utilized in a separate study to trace this restricted progenitor population throughout pubertal development [24]. Elf5-expressing cells exclusively produced mammary epithelial cells with a luminal identity and were a major driver of branching morphogenesis [24]. In 2014, Rios et al. confirmed that these Elf5-expressing cells were short-lived and restricted progenitors, as the positive cells could not be detected in the mammary glands of lineage tracer mice after 20 weeks [24]. Combined, these findings show that there may exist both short- and long-lived progenitor cells that exclusively mature into luminal subtypes.

Lineage tracing studies were performed in order to hone-in on the exact nature of mammary progenitor populations. In 2011, van Keymeulen et al. established that all mammary epithelial lineages are derived from cytokeratin-14 (K14) expressing embryonic progenitors [23]. Following this population throughout puberty revealed that K14+ MaSCs promote basal expansion and maintenance. MaSCs expressing K8 promoted luminal cell expansion and maintenance throughout puberty. When cultured in vitro these restricted progenitors maintain their identity, while only basal cells display multipotency in transplantation and reconstitution assays [23]. Rios et al. used lineage-tracing experiments to identify a cytokeratin 5 (K5) expressing bipotent progenitor population [24]. K5-positive cells labeled at the onset of puberty contributed to the formation of both mature luminal and myoepithelial cells.

5. Three-Dimensional Spheroid Cultures

In the late 1980s and early '90s, three-dimensional (3D) cultures were instrumental in the discovery of the cell biology of mammary gland development and breast cancer. We term these classical three-dimensional spheroid cultures in our review, as these did not yet focus so much on the function and preservation of stem cells through Wnt signaling. We will cover more on Wnt signals and organoids later. For an excellent overview with historic perspectives on the development of these 3D culture platforms we refer you to a review by Drs Simian and Bissell [25]. Essential for these revolutionary in vitro approaches was the isolation of gel from the matrix of chondrosarcomas in 1977 by Orkin and colleagues [26] that is now commonly known as Matrigel (Figure 2). For example, these classical 3D spheroid cultures revealed that a 3D basement membrane [27] impacts the response of a series of human breast-tumor cell lines at different stages of progression, cultured within a physiological context [28]. Importantly, the 3D aspect of these cultures revealed new discoveries, such as bidirectional cross-modulation of integrin and EGFR (Epidermal Growth Factor Receptor) signaling, that were not present in artificial 2D cultures [29].

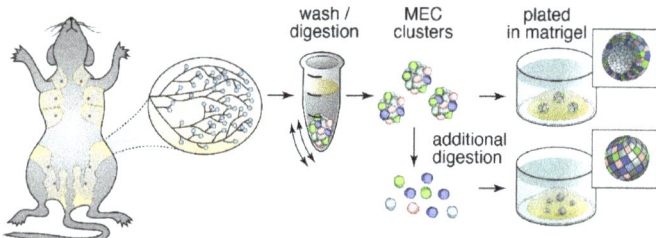

Figure 2. Schematic of three-dimensional spheroid cultures of mammary gland tissue. The discovery of Matrigel by Orkin and colleagues [26] enabled cell biological studies by many research groups with three-dimensional (3D) spheroid cultures of mammary gland tissue in vitro. Plating of digested MEC clusters aided the identification of restricted luminal- or basal-cells and bipotent progenitors in 3D, while further digestion into single mammary epithelial cells and plating into colony-forming assays provided information on the proliferative capacity.

Classical 3D spheroid cultures also aided identification of restricted luminal- or basal-cells and bipotent progenitors. In vitro experimentation confirmed that, the restricted differentiation potential of both luminal cells and basal, myoepithelial cells can be maintained, given specific culture conditions [30]. In mammosphere assays, single MECs can be cultured short-term in ultra-low adherence plates to generate mammospheres. These assays interrogate the function and clonogenic capacity of MaSCs. Mammosphere cultures could generate MEC colonies with either restricted unipotent differentiation potential or a bipotent stem-like phenotype, suggesting the existence of unipotent- and bipotent-progenitors [31]. Isolated single mammary epithelial cells can also be plated in Matrigel pellets in a colony-forming assay (Figure 2). Single MECs are able to seed into the surrounding matrix and clonally expand. The number of colonies that are able to form, as well as the size of the colonies, provides a representation of the proliferative capacity of progenitor cells within the total MEC population. Similarly, only MaSCs with self-renewal potential are able to survive non-adherent conditions. The number of mammospheres that are able to form can be used as a proxy to quantify MaSC activity. Use of these platforms has allowed for new insights into the mechanisms by which ductal morphogenesis is directed, particularly with regard to the role of different growth factor receptors, which we discuss next.

6. EGFR Family and Ligands

The EGFR family consists of EGFR (ErbB1/Her1), ErbB2/Her2, ErbB3/Her3, and ErbB4/Her4. ErbB receptors can both homo- and heterodimerize, with 10 possible combinations-six heterodimers and four homodimers. There is a high level of homology between kinase domains of the four EGFRs (~60–80%) with divergence occurring predominantly in the C terminus (shared identity is only ~10–25%). ErbB proteins have tissue specific expression, though they are commonly expressed together. EGFRs are found in several epithelial cell types such as the lung, intestine, and the breast. ErbB2 has no known ligands (Table 1), but frequently dimerizes with the other three EGFR members because of its unique and extended interaction loop [32]. ErbB3 is kinase dead, its cytoplasmic domain unable to initiate phosphorylation cascades. ErbB3 is able to trans phosphorylate its own intracellular domain to assist heterodimerization, as well as allosterically activate other EGFRs, however [33].

Table 1. The EGFR family members and their interacting ligands. Adapted from Hynes and Watson [34].

EGFR Family	EGFR (ErbB1/Her1)	EGFR2 (ErbB2/Her2)	EGFR3 (ErbB3/Her3)	EGFR4 (ErbB4/Her4)
EGF	X			
TGF	X			
AREG	X			
EPG	X			
BTC	X			X
HB-EGF	X			X
EPR	X			X
NRG1			X	X
NRG2			X	X
NRG3				X

EGF: Epidermal Growth Factor; TGF: Transforming Growth Factor; AREG: Amphiregulin; EPG: Epigen; BTC: Betacellulin; HB-EGF: Heparin-binding EGF-like growth factor; EPR: Epiregulin; NRG: Neuregulin; EGFR: Epidermal Growth Factor Receptor; ErbB: Erythroblastic leukemia viral oncogene homolog; Her: Human epidermal growth factor receptor.

Up to 13 different ligands have been found to bind EGFR family proteins: EGF, HB-EGF, transforming growth factor (TGF), amphiregulin (AREG), epiregulin (EREG), epigen (EPG), betacellulin (BTC), and neuregulins 1–6 (NRG) [34–36]. Ligand binding induces phosphorylation at tyrosine residues on the cytoplasmic domain [37]. EGF and TGF are the key ligands for EGFR and ErbB3/B4 preferentially bind neuregulins. The EGFR family members and their preferred ligands can be found in Table 1. Evidence suggests that EGFR phosphorylation and the duration and amplitude of signaling events are influenced by the binding of different ligands. This results in divergent cellular responses. For example, AREG is more potent in stimulating ductal elongation compared to EGF [38]. These ligand-specific nuances are important during development and cancer and we will cover some of the cancer-specific nuances of EGFR signaling in Section 10.

7. EGFR during Mammary Gland Development

The vast majority of what is understood about the EGFR family's role in mammary development comes through the use of genetic mouse models. *Egfr*-deficient mice perish just after birth, which complicated deciphering the exact nature of EGFR during mammary organogenesis [39,40]. Luetteke et al. generated *Waved-2* mice to circumvent this problem. The *Waved-2* allele has a point mutation near EGFR's cytoplasmic kinase domain that reduces activity; it is hypomorphic [41]. *Waved-2* mice have defective mammary development with diminished branching and a reduction in ductal invasion [42,43]. Use of a dominant negative EGFR protein using the mammary-specific MMTV promoter confirmed its role during pubertal development. Mice with the dominant negative EGFR display reduced proliferation and inhibited duct maturation [44]. *Egfr*'s importance in the stroma was confirmed via the generation of mixed tissue recombinants from transplanting neonatal epithelial cells from wild type or *egfr*-deficient mice [43,45,46].

Perturbations in other EGFR family genes also result in dramatic mammary developmental phenotypes. Specifically, deficiency in the *ErbB2–4* results in impaired ductal outgrowth during puberty. Deletion of *ErbB2* shunts ductal outgrowth [47,48]. ErbB2 also controls terminal end bud (TEB) formation through its regulation of cellular compartmentalization. In summary, despite many studies into the role of EGFR proteins in the mammary gland, the exact nature of each member has not been fully elucidated. Stromal and epithelial expression of the EGFR family is critically important at all stages of mammary development. A better understanding of EGFR and its downstream effectors is needed to create a clearer picture of the signals and processes that regulate the complex process of mammary organogenesis.

8. EGFR Signal Strength, Downstream Effector Kinases, Cell Fate

Mammary epithelial cells are organized into a developmental hierarchy based on extracellular receptor and gene expression patterns. The exact nature of these populations, and the factors that balance their proliferation with differentiation, are not well understood. Recent evidence has emerged, however, that EGFR signaling in MECs may be a key player in better defining this hierarchy as depicted in Figure 3.

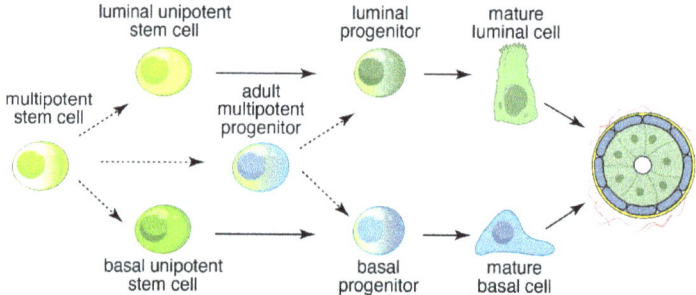

Figure 3. Schematic of the developmental hierarchy in the mammary gland. It should be explicitly stressed that Figure 3 is a model. In this hierarchy, mature luminal cells and mature basal cells are maintained by lineage-restricted, unipotent progenitors, which are replenished by multipotent stem cells that are present during embryogenesis.

In 2011, a report by Pasic et al. began to decipher EGFR's potential role in controlling MEC fate decisions during development. An ex vivo organoid model was utilized using cells taken from normal human breast tissue. They observed that different EGFR ligands could elicit discrete cell fate decisions. EGF stimulation of human breast organoids initiated a significant expansion of the basal (myoepithelial) population. Conversely, AREG stimulation drove organoids towards a luminal (ductal) cell fate. Interrogation of the downstream effector revealed that this deviance in cell fate decisions was due in part to the strength of downstream MEK-ERK signals, in which stronger activation EGFR-Ras-MEK-ERK selectively expanded the basal cell population and weaker activation drives luminal expansion [49].

Mukhopadhyay et al. expanded our insights into this initial model in 2013 [50]. Using an hTERT-immortalized human stem/progenitor cell pool, they observed similar cell fate decision changes that were dependent on the strength and duration of EGFR signals. Once more, it was observed that stimulation with the weak agonist AREG promoted luminal cell fate and a strong agonist (TGFα) drove cells towards a basal cell identity. In contrast to the data presented in Pasic et al. [49], however, Mukhopadhyay et al. found that EGF stimulation did not drive MaSCs down a specific lineage [50]. The addition of U0126, an inhibitor against the MEK-ERK pathway, significantly reduced differentiation into CD49f^{lo}EpCAM^{hi} and EpCAM^{lo} cells [50]. Taken together, it appears that the duration and amplitude of EGFR signals affects MEC fate choices.

Since many of the signaling effectors triggered by the EGFR lay downstream of Ras, it is of interest to consider the strength and duration of Ras activation as the cell fate determination factor. A historic study reported that nuances in receptor-Ras signaling can affect cell fate in a PC-12 cell line system. Stimulation of rat adrenal carcinoma cells (PC-12) with different EGFR ligands produced altered cell fate. In the PC-12 system, EGF is a weaker agonist compared to the strong nerve growth factor (NGF). EGF stimulation led to a short pulse of Ras-MEK-ERK activation and cell proliferation, while NGF stimulation elicited prolonged Ras-MEK-ERK signals, exit from the cell cycle and differentiation [51]. Since that report in 1995, very little work has followed up on this, perhaps because it is challenging to couple quantitative biochemical measurements to cell fate decisions, especially in in vivo studies.

9. EGFR and Other Receptor Tyrosine Kinases Signaling and Ductal Morphogenesis

Ductal morphogenesis is the process in which the mammary epithelium invades the fat pad during puberty to form a fully branched ductal epithelial tree. It is known to occur in a somewhat stochastic process, regulated by the combinatorial input of diverse signals. The stochastic aspect is perhaps best exemplified by the fact that there are substantial differences between mammary glands of mouse littermates. This has led the field to conclude that predetermined genetic control of pubertal development is not a possibility, unlike in the development of other epithelial tissues [52]. Development is dictated by mechanical factors and molecular signals from the surrounding stroma [53]. As a result, maturation of the breast is context-dependent.

The pubertal developmental process is initiated in large part by the expression of ovarian and pituitary hormones [54]. These signals cooperate to facilitate growth and communication between epithelial and stromal cells. Genetic knockout of estrogen receptor alpha (ERα) leads to incompletely developed mammary ductal trees, and exogenous administration of estrogen in mice lacking ovaries rescues ductal morphogenesis [55,56]. Estrogen facilitates stromal cell expression of hepatocyte growth factor (HGF) and epithelial expression of amphiregulin (AREG) [57,58]. AREG can communicate with the epidermal growth factor receptor (EGFR), whose expression is essential on mammary stromal cells [46]. Estrogen's collective functions serve to regulate local cell growth during pubertal development.

Estrogen is not the only steroid hormone important for pubertal mammary gland development, however. In fact, estrogen alone is insufficient to restore ductal morphogenesis when other input (like from the pituitary gland) is missing. Exogenous administration of growth hormone, normally produced by the pituitary gland, can restore the impaired branching phenotype of pituitary gland-deficient mice [59]. Growth hormone induces stromal insulin-like growth factor 1 (IGF1) expression, which binds to IGFR on epithelial cells [60]. Together growth factor and IGF1 act as global regulators of ductal morphogenesis.

Several growth factor receptors and receptor tyrosine kinases (RTKs) are involved in the integrated signaling environment that directs mammary morphogenesis. Fibroblast growth factors (FGF) and their receptors (FGFRs) are critically important for growth and branching. FGF2 and FGFR2 in particular shape the profile of ductal outgrowth and MEC proliferation. Genetic deletion of *fgfr2* disrupts ectodermal and placode formation during embryonic mammary organogenesis [61]. Mammary epithelial cells lacking *fgfr2* have a proliferative disadvantage when compared to their wild-type and *fgfr2*-heterozygous counterparts, and are depleted within TEBs [62]. Mice with inducible deletion of *fgfr2*$^{-/-}$ reveal a similar phenotype; proliferation is significantly attenuated and TEBs are completely absent from the glands [63]. In summary, *fgfr2* is a key regulator of luminal epithelial cells and it plays a specific role in the TEBs of elongating ducts.

The EGFR family of signaling proteins plays a pivotal role in directing pubertal mammary gland development in conjunction with FGF and FGF2. In brief, perturbations to each of the four EGFR family members result in developmental defects. In ex vivo culture, FGF2 addition can rescue growth and branching in EGFR-null 3D spheroids [45]. Mice with dominant negative EGFR display reduced proliferation and inhibited duct maturation [44]. Deletion of *ErbB2* shunts ductal outgrowth [47,48]. *ErbB2* also controls TEB formation through its regulation of cellular compartmentalization. *ErbB3* deficiency results in small TEBs and increased branch density with decreased TEB size as a result in an increase in apoptosis, controlled via observed changes in the PI3K (Phosphoinositide 3-kinase) signaling pathway. Anti-apoptotic transcription factor Bcl-2 is reduced in $ErbB3^{-/-}$ mice [64]. Mice deficient for *ErbB4* have defect occurring later in breast development, specifically during the formation of milk-producing luminal cells [65].

10. ERFR in Breast Cancer and Oncogenic PI3K Signals That Switch Fate

Dr Schlessinger put forth an elegant and simple model for EGFR activation with EGF as an external signal leading to the conversion of a monomeric receptor to a ligand-induced dimer [66], which served as a framework for further studies. The EGFR dimer turned out to be an asymmetric structure in which one EGFR kinase domain in a dimer acts as an allosteric activator for the other [67], which subsequently paved the way to mechanistically understand how a catalytically inactive Her3 can facilitate the activation of other EGFRs, such as Her2 [68]. Her2 overexpression is frequently found in breast cancer and typically associated with poor prognosis; a Her2/Her3 heterodimer operates as an oncogenic unit that drives breast cancer proliferation [69], with the phosphorylated tyrosines in the intracellular tail of the catalytically inactive Her3 functioning as adapter scaffolds for intracellular kinases such as PI3K (Phosphoinositide 3-kinase) and PLC (Phospholipase C).

Whereas it is clear that the EGFR family plays a role in mammary gland development and maturation as well as breast cancer, a lot less is known about the specific effector kinase pathways that lie downstream of the receptor families such as the EGFR. Elegant imaging studies revealed that levels of phosphorylated ERK kinases (a type of MAPK) are highest in MECs near the front of elongating ducts whereas levels of phosphorylated Akt kinase were equal throughout and Huebner et al. proposed a model of receptor-induced proliferation leading to highly motile cells with high phospho-ERK [70]. Two thought-provoking studies relate cell fate choices to aberrant PI3K signals in the context of breast cancer. Cell fate, heterogeneity, and cell lineage conversions are aspects that are of great relevance to cancer as these impact the tumor type and also often responses to therapy [71]. PIK3CA (Phosphoinositide 3-kinase p110 alpha) with a histidine to arginine mutation at position 1047 (H1047R) is a frequent mutation occurring in human breast cancer and expression of PIK3CA(H1047R) in lineage-committed basal Lgr5-positive and luminal keratin-8-positive cells led to dedifferentiation into a multipotent stem-like state [72]. Furthermore, the tumor cell of origin influenced the frequency of malignant breast tumors, linking (heterogeneous) cell fate to cancer aggressiveness [72]. Van Keymeulen et al. reported similar results in their studies in the context of loss of the tumor suppressor p53; expression of PIK3CA(H1047R) in basal cells (keratin K5-CreERT2 driver) gave rise to luminal-like cells and expression in luminal cells (K8-CReERT2) resulted in basal-like cells before progressing into invasive tumors [73]. Therefore, the rules that are thought to exist in normal unipotent progenitors (see Figure 3) appear alter when cells express PIK3CA(H1047R), which brings up a bigger question. What aberrant biochemical signals are capable to induce crossover of basal- and luminal-cell fates and drive further increases in heterogeneity and fluidity between mammary epithelial cells?

11. The Mammary Stem Cell Conundrum: More Questions than Answers

While there is a general consensus about some of the factors that mark and or regulate the MaSC population, the field has been left with more questions than answers when trying to specifically define MaSCs [74]. For example, the estimates for stem cell frequency, derived from calculating the number of mammary repopulating units, varies dramatically. Estimates for MaSC frequency range from 1 in every 100 total cells to 1 in every 4900 [75–77]. Extracellular markers used to sort MaSCs have proven insufficient to exclusively identify MaSC populations, but rather, only identify populations within which MaSCs are enriched [78–80]. The embryonic stem cell marker Oct4 (Octamer-binding transcription factor 4) has been found to label human mammary stem cells, but is insufficient to specifically separate MaSCs from other progenitor cells [81,82].

Some progress has been made towards separating MaSCs from mature myoepithelial and basal progenitors by using transgenic mouse models. MaSCs residing in the terminal end bud (TEB) cap cells exclusively express the phosphatase s-Ship [83], but MaSCs during pubertal development are not just found in cap cell populations. Lgr5, given its well-known role in intestinal epithelial populations, became of interest as a potential marker of the MaSC population [84]. Again, the Lgr5 story is unclear with opposing results of studies that use slightly different approaches. Whether Lgr5$^+$ cells have increased repopulating activity and whether they trend towards quiescence or self-renewal has not been clearly delineated. The exact nature and potential of Lgr5$^+$ and Lgr5-negative MaSC populations is an ongoing field of research [85–87]. The Lgr5 question is emblematic of the larger picture that MaSCs are a highly heterogeneous population. Isolating a basal population enriched for MaSCs from fetal mice revealed a distinct stem cell identity. Fetal-derived MaSCs display augmented clonogenic potency and repopulating efficiency when compared to their adult stem cell counterparts [88]. Further, these fetal MaSCs expressed unique extracellular receptor pattern, one that has features of both basal and luminal cells, which was also different from pubertal MaSCs [89]. The heterogeneity is further compounded when looking at adult mammary glands. Adults MaSCs have been found to display "lineage priming," in which restricted differentiation programs exist within seemingly pluripotent and self-renewal competent stem cells [90,91]. Recent RNAseq studies have begun to further subdivide the MaSC pool. In 2017, Pal et al. found an early progenitor subset marked by CD55 that exists between basal and luminal cells [92]. In sum, the spatial-, temporal-, and functional-heterogeneity of MaSCs has made their study complicated and bolstered the importance of finding new regulatory factors.

In summary, in vitro and in vivo findings suggest that breast epithelial cells can be arranged into a developmental hierarchy (Figure 3), but it should be explicitly stressed that this is just a model. In this hierarchy, mature luminal and myoepithelial cells are maintained by lineage-restricted progenitors, which is replenished by the MaSC population [93]. Bipotent progenitors exist within this hierarchy, but the exact placement is unclear and has therefore been excluded. Extracellular ligand expression and transcription factor regulation has served as the basis for the construction of this model. The extraordinary complexity of the mammary stem cell population has complicated a clear understanding of the drivers for epithelial cell fate decisions.

12. Organoids to Assess Stem- and Progenitor-Potential

Organoids are miniature, three-dimensional, in vitro tissue cultures that retain stem cell function, and are generated from pieces of tissue (Figure 4). Organoids have been instrumental to study stem cell biology of epithelial cell lineages [94,95]. They have gained traction as ideal platforms to screen for biomarkers, obtain personalized predictive-/prognostic information, and test novel therapeutic strategies and rational drug design [96–98]. Organoids and classical mammosphere cultures are similar in that both are in vitro 3D cultures of cells (Figures 2 and 4). However, organoids typically depend more on the extracellular matrix and may display more self-organization and spatially restricted lineage commitment [99].

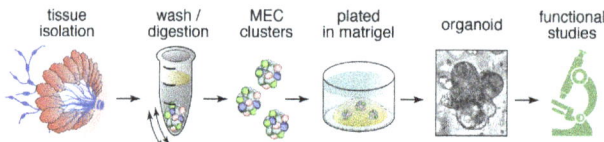

Figure 4. Pipeline of mammary gland organoid cultures. Submerging the Matrigel droplet with growth medium containing Wnt and R-Spondin ligands enables sustained maintenance of stem cell function and allows for functional studies on mammary stem cells (MaSCs) in these 3D cultures.

Furthermore, organoids can be cultured indefinitely and can be cryopreserved, whereas classical mammosphere cultures generally survive for shorter time periods [100]. Indeed, several different mammosphere cultures media cocktails have been applied in the past, but for many of these studies the goal was not to sustain growth long term. For example, Mroue and Bissell used growth media containing insulin transferrin selenium (ITS) and fetal bovine serum (FBS) for mammospheres generated from mouse mammary glands, but cultures were not sustained for long periods of time in this study [101]. It should be noted that the use of FBS in organoid culture is challenging since the exact composition is unknown and components can vary from batch-to-batch. Ewald et al., used growth media containing ITS supplemented with FGF2 and cultures were grown and assessed for a couple of days [102].

A crucial part of successfully culturing organoids (Figure 4) is to preserve stem cell function over long periods of time. The Wnt pathway has been shown to play an important role in stem cell maintenance [103]. In the canonical Wnt pathway, Wnt proteins bind to Frizzled (FZD) and LRP (lipoprotein receptor-related protein) receptors. Dickkopf (DKK) is a ligand that binds to LRP6 with high affinity [104]. Wnt binding to FZD and LRP receptors results in increased levels of β-catenin, which translocate into the nucleus to form a transcriptionally active complex with Tcf factors (T cell factor) [105,106]. In the absence of Wnt signals, Tcf transcription factors bind to Groucho repressors [107–109] and as such Tcf factors act as switches to turn on Wnt target genes [110]. Intriguingly, one of the β-catenin/Tcf target genes is the extracellular receptor *Lgr5* [111]. R-spondins are ligands for Lgr5 (Leucine-rich repeat-containing G-protein coupled receptor 5), and can associate with the Frizzled/LRP Wnt receptor complex to enhance the Wnt signal [112]. Structure-based design and subsequent production of surrogate Wnt ligands that are hybrid molecules combining the DKK and Wnt ligands proved clever tools to sustain canonical Wnt signaling in combination with R-spondin ligands and support efficient organoid growth [113].

In addition to surrogate Wnt and R-spondin ligands, EGF and Noggin are required to indefinitely expand organoids [114]. Furthermore, additional components can be added to the organoid medium to help maintain organoid cultures. These include fibroblast growth factor (FGF) 7, FGF10, Activin like kinase inhibitor (A83-01), SB202190 (p38 mitogen-activated protein kinase inhibitor), and nicotinamide [115]. Neuregulin 1 (Nrg1) is required for morphogenesis and differentiation of the mammary gland [116]. Addition of Nrg1 to organoid culture medium resulted in higher efficiency of mammary organoid generation [114]. Rho kinase inhibitor (Y-27632) was found to induce indefinite proliferation in vitro in normal and tumor epithelial cells [117] and addition of Y-27632 to organoid culture medium improved organoid culture conditions [114]. In Section 6 we discussed the heterogeneity and complexity of the stem- and progenitor- cell population in the mammary gland with Lgr5+ and Lgr5− cells and different characteristics in fetal-, puberty-, and adult-stages. We anticipate that successful mammary gland organoids will require complex but clearly defined (growth) factor medium and that systematic application of standard operating protocols (SOPs) will propel the field's efforts of organoid and cell heterogeneity forward.

13. Reconstructing Mammary Epithelial Cell Types and States Using Single-Cell Genomics

Advances in next generation sequencing and microfluidic-based handling of cells and reagents now enable us to explore cellular heterogeneity in an unbiased manner using various single-cell genomics modalities to profile genomic features in individual cells [118]. The current scientific knowledge about the MEC system is largely limited to data generated by bulk profiling methods, which only provide averaged read-outs that generally mask cellular heterogeneity. This averaged approach is particularly problematic when the biological effect of interest is limited to only a subpopulation of cells such as stem/progenitor cells, which may comprise only minor subsets of the total number of cells in a tissue. However, over the very recent years several studies emerged that utilized single-cell genomics approaches for unbiased identification of the cell types and states within the MEC compartment.

Among the genomics modalities available to date, single-cell RNA sequencing (scRNAseq) is the most advanced and most widely accessible to the research community, and has recently been applied to both human and mouse mammary epithelial samples (Figure 5). A recent study using a combination of microfluidic- and droplet-enabled single-cell transcriptomics pipelines revealed that the human breast epithelium contains three very distinct types of cells that each contain additional distinct cell states [119]. Based on these data, the human epithelium contains one basal and two luminal cell types, namely a hormone-responsive and a secretory type of luminal cells. The secretory luminal cell type was previously called luminal progenitors and generally expresses markers such as ELF5 (E74-like Facotr 5) and KIT (v-kit Hardy-Zuckerman 4 feline sarcoma viral oncogene homolog, CD117). Within basal cells, further distinctions can be made based on expression of myoepithelial markers (e.g., ACTA2, Actin Alpha 2, Smooth Muscle). Pseudo temporal analysis of the differentiation trajectories in this dataset defined a continuous lineage that seamlessly connected the basal and two luminal cell types, which is in line with the concept that basal and luminal cell types are maintained by an integrated system of stem and progenitor cells.

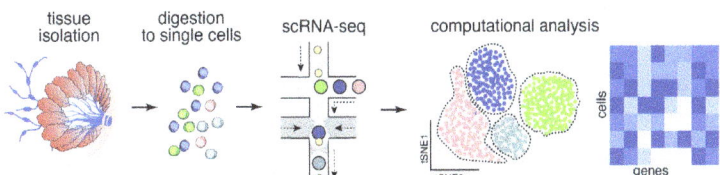

Figure 5. Pipeline of scRNAseq to resolve cellular heterogeneity with novel sequencing techniques. Processing mammary gland tissue of breast cancers into single-cell droplets coupled to single-cell RNA sequencing (scRNAseq) and data analysis (e.g., tSNE plots) allows for high resolution investigation of different cell types on the basis of individual cell transcriptome.

The mouse mammary epithelium at post-pubertal stage generally revealed a comparable cell type and state composition with some differences in terms of marker genes expressed in each cell type. Pal et al. [92] used scRNAseq of isolated mouse MECs to define three main cell types, namely basal (marked by Krt14, Keratin 14), secretory luminal or also called luminal progenitors (L-sec; marked by *Elf5*) and mature, hormone-responsive luminal cells (L-HR; marked by Prlr, Prolactin receptor). In addition to the main cell types, intermediate states were identified marked by expression of both luminal and basal genes, which could be indicative of transitional cell states between luminal and basal cells and thus support the notion of one continuous lineage trajectory that maintains all MEC cell types. Another similar study focused on the differentiation dynamics of the mouse mammary epithelium during various developmental stages of adult virgin, pregnant, lactating and involuting mammary gland using scRNAseq, which defined the lineage hierarchies as a differentiation continuum rather that discrete differentiation stages [120]. The most elusive cell type remains the MaSC, which so far did not emerge as a distinct cluster in either human or mouse single-cell transcriptomics analyses, although a subset of basal cells in both human and mouse cells expresses the putative MaSC markers PROCR (Protein Coding, CD201) or LGR5 [119,120]. It remains to be determined whether more sophisticated analysis tools such as single-cell potency analysis [121], or higher sequencing depth per cell and larger cell numbers are required to unambiguously define the MaSC as a distinct cell type (Figure 5). Recent years have also seen the emergence of studies that applied scRNAseq to unravel complexity of breast cancer [122,123], including the immune environment of breast tumors [124,125], and response to Herceptin therapy that targets EGFR2 (Her2) [126]. More is certainly to come as scRNAseq and its analysis becomes more mainstream and affordable.

In addition to gene expression programs, the epigenetic makeup of the cell is a critical determinant of cellular identity that is not detectable in scRNAseq data. Recent technological advances now allow for profiling chromatin accessibility using the Assay for Transposase-Accessible Chromatin using sequencing (ATACseq) to reconstruct cis/trans regulatory elements associated with cellular identity [127]. Further adaptation of this pipeline enabled single-cell-level ATACseq to profile cellular heterogeneity on an epigenetic level both using massively parallel [128] and combinatorial indexing methods [129]. This approach has recently been applied to elucidate transcriptional regulators of the fetal mammary gland developmental lineages showing that fetal MaSCs can be separated into basal-like and luminal-like lineages, suggesting an early lineage segregation prior to birth [130]. Another study utilized a combination of single-cell ATAC and RNA sequencing isolated mammary epithelial cells to reveal the spectrum of heterogeneity within the MEC system in the adult stage [131] Interestingly, a distinct luminal progenitor cell state within the secretory luminal cell type emerged in chromatin accessibility analysis that was clustering separately in transcriptomics data. By integrating single-cell transcriptomics and chromatin accessibility landscapes, this work further identified novel cis- and trans-regulatory elements that are differentially activated in the epithelial cell types and the newly defined progenitor cell state. Taken together, these single-cell genomics studies provide invaluable resources that may serve as reference atlases to map out how the system goes awry during diseases such as cancer in unprecedented resolution.

14. Conclusions

In summary, cartoons such as the one depicted in Figure 3 in our review give the impression of simple and clean cell lineage choices with well-defined trajectories of cell development in unipotent manners. In reality the mammary gland, and therefore breast cancer, is much more complex and cellular heterogeneity is obvious. The pair of studies using expression of oncogenic PIK3CA(H1047R) in different mammary epithelium cell subsets give particularly striking examples of crossover between basal- and luminal- cell fates and the possibility of dedifferentiation into a multipotent stem-like state [71,72]. It is not difficult to imagine how such fluidity in cell identity may greatly impact how breast cancer patients respond to specific types of therapy in the clinic. Fortunately, technology is constantly evolving. For example, studies that assess the potential of cell populations with organoids coupled to characterization of the transcriptional landscape at the single-cell level are starting to emerge (Figure 6). Intelligent combination of organoids, mouse models, scRNAseq, ATACseq, lineage tracing, CyTOF (mass cytometry by time-of-flight), and other novel technology platforms will be required to comprehensively understand cell heterogeneity in the mammary gland and breast cancer.

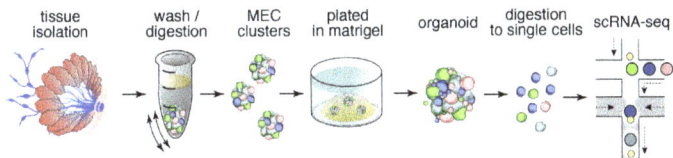

Figure 6. Organoids, scRNAseq, and other technologies to resolve cellular heterogeneity. Combination of different platforms such as organoids and scRNAseq but also mouse models, lineage tracing, and patient-centric assays will likely each make important contributions to resolve cellular heterogeneity in the mammary gland and in breast cancer.

Author Contributions: Writing—original draft preparation, A.S., H.D., K.K., J.P.R.; writing—review and editing, J.P.R.; funding acquisition, K.K. and J.P.R. The authors thank freelance illustrator Anna Hupalowska for the graphics.

Funding: The authors thank support through NIH grants. Specifically, NIH F31 CA200342 to AS, NIAID P01-AI091580 to JPR, and NCI R01CA234496 and R00CA181490 to KK. We also thank the American Cancer Society (132551-RSG-18-194-01-DDC to K.K.) and support from the Mark Foundation for Cancer Research for the Roose lab.

Conflicts of Interest: Jeroen Roose is a co-founder and scientific advisor of Seal Biosciences, Inc. and on the scientific advisory committee for the Mark Foundation for Cancer Research. The authors declare no conflict of interest.

References

1. Macias, H.; Hinck, L. Mammary gland development. *Wiley Interdiscip. Rev. Dev. Biol.* **2012**, *1*, 533–557. [CrossRef] [PubMed]
2. Hogg, N.A.; Harrison, C.J.; Tickle, C. Lumen formation in the developing mouse mammary gland. *J. Embryol. Exp. Morphol.* **1983**, *73*, 39–57. [PubMed]
3. Visvader, J.E. Keeping abreast of the mammary epithelial hierarchy and breast tumorigenesis. *Genes Dev.* **2009**, *23*, 2563–2577. [CrossRef] [PubMed]
4. Hinck, L.; Silberstein, G.B. Key stages in mammary gland development: the mammary end bud as a motile organ. *Breast Cancer Res.* **2005**, *7*, 245–251. [CrossRef] [PubMed]
5. Sternlicht, M.D.; Kouros-Mehr, H.; Lu, P.; Werb, Z. Hormonal and local control of mammary branching morphogenesis. *Differentiation* **2006**, *74*, 365–381. [CrossRef] [PubMed]
6. Williams, J.M.; Daniel, C.W. Mammary ductal elongation: differentiation of myoepithelium and basal lamina during branching morphogenesis. *Dev. Biol.* **1983**, *97*, 274–290. [CrossRef]
7. Visvader, J.E.; Stingl, J. Mammary stem cells and the differentiation hierarchy: Current status and perspectives. *Genes Dev.* **2014**, *28*, 1143–1158. [CrossRef] [PubMed]
8. Oakes, S.R.; Naylor, M.J.; Asselin-Labat, M.L.; Blazek, K.D.; Gardiner-Garden, M.; Hilton, H.N.; Kazlauskas, M.; Pritchard, M.A.; Chodosh, L.A.; Pfeffer, P.L.; et al. The Ets transcription factor Elf5 specifies mammary alveolar cell fate. *Genes Dev.* **2008**, *22*, 581–586. [CrossRef]
9. Chakrabarti, R.; Wei, Y.; Romano, R.A.; DeCoste, C.; Kang, Y.; Sinha, S. Elf5 regulates mammary gland stem/progenitor cell fate by influencing notch signaling. *Stem Cells* **2012**, *30*, 1496–1508. [CrossRef]
10. Lee, H.J.; Gallego-Ortega, D.; Ledger, A.; Schramek, D.; Joshi, P.; Szwarc, M.M.; Cho, C.; Lydon, J.P.; Khokha, R.; Penninger, J.M.; et al. Progesterone drives mammary secretory differentiation via RankL-mediated induction of Elf5 in luminal progenitor cells. *Development* **2013**, *140*, 1397–1401. [CrossRef]
11. Kouros-Mehr, H.; Slorach, E.M.; Sternlicht, M.D.; Werb, Z. GATA-3 maintains the differentiation of the luminal cell fate in the mammary gland. *Cell* **2006**, *127*, 1041–1055. [CrossRef] [PubMed]
12. Yamaji, D.; Na, R.; Feuermann, Y.; Pechhold, S.; Chen, W.; Robinson, G.W.; Hennighausen, L. Development of mammary luminal progenitor cells is controlled by the transcription factor STAT5A. *Genes Dev.* **2009**, *23*, 2382–2387. [CrossRef] [PubMed]

13. Asselin-Labat, M.L.; Sutherland, K.D.; Barker, H.; Thomas, R.; Shackleton, M.; Forrest, N.C.; Hartley, L.; Robb, L.; Grosveld, F.G.; van der Wees, J.; et al. Gata-3 is an essential regulator of mammary-gland morphogenesis and luminal-cell differentiation. *Nat. Cell Biol.* **2007**, *9*, 201–209. [CrossRef] [PubMed]
14. Shehata, M.; Teschendorff, A.; Sharp, G.; Novcic, N.; Russell, I.A.; Avril, S.; Prater, M.; Eirew, P.; Caldas, C.; Watson, C.J.; et al. Phenotypic and functional characterisation of the luminal cell hierarchy of the mammary gland. *Breast Cancer Res.* **2012**, *14*, e134. [CrossRef] [PubMed]
15. Regan, J.L.; Kendrick, H.; Magnay, F.A.; Vafaizadeh, V.; Groner, B.; Smalley, M.J. c-Kit is required for growth and survival of the cells of origin of Brca1-mutation-associated breast cancer. *Oncogene* **2012**, *31*, 869–883. [CrossRef] [PubMed]
16. Asselin-Labat, M.L.; Sutherland, K.D.; Vaillant, F.; Gyorki, D.E.; Wu, D.; Holroyd, S.; Breslin, K.; Ward, T.; Shi, W.; Bath, M.L.; et al. Gata-3 negatively regulates the tumor-initiating capacity of mammary luminal progenitor cells and targets the putative tumor suppressor caspase-14. *Mol. Cell Biol.* **2011**, *31*, 4609–4622. [CrossRef] [PubMed]
17. Nassour, M.; Idoux-Gillet, Y.; Selmi, A.; Come, C.; Faraldo, M.L.; Deugnier, M.A.; Savagner, P. Slug controls stem/progenitor cell growth dynamics during mammary gland morphogenesis. *PLoS ONE* **2012**, *7*, e53498. [CrossRef] [PubMed]
18. Guo, W.; Keckesova, Z.; Donaher, J.L.; Shibue, T.; Tischler, V.; Reinhardt, F.; Itzkovitz, S.; Noske, A.; Zurrer-Hardi, U.; Bell, G.; et al. Slug and Sox9 cooperatively determine the mammary stem cell state. *Cell* **2012**, *148*, 1015–1028. [CrossRef]
19. Mills, A.A.; Zheng, B.; Wang, X.J.; Vogel, H.; Roop, D.R.; Bradley, A. p63 is a p53 homologue required for limb and epidermal morphogenesis. *Nature* **1999**, *398*, 708–713. [CrossRef]
20. Yalcin-Ozuysal, O.; Fiche, M.; Guitierrez, M.; Wagner, K.U.; Raffoul, W.; Brisken, C. Antagonistic roles of Notch and p63 in controlling mammary epithelial cell fates. *Cell Death Differ.* **2010**, *17*, 1600–1612. [CrossRef]
21. Bouras, T.; Pal, B.; Vaillant, F.; Harburg, G.; Asselin-Labat, M.L.; Oakes, S.R.; Lindeman, G.J.; Visvader, J.E. Notch signaling regulates mammary stem cell function and luminal cell-fate commitment. *Cell Stem Cell* **2008**, *3*, 429–441. [CrossRef]
22. Cicalese, A.; Bonizzi, G.; Pasi, C.E.; Faretta, M.; Ronzoni, S.; Giulini, B.; Brisken, C.; Minucci, S.; Di Fiore, P.P.; Pelicci, P.G. The tumor suppressor p53 regulates polarity of self-renewing divisions in mammary stem cells. *Cell* **2009**, *138*, 1083–1095. [CrossRef] [PubMed]
23. Van Keymeulen, A.; Rocha, A.S.; Ousset, M.; Beck, B.; Bouvencourt, G.; Rock, J.; Sharma, N.; Dekoninck, S.; Blanpain, C. Distinct stem cells contribute to mammary gland development and maintenance. *Nature* **2011**, *479*, 189–193. [CrossRef] [PubMed]
24. Rios, A.C.; Fu, N.Y.; Lindeman, G.J.; Visvader, J.E. In situ identification of bipotent stem cells in the mammary gland. *Nature* **2014**, *506*, 322–327. [CrossRef] [PubMed]
25. Simian, M.; Bissell, M.J. Organoids: A historical perspective of thinking in three dimensions. *J. Cell Biol.* **2017**, *216*, 31–40. [CrossRef] [PubMed]
26. Orkin, R.W.; Gehron, P.; McGoodwin, E.B.; Martin, G.R.; Valentine, T.; Swarm, R. A murine tumor producing a matrix of basement membrane. *J. Exp. Med.* **1977**, *145*, 204–220. [CrossRef]
27. Barcellos-Hoff, M.H.; Aggeler, J.; Ram, T.G.; Bissell, M.J. Functional differentiation and alveolar morphogenesis of primary mammary cultures on reconstituted basement membrane. *Development* **1989**, *105*, 223–235. [PubMed]
28. Petersen, O.W.; Ronnov-Jessen, L.; Howlett, A.R.; Bissell, M.J. Interaction with basement membrane serves to rapidly distinguish growth and differentiation pattern of normal and malignant human breast epithelial cells. *Proc. Natl. Acad. Sci. USA* **1992**, *89*, 9064–9068. [CrossRef]
29. Wang, F.; Weaver, V.M.; Petersen, O.W.; Larabell, C.A.; Dedhar, S.; Briand, P.; Lupu, R.; Bissell, M.J. Reciprocal interactions between beta1-integrin and epidermal growth factor receptor in three-dimensional basement membrane breast cultures: a different perspective in epithelial biology. *Proc. Natl. Acad. Sci. USA* **1998**, *95*, 14821–14826. [CrossRef]
30. Pechoux, C.; Gudjonsson, T.; Ronnov-Jessen, L.; Bissell, M.J.; Petersen, O.W. Human mammary luminal epithelial cells contain progenitors to myoepithelial cells. *Dev. Biol.* **1999**, *206*, 88–99. [CrossRef]
31. Dontu, G.; Abdallah, W.M.; Foley, J.M.; Jackson, K.W.; Clarke, M.F.; Kawamura, M.J.; Wicha, M.S. In vitro propagation and transcriptional profiling of human mammary stem/progenitor cells. *Genes Dev.* **2003**, *17*, 1253–1270. [CrossRef]

32. Eccles, S.A. The epidermal growth factor receptor/Erb-B/HER family in normal and malignant breast biology. *Int. J. Dev. Biol.* **2011**, *55*, 685–696. [CrossRef]
33. Shi, F.; Telesco, S.E.; Liu, Y.; Radhakrishnan, R.; Lemmon, M.A. ErbB3/HER3 intracellular domain is competent to bind ATP and catalyze autophosphorylation. *Proc. Natl. Acad. Sci. USA* **2010**, *107*, 7692–7697. [CrossRef]
34. Hynes, N.E.; Watson, C.J. Mammary gland growth factors: roles in normal development and in cancer. *Cold Spring Harb. Perspect. Biol.* **2010**, *2*, e003186. [CrossRef]
35. Normanno, N.; Bianco, C.; De Luca, A.; Salomon, D.S. The role of EGF-related peptides in tumor growth. *Front. Biosci.* **2001**, *6*, 685–707. [CrossRef]
36. Riese, D.J.; Kim, E.D.; Elenius, K.; Buckley, S.; Klagsbrun, M.; Plowman, G.D.; Stern, D.F. The epidermal growth factor receptor couples transforming growth factor-alpha, heparin-binding epidermal growth factor-like factor, and amphiregulin to Neu, ErbB-3, and ErbB-4. *J. Biol. Chem.* **1996**, *271*, 20047–20052. [CrossRef]
37. Moriki, T.; Maruyama, H.; Maruyama, I.N. Activation of preformed EGF receptor dimers by ligand-induced rotation of the transmembrane domain. *J. Mol. Biol.* **2001**, *311*, 1011–1026. [CrossRef]
38. Sternlicht, M.D.; Sunnarborg, S.W. The ADAM17-amphiregulin-EGFR axis in mammary development and cancer. *J. Mammary Gland Biol. Neoplasia* **2008**, *13*, 181–194. [CrossRef]
39. Miettinen, P.J.; Berger, J.E.; Meneses, J.; Phung, Y.; Pedersen, R.A.; Werb, Z.; Derynck, R. Epithelial immaturity and multiorgan failure in mice lacking epidermal growth factor receptor. *Nature* **1995**, *376*, 337–341. [CrossRef]
40. Threadgill, D.W.; Dlugosz, A.A.; Hansen, L.A.; Tennenbaum, T.; Lichti, U.; Yee, D.; LaMantia, C.; Mourton, T.; Herrup, K.; Harris, R.C.; et al. Targeted disruption of mouse EGF receptor: effect of genetic background on mutant phenotype. *Science* **1995**, *269*, 230–234. [CrossRef]
41. Luetteke, N.C.; Phillips, H.K.; Qiu, T.H.; Copeland, N.G.; Earp, H.S.; Jenkins, N.A.; Lee, D.C. The mouse waved-2 phenotype results from a point mutation in the EGF receptor tyrosine kinase. *Genes Dev.* **1994**, *8*, 399–413. [CrossRef]
42. Fowler, K.J.; Walker, F.; Alexander, W.; Hibbs, M.L.; Nice, E.C.; Bohmer, R.M.; Mann, G.B.; Thumwood, C.; Maglitto, R.; Danks, J.A.; et al. A mutation in the epidermal growth factor receptor in waved-2 mice has a profound effect on receptor biochemistry that results in impaired lactation. *Proc. Natl. Acad. Sci. USA* **1995**, *92*, 1465–1469. [CrossRef]
43. Sebastian, J.; Richards, R.G.; Walker, M.P.; Wiesen, J.F.; Werb, Z.; Derynck, R.; Hom, Y.K.; Cunha, G.R.; DiAugustine, R.P. Activation and function of the epidermal growth factor receptor and erbB-2 during mammary gland morphogenesis. *Cell Growth Differ.* **1998**, *9*, 777–785.
44. Xie, W.; Paterson, A.J.; Chin, E.; Nabell, L.M.; Kudlow, J.E. Targeted expression of a dominant negative epidermal growth factor receptor in the mammary gland of transgenic mice inhibits pubertal mammary duct development. *Mol. Endocrinol.* **1997**, *11*, 1766–1781. [CrossRef]
45. Sternlicht, M.D.; Sunnarborg, S.W.; Kouros-Mehr, H.; Yu, Y.; Lee, D.C.; Werb, Z. Mammary ductal morphogenesis requires paracrine activation of stromal EGFR via ADAM17-dependent shedding of epithelial amphiregulin. *Development* **2005**, *132*, 3923–3933. [CrossRef]
46. Wiesen, J.F.; Young, P.; Werb, Z.; Cunha, G.R. Signaling through the stromal epidermal growth factor receptor is necessary for mammary ductal development. *Development* **1999**, *126*, 335–344.
47. Andrechek, E.R.; White, D.; Muller, W.J. Targeted disruption of ErbB2/Neu in the mammary epithelium results in impaired ductal outgrowth. *Oncogene* **2005**, *24*, 932–937. [CrossRef]
48. Jackson-Fisher, A.J.; Bellinger, G.; Ramabhadran, R.; Morris, J.K.; Lee, K.F.; Stern, D.F. ErbB2 is required for ductal morphogenesis of the mammary gland. *Proc. Natl. Acad. Sci. USA* **2004**, *101*, 17138–17143. [CrossRef]
49. Pasic, L.; Eisinger-Mathason, T.S.; Velayudhan, B.T.; Moskaluk, C.A.; Brenin, D.R.; Macara, I.G.; Lannigan, D.A. Sustained activation of the HER1-ERK1/2-RSK signaling pathway controls myoepithelial cell fate in human mammary tissue. *Genes Dev.* **2011**, *25*, 1641–1653. [CrossRef]
50. Mukhopadhyay, C.; Zhao, X.; Maroni, D.; Band, V.; Naramura, M. Distinct effects of EGFR ligands on human mammary epithelial cell differentiation. *PLoS ONE* **2013**, *8*, e75907. [CrossRef]
51. Marshall, C.J. Specificity of receptor tyrosine kinase signaling: transient versus sustained extracellular signal-regulated kinase activation. *Cell* **1995**, *80*, 179–185. [CrossRef]
52. Metzger, R.J.; Klein, O.D.; Martin, G.R.; Krasnow, M.A. The branching programme of mouse lung development. *Nature* **2008**, *453*, 745–750. [CrossRef]

53. Schedin, P.; Keely, P.J. Mammary gland ECM remodeling, stiffness, and mechanosignaling in normal development and tumor progression. *Cold Spring Harb. Perspect. Biol.* **2011**, *3*, e003228. [CrossRef]
54. Brisken, C.; O'Malley, B. Hormone action in the mammary gland. *Cold Spring Harb. Perspect. Biol.* **2010**, *2*, e003178. [CrossRef]
55. Bocchinfuso, W.P.; Korach, K.S. Mammary gland development and tumorigenesis in estrogen receptor knockout mice. *J. Mammary Gland Biol. Neoplasia* **1997**, *2*, 323–334. [CrossRef]
56. Daniel, C.W.; Silberstein, G.B.; Strickland, P. Direct action of 17 beta-estradiol on mouse mammary ducts analyzed by sustained release implants and steroid autoradiography. *Cancer Res.* **1987**, *47*, 6052–6057.
57. Zhang, H.Z.; Bennett, J.M.; Smith, K.T.; Sunil, N.; Haslam, S.Z. Estrogen mediates mammary epithelial cell proliferation in serum-free culture indirectly via mammary stroma-derived hepatocyte growth factor. *Endocrinology* **2002**, *143*, 3427–3434. [CrossRef]
58. Coleman, S.; Silberstein, G.B.; Daniel, C.W. Ductal morphogenesis in the mouse mammary gland: evidence supporting a role for epidermal growth factor. *Dev. Biol.* **1988**, *127*, 304–315. [CrossRef]
59. Gallego, M.I.; Binart, N.; Robinson, G.W.; Okagaki, R.; Coschigano, K.T.; Perry, J.; Kopchick, J.J.; Oka, T.; Kelly, P.A.; Hennighausen, L. Prolactin, growth hormone, and epidermal growth factor activate Stat5 in different compartments of mammary tissue and exert different and overlapping developmental effects. *Dev. Biol.* **2001**, *229*, 163–175. [CrossRef]
60. Kleinberg, D.L.; Feldman, M.; Ruan, W. IGF-I: an essential factor in terminal end bud formation and ductal morphogenesis. *J. Mammary Gland Biol. Neoplasia* **2000**, *5*, 7–17. [CrossRef]
61. Xu, X.; Weinstein, M.; Li, C.; Naski, M.; Cohen, R.I.; Ornitz, D.M.; Leder, P.; Deng, C. Fibroblast growth factor receptor 2 (FGFR2)-mediated reciprocal regulation loop between FGF8 and FGF10 is essential for limb induction. *Development* **1998**, *125*, 753–765.
62. Lu, P.; Ewald, A.J.; Martin, G.R.; Werb, Z. Genetic mosaic analysis reveals FGF receptor 2 function in terminal end buds during mammary gland branching morphogenesis. *Dev. Biol.* **2008**, *321*, 77–87. [CrossRef]
63. Parsa, S.; Ramasamy, S.K.; De Langhe, S.; Gupte, V.V.; Haigh, J.J.; Medina, D.; Bellusci, S. Terminal end bud maintenance in mammary gland is dependent upon FGFR2b signaling. *Dev. Biol.* **2008**, *317*, 121–131. [CrossRef]
64. Jackson-Fisher, A.J.; Bellinger, G.; Breindel, J.L.; Tavassoli, F.A.; Booth, C.J.; Duong, J.K.; Stern, D.F. ErbB3 is required for ductal morphogenesis in the mouse mammary gland. *Breast Cancer Res.* **2008**, *10*, e96. [CrossRef]
65. Tidcombe, H.; Jackson-Fisher, A.; Mathers, K.; Stern, D.F.; Gassmann, M.; Golding, J.P. Neural and mammary gland defects in ErbB4 knockout mice genetically rescued from embryonic lethality. *Proc Natl. Acad. Sci. USA* **2003**, *100*, 8281–8286. [CrossRef]
66. Schlessinger, J. Ligand-induced, receptor-mediated dimerization and activation of EGF receptor. *Cell* **2002**, *110*, 669–672. [CrossRef]
67. Zhang, X.; Gureasko, J.; Shen, K.; Cole, P.A.; Kuriyan, J. An allosteric mechanism for activation of the kinase domain of epidermal growth factor receptor. *Cell* **2006**, *125*, 1137–1149. [CrossRef]
68. Jura, N.; Shan, Y.; Cao, X.; Shaw, D.E.; Kuriyan, J. Structural analysis of the catalytically inactive kinase domain of the human EGF receptor 3. *Proc. Natl. Acad. Sci. USA* **2009**, *106*, 21608–21613. [CrossRef]
69. Holbro, T.; Beerli, R.R.; Maurer, F.; Koziczak, M.; Barbas, C.F.; Hynes, N.E. The ErbB2/ErbB3 heterodimer functions as an oncogenic unit: ErbB2 requires ErbB3 to drive breast tumor cell proliferation. *Proc. Natl. Acad. Sci. USA* **2003**, *100*, 8933–8938. [CrossRef]
70. Huebner, R.J.; Neumann, N.M.; Ewald, A.J. Mammary epithelial tubes elongate through MAPK-dependent coordination of cell migration. *Development* **2016**, *143*, 983–993. [CrossRef]
71. Koren, S.; Bentires-Alj, M. Breast tumor heterogeneity: Source of fitness, hurdle for therapy. *Mol. Cell* **2015**, *60*, 537–546. [CrossRef]
72. Koren, S.; Reavie, L.; Couto, J.P.; De Silva, D.; Stadler, M.B.; Roloff, T.; Britschgi, A.; Eichlisberger, T.; Kohler, H.; Aina, O.; et al. PIK3CA(H1047R) induces multipotency and multi-lineage mammary tumours. *Nature* **2015**, *525*, 114–118. [CrossRef]
73. Van Keymeulen, A.; Lee, M.Y.; Ousset, M.; Brohee, S.; Rorive, S.; Giraddi, R.R.; Wuidart, A.; Bouvencourt, G.; Dubois, C.; Salmon, I.; et al. Reactivation of multipotency by oncogenic PIK3CA induces breast tumour heterogeneity. *Nature* **2015**, *525*, 119–123. [CrossRef]
74. Kaimala, S.; Bisana, S.; Kumar, S. Mammary gland stem cells: More puzzles than explanations. *J. Biosci.* **2012**, *37*, 349–358. [CrossRef]

75. Moraes, R.C.; Zhang, X.; Harrington, N.; Fung, J.Y.; Wu, M.F.; Hilsenbeck, S.G.; Allred, D.C.; Lewis, M.T. Constitutive activation of smoothened (SMO) in mammary glands of transgenic mice leads to increased proliferation, altered differentiation and ductal dysplasia. *Development* **2007**, *134*, 1231–1242. [CrossRef]
76. Shackleton, M.; Vaillant, F.; Simpson, K.J.; Stingl, J.; Smyth, G.K.; Asselin-Labat, M.L.; Wu, L.; Lindeman, G.J.; Visvader, J.E. Generation of a functional mammary gland from a single stem cell. *Nature* **2006**, *439*, 84–88. [CrossRef]
77. Lim, E.; Vaillant, F.; Wu, D.; Forrest, N.C.; Pal, B.; Hart, A.H.; Asselin-Labat, M.L.; Gyorki, D.E.; Ward, T.; Partanen, A.; et al. Aberrant luminal progenitors as the candidate target population for basal tumor development in BRCA1 mutation carriers. *Nat. Med.* **2009**, *15*, 907–913. [CrossRef]
78. Sleeman, K.E.; Kendrick, H.; Ashworth, A.; Isacke, C.M.; Smalley, M.J. CD24 staining of mouse mammary gland cells defines luminal epithelial, myoepithelial/basal and non-epithelial cells. *Breast Cancer Res.* **2006**, *8*, e7. [CrossRef]
79. Jones, C.; Mackay, A.; Grigoriadis, A.; Cossu, A.; Reis-Filho, J.S.; Fulford, L.; Dexter, T.; Davies, S.; Bulmer, K.; Ford, E.; et al. Expression profiling of purified normal human luminal and myoepithelial breast cells: identification of novel prognostic markers for breast cancer. *Cancer Res.* **2004**, *64*, 3037–3045. [CrossRef]
80. Kawase, Y.; Yanagi, Y.; Takato, T.; Fujimoto, M.; Okochi, H. Characterization of multipotent adult stem cells from the skin: Transforming growth factor-beta (TGF-beta) facilitates cell growth. *Exp. Cell Res.* **2004**, *295*, 194–203. [CrossRef]
81. Tai, M.H.; Chang, C.C.; Kiupel, M.; Webster, J.D.; Olson, L.K.; Trosko, J.E. Oct4 expression in adult human stem cells: evidence in support of the stem cell theory of carcinogenesis. *Carcinogenesis* **2005**, *26*, 495–502. [CrossRef]
82. Liu, B.Y.; McDermott, S.P.; Khwaja, S.S.; Alexander, C.M. The transforming activity of Wnt effectors correlates with their ability to induce the accumulation of mammary progenitor cells. *Proc. Natl. Acad. Sci. USA* **2004**, *101*, 4158–4163. [CrossRef]
83. Bai, L.; Rohrschneider, L.R. s-SHIP promoter expression marks activated stem cells in developing mouse mammary tissue. *Genes Dev.* **2010**, *24*, 1882–1892. [CrossRef]
84. Barker, N.; Tan, S.; Clevers, H. Lgr proteins in epithelial stem cell biology. *Development* **2013**, *140*, 2484–2494. [CrossRef]
85. Plaks, V.; Brenot, A.; Lawson, D.A.; Linnemann, J.R.; Van Kappel, E.C.; Wong, K.C.; de Sauvage, F.; Klein, O.D.; Werb, Z. Lgr5-expressing cells are sufficient and necessary for postnatal mammary gland organogenesis. *Cell Rep.* **2013**, *3*, 70–78. [CrossRef]
86. de Visser, K.E.; Ciampricotti, M.; Michalak, E.M.; Tan, D.W.; Speksnijder, E.N.; Hau, C.S.; Clevers, H.; Barker, N.; Jonkers, J. Developmental stage-specific contribution of LGR5(+) cells to basal and luminal epithelial lineages in the postnatal mammary gland. *J. Pathol.* **2012**, *228*, 300–309. [CrossRef]
87. Fu, N.Y.; Rios, A.C.; Pal, B.; Law, C.W.; Jamieson, P.; Liu, R.; Vaillant, F.; Jackling, F.; Liu, K.H.; Smyth, G.K.; et al. Identification of quiescent and spatially restricted mammary stem cells that are hormone responsive. *Nat. Cell Biol.* **2017**, *19*, 164–176. [CrossRef]
88. Makarem, M.; Kannan, N.; Nguyen, L.V.; Knapp, D.J.; Balani, S.; Prater, M.D.; Stingl, J.; Raouf, A.; Nemirovsky, O.; Eirew, P.; et al. Developmental changes in the in vitro activated regenerative activity of primitive mammary epithelial cells. *PLoS Biol.* **2013**, *11*, e1001630. [CrossRef]
89. Spike, B.T.; Engle, D.D.; Lin, J.C.; Cheung, S.K.; La, J.; Wahl, G.M. A mammary stem cell population identified and characterized in late embryogenesis reveals similarities to human breast cancer. *Cell Stem Cell* **2012**, *10*, 183–197. [CrossRef]
90. Pal, B.; Bouras, T.; Shi, W.; Vaillant, F.; Sheridan, J.M.; Fu, N.; Breslin, K.; Jiang, K.; Ritchie, M.E.; Young, M.; et al. Global changes in the mammary epigenome are induced by hormonal cues and coordinated by Ezh2. *Cell Rep.* **2013**, *3*, 411–426. [CrossRef]
91. Kaanta, A.S.; Virtanen, C.; Selfors, L.M.; Brugge, J.S.; Neel, B.G. Evidence for a multipotent mammary progenitor with pregnancy-specific activity. *Breast Cancer Res.* **2013**, *15*, e65. [CrossRef]
92. Pal, B.; Chen, Y.; Vaillant, F.; Jamieson, P.; Gordon, L.; Rios, A.C.; Wilcox, S.; Fu, N.; Liu, K.H.; Jackling, F.C.; et al. Construction of developmental lineage relationships in the mouse mammary gland by single-cell RNA profiling. *Nat. Commun.* **2017**, *8*, e1627. [CrossRef]
93. Raouf, A.; Sun, Y.; Chatterjee, S.; Basak, P. The biology of human breast epithelial progenitors. *Semin. Cell Dev. Biol.* **2012**, *23*, 606–612. [CrossRef]

94. Clevers, H. Modeling Development and disease with organoids. *Cell* **2016**, *165*, 1586–1597. [CrossRef]
95. Sato, T.; Clevers, H. Growing self-organizing mini-guts from a single intestinal stem cell: mechanism and applications. *Science* **2013**, *340*, 1190–1194. [CrossRef]
96. Muranen, T.; Selfors, L.M.; Worster, D.T.; Iwanicki, M.P.; Song, L.; Morales, F.C.; Gao, S.; Mills, G.B.; Brugge, J.S. Inhibition of PI3K/mTOR leads to adaptive resistance in matrix-attached cancer cells. *Cancer Cell* **2012**, *21*, 227–239. [CrossRef]
97. Schwank, G.; Clevers, H. *Gastrointestinal Physiology and Diseases*; Humana Press: New York, NY, USA, 2016; pp. 3–11.
98. Takebe, T.; Sekine, K.; Enomura, M.; Koike, H.; Kimura, M.; Ogaeri, T.; Zhang, R.R.; Ueno, Y.; Zheng, Y.W.; Koike, N.; et al. Vascularized and functional human liver from an iPSC-derived organ bud transplant. *Nature* **2013**, *499*, 481–484. [CrossRef]
99. Lancaster, M.A.; Knoblich, J.A. Organogenesis in a dish: Modeling development and disease using organoid technologies. *Science* **2014**, *345*, e1247125. [CrossRef]
100. Fatehullah, A.; Tan, S.H.; Barker, N. Organoids as an in vitro model of human development and disease. *Nat. Cell Biol.* **2016**, *18*, 246–254. [CrossRef]
101. Mroue, R.; Bissell, M.J. *Epithelial Cell Culture Protocols*; Humana Press: Totowa, NJ, USA, 2012; pp. 221–250.
102. Ewald, A.J.; Brenot, A.; Duong, M.; Chan, B.S.; Werb, Z. Collective epithelial migration and cell rearrangements drive mammary branching morphogenesis. *Dev. Cell* **2008**, *14*, 570–581. [CrossRef]
103. Nusse, R. Wnt signaling and stem cell control. *Cell Res.* **2008**, *18*, 523–527. [CrossRef]
104. Mao, B.; Wu, W.; Li, Y.; Hoppe, D.; Stannek, P.; Glinka, A.; Niehrs, C. LDL-receptor-related protein 6 is a receptor for Dickkopf proteins. *Nature* **2001**, *411*, 321–325. [CrossRef]
105. Behrens, J.; von Kries, J.P.; Kuhl, M.; Bruhn, L.; Wedlich, D.; Grosschedl, R.; Birchmeier, W. Functional interaction of beta-catenin with the transcription factor LEF-1. *Nature* **1996**, *382*, 638–642. [CrossRef]
106. Molenaar, M.; van de Wetering, M.; Oosterwegel, M.; Peterson-Maduro, J.; Godsave, S.; Korinek, V.; Roose, J.; Destree, O.; Clevers, H. XTcf-3 transcription factor mediates beta-catenin-induced axis formation in Xenopus embryos. *Cell* **1996**, *86*, 391–399. [CrossRef]
107. Roose, J.; Molenaar, M.; Peterson, J.; Hurenkamp, J.; Brantjes, H.; Moerer, P.; van de Wetering, M.; Destree, O.; Clevers, H. The Xenopus Wnt effector XTcf-3 interacts with Groucho-related transcriptional repressors. *Nature* **1998**, *395*, 608–612. [CrossRef]
108. Cavallo, R.A.; Cox, R.T.; Moline, M.M.; Roose, J.; Polevoy, G.A.; Clevers, H.; Peifer, M.; Bejsovec, A. Drosophila Tcf and groucho interact to repress wingless signalling activity. *Nature* **1998**, *395*, 604–608. [CrossRef]
109. Waltzer, L.; Bienz, M. The control of beta-catenin and TCF during embryonic development and cancer. *Cancer Metastasis Rev.* **1999**, *18*, 231–246. [CrossRef]
110. Roose, J.; Clevers, H. TCF transcription factors: molecular switches in carcinogenesis. *Biochim. Biophys. Acta* **1999**, *1424*, M23–M37. [CrossRef]
111. Leung, C.; Tan, S.H.; Barker, N. Recent advances in Lgr5(+) stem cell research. *Trends Cell Biol.* **2018**, *28*, 380–391. [CrossRef]
112. De Lau, W.; Barker, N.; Low, T.Y.; Koo, B.K.; Li, V.S.; Teunissen, H.; Kujala, P.; Haegebarth, A.; Peters, P.J.; van de Wetering, M.; et al. Lgr5 homologues associate with Wnt receptors and mediate R-spondin signalling. *Nature* **2011**, *476*, 293–297. [CrossRef]
113. Janda, C.Y.; Dang, L.T.; You, C.; Chang, J.; de Lau, W.; Zhong, Z.A.; Yan, K.S.; Marecic, O.; Siepe, D.; Li, X.; et al. Surrogate Wnt agonists that phenocopy canonical Wnt and beta-catenin signalling. *Nature* **2017**, *545*, 234–237. [CrossRef]
114. Sachs, N.; de Ligt, J.; Kopper, O.; Gogola, E.; Bounova, G.; Weeber, F.; Balgobind, A.V.; Wind, K.; Gracanin, A.; Begthel, H.; et al. A living biobank of breast cancer organoids captures disease heterogeneity. *Cell* **2018**, *172*, 373–386.e10. [CrossRef]
115. Sato, T.; Clevers, H. SnapShot: Growing organoids from stem cells. *Cell* **2015**, *161*, 1700–1701. [CrossRef]
116. Yang, Y.; Spitzer, E.; Meyer, D.; Sachs, M.; Niemann, C.; Hartmann, G.; Weidner, K.M.; Birchmeier, C.; Birchmeier, W. Sequential requirement of hepatocyte growth factor and neuregulin in the morphogenesis and differentiation of the mammary gland. *J. Cell Biol.* **1995**, *131*, 215–226. [CrossRef]
117. Liu, X.; Ory, V.; Chapman, S.; Yuan, H.; Albanese, C.; Kallakury, B.; Timofeeva, O.A.; Nealon, C.; Dakic, A.; Simic, V.; et al. ROCK inhibitor and feeder cells induce the conditional reprogramming of epithelial cells. *Am. J. Pathol.* **2012**, *180*, 599–607. [CrossRef]

118. Tanay, A.; Regev, A. Scaling single-cell genomics from phenomenology to mechanism. *Nature* **2017**, *541*, 331–338. [CrossRef]
119. Nguyen, Q.H.; Pervolarakis, N.; Blake, K.; Ma, D.; Davis, R.T.; James, N.; Phung, A.T.; Willey, E.; Kumar, R.; Jabart, E.; et al. Profiling human breast epithelial cells using single cell RNA sequencing identifies cell diversity. *Nat. Commun.* **2018**, *9*, e2028. [CrossRef]
120. Bach, K.; Pensa, S.; Grzelak, M.; Hadfield, J.; Adams, D.J.; Marioni, J.C.; Khaled, W.T. Differentiation dynamics of mammary epithelial cells revealed by single-cell RNA sequencing. *Nat. Commun.* **2017**, *8*, e2128. [CrossRef]
121. Chen, W.; Morabito, S.J.; Kessenbrock, K.; Enver, T.; Meyer, K.B.; Teschendorff, A.E. Teschendorff. Single-cell landscape in mammary epithelium reveals bipotent-like cells associated with breast cancer risk and outcome. *Commun. Biol.* **2019**, 1–13.
122. Chung, W.; Eum, H.H.; Lee, H.O.; Lee, K.M.; Lee, H.B.; Kim, K.T.; Ryu, H.S.; Kim, S.; Lee, J.E.; Park, Y.H.; et al. Single-cell RNA-seq enables comprehensive tumour and immune cell profiling in primary breast cancer. *Nat. Commun.* **2017**, *8*, e15081. [CrossRef]
123. Gao, R.; Kim, C.; Sei, E.; Foukakis, T.; Crosetto, N.; Chan, L.K.; Srinivasan, M.; Zhang, H.; Meric-Bernstam, F.; Navin, N. Nanogrid single-nucleus RNA sequencing reveals phenotypic diversity in breast cancer. *Nat. Commun.* **2017**, *8*, e228. [CrossRef]
124. Azizi, E.; Carr, A.J.; Plitas, G.; Cornish, A.E.; Konopacki, C.; Prabhakaran, S.; Nainys, J.; Wu, K.; Kiseliovas, V.; Setty, M.; et al. Single-cell map of diverse immune phenotypes in the breast tumor microenvironment. *Cell* **2018**, *174*, 1293–1308.e136. [CrossRef]
125. Hu, Q.T.; Hong, Y.; Qi, P.; Lu, G.Q.; Mai, X.Y.; Xu, S.; He, X.Y.; Guo, Y.; Gao, L.L.; Jing, Z.Y.; et al. An atlas of infiltrated B-lymphocytes in breast cancer revealed by paired single-cell RNA-sequencing and antigen receptor profiling. *BioRxiv* **2019**, e695601.
126. Wang, J.; Xu, R.; Yuan, H.; Zhang, Y.; Cheng, S. Single-cell RNA sequencing reveals novel gene expression signatures of trastuzumab treatment in HER2+ breast cancer: A pilot study. *Medicine* **2019**, *98*, e15872. [CrossRef]
127. Buenrostro, J.D.; Wu, B.; Chang, H.Y.; Greenleaf, W.J. ATAC-seq: A method for assaying chromatin accessibility genome-wide. *Curr. Protoc. Mol. Biol.* **2015**, *109*, 21–29. [CrossRef]
128. Buenrostro, J.D.; Wu, B.; Litzenburger, U.M.; Ruff, D.; Gonzales, M.L.; Snyder, M.P.; Chang, H.Y.; Greenleaf, W.J. Single-cell chromatin accessibility reveals principles of regulatory variation. *Nature* **2015**, *523*, 486–490. [CrossRef]
129. Cusanovich, D.A.; Daza, R.; Adey, A.; Pliner, H.A.; Christiansen, L.; Gunderson, K.L.; Steemers, F.J.; Trapnell, C.; Shendure, J. Multiplex single cell profiling of chromatin accessibility by combinatorial cellular indexing. *Science* **2015**, *348*, 910–914. [CrossRef]
130. Chung, C.Y.; Ma, Z.; Dravis, C.; Preissl, S.; Poirion, O.; Luna, G.; Hou, X.M.; Giraddi, R.R.; Ren, B.; Wahl, G.M. Single-cell chromatin accessibility analysis of mammary gland development reveals cell state transcriptional regulators and cellular lineage relationships. *BioRxiv* **2019**, e624957.
131. Pervolarakis, N.; Sun, P.; Gutierrez, G.; Nguyen, Q.H.; Jhutty, D.; Zheng, G.X.Y.; Nemec, C.M.; Dai, X.; Watanabe, K.; Kessenbrock, K. Integrated single-cell transcriptomics and chromatin accessibility analysis reveals novel regulators of mammary epithelial cell identity. *Cell Rep.* **2019**, 1–39. [CrossRef]

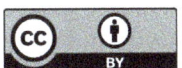

© 2019 by the authors. Licensee MDPI, Basel, Switzerland. This article is an open access article distributed under the terms and conditions of the Creative Commons Attribution (CC BY) license (http://creativecommons.org/licenses/by/4.0/).

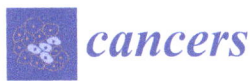

Review

Targeting Epithelial Mesenchymal Plasticity in Pancreatic Cancer: A Compendium of Preclinical Discovery in a Heterogeneous Disease

James H. Monkman [1,2,3,*], Erik W. Thompson [1,2,3] and Shivashankar H. Nagaraj [1,2,3,*]

1. Institute of Health and Biomedical Innovation, Queensland University of Technology, Brisbane, QLD 4059, Australia; e2.thompson@qut.edu.au
2. School of Biomedical Sciences, Queensland University of Technology, Brisbane, QLD 4059, Australia
3. Translational Research Institute, Brisbane, QLD 4102, Australia
* Correspondence: james.monkman@qut.edu.au (J.H.M.); shiv.nagaraj@qut.edu.au (S.H.N.)

Received: 8 August 2019; Accepted: 30 October 2019; Published: 7 November 2019

Abstract: Pancreatic Ductal Adenocarcinoma (PDAC) is a particularly insidious and aggressive disease that causes significant mortality worldwide. The direct correlation between PDAC incidence, disease progression, and mortality highlights the critical need to understand the mechanisms by which PDAC cells rapidly progress to drive metastatic disease in order to identify actionable vulnerabilities. One such proposed vulnerability is epithelial mesenchymal plasticity (EMP), a process whereby neoplastic epithelial cells delaminate from their neighbours, either collectively or individually, allowing for their subsequent invasion into host tissue. This disruption of tissue homeostasis, particularly in PDAC, further promotes cellular transformation by inducing inflammatory interactions with the stromal compartment, which in turn contributes to intratumoural heterogeneity. This review describes the role of EMP in PDAC, and the preclinical target discovery that has been conducted to identify the molecular regulators and effectors of this EMP program. While inhibition of individual targets may provide therapeutic insights, a single 'master-key' remains elusive, making their collective interactions of greater importance in controlling the behaviours' of heterogeneous tumour cell populations. Much work has been undertaken to understand key transcriptional programs that drive EMP in certain contexts, however, a collaborative appreciation for the subtle, context-dependent programs governing EMP regulation is needed in order to design therapeutic strategies to curb PDAC mortality.

Keywords: pancreatic cancer; epithelial mesenchymal plasticity; target discovery; review

1. Pancreatic Cancer, Tumour Heterogeneity, and Carcinoma Vulnerabilities

Pancreatic cancer (PC) is the fourth most common cause of cancer-related deaths in Western societies, with 57,000 new cases annually, resulting in nearly 46,000 deaths in North America alone [1]. The most common type of PC is Pancreatic Ductal Adenocarcinoma (PDAC), which arises in the ductal epithelium of the exocrine tissue responsible for secreting pancreatic digestive juices. Late detection combined with early metastatic spread have limited gains in overall survival relative to other cancers such that PDAC mortality has the potential to surpass that of both colorectal and breast cancers by 2030 [2]. PDAC research therefore aims to define better diagnostic markers and novel therapeutic avenues, however is significantly complicated by the clinical heterogeneity present both within and between patient tumours. This emphasises the need for more integrative approaches aimed at developing a better understanding of targetable processes in PDAC tumourigenesis.

Cancer is a genetic disease caused by the accumulation of somatic mutations, resulting in a functional imbalance between tumour suppressive and oncogenic signals [3]. While transformed cells retain characteristics of the host to efficiently avoid being detected as foreign by the immune system, many aberrant phenotypes caused by genetic mutations and dysregulated signaling potentially render these cells susceptible to selective therapeutic interventions. Extensive examinations of the molecular traits of PDAC aimed at identifying such vulnerabilities have been conducted to date. Indeed, genomic and transcriptional profiling of patient tumours as part of large-scale studies by the The Cancer Genome Atlas (TCGA) and International Cancer Genome Consortium (ICGC) have allowed for insights into the scale of inter-tumour heterogeneity in a breadth of patient cohorts [4–6].

These studies have identified four major genetic aberrations common to pancreatic tumours [7–9]. 90% of tumours carry gain-of-function mutations in KRAS2, activating proliferative and cell survival pathways, whilst 95% contain either partial or complete inactivating mutations in CDKN2A, contributing to loss of cell cycle regulation, furthering proliferation. TP53, responsible for responding to DNA damage and inducing apoptosis, is altered in 60% of cases. SMAD4 inactivation is also common in pancreatic cancer development, and is found in 50% of patient cancers, disrupting the tumour suppressive signals of TGFβ, aiding proliferation [10]. As well as these four common driver mutations, genomic sequencing of tumours has identified an additional panel of consistently mutated genes [6]. These genetic mutations implicate pathways often dysregulated in cancer, including KRAS, TGFβ, WNT, NOTCH, ROBO/SLT, G1/S, SWI-SNF, and chromatin/DNA/RNA modification and repair.

Transcriptional profiling of PDAC tumours has allowed researchers to define discrete regulatory mechanisms within these networks that are associated with particular prognostic indices in different molecular subtypes of PDAC, which include squamous, pancreatic progenitor, immunogenic and aberrantly differentiated endocrine/ exocrine tumours [6]. Such classification schemes may provide clinical value by aiding in patient treatment regimen selection and planning [11], however, to date they have provided limited clinical value due to lack of targetable phenomena. It is important to note that while these studies have aimed to characterise changes within carcinoma cells, the excessive presence of desmoplastic stroma may confound these results. Indeed, microdissection of the tumour from its associated stroma has allowed the retrospective re-evaluation of large-scale transcriptional profiling efforts, highlighting the overwhelming contribution of stromal contamination to many such studies. Deconvolution based on laser capture microdissection and RNASeq profiling of 60 matched tumour/stroma pairs suggested that ICGC and TCGA samples contained stromal fractions of 46% and 55%, respectively, highlighting difficulties in deriving definitive conclusions from whole tumour analyses [12].

Such studies are invaluable as a means of understanding the intertumoural heterogeneity that exists between patients, and they form a strong set of public data that have been analysed to better appreciate the diversity of tumour presentation [13]. An increasing focus on single cell analytic technologies has yielded exciting opportunities to understand the contributions that individual cells make towards intratumoural heterogeneity, tumour progression, and patient outcomes [14,15]. These studies highlight the need for efforts aimed at distinguishing the heterogeneous nature of a tumour's biology from that of the surrounding host tissue in which it propagates, so as to be better able to exploit cancer specific vulnerabilities [16].

As such, it is not surprising that the interactions between neoplastic epithelial cells and host myofibroblast and stellate populations, which can promote stromal inflammation, are increasingly being recognised. This desmoplastic reaction, which accounts for up to 90% of PDAC tumour volume, has pro-tumourigenic properties by leading to increased tissue stiffness and hypoxia as well as by providing physical barriers to both immune surveillance and chemotherapeutic penetrance [17–19]. The fibrillar collagen, hyaluronic acid and fibronectin rich extracellular matrix (ECM) deposited by stromal cells contains many soluble cytokines and growth factors secreted by both cancer and stromal compartments and contributes to both tumour initiation and progression [20–23]. Resident cells are forced to interact within this dynamic tumour microenvironment and are subject to stimuli that influence cell phenotypes in both stromal and carcinoma components. Such stimuli may propagate the invasion and dissemination of carcinoma cells by inducing epithelial mesenchymal plasticity (EMP), and thus this process is considered an important vulnerability that, when effectively targeted, may curb tumour progression [24,25].

2. EMP and PDAC Progression

EMP is often separated into two distinct but related processes—the forward process of epithelial-mesenchymal transition (EMT), and the reverse process of mesenchymal-epithelial transition (MET) [26]. These programs serve to describe the plasticity within epithelial cells that enables them to dedifferentiate into a more motile mesenchymal state, thereby allowing them to more effectively migrate. EMP is thought to play a significant role in several stages of tumour formation [27] and progression [28]. Initially, this plasticity allows tumour cells to detach and migrate from their site of origin (invasion), gaining access to lymphatic and blood vessels (intravasation), and then penetrating distant sites (extravasation), to form metastases.

A litany of reviews regarding different facets of EMP in PDAC, have been written, including those focused on molecular mechanisms of EMP regulation and metastasis [29–36], the role of epigenetic regulation [37], therapy development and resistance [38–42], microRNA regulation [43,44], and cancer stem cell generation [45–49]. This review thus focuses on some of the ongoing controversy surrounding in vivo evidence of EMP and the limitations of current approaches, highlighting the need to integrate a greater diversity of published EMP molecular regulators.

Development of PDAC frequently progresses undetected, remaining asymptomatic until it becomes an advanced stage of disease. Non-invasive precursor lesions formed either by epithelial proliferations or mucinous cysts in the pancreatic ducts, termed pancreatic intraepithelial neoplasia (PanINs), or intraductal papillary mucinous neoplasms (IPMNs), respectively, mark the onset of a histologically definable neoplasm in PDAC [50]. Such neoplasms, namely PanINs, progress through stages of dysplasia within the ductal epithelium, giving rise to the most common form of PDAC, pancreatic ductal adenocarcinoma (PDAC). The full breadth of factors that contribute to the invasive and metastatic behaviour of PDAC are vast. In this form of PDAC, there is very little latency between primary tumour formation and local and distant metastasis, implying that PDAC carcinoma cells may be readily equipped to invade and disseminate from a very early stage of development [51,52].

Invasive regions of human carcinomas are typically characterised by the presence of tumour-derived, fibroblast-like cells expressing mesenchymal markers such as vimentin, fibronectin and N-cadherin, with decreased expression of epithelial adhesion molecule E-Cadherin and increased nuclear beta-catenin relative to surrounding cells [53–57]. Decreased expression of E-cadherin has been shown to correlate with invasive and undifferentiated PDAC [58]. Furthermore, PDAC patients with tumour cells that express decreased E-cadherin and higher amounts of vimentin, s100A4, fibronectin and SNAI1 are more likely to have distant metastases, lymph node invasion and lower overall survival [54,59–62]. The EMP inducing transcription factor (TF) *TWIST1* has been shown to be upregulated in PDAC compared to match normal tissues [63], and *SNAI1* mRNA levels in PDAC fine needle aspirates are significantly correlated with lymph node and perineural invasion as well as with poorer survival [64]. A mediator of transforming growth factor beta (TGFβ) signaling, SMAD3, was also shown to accumulate in the nucleus of PDAC samples, and was correlated with higher grade tumours and lymph node metastasis, indicating a role for TGFβ in driving EMP in vivo [65]. Solitary infiltrating cancer cells displaying low E-cadherin and increased vimentin expression have proven to be significant prognostic indicators in resected clinical specimens from PDAC patients [66]. Tumour budding cells in PDAC have been observed with increased levels of *ZEB1* and *ZEB2*, and reduced levels of E-cadherin and β-catenin, indicative of EMP mediated local invasion. *ZEB2* overexpression in tumour-stroma associated cells also correlated with pathological assessment of tumour size, and lymph node metastasis [67]. Such striking pathology provides some of the clearest evidence for the role of EMP in PDAC progression.

While this clinical evidence strongly supports a role for EMP in mediating cancer invasion, the inability to accurately follow carcinoma epithelial dedifferentiation in vivo has led to some debate surrounding the extent of its role in tumour progression [68,69]. Such debate has necessitated the use of genetically engineered mouse models (GEMMs) to trace the role of EMP in cancer progression, specifically the pancreatic epithelium conditional *Kras/P53* mutant (PKCY) mice Lineage labelling of epithelial cells in this spontaneous PDAC model has allowed researchers to track these cells as they adopt mesenchymal properties and migrate away from the primary tumour into the circulation, seeding liver metastases [70]. In one study, EMP was detected in 42% of labelled PDAC epithelial cells, as assessed by the expression of EMP markers Zeb1 or Fsp1 and/or lack of E-cadherin. These cells were mostly observed in regions of inflammation, supporting the idea that EMP is driven by inflammatory interactions within the tissue microenvironment. Interestingly, some labelled epithelial cells that had undergone EMP displayed evidence of delamination and fibroblast morphology prior to tumour formation, and were otherwise indistinguishable from host stromal cells [70]. This is supportive of the very early, integral role that EMP may play in PanIN formation prior to tumour development.

Further studies in this same PDAC mouse model have shown that suppression of EMP via the knock-out of *Twist1* or *Snail* TFs does not reduce metastasis, despite the decreased expression of EMP markers and increased cell proliferation as evidence for EMP ablation [71]. Equivalent numbers of lineage labelled epithelial cells were found in circulation and in metastases regardless of *Twist/ Snail* knockout, suggesting that other mechanisms are involved in PDAC cellular invasion. PDAC cells do not possess a strong epithelial phenotype however, and may thus be insensitive to the loss of *Snail* TFs, which are potent repressors of epithelial programs but are less efficient in inducing mesenchymal properties. This possibly explains why *Snail* is dispensable for EMP and metastatic progression in this model [71,72], and points towards alternative mechanisms of EMP induction that may be driving factors in this PDAC system.

Indeed, there is evidence that the *Zeb1* TF is largely responsible for driving EMP in this GEMM model of PDAC development [73]. *Zeb1* ablation in PDAC cells was not found to affect *Twist1* expression, however it was associated with decreased *Zeb2*, *Slug* and a slight reduction in *Snail* expression. *Zeb1* depleted tumours were better differentiated, indicating less local invasion, and showed significantly reduced metastasis when compared to control PDAC mice [73]. This is in direct contrast to depletion of *Twist1* or *Snail*, which did not affect metastasis in this model system, highlighting the importance of recognising the context and tissue specific drivers of EMP.

Subsequent investigations aimed at overcoming the limitations of identifying single EMP regulatory TFs has shown that lineage labelled cancer cells are able to metastasize without expression of αSma or Fsp1, both of which are thought to be robust markers of EMP activation in this model [74]. Indeed, larger metastatic nodules were found containing exclusively cells that had never expressed αSma or Fsp1, while micrometastatic clusters of 3–5 cells were shown to have undergone EMP. Such evidence, combined with the fact that *Zeb1* depletion in previous studies resulted in only a 50% reduction in metastasis underscores the pitfalls of seeking to identify individual master regulators and markers of such a complex process. Adding to this complexity, the emerging importance of hybrid EMP phenotypes, in which the expression of both epithelial and mesenchymal markers may occur at levels that are insufficient to drive the reporter constructs used in such lineage tracing models, adds a further technical challenge [75–77].

More recent attempts to understand EMP in individual PDAC cells has shown the activation of EMP transcriptional programs within certain subsets of tumour cell populations [14]. This study highlighted a clear role for cytokines from the stromal compartment in inducing EMP in certain PDAC cell lines, and indicated that EMP activation could be observed in discrete tumour gland subunits with prognostic utility. These models have provided considerable insights into the diverse mechanisms of PDAC development, and highlight that there are context-dependent EMP programs involved in both local invasion and metastatic dissemination that require further examination [72,78].

3. In Vitro EMP Models and Exogenous Stimuli

While GEMMS, in particular the PKCY model of spontaneous PDAC formation, are currently the gold standard for studies of the biology of EMP in tumourigenesis, *in vitro* studies form the basis for the majority of our current molecular understanding of intracellular events which occur in EMP. Many publicly available and in-house generated cell lines are used to study PDAC, but only a very limited number of these undergo well-characterised, stimulus-driven transitions that mimic the pathophysiological induction of EMP. This is perhaps consistent with the limited number of EMP events witnessed in in vivo models, highlighting the difficulties of studying such a dynamic process.

EMP is modulated by TGFβ, receptor tyrosine kinases (RTK) ligands, WNT ligands, interleukins, hypoxia via HIF1α signaling, as well as HIPPO, NOTCH signaling. Their mechanisms and specific impact on downstream EMP targets have been comprehensively reviewed elsewhere, however our understanding of their subtleties is on-going [79,80]. TGFβ acts as a tumour suppressor in normal tissue and early stage disease by regulating cell proliferation and inducing apoptosis through canonical signaling pathways, however this activity is lost as cellular transformation progresses [81–85]. Indeed, TGFβ is a potent activator of EMP in PDAC cells when its tumour suppressive signals are disrupted through SMAD4 mutations, found in 50% of PDAC tumours [81,86]. Similarly, activating *KRAS* mutations found almost ubiquitously in PDAC cooperate with TGFβ signaling to hyperactivate downstream RAS/RAF MAPK pathways to induce EMP [87]. While TGFB activates the greatest number of EMP signaling pathways, and may thus be considered a major driver in PDAC, the activation of additional pathways shown in Figure 1 by RTK, WNT and interleukin ligands may provide additional layers of crosstalk. Activation of SMAD, MAPK, PI3K, STAT, and NFκB pathways are commonly demonstrated in PDAC EMP research, however the relative extent to which each pathway governs EMP is unclear, as many studies evaluate these pathways independently [29,88–94].

These complex pathways ultimately serve to influence transcriptional programs that co-operate directly and indirectly to control the plasticity that exists between epithelial and mesenchymal phenotypes of carcinoma cells (Figure 1). Of note is the increasing recognition for the role of long non-coding RNAs (LncRNA) and micro-RNAs (miRNA) in EMP regulation. Among the cells that do undergo EMP-like transitions, there is a degree of selectivity for the ligands that are able to activate these EMP programs, and this is reflected in the limited number of commercial cell lines that are commonly manipulated within the field. This is consistent with the level of heterogeneity reported in PDAC, and suggests discrete differences in steady state signaling, which may predispose a given cell's response or resistance to exogenous stimuli.

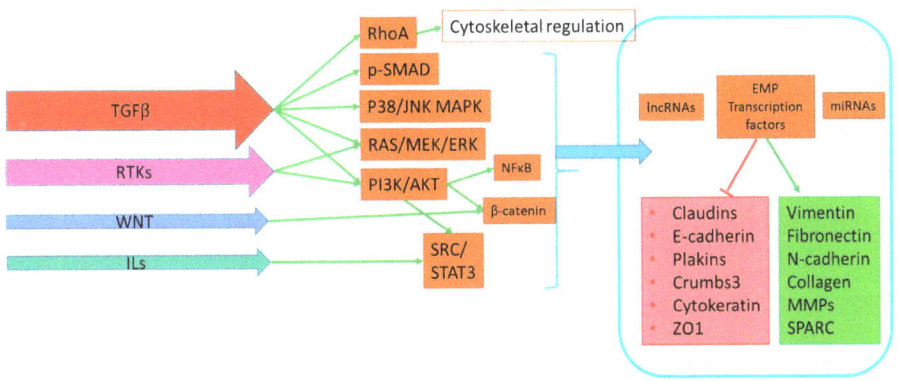

Figure 1. Simplified overview of cooperating signaling pathways in EMP.

EMP is induced by stimuli shown within arrows on the left in order of potency. These signals activate signal transduction pathways that cooperate directly and indirectly to translocate signals to the nucleus (braced) to regulate EMP transcription factors, long non-coding RNAs (LncRNA), and micro RNAs (miRNAs).These factors then modulate EMP by discrete regulation of epithelial (Red Box) and mesenchymal (Green box) cellular properties, which in turn influence migration and invasion. Transforming growth factor (TGFB) activates the greatest number of these pathways, including direct cytoskeletal regulation by RhoA, aswell as canonical SMAD and non-canonical p38/JNK, MEK/ERK MAPK pathways and PI3K/AKT. Receptor tyrosine kinase (RTK) signaling is induced by binding of growth factor (GF) ligands such as EGF, IGF, FGF, HGF or VEGF and activates RAS/MEK/ERK, PI3K/AKT/NFκB and downstream SRC pathways. WNT signaling also modulates EMP by downstream stabilisation of B-catenin and subsequent nuclear translocation for EMP program activation by TCF/LEF transcription factors. Interleukins (ILs) can also induce EMP programs via STAT3 signaling. Additional mediators of EMP include Hypoxia, Hedgehog, Notch and Integrin signaling (not shown), and highlight the context dependent activation of EMP from micro-environmental cues.

While most studies rely upon knockdown and over-expression approaches to demonstrate the function of proteins in the context of cell migration, proliferation and EMP transitions, relatively few studies have investigated these targets in the context of the physiological induction of EMP in response to exogenous stimuli. Among PDAC cell lines, L3.6pl cells have been shown to respond to VEGF treatment [95], while the inflammatory cytokines TNF-α and IL-1β drive EMP in PaTu 8988T and AsPC-1 cells via Hedgehog signaling [96]. Collagen 1 also stimulated L3.6pl and BxPC-3 cells to become more invasive through interaction with DDR1 [97], and BMP2 was able to elicit a similar response in BxPC-3 cells [98]. PANC-1 cells are a well characterised model of inducible EMP, first shown by Ellenrieder et al to undergo a bidirectional change in response to TGFβ alongside CAPAN-1, COLO-357, IMIM-PC1 [99], HPAF-II, and CAPAN-2 cells [100]. PANC-1 cells have since been repeatedly modelled with regard to their EMP response, which has been shown to be inducible in response to TGFβ, TNF-α, HGF, or hypoxia through differing mechanisms [101–104]. *SNAI1* appears to be a major driver in this model, being heavily regulated at the transcript and protein level, despite modest changes in E-cadherin and Vimentin proteins [105]. EMP is thus invariably the result of exogenous stimuli that activate discrete but conserved cellular pathways through novel intermediates that are an ongoing focus of basic cancer cell biology research.

4. Pre-Clinical Discovery of EMP Targets

As a result of the complexities of discerning cancer biology from native processes in vivo, the use of cell lines derived from primary tumours are a valuable means of modelling the molecular and phenotypic properties of cancers. Extensive investigation has been performed using gene silencing and overexpression approaches to evaluate the role that particular molecules have in regulating or effecting the EMP phenotypes of PDAC cells, however a concise summary of novel targets in the PDAC EMP field has to date been lacking. Thus, this review provides an exhaustive overview of such research as a platform for their integration, and progressive evaluation. The function of these candidate molecules can be broadly separated into secreted/soluble products (Table 1), receptors (Table 2), other membrane associated proteins (Table 3), cytoskeletal adaptors (Table 4), kinases (Table 5), intracellular mediators (Table 6), transcription factors (Table 7) and post transcriptional controllers (Table 8). The candidates shown were selected by searching Pubmed for the terms 'pancreatic' and 'epithelial', and articles investigating a novel candidate's impact on EMP phenotypes were manually curated. These effectors have been characterised to varying extents for their influence on invasion, migration, xenograft tumour growth, prognostic associations, and impact on known EMP signaling pathways. The proposed mechanisms of candidates and assays used to assess such effects are shown within tables and may be used to gauge where further support may be warranted to confirm and extend such findings. Due to the inherent variation in models used, the statistical power granted by IHC for varying sized patient cohorts with accompanying clinical information, and the level of EMP as a primary context, it is difficult to draw direct conclusions regarding pivotal significance within the field and clinical importance from such singular studies. Candidate expression in primary patient material that correlated with lymph-node metastasis are shown in bold within tables, and provide the best surrogate for their role in EMP mediated invasion, and include membrane bound proteins IGFBP2, ITGB4, CEACAM6 [106–108]. The use of IHC to capture dynamic EMP processes may be limited however, as shown in the case of LIN28B, where its expression is both induced by TGFβ and high in PDAC tissue, despite its role to suppress the pro-EMP non-coding RNA LET7a [109,110]. Such studies highlight both the utility and limitations of the links between in vitro assays and clinical material, and emphasise the need for both wider cohorts of patient material for validation and the development of GEMM models to strengthen findings in a standardized manner.

Figure 2 illustrates the proposed activity of some of these novel candidates, and how they may positively or negatively regulate discrete EMP signaling pathways. Of note are several candidates that converge to positively regulate EMP migratory phenotypes through FAK/Src and FAK/PI3K signaling, including the 5HT receptor and mucins, as well as EEF2K, USP22, and ZIP4. Their complete mechanisms of action and prevalence in PDAC tissue remain to be elucidated, however their inhibition may curb carcinoma invasion by blocking FAK activation and subsequent EMP modulation. Similarly, candidates participating in stability of EMP signaling and TF activity provide targets to modulate the EMP process specific for carcinoma cells. AURKA kinase has been shown to participate in a positive feedback loop with stabilization and activity of TWIST1, while PEAK1 and NES have been implicated in stabilization YAP/TAZ and SMAD TF activity. The discovery of discrete EMP regulation and development of combinatorial inhibitors may provide the opportunity for more personalized therapeutic approaches to curb metastatic disease.

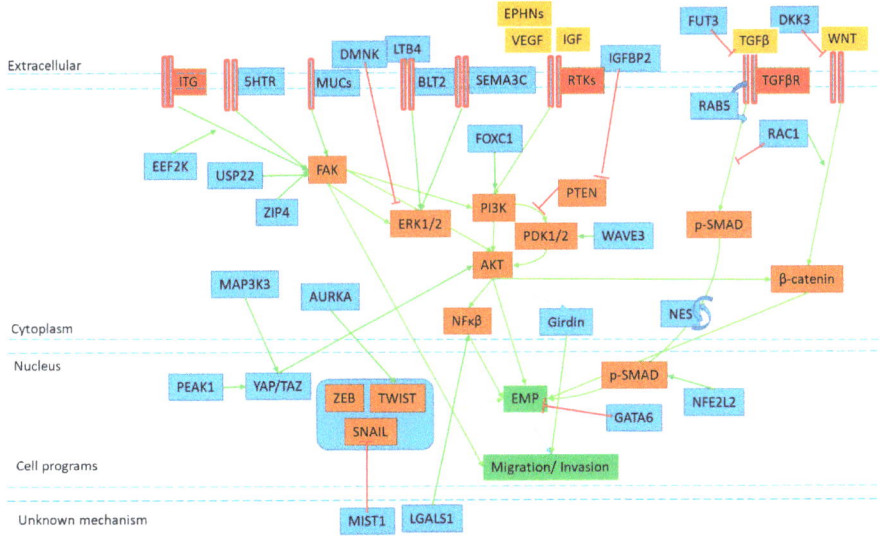

Figure 2. Simplified overview of the proposed mechanisms of novel candidates.

EMP and cell migration (GREEN boxes) is induced through cell surface proteins (ITG, 5HTR, MUC, BLT2, SEMA3C, RTK, TGFβR) (RED) to activate signaling pathways (ORANGE boxes, blue arrows). These pathways are influenced by novel mediators (BLUE boxes) through activation (GREEN arrows) or inhibition (RED T) of known signaling members, however complete mechanisms of action remain to be elucidated. For full details, evidence of proposed mechanism and references of novel mediators, see tables below. Note signaling pathways shown have had intermediates removed for ease of visualisation.

Table 1. Soluble and secreted factors that influence EMP. This table describes novel candidates that may be secreted within the ECM and act either directly through ligand-receptor interactions, or through mechanisms that remain to be demonstrated. Candidates that exhibit clinical correlation with lymph node metastasis are shown in bold.

Cell Line	Target	EMT Regulation (Direct or Indirect Observation)	KD/KO/Over-expression	Pathway/Mechanism	Functional Assay	Human Prognostic Association	EMT Activator	Reference
BxPC-3	DKK3	Negative, Direct	Over-expression	DKK3 is overexpressed in tumour and is antagonist of WNT ligand activity, preventing nuclear translocation of β-catenin and EMP under hypoxia	Transwell assays, chemo-resistance, IHC in 75 matched PDAC v normal samples, xenograft growth	Not performed	Hypoxia	[111]
ASPC-1, PANC-1	**IGFBP2**	**Positive, Direct**	**siRNA/Over-expression**	**IGFBP2 activated NF-κB through PI3K/AKT/IKK, inhibited by PTEN**	**WB, Transwell assays, orthotopic growth, IHC in 80 patient PDAC and lymph node samples**	**Survival and lymph node metastasis**	-	**[106]**
PANC-1	LTB4	Positive, Direct	siRNA	LTB4 induced EMT through receptor BLT2 and ERK1/2 activation	WB, Transwell assays	Not performed	LTB4	[112]
Patu8988, PANC-1	DMKN	Positive, Indirect	shRNA	Knockdown reduced p-STAT3 and EMT increased ERK1/2, AKT	Proliferation, Transwell assays, Xenograft, IHC in 44 patient PDAC tumours	Correlated with T stage	-	[113]
PANC-1	LGALS1	Positive, Direct	shRNA/Over-expression	LGALS1 IHC expression correlated with MMP9 and Vimentin in PDAC. PSC LGALS1 promoted cancer cell EMT and activation of NF-κB	Xenograft, Proliferation, Invasion, IHC in 66 PDAC tumours	Not performed	-	[114]
BxPC-3, CFPAC	SEMA3C	Positive, Indirect	shRNA/Over-expression	SEMA3C knockdown suppressed EMT and tumourigenesis, and activation of ERK1/2 signaling	Proliferation, migration, Scratch wound, Xenograft, IHC in 118 PDAC tumours	Stage, survival, recurrence	-	[115]
Capan-1	FUT3	Positive, Direct	shRNA/Over-expression	FUT3 knockdown impeded proliferation, migration, tumour growth and TGFβ induced EMT	Proliferation, Scratch wound, Transwell assays, Xenograft	Not performed	TGFβ	[116]
PANC-1, MIAPaCa-2, Capan-2	**MIF/ NR3C2**	**Positive, Indirect**	**siRNA/Over-expression**	**MIF induces miR-301b, targeting NR3C2, inducing EMT and chemo sensitivity**	**PDAC transcriptome by array, IHC of 173 PDAC, Proliferation, Colony formation, Transwell assays, chemo-resistance**	**NR3C2 inversely prognostic by RNA and IHC**	-	**[117]**

Table 1. Cont.

Cell Line	Target	EMT Regulation (Direct or Indirect Observation)	KD/KO/Over-expression	Pathway/Mechanism	Functional Assay	Human Prognostic Association	EMT Activator	Reference
PANC-1, BxPC-3	WNT5A	Positive, Direct	siRNA, Over-expression	Wnt5a expression induced EMT and invasion and was elevated in PDAC by IHC	Scratch wound, Transwell assays, WB, orthotopic growth, IHC of 134 PDAC v normal	No	-	[118]
PANC-1	LCN2	Negative, Indirect	Over-expression	LCN2 expression correlated with better survival and lower EMT state	IHC of 60 PDAC tumours, Transwell assays	Protective by IHC	-	[119]
MIAPaca-2, BxPC-3, SUIT-2	NOV	Positive, Indirect	shRNA/Over-expression	NOV expression high in PDAC by IHC, and induced EMT phenotypes in vitro/in vivo	Colony formation, soft agar, Proliferation, Transwell assays, in vivo metastasis	Not performed	-	[120]
PANC-1, BxPC-3	CCL18	Positive, Direct		CCL18 expressed in mesenchymal and cancer cells, and induced EMT	WB, Transwell assays, IHC of 62 PDAC tumours, serum ELISA from PDAC patients	Survival	-	[121]
PANC-1, BxPC-3	TUFT1	Positive, Indirect	siRNA/Over-expression	TUFT1 expression correlated with T stage and lymph node metastasis by IHC, RNA expression correlated with HIF1a, SNAI1 and VIM	WB, Proliferation, scratch wound, Transwell assays, Xenograft, IHC of 63 PDAC tumours	Yes in TCGA by RNA	-	[122]
SW1990, ASPC-1	OLR1	Positive, Direct	siRNA/Over-expression	OLR1 overexpressed in tumours and correlates with metastasis and poor survival, overexpression induced EMT	Transwell assays, scratch wound, Proliferation/apoptosis, IHC of 98 PDAC tumours	Yes survival by IHC and TCGA	-	[123]
MIAPaCa-2, PANC-1, ASPC-1, BxPC-3	LOXL2	Positive, Indirect	siRNA/Over-expression	LOXL2 IHC expression correlated with recurrence, depth of invasion and poor survival, and enhanced EMT in vitro	Transwell assays, IHC of 80 PDAC tumours	Yes by IHC	-	[124]
PANC-1, PK9	TFF1	Negative, Direct	siRNA	TFF only expressed in PanIN and intraductal neoplasia, not normal or invasive PDAC, knockdown activated EMT, loss of TFF in GEMM drove PanIN, PDAC and CAF infiltration	Transwell Invasion, Scratch wound, KC GEMM, IHC on small number of samples	Not performed	-	[125]

Table 2. Receptors. This table describes known receptors that may be activated to transduce signals required for EMP modulation. Candidates that exhibit clinical correlation with lymph node metastasis are shown in bold.

Cell Line	Target	EMT Regulation	KD/KO/Over-expression	Pathway/Mechanism	Functional Assay	Prognostic Association	EMT Activator	Reference
L3.6pl	VEGFR1 activation	Positive, Direct		RTK VEGFR-1 activation induced SNAI1/2, TWIST	E-cadherin/β-catenin localization/WB	Not performed	VEGF	[95]
PANC-1, MiaPaCa-2	HTR1B, HTR1D	Positive, Indirect	siRNA	5-HT receptor knockdown reduced uPAR and Src/FAK signaling and EMT	Scratch wound, Transwell, Colony formation	Not performed	-	[126]
PANC-1 HPAC	IGF1R	Positive, Indirect	siRNA	IGF1R overexpressed in PDAC by IHC, silencing inhibits AKT/PI3K, MAPK, JAK/STAT signaling pathways	Transwell assays, soft agar, Proliferation, apoptosis, IHC of TMA	Not performed	-	[127]
L3.6pl, BxPC-3	DDR1	Positive, Direct	siRNA/Over-expression	DDR1 expression correlates with CHD2 expression by IHC, DDR1-b signals through SHC1 adapter to PYK2 to induce CDH2	Invasion, IHC of PDAC TMA	Not performed	COL1A	[97]
PANC-1	SMO	Positive, Indirect	siRNA	Hedgehog activated in tumourspheres, SMO knockdown inhibited CSC/EMT features properties	Proliferation, sphere formation, Transwell assays, Xenograft	Not performed	-	[128]
PANC-1, BxPC-3	EPHA4	Positive, Direct	siRNA	EPHA4 knockdown suppressed EMT, MMP2 activity	Gelatin zymography, Transwell assays, scratch wound, WB	Not performed	-	[129]
CFPAC-1, AsPC-1	**ITGB4**	**Positive, Direct**	**siRNA/Over-expression**	**ITGB4 IHC expression correlated with T stage, knockdown inhibited EMP**	**Transwell assays, WB, IHC of 134 PDAC tumours**	**Survival lymph node metastasis by IHC**	**TGFβ**	**[107]**
PANC-1, MiaPaCa2, Capan2	F2R	Positive, Indirect	shRNA	F2R (PAR1) expression associated with mesenchymal gene signature	Xenograft, Scratch wound	Not performed	-	[130]

Table 3. Membrane associated proteins. This table describes membrane bound proteins that may interact with other cells and the extracellular environment to sense cues that modulate EMP in a context dependent fashion. Candidates that exhibit clinical correlation with lymph node metastasis are shown in bold.

Cell Line	Target	EMT Regulation	KD/KO/Over-expression	Pathway/Mechanism	Functional Assay	Prognostic Association	EMT Activator	Reference
PANC-1	CDCP1	Positive, Indirect	siRNA	CDCP1 expression high in PDAC, induced by BMP4/ERK signaling, and knockdown inhibited EMT phenotypes	Scratch wound, Transwell, spheroid formation, chemo-resistance, IHC on 42 PDAC tumours	Not performed	-	[131]
Colo-357, Capan-1	MUC16	Positive, Indirect	siRNA, CRISPR/Cas9	MUC16 knockdown decreased FAK mediated AKT/ERK/MAPK activation, and EMT	Proliferation, migration, Colony formation, Xenograft	Not performed	-	[132]
MiaPaCa2	ANXA1	Positive, Indirect	CRISPR	ANXA1 KO downregulated miR196a, effected cell motility and liver metastases in vivo	Scratch wound, Transwell migration, Invasion, Xenograft	Not performed	-	[133,134]
CFPAC-1, PANC-1	**CEACAM6**	**Positive, Direct**	**shRNA, Over-expression**	**CEACAM6, regulated by miR-29a/b/c, required for EMT**	**Transwell assays, Xenograft, WB, IHC in 99 PDAC tumours**	**Lymph node metastasis**	-	**[108]**
SUIT-2, CAPAN-2	TM4SF1	Negative, Indirect	siRNA	TM4SF1 IHC expression protective, knockdown induced migration and decreased E-cadherin	Transwell assays, IHC in 74 PDAC tumours	Yes inversely prognostic by IHC	TGFβ	[135]
PANC-1, SW1990	DPP4	Positive, Indirect	siRNA/Over-expression	DPP4 (CD26) knockdown suppressed EMT, in vivo growth	Proliferation, Transwell assays, Xenograft, WB	Not performed	-	[136]
PANC-1, AsPC-1	SLC39A4	Positive, Indirect	siRNA/overexpression	SLC39A4 (ZIP4) IHC expression correlated with ZEB1 and EMT, increasing FAK and paxillin phosphorylation	Xenograft, Scratch wound, Transwell migration, Invasion, IHC of 72 paired PDAC v normal	Not performed	-	[137]

Table 4. Cytoskeletal adaptors. This table describes intracellular adapter proteins that may participate in and be required protein complex localization and transduction of signals that modulate EMP. Candidates that exhibit clinical correlation with lymph node metastasis are shown in bold.

Cell Line	Target	EMT Regulation	KD/KO/Over-expression	Pathway/Mechanism	Functional Assay	Prognostic Association	EMT Activator	Reference
PANC-1, CFPAC-1	**WASF3**	**Positive, Indirect**	**siRNA,**	**WASF3 (WAVE3) knockdown suppressed PDK2, downregulating PI3K/AKT pathway and EMT**	**Proliferation, migration, Invasion, Scratch wound, IHC of 87 paired PDAC v normal**	**Lymph node metastasis**	**-**	**[138]**
PANC-1, AsPC-1, MiaPaCa-2	NES	Positive, Direct	shRNA/Over-expression	NES (Nestin) required for EMT and induced by TGFβ in positive feedback loop promoting p-smad2	Xenograft, Transwell assays, IHC of GEMM	Not performed	TGFβ	[139,140]
HPAF-II, PANC-04.03 PANC-1	DNM2	Positive, Indirect	siRNA, Over-expression	Upregulated by IHC in PDAC, DNM2/VAV1 interaction required for RAC-1 induced lamellipodia formation	Transwell assays, lamellipodia formation, xenograft, IHC of 85 PDAC tumours	Not performed	EGF (HPAF-II)	[141,142]
SUIT-2	RAB5A	Positive, Indirect	siRNA	RAB5 IHC expression correlated with invasion and CDH1, aids TGFβR endocytosis, stimulates FA turnover, prognostic in PDAC, breast, ovarian	Morphology, Proliferation, Transwell assays, IHC of 111 PDAC tumours	Survival IHC	-	[143]

Table 5. Kinases and Phosphatases. This table describes proteins with activity that may directly participate in signal transduction by phospho-regulation of intracellular substrates. Candidates that exhibit clinical correlation with lymph node metastasis are shown in bold.

Cell Line	Target	EMT Regulation	KD/KO/Over-expression	Pathway/Mechanism	Functional Assay	Prognostic Association	EMT Activator	Reference
PANC-1, MIAPaCa-2	EEF2K	Positive, Direct	siRNA/Over-expression	EEF2K promotes EMT through TG2/β1 integrin/SRC/uPAR/MMP2 signaling	Scratch wound, Transwell assays, WB	Not performed	-	[144]
Patu8988, PANC-1, BxPC-3, Capan-1	CDK14	Positive, Direct	siRNA	Suppression of CDK14 reduced PI3K/AKT activation and EMT	Proliferation, Colony formation, Transwell assays	Not performed	-	[145]
HDPE	PRAG1	Positive, Indirect	siRNA/Over-expression	Phosphorylation of PRAG1 found in malignant cells, Over-expression induced JAK1/STAT3 mediated EMT	Transwell assays, phospho-WB	Not performed	-	[146]
BxPC-3, PANC-1	AURKA	Positive, Direct	shRNA	AURKA IHC expression high in PDAC, phosphorylates and stabilizes TWIST1 in positive feedback loop, promoting EMT	Sphere formation, migration, Proliferation, Xenograft, IHC on small PDAC cohort	Not performed	-	[63]
PANC-1, ASPC-1	MAP3K3	Positive, Direct	CRISPR	MAP3K3 (MEKK3) KO reduced EMT, CSC and migration, and YAP/TAZ transcriptional activity on AXL, DKK1, FosL1, CTGF	Transwell migration Invasion, Proliferation, Xenograft, ChIP	Not performed	-	[147]
PANC-1, COLO357	RAC1	Negative, Direct	siRNA/Over-expression	RAC1b inhibits canonical and non-canonical TGFβ signaling, effecting MKK6-p38 and MEK-ERK-MAPK EMT activation	Migration, qPCR	Not performed	TGFβ	[90,148]
HPAF-II, CAPAN-2	PTPN11	Positive, Direct	shRNA/Over-expression	PTPN11 (SHP2) activity enhances the effect of EGF on TGFβ induced EMT, resulting in more complete EMT	Cell scatter, scratch wound, WB	Not performed	TGFβ/EGF	[100]

Table 6. Enzymes and Co-factors. This table describes intracellular proteins that may directly or indirectly participate in pathways required for EMP modulation by other enzymatic control of substrate proteins. Candidates that exhibit clinical correlation with lymph node metastasis are shown in bold.

Cell Line	Target	EMT Regulation	KD/KO/Over-expression	Pathway/Mechanism	Functional Assay	Prognostic Association	EMT Activator	Reference
PANC-1	USP22	Positive, Direct	shRNA/Over-expression	USP22 expression correlated with Ezrin and FAK phosphorylation and EMT	Scratch wound, Transwell assays, WB	Not performed	-	[149]
779E, 1334 PDCL	EIF5A	Positive, Indirect	shRNA/Over-expression	Mutant KRAS induces EIF5A, stimulating PEAK1 mediated FCM signaling. PEAK1 binds YAP/TAZ driving stem TFs	Sphere formation, IP, WB	Not performed	-	[150]
AsPC-1, PANC-1	EIF4E	Negative, Indirect	siRNA	Knockdown of MNK effector, EIF4E, induced ZEB1 through repression of miR-200c, miR-141, MNK inhibitors induce MET	Collagen 3D, qPCR	Not performed	-	[94]
BxPC-3	RGCC	Positive, Direct	siRNA	RGCC regulated by HIF1α and required for hypoxia induced EMT	qPCR, WB	Not performed	hypoxia	[151]
PANC-1 MIA PaCa-2	SET	Positive, Direct	shRNA/ Over-expression	SET over-expression activated Rac1/JNK/c-Jun pathway and decreased PP2A activity, N-cadherin and EMT TFs up GPX1 IHC expression lower in	Transwell assays, Colony formation, Xenograft tumour growth and liver metastases	Not performed	-	[152]
MiaPaCa2, SW1990, PANC-1, CFPAC1	GPX1	Negative, Direct	shRNA/Over-expression	PDAC, silencing induced EMT and gemcitabine resistance through ROS activated PI3K/Akt/GSK3B/SNAIL, Over-expression sensitized in vivo	Transwell migration, chemo-resistance, Xenografts, IHC of 281 PDAC tumours, and 42 paired PDAC v normal	Yes inversely prognostic by IHC	-	[153]
BxPC-3, PANC-1, MiaPaCa2, PSN1	HDAC1	Positive, Indirect	siRNA	HDAC IHC expression and activity correlated with EMT phenotype	IHC, Transwell Invasion, IHC of 103 PDAC tumours	Survival by IHC	-	[154]
PANC-1 BxPC-3	Class I HDAC	Positive, Indirect	4SC-202 small inhibitor	HDACi (inhibition) blocked TGFβ induced EMT in PANC-1, requiring BRD4 and MYC for effect of HDACi	Migration, sphere formation, Xenograft	Not performed	TGFβ (PANC-1)	[155]
CFPAC-1, L3.7-2	PAFAH1B2	Positive, Direct	siRNA/Over-expression	PAFAH1B2 IHC expression higher in PDAC, HIF1a expression regulated PAFAH1B2 via direct promoter binding	Transwell migration, Invasion, orthotopic Xenograft/ liver metastases, HIF1a/PAFAH1B2 co-localization in PDAC, IHC of 124 PDAC tumours and 70 normal	Survival by IHC and TCGA	hypoxia	[156]

Table 6. Cont.

Cell Line	Target	EMT Regulation	KD/KO/Over-expression	Pathway/Mechanism	Functional Assay	Prognostic Association	EMT Activator	Reference
PANC-1, MIAPaCa-2	KDM4B	Positive, Direct	siRNA	KDM4B IHC expression correlated with ZEB1 in PDAC, knockdown inhibited TGFβ induced EMT in PANC-1 by regulating ZEB1 methylation	CHIP, scratch wound, Transwell assays, IHC of 49 PDAC tumours	Not performed	TGFβ	[157]
HPAC, BxPC-3, Colo357 PANC-1, MiaPaCa-2	SMURF2	Negative, Direct		SMURF negative regulator of TGFβ induced EMT, suppressed by miR-15b	Scratch wound, Transwell assays, WB	Not performed	TGFβ	[158]
CAPAN-1 PANC-1	CUL4B	Positive, Direct	miRNA	CUL4B IHC expression higher in PDAC, regulated by miR-300, required for Wnt/β-catenin induced EMP	qPCR, Transwell assays, Xenograft, IHC of 110 PDAC v normal	Not performed	-	[159]
PANC-1	KMT5C	Positive, Direct	siRNA	KMT5C (SUV420H2) expression higher in PanIN and PDAC, methylates H4K20me3, suppresses epithelial drivers FOXA1, OVOL2, OVOL2	Transwell assays, chemo-resistance, sphere formation,	Not performed	-	[160]
PANC-1	NOX4	Positive, Direct	siRNA	NOX4 IHC expression elevated in PDAC, aids ROS generation and TGFβ induced EMT	Transwell assays, WB	Not performed	TGFβ	[161]
BxPC-3	PAWR	Negative, Indirect	siRNA, Over-expression	PAWR (PAR4) suppressed in cisplatin resistant EMT cells, required PI3K/AKT signaling	Transwell assays, Proliferation, WB, Xenograft	Not performed	-	[162]
BxPC-3	PPM1H	Negative, Indirect	siRNA	PPM1H expression decreased by TGFβ/BMP2 treatment, knockdown induced EMT	Proliferation, Transwell assays, WB, apoptosis	Not performed	TGFβ, BMP2	[98]
PANC-1	HMGN5	Positive, Indirect	shRNA	HMNG5 silencing reduced Wnt expression	Xenograft, Transwell migration Invasion, WB,	Not performed	-	[163]
PANC-1	GOLM1	Positive, Direct	siRNA/overexpression	GOLM1 (GP73) overexpression induced EMT and correlated with human metastasis and Xenograft growth	Xenograft, Transwell migration Invasion, Scratch wound, WB	Not performed	-	[164]

Table 7. Transcription Factors and Cofactors. This table describes transcription factors and cofactors that influence gene expression required for actions of EMP in their respective systems. Candidates that exhibit clinical correlation with lymph node metastasis are shown in bold.

Cell Line	Target	EMT Regulation	KD/KO/Over-expression	Pathway/Mechanism	Functional Assay	Prognostic Association	EMT Activator	Reference
PaTu 8988T, AsPC1	GLI1	Positive, Direct	siRNA	GLI1 component of HH signaling, induced EMT by TNF-α/IL-1β, mediated through NF-κB pathway	Transwell assays, WB	Not performed	TNF-α/IL-1β	[96,165–168]
Colo-357, L3.7	FOXM1	Positive, Indirect	siRNA/Over-expression	FOXM1c activates uPAR promoter directly, inducing EMT	Scratch wound, Transwell migration, IHC of PDAC TMA v normal	Elevated in metastatic PDAC	-	[169]
BxPC-3, ASPC-1, PANC-1	TAZ	Negative, Direct	shRNA, Over-expression	TAZ required for EMT through TEA/ATTS TFs, activation correlates with suppression of Nf2	Colony formation, Xenograft, Transwell assays, IHC of 57 PDAC v normal	Correlated with PDAC differentiation	-	[170]
PANC-1, CAPAN-1	YAP	Positive, Direct	shRNA/Over-expression	YAP expression associated with activation of AKT cascade and EMT	Transwell assays, chemo-resistance, WB	Not performed	-	[171]
PANC-1, BxPC-3	HSF1	Positive, Indirect	siRNA	p-HSF1 IHC elevated in PDAC, promotes invasion and is downregulated by p-AMPK IGFR1 positively regulates	Transwell assays, scratch, WB, GEMM	Not performed	-	[172]
HPAC, MiaPaCa2	FOXC1	Positive, Indirect	siRNA/Over-expression	FOXC1, activating PI3K/Akt/ERK, promoting migration, and EMT, and tumour growth BHLHA15 (MIST1)	Xenograft, Transwell migration Invasion, soft agar	Not performed	IGF	[173]
PANC-1, SW1990	**BHLHA15, Direct**	Negative, Direct	Over-expression	Over-expression suppressed tumour growth & metastases. Caused MET by suppressing SNAIL indirectly	Transwell migration, Invasion, Xenograft and liver met	Not performed	-	[174]

Table 7. Cont.

Cell Line	Target	EMT Regulation	KD/KO/Over-expression	Pathway/Mechanism	Functional Assay	Prognostic Association	EMT Activator	Reference
PANC-1	KLF8, Indirect	Positive, Direct	siRNA, Over-expression	KLF8 IHC elevated in PDAC, directly induces FHL2 transcription via promoter binding	WB, Invasion	Not performed	-	[175]
GEMM	P73, Direct	Negative, Direct	GEMM	P73 deficiency led to stromal deposition and EMT in PDAC tumours, decreased BGN secretion, required for tumour suppressive functions of TGFβ	GEMM, Transwell assays	Not performed	-	[176]
GEMM	PRRX1	Positive, Direct	Overexpression	PRRX1 a/b have discrete functions in MET/EMT, knockdown suppresses tumour growth and EMT	GEMM tumour model, Xenograft	Not performed	-	[177]
Capan-2	TRIM28	Positive, Indirect	Overexpression	TRIM28 Overexpression drove EMT and Invasion, correlated with T stage	Transwell assays, WB, Xenograft, IHC of 91 PDAC	Lymph node metastasis and survival	-	[178]
PANC-1	ETS1	Positive, Direct	shRNA	ETS1 knockdown epithelialized PANC-1 cells	Scratch wound, adhesion, qPCR for EMT markers	Not performed	-	[179]
HDPE, COLO-357	NFE2L2	Positive, Direct	siRNA/Over-expression	NFE2L2 activation enhanced TGFβ induced EMT in both premalignant and malignant cells	Scratch wound, Transwell assays, WB, qPCR	Not performed	TGFβ	[180]
PANC-1, HPAF-II	PDX1	Positive, Indirect	shRNA, GEMM	PDX1 has dual roles in premalignant and transformed cells. PDX1 expression is reduced in tumours and EMT	Colony formation, GEMMs, IHC of 183 PDAC	Inversely prognostic for survival	TGFβ (PANC-1), HGF (HPAF-II)	[181]

Table 7. Cont.

Cell Line	Target	EMT Regulation	KD/KO/Over-expression	Pathway/Mechanism	Functional Assay	Prognostic Association	EMT Activator	Reference
PANC-1	BCL9L	Positive, Direct	siRNA/Over-expression	BCL9L knockdown prevented EMT and inhibited in vivo growth	Proliferation, Transwell assays, Xenograft	Not performed	TGFβ	[182]
GEMM	ETV1	Positive, Direct	Overexpression	ETV1 induces SPARC, required for tumour growth and metastasis in vivo, EMT in vitro	Xenograft, Invasion	Not performed	-	[183]
ASPC-1, SW1990	EPAS1	**Positive, Direct**	siRNA	**EPAS1 (HIF2α) IHC expression high in PDAC, and knockdown inhibited EMT**	**CHIP, Transwell assays, IHC of 70 PDAC**	**Lymph node metastasis, differentiation**	-	[184]
PANC-1 BxPC-3	SIX1	Positive, Indirect	siRNA/shRNA	SIX1 IHC expression elevated in PDAC, knockdown reduced migration and tumour size	Migration, EMT markers, PANC-1 Xenograft, CD44-/CD24+, IHC of 139 PDAC	No	-	[185]
Cfpac-1	GRHL2	Negative, Direct	siRNA	GRHL2 IHC expression elevated in normal duct and liver metastases, drives epithelial phenotype.	Proliferation, EMT markers, Colony and sphere formation, drug resistance, IHC of 155 PDAC	No	-	[186]
PaTu8988S	GATA6	Negative, Direct	shRNA/Over-expression	GATA6 IHC expression low in PDAC, Silencing induced EMT	chemo-resistance, IF, Invasion, Xenograft, IHC of 58 PDAC	Inversely prognostic for survival	-	[187]

Table 8. Post transcriptional effectors. This table describes factors that may post transcriptionally modulate EMP by controlling stability of mRNA and hence expression of effector proteins. Candidates that exhibit clinical correlation with lymph node metastasis are shown in bold.

Cell Line	Target	EMT Regulation	KD/KO/Over-expression	Pathway/Mechanism	Functional Assay	Prognostic Association	EMT Activator	Reference
Miapaca-2, PANC-1, Patu-8988	HNRNPA2B1	Positive, Direct	shRNA/Over-expression	Knockdown epithelialized cells, Over-expression drove EMT through ERK/SNAI1 pathway	Cell viability, Transwell assays, PANC-1 Xenograft, EMT markers	Not performed	-	[188]
SW1990, BxPC-3	YTHDF2	Negative, Direct	shRNA	Knockdown reduced p-AKT, p-GSK-3b, promoted EMT, YAP knockdown reversed effect	Proliferation, Colony formation, Invasion, adhesion	Not performed	-	[189]
Panc-1, Patu8988	Lnc TUG1	Positive, Direct	shRNA	Lnc TUG1 sponges miR-382, preventing repression of ezh2	Colony formation, Transwell assays, WB	Not performed	-	[190]
Gemcitabine resistant BxPC-3	DYNC2H1-4	Positive, Direct	siRNA	Lnc DYNC2H1-4 sponges miR-145, upregulating ZEB1, MMP3 and other CSC markers	Transwell assays, CSC markers, Xenograft	Not performed	-	[191]
ASPC-1, BxPC-3, PANC-1	miR-23	Positive, Direct	miRNAs	miR-23 promotes EMT by regulating ESRP1, miR-23 required for TGFβ induced EMT	WB, Transwell assays, Xenograft, qPCR of 52 paired PDAC tumour v normal	Survival by RNA	TGFβ	[192]
SW1990, PANC-1, BxPC-3, CAPAN-1	NORAD	Positive, Direct	shRNA/Over-expression	Lnc NORAD acts as ceRNA of miR-125a-3p, enhancing RHOa and EMT	Scratch wound, Transwell assays, Xenograft	Not performed	Hypoxia	[193]
Panc-1	Lnc H19	Positive, Direct	siRNA	H19 antagonised LET-7, inducing HMGA-2 mediated EMT	Transwell assays, scratch wound, WB	Not performed	-	[194]
ASPC-1, BxPC-3	LncRNA-ROR	Positive, Direct	shRNA/Over-expression	LncRNA-ROR expression induces ZEB1 and EMT	Scratch wound, Transwell assays, Xenograft	Not performed	-	[195]

Table 8. Cont.

Cell Line	Target	EMT Regulation	KD/KO/Over-expression	Pathway/Mechanism	Functional Assay	Prognostic Association	EMT Activator	Reference
PANC-1, BxPC-3, COLO357	miR-100, miR-125b	Positive, Indirect	siRNA/CRISPR/Over-expression	TGFβ induced lnc-miR100HG, which codes for tumourigenic miR 100, miR125b and LET-7a. LIN28B also induced by TGFβ, suppresses LET-7a activity	miR Over-expression, Xenograft, Scratch wound, sphere formation, RNAseq, RIPseq	Survival by RNA	TGFβ	[109]
BxPC-3, PANC-1, CFPAC-1, SW1990	miR-361-3p	Positive, Direct	Over-expression	miR-361-3p downregulates DUSP2, preventing inactivation of ERK1/2	Orthotopic metastasis, Transwell assays	Survival by RNA	-	[196]
Sw1990	miR-1271	Negative, Direct	miR Mimics, Inhibitors	miR -1271 inhibited EMT and migration	Proliferation, Transwell migration invasion, xenograft	Not performed	-	[197]
Panc-1	LSM1	Positive, Indirect	Over-expression	Lsm1 (CaSm) induction induced EMT and proliferation, effecting apoptotic and metastasis gene expression	Proliferation, anoikis, Transwell assays, chemo-resistance, xenograft	Not performed	-	[198]
KPCY	MTDH	Positive, Indirect	siRNA	MTDH expression promoted CSC and metastasis, high cytoplasmic expression by IHC	Spheroid formation, orthotopic and metastatic xenograft models, IHC of 134 PDAC	Survival	-	[199]
ASPC-1, HS766t, BxPC-3	LIN28B	Positive, Direct	shRNA	LIN28B IHC expression high in PDAC, suppression inhibited proliferation and EMT	Colony formation, Proliferation, migration, IHC of 185 PDAC tumours	Survival, stage, metastasis	-	[110]

5. Conclusions

Overall, investigation of the fundamental biology of EMP aims to combat local and metastatic invasion by providing a better understanding of the processes that allow cancer cells to dissociate from their epithelial adhesions to spread. EMP is a prominent driver of PDAC progression, thus highlighting the importance of our understanding of the subtleties of its regulation. The ability of EMP programs to direct cancer cells towards a drug resistant and migratory lineage capable of seeding local and distant recurrence presents a significant barrier to current treatment regimens. Therefore, the identification of new candidate molecules regulating these processes are crucial to inform targeted therapies and provide insights into the vulnerabilities of heterogeneous populations of tumour cells present in PDAC.

It is clear from this ever-growing list of EMP effectors in PDAC cells alone, that much work remains to delineate their collective interactions within and beyond our current understanding on EMP signaling pathways. While candidates have been shown to play roles in aspects of EMP signaling and associated phenotypes, significant support is required for their mechanisms of action to make concrete conclusions about their directive actions in cancer. Our understanding of receptor mediated canonical signaling through PI3K/AKT, MAPK, NFκB and other well studied cell cycle pathways has required decades to tease apart, and the subtleties of EMP programs provides a similar challenge. Open source integrative tools such as Reactome [200], WikiPathways [201], String [202], and Cytoscape [203] provide platforms for researchers to combine such analyses to build upon our current understanding and fill knowledge gaps in the field of cancer biology. In this way, progress may be made to better understand and discover properties that may be modulated in concert to control EMP in cancer.

In vitro and xenograft tumour modelling and manipulation of target molecules often demonstrates a role in cancer cell migration and tumour formation, however stronger evidence for their physiological role in regulating EMP, metastasis and therapy resistance may require GEMMs. The use of *in vivo* manipulation of PDAC GEMM models using targeted CRISPR approaches may be such a route towards a system that better recapitulates the spontaneity and heterogeneity of human tumours [204].

Conflicts of Interest: The authors declare no conflict of interest.

References

1. Siegel, R.L.; Miller, K.D.; Jemal, A. Cancer statistics, 2019. *CA Cancer J. Clin.* **2019**, *69*, 7–34. [CrossRef] [PubMed]
2. Rahib, L.; Smith, B.D.; Aizenberg, R.; Rosenzweig, A.B.; Fleshman, J.M.; Matrisian, L.M. Projecting cancer incidence and deaths to 2030: The unexpected burden of thyroid, liver, and pancreas cancers in the united states. *Cancer Res.* **2014**, *74*, 2913–2921. [CrossRef] [PubMed]
3. Vogelstein, B.; Papadopoulos, N.; Velculescu, V.E.; Zhou, S.; Diaz, L.A., Jr.; Kinzler, K.W. Cancer genome landscapes. *Science* **2013**, *339*, 1546–1558. [CrossRef] [PubMed]
4. Weinstein, J.N.; Collisson, E.A.; Mills, G.B.; Shaw, K.R.; Ozenberger, B.A.; Ellrott, K.; Shmulevich, I.; Sander, C.; Stuart, J.M. The cancer genome atlas pan-cancer analysis project. *Nat. Genet.* **2013**, *45*, 1113–1120. [CrossRef]
5. Waddell, N.; Pajic, M.; Patch, A.M.; Chang, D.K.; Kassahn, K.S.; Bailey, P.; Johns, A.L.; Miller, D.; Nones, K.; Quek, K.; et al. Whole genomes redefine the mutational landscape of pancreatic cancer. *Nature* **2015**, *518*, 495–501. [CrossRef]
6. Bailey, P.; Chang, D.K.; Nones, K.; Johns, A.L.; Patch, A.-M.; Gingras, M.-C.; Miller, D.K.; Christ, A.N.; Bruxner, T.J.C.; Quinn, M.C.; et al. Genomic analyses identify molecular subtypes of pancreatic cancer. *Nature* **2016**, *531*, 47–52. [CrossRef]
7. Maitra, A.; Hruban, R.H. Pancreatic cancer. *Annu. Rev. Pathol.* **2008**, *3*, 157–188. [CrossRef]
8. Jones, S.; Zhang, X.; Parsons, D.W.; Lin, J.C.; Leary, R.J.; Angenendt, P.; Mankoo, P.; Carter, H.; Kamiyama, H.; Jimeno, A.; et al. Core signaling pathways in human pancreatic cancers revealed by global genomic analyses. *Science* **2008**, *321*, 1801–1806. [CrossRef]

9. Benjamin, J.; Hruban, H.R.R.; Aguirre, A.J.; Moffitt, R.A.; Yeh, J.J.; Chip, S.A.; Robertson, G.; Cherniack, A.D.; Gupta, M.; Getz, G.; et al. Integrated genomic characterization of pancreatic ductal adenocarcinoma. *Cancer Cell* **2017**, *32*, 185–203.e113. [CrossRef]
10. Hruban, R.H.; Maitra, A.; Schulick, R.; Laheru, D.; Herman, J.; Kern, S.E.; Goggins, M. Emerging molecular biology of pancreatic cancer. *Gastrointest. Cancer Res. GCR* **2008**, *2*, S10–S15.
11. Collisson, E.A.; Sadanandam, A.; Olson, P.; Gibb, W.J.; Truitt, M.; Gu, S.; Cooc, J.; Weinkle, J.; Kim, G.E.; Jakkula, L.; et al. Subtypes of pancreatic ductal adenocarcinoma and their differing responses to therapy. *Nat. Med.* **2011**, *17*, 500–503. [CrossRef] [PubMed]
12. Maurer, C.; Holmstrom, S.R.; He, J.; Laise, P.; Su, T.; Ahmed, A.; Hibshoosh, H.; Chabot, J.A.; Oberstein, P.E.; Sepulveda, A.R.; et al. Experimental microdissection enables functional harmonisation of pancreatic cancer subtypes. *Gut* **2019**, *68*, 1034–1043. [CrossRef] [PubMed]
13. Zhao, L.; Zhao, H.; Yan, H. Gene expression profiling of 1200 pancreatic ductal adenocarcinoma reveals novel subtypes. *BMC Cancer* **2018**, *18*, 603. [CrossRef] [PubMed]
14. Ligorio, M.; Sil, S.; Malagon-Lopez, J.; Nieman, L.T.; Misale, S.; Di Pilato, M.; Ebright, R.Y.; Karabacak, M.N.; Kulkarni, A.S.; Liu, A.; et al. Stromal microenvironment shapes the intratumoral architecture of pancreatic cancer. *Cell* **2019**, *178*, 160–175.e27. [CrossRef] [PubMed]
15. Peng, J.; Sun, B.-F.; Chen, C.-Y.; Zhou, J.-Y.; Chen, Y.-S.; Chen, H.; Liu, L.; Huang, D.; Jiang, J.; Cui, G.-S.; et al. Single-cell RNA-seq highlights intra-tumoral heterogeneity and malignant progression in pancreatic ductal adenocarcinoma. *Cell Res.* **2019**, *29*, 725–738. [CrossRef]
16. Moffitt, R.A.; Marayati, R.; Flate, E.L.; Volmar, K.E.; Loeza, S.G.H.; Hoadley, K.A.; Rashid, N.U.; Williams, L.A.; Eaton, S.C.; Chung, A.H.; et al. Virtual microdissection identifies distinct tumor- and stroma-specific subtypes of pancreatic ductal adenocarcinoma. *Nat. Genet.* **2015**, *47*, 1168–1178. [CrossRef]
17. Spivak-Kroizman, T.R.; Hostetter, G.; Posner, R.; Aziz, M.; Hu, C.; Demeure, M.J.; Von Hoff, D.; Hingorani, S.R.; Palculict, T.B.; Izzo, J.; et al. Hypoxia triggers hedgehog-mediated tumor-stromal interactions in pancreatic cancer. *Cancer Res.* **2013**, *73*, 3235–3247. [CrossRef]
18. Moir, J.A.; Mann, J.; White, S.A. The role of pancreatic stellate cells in pancreatic cancer. *Surg. Oncol.* **2015**, *24*, 232–238. [CrossRef]
19. Feig, C.; Gopinathan, A.; Neesse, A.; Chan, D.S.; Cook, N.; Tuveson, D.A. *The Pancreas Cancer Microenvironment*; AACR: Philadelphia, PA, USA, 2012.
20. Neesse, A.; Michl, P.; Frese, K.K.; Feig, C.; Cook, N.; Jacobetz, M.A.; Lolkema, M.P.; Buchholz, M.; Olive, K.P.; Gress, T.M. Stromal biology and therapy in pancreatic cancer. *Gut* **2011**, *60*, 861–868. [CrossRef]
21. Korc, M. Pancreatic cancer–associated stroma production. *Am. J. Surg.* **2007**, *194*, S84–S86. [CrossRef]
22. Hanahan, D.; Weinberg, R.A. Hallmarks of cancer: The next generation. *Cell* **2011**, *144*, 646–674. [CrossRef] [PubMed]
23. Xu, Z.; Pothula, S.P.; Wilson, J.S.; Apte, M.V. Pancreatic cancer and its stroma: A conspiracy theory. *World J. Gastroenterol. WJG* **2014**, *20*, 11216–11229. [CrossRef] [PubMed]
24. Mahadevan, D.; Von Hoff, D.D. Tumor-stroma interactions in pancreatic ductal adenocarcinoma. *Mol. Cancer Therap.* **2007**, *6*, 1186–1197. [CrossRef] [PubMed]
25. Thomas, D.; Radhakrishnan, P. Tumor-stromal crosstalk in pancreatic cancer and tissue fibrosis. *Mol. Cancer* **2019**, *18*, 14. [CrossRef] [PubMed]
26. Trelstad, R.L.; Hay, E.D.; Revel, J.D. Cell contact during early morphogenesis in the chick embryo. *Dev. Biol.* **1967**, *16*, 78–106. [CrossRef]
27. Huber, M.A.; Kraut, N.; Beug, H. Molecular requirements for epithelial-mesenchymal transition during tumor progression. *Curr. Opin. Cell Biol.* **2005**, *17*, 548–558. [CrossRef]
28. Tsai, J.H.; Yang, J. Epithelial-mesenchymal plasticity in carcinoma metastasis. *Genes Dev.* **2013**, *27*, 2192–2206. [CrossRef]
29. Giovannetti, E.; van der Borden, C.L.; Frampton, A.E.; Ali, A.; Firuzi, O.; Peters, G.J. Never let it go: Stopping key mechanisms underlying metastasis to fight pancreatic cancer. *Semin. Cancer Biol.* **2017**, *44*, 43–59. [CrossRef]
30. Du, Y.X.; Liu, Z.W.; You, L.; Wu, W.M.; Zhao, Y.P. Advances in understanding the molecular mechanism of pancreatic cancer metastasis. *Hepatobiliary Pancreat. Dis. Int.* **2016**, *15*, 361–370. [CrossRef]

31. Beuran, M.; Negoi, I.; Paun, S.; Ion, A.D.; Bleotu, C.; Negoi, R.I.; Hostiuc, S. The epithelial to mesenchymal transition in pancreatic cancer: A systematic review. *Pancreatol. Off. J. Int. Assoc. Pancreatol.* **2015**, *15*, 217–225. [CrossRef]
32. Satoh, K.; Hamada, S.; Shimosegawa, T. Involvement of epithelial to mesenchymal transition in the development of pancreatic ductal adenocarcinoma. *J. Gastroenterol.* **2015**, *50*, 140–146. [CrossRef] [PubMed]
33. Hamada, S.; Satoh, K.; Masamune, A.; Shimosegawa, T. Regulators of epithelial mesenchymal transition in pancreatic cancer. *Front. Physiol.* **2012**, *3*, 254. [CrossRef] [PubMed]
34. Bailey, J.M.; Leach, S.D. Signaling pathways mediating epithelial-mesenchymal crosstalk in pancreatic cancer: Hedgehog, Notch and TGFBeta. In *Pancreatic Cancer and Tumor Microenvironment*; Grippo, P.J., Munshi, H.G., Eds.; Transworld Research Network: Trivandrum, India, 2012.
35. Dangi-Garimella, S.; Krantz, S.B.; Shields, M.A.; Grippo, P.J.; Munshi, H.G. Epithelial-mesenchymal transition and pancreatic cancer progression. In *Pancreatic Cancer and Tumor Microenvironment*; Grippo, P.J., Munshi, H.G., Eds.; Transworld Research Network: Trivandrum, India, 2012.
36. Chaffer, C.L.; San Juan, B.P.; Lim, E.; Weinberg, R.A. EMT, cell plasticity and metastasis. *Cancer Metastasis Rev.* **2016**, *35*, 645–654. [CrossRef] [PubMed]
37. Trager, M.M.; Dhayat, S.A. Epigenetics of epithelial-to-mesenchymal transition in pancreatic carcinoma. *Int. J. Cancer* **2017**, *141*, 24–32. [CrossRef] [PubMed]
38. Elaskalani, O.; Razak, N.B.; Falasca, M.; Metharom, P. Epithelial-mesenchymal transition as a therapeutic target for overcoming chemoresistance in pancreatic cancer. *World J. Gastrointest. Oncol.* **2017**, *9*, 37–41. [CrossRef] [PubMed]
39. Gaianigo, N.; Melisi, D.; Carbone, C. EMT and treatment resistance in pancreatic cancer. *Cancers* **2017**, *9*, 122. [CrossRef]
40. Ishiwata, T. Cancer stem cells and epithelial-mesenchymal transition: Novel therapeutic targets for cancer. *Pathol. Int.* **2016**, *66*, 601–608. [CrossRef] [PubMed]
41. Kyuno, D.; Yamaguchi, H.; Ito, T.; Kono, T.; Kimura, Y.; Imamura, M.; Konno, T.; Hirata, K.; Sawada, N.; Kojima, T. Targeting tight junctions during epithelial to mesenchymal transition in human pancreatic cancer. *World J. Gastroenterol. WJG* **2014**, *20*, 10813–10824. [CrossRef]
42. Shibue, T. EMT, CSCs, and drug resistance: The mechanistic link and clinical implications. *Nat. Rev. Clin. Oncol.* **2017**, *14*, 611–629. [CrossRef]
43. Hawa, Z.; Haque, I.; Ghosh, A.; Banerjee, S.; Harris, L.; Banerjee, S.K. The miRacle in pancreatic cancer by miRNAs: Tiny angels or devils in disease progression. *Int. J. Mol. Sci.* **2016**, *17*, 809. [CrossRef]
44. Brabletz, S.; Brabletz, T. The ZEB/miR-200 feedback loop—A motor of cellular plasticity in development and cancer? *EMBO Rep.* **2010**, *11*, 670–677. [CrossRef] [PubMed]
45. Rhim, A.D. Epithelial to mesenchymal transition and the generation of stem-like cells in pancreatic cancer. *Pancreatology* **2013**, *13*, 114–117. [CrossRef] [PubMed]
46. Zhan, H.X.; Xu, J.W.; Wu, D.; Zhang, T.P.; Hu, S.Y. Pancreatic cancer stem cells: New insight into a stubborn disease. *Cancer Lett.* **2015**, *357*, 429–437. [CrossRef] [PubMed]
47. Vaz, A.P.; Ponnusamy, M.P.; Seshacharyulu, P.; Batra, S.K. A concise review on the current understanding of pancreatic cancer stem cells. *J. Cancer Stem Cell Res.* **2014**, *2*, e1004. [CrossRef] [PubMed]
48. Castellanos, J.A.; Merchant, N.B.; Nagathihalli, N.S. Emerging targets in pancreatic cancer: Epithelial-mesenchymal transition and cancer stem cells. *Onco Targets Ther.* **2013**, *6*, 1261–1267. [CrossRef] [PubMed]
49. Karamitopoulou, E. Tumor budding cells, cancer stem cells and epithelial-mesenchymal transition-type cells in pancreatic cancer. *Front. Oncol.* **2012**, *2*, 209. [CrossRef]
50. Chuai, G.; Yang, F.; Yan, J.; Chen, Y.; Ma, Q.; Zhou, C.; Zhu, C.; Gu, F.; Liu, Q. Deciphering relationship between microhomology and in-frame mutation occurrence in human CRISPR-based gene knockout. *Mol. Ther. Nucleic Acids* **2016**, *5*, e323. [CrossRef]
51. Nguyen, D.X.; Bos, P.D.; Massague, J. Metastasis: from dissemination to organ-specific colonization. *Nat Rev Cancer* **2009**, *9*, 274–284. [CrossRef]
52. Nieto, J.; Grossbard, M.L.; Kozuch, P. Metastatic pancreatic cancer 2008: Is the glass less empty? *Oncologist* **2008**, *13*, 562–576. [CrossRef]

53. Schmalhofer, O.; Brabletz, S.; Brabletz, T. E-cadherin, beta-catenin, and ZEB1 in malignant progression of cancer. *Cancer Metastasis Rev.* **2009**, *28*, 151–166. [CrossRef]
54. Nakajima, S.; Doi, R.; Toyoda, E.; Tsuji, S.; Wada, M.; Koizumi, M.; Tulachan, S.S.; Ito, D.; Kami, K.; Mori, T.; et al. N-cadherin expression and epithelial-mesenchymal transition in pancreatic carcinoma. *Clin. Cancer Res. Off. J. Am. Assoc. Cancer Res.* **2004**, *10*, 4125–4133. [CrossRef] [PubMed]
55. Peinado, H.; Portillo, F.; Cano, A. Transcriptional regulation of cadherins during development and carcinogenesis. *Int. J. Dev. Biol.* **2004**, *48*, 365–375. [CrossRef] [PubMed]
56. Hotz, B.; Arndt, M.; Dullat, S.; Bhargava, S.; Buhr, H.J.; Hotz, H.G. Epithelial to mesenchymal transition: Expression of the regulators snail, slug, and twist in pancreatic cancer. *Clin. Cancer Res. Off. J. Am. Assoc. Cancer Res.* **2007**, *13*, 4769–4776. [CrossRef] [PubMed]
57. Brabletz, T.; Jung, A.; Reu, S.; Porzner, M.; Hlubek, F.; Kunz-Schughart, L.A.; Knuechel, R.; Kirchner, T. Variable beta-catenin expression in colorectal cancers indicates tumor progression driven by the tumor environment. *Proc. Natl. Acad. Sci. USA* **2001**, *98*, 10356–10361. [CrossRef]
58. Joo, Y.E.; Rew, J.S.; Park, C.S.; Kim, S.J. Expression of E-cadherin, alpha- and beta-catenins in patients with pancreatic adenocarcinoma. *Pancreatol. Off. J. Int. Assoc. Pancreatol.* **2002**, *2*, 129–137. [CrossRef]
59. Yin, T.; Wang, C.; Liu, T.; Zhao, G.; Zha, Y.; Yang, M. Expression of snail in pancreatic cancer promotes metastasis and chemoresistance. *J. Surg. Res.* **2007**, *141*, 196–203. [CrossRef]
60. Oida, Y.; Yamazaki, H.; Tobita, K.; Mukai, M.; Ohtani, Y.; Miyazaki, N.; Abe, Y.; Imaizumi, T.; Makuuchi, H.; Ueyama, Y.; et al. Increased S100A4 expression combined with decreased E-cadherin expression predicts a poor outcome of patients with pancreatic cancer. *Oncol. Rep.* **2006**, *16*, 457–463. [CrossRef]
61. Javle, M.M.; Gibbs, J.F.; Iwata, K.K.; Pak, Y.; Rutledge, P.; Yu, J.; Black, J.D.; Tan, D.; Khoury, T. Epithelial-mesenchymal transition (EMT) and activated extracellular signal-regulated kinase (p-Erk) in surgically resected pancreatic cancer. *Ann. Surg. Oncol.* **2007**, *14*, 3527–3533. [CrossRef]
62. Yamada, S.; Fuchs, B.C.; Fujii, T.; Shimoyama, Y.; Sugimoto, H.; Nomoto, S.; Takeda, S.; Tanabe, K.K.; Kodera, Y.; Nakao, A. Epithelial-to-mesenchymal transition predicts prognosis of pancreatic cancer. *Surgery* **2013**, *154*, 946–954. [CrossRef]
63. Wang, J.; Nikhil, K.; Viccaro, K.; Chang, L.; Jacobsen, M.; Sandusky, G.; Shah, K. The Aurora-A-Twist1 axis promotes highly aggressive phenotypes in pancreatic carcinoma. *J. Cell Sci.* **2017**, *130*, 1078–1093. [CrossRef]
64. Wang, Z.; Zhao, L.; Xiao, Y.; Gao, Y.; Zhao, C. Snail transcript levels in diagnosis of pancreatic carcinoma with fine-needle aspirate. *Br. J. Biomed. Sci.* **2015**, *72*, 107–110. [CrossRef] [PubMed]
65. Yamazaki, K.; Masugi, Y.; Effendi, K.; Tsujikawa, H.; Hiraoka, N.; Kitago, M.; Shinoda, M.; Itano, O.; Tanabe, M.; Kitagawa, Y.; et al. Upregulated SMAD3 promotes epithelial-mesenchymal transition and predicts poor prognosis in pancreatic ductal adenocarcinoma. *Lab. Investig. J. Tech. Methods Pathol.* **2014**, *94*, 683–691. [CrossRef] [PubMed]
66. Masugi, Y.; Yamazaki, K.; Hibi, T.; Aiura, K.; Kitagawa, Y.; Sakamoto, M. Solitary cell infiltration is a novel indicator of poor prognosis and epithelial-mesenchymal transition in pancreatic cancer. *Hum. Pathol.* **2010**, *41*, 1061–1068. [CrossRef] [PubMed]
67. Galvan, J.A.; Zlobec, I.; Wartenberg, M.; Lugli, A.; Gloor, B.; Perren, A.; Karamitopoulou, E. Expression of E-cadherin repressors SNAIL, ZEB1 and ZEB2 by tumour and stromal cells influences tumour-budding phenotype and suggests heterogeneity of stromal cells in pancreatic cancer. *Br. J. Cancer* **2015**, *112*, 1944–1950. [CrossRef] [PubMed]
68. Tarin, D.; Thompson, E.W.; Newgreen, D.F. The fallacy of epithelial mesenchymal transition in neoplasia. *Cancer Res.* **2005**, *65*, 5996–6000. [CrossRef]
69. Ledford, H. Cancer theory faces doubts. *Nature* **2011**, *472*, 273. [CrossRef]
70. Rhim, A.D.; Mirek, E.T.; Aiello, N.M.; Maitra, A.; Bailey, J.M.; McAllister, F.; Reichert, M.; Beatty, G.L.; Rustgi, A.K.; Vonderheide, R.H.; et al. EMT and dissemination precede pancreatic tumor formation. *Cell* **2012**, *148*, 349–361. [CrossRef]
71. Zheng, X.; Carstens, J.L.; Kim, J.; Scheible, M.; Kaye, J.; Sugimoto, H.; Wu, C.C.; LeBleu, V.S.; Kalluri, R. Epithelial-to-mesenchymal transition is dispensable for metastasis but induces chemoresistance in pancreatic cancer. *Nature* **2015**, *527*, 525–530. [CrossRef]

72. Aiello, N.M.; Brabletz, T.; Kang, Y.; Nieto, M.A.; Weinberg, R.A.; Stanger, B.Z. Upholding a role for EMT in pancreatic cancer metastasis. *Nature* **2017**, *547*, E7–E8. [CrossRef]
73. Krebs, A.M.; Mitschke, J.; Lasierra Losada, M.; Schmalhofer, O.; Boerries, M.; Busch, H.; Boettcher, M.; Mougiakakos, D.; Reichardt, W.; Bronsert, P.; et al. The EMT-activator Zeb1 is a key factor for cell plasticity and promotes metastasis in pancreatic cancer. *Nat. Cell Biol.* **2017**, *19*, 518–529. [CrossRef]
74. Chen, Y.; LeBleu, V.S.; Carstens, J.L.; Sugimoto, H.; Zheng, X.; Malasi, S.; Saur, D.; Kalluri, R. Dual reporter genetic mouse models of pancreatic cancer identify an epithelial-to-mesenchymal transition-independent metastasis program. *EMBO Mol. Med.* **2018**, *10*, e9085. [CrossRef] [PubMed]
75. Thompson, E.W.; Nagaraj, S.H. Transition states that allow cancer to spread. *Nature* **2018**, *556*, 442–444. [CrossRef] [PubMed]
76. Pastushenko, I.; Brisebarre, A.; Sifrim, A.; Fioramonti, M.; Revenco, T.; Boumahdi, S.; Van Keymeulen, A.; Brown, D.; Moers, V.; Lemaire, S.; et al. Identification of the tumour transition states occurring during EMT. *Nature* **2018**, *556*, 463–468. [CrossRef] [PubMed]
77. Pastushenko, I.; Blanpain, C. EMT Transition states during tumor progression and metastasis. *Trends Cell Biol.* **2019**, *29*, 212–226. [CrossRef] [PubMed]
78. Brabletz, S.; Brabletz, T.; Stemmler, M.P. Road to perdition: Zeb1-dependent and -independent ways to metastasis. *Cell Cycle* **2017**, *16*, 1729–1730. [CrossRef] [PubMed]
79. Lamouille, S.; Xu, J.; Derynck, R. Molecular mechanisms of epithelial–mesenchymal transition. *Nat. Rev. Mol. Cell Biol.* **2014**, *15*, 178–196. [CrossRef] [PubMed]
80. Gonzalez, D.M.; Medici, D. Signaling mechanisms of the epithelial-mesenchymal transition. *Sci. Signal.* **2014**, *7*, re8. [CrossRef]
81. David, C.J.; Huang, Y.-H.; Chen, M.; Su, J.; Zou, Y.; Bardeesy, N.; Iacobuzio-Donahue, C.A.; Massagué, J. TGF-β Tumor Suppression through a Lethal EMT. *Cell* **2016**, *164*, 1015–1030. [CrossRef]
82. Glazer, E.S.; Welsh, E.; Pimiento, J.M.; Teer, J.K.; Malafa, M.P. TGFβ1 overexpression is associated with improved survival and low tumor cell proliferation in patients with early-stage pancreatic ductal adenocarcinoma. *Oncotarget* **2017**, *8*, 999. [CrossRef]
83. Rowland-Goldsmith, M.A.; Maruyama, H.; Kusama, T.; Ralli, S.; Korc, M. Soluble type II transforming growth factor-beta (TGF-beta) receptor inhibits TGF-beta signaling in COLO-357 pancreatic cancer cells in vitro and attenuates tumor formation. *Clin. Cancer Res. Off. J. Am. Assoc. Cancer Res.* **2001**, *7*, 2931–2940.
84. Wagner, M.; Kleeff, J.; Friess, H.; Buchler, M.W.; Korc, M. Enhanced expression of the type II transforming growth factor-beta receptor is associated with decreased survival in human pancreatic cancer. *Pancreas* **1999**, *19*, 370–376. [CrossRef] [PubMed]
85. Chuvin, N.; Vincent, D.F.; Pommier, R.M.; Alcaraz, L.B.; Gout, J.; Caligaris, C.; Yacoub, K.; Cardot, V.; Roger, E.; Kaniewski, B.; et al. Acinar-to-Ductal Metaplasia Induced by Transforming Growth Factor Beta Facilitates KRAS(G12D)-driven Pancreatic Tumorigenesis. *Cell. Mol. Gastroenterol. Hepatol.* **2017**, *4*, 263–282. [CrossRef] [PubMed]
86. Subramanian, G.; Schwarz, R.E.; Higgins, L.; McEnroe, G.; Chakravarty, S.; Dugar, S.; Reiss, M. Targeting endogenous transforming growth factor beta receptor signaling in SMAD4-deficient human pancreatic carcinoma cells inhibits their invasive phenotype1. *Cancer Res.* **2004**, *64*, 5200–5211. [CrossRef] [PubMed]
87. Janda, E.; Lehmann, K.; Killisch, I.; Jechlinger, M.; Herzig, M.; Downward, J.; Beug, H.; Grunert, S. Ras and TGF[beta] cooperatively regulate epithelial cell plasticity and metastasis: Dissection of Ras signaling pathways. *J. Cell Biol.* **2002**, *156*, 299–313. [CrossRef] [PubMed]
88. Al-Ismaeel, Q.; Neal, C.P.; Al-Mahmoodi, H.; Almutairi, Z.; Al-Shamarti, I.; Straatman, K.; Jaunbocus, N.; Irvine, A.; Issa, E.; Moreman, C.; et al. ZEB1 and IL-6/11-STAT3 signaling cooperate to define invasive potential of pancreatic cancer cells via differential regulation of the expression of S100 proteins. *Br. J. Cancer* **2019**, *121*, 65–75. [CrossRef] [PubMed]
89. Ram Makena, M.; Gatla, H.; Verlekar, D.; Sukhavasi, S.; Pandey, M.K.; Pramanik, K.C. Wnt/beta-Catenin signaling: The culprit in pancreatic carcinogenesis and therapeutic resistance. *Int. J. Mol. Sci.* **2019**, *20*, 4242. [CrossRef]
90. Witte, D.; Otterbein, H.; Forster, M.; Giehl, K.; Zeiser, R.; Lehnert, H.; Ungefroren, H. Negative regulation of TGF-beta1-induced MKK6-p38 and MEK-ERK signaling and epithelial-mesenchymal transition by Rac1b. *Sci. Rep.* **2017**, *7*, 17313. [CrossRef]

91. Wang, G.; Yu, Y.; Sun, C.; Liu, T.; Liang, T.; Zhan, L.; Lin, X.; Feng, X.H. STAT3 selectively interacts with Smad3 to antagonize TGF-beta signaling. *Oncogene* **2016**, *35*, 4388–4398. [CrossRef]
92. Sheng, W.; Chen, C.; Dong, M.; Wang, G.; Zhou, J.; Song, H.; Li, Y.; Zhang, J.; Ding, S. Calreticulin promotes EGF-induced EMT in pancreatic cancer cells via Integrin/EGFR-ERK/MAPK signaling pathway. *Cell Death Dis.* **2017**, *8*, e3147. [CrossRef]
93. Witte, D.; Bartscht, T.; Kaufmann, R.; Pries, R.; Settmacher, U.; Lehnert, H.; Ungefroren, H. TGF-beta1-induced cell migration in pancreatic carcinoma cells is RAC1 and NOX4-dependent and requires RAC1 and NOX4-dependent activation of p38 MAPK. *Oncol. Rep.* **2017**, *38*, 3693–3701. [CrossRef]
94. Kumar, K.; Chow, C.R.; Ebine, K.; Arslan, A.D.; Kwok, B.; Bentrem, D.J.; Eckerdt, F.D.; Platanias, L.C.; Munshi, H.G. Differential regulation of ZEB1 and EMT by MAPK-interacting protein Kinases (MNK) and eIF4E in pancreatic cancer. *Mol. Cancer Res. MCR* **2016**, *14*, 216–227. [CrossRef] [PubMed]
95. Yang, A.D.; Camp, E.R.; Fan, F.; Shen, L.; Gray, M.J.; Liu, W.; Somcio, R.; Bauer, T.W.; Wu, Y.; Hicklin, D.J.; et al. Vascular endothelial growth factor receptor-1 activation mediates epithelial to mesenchymal transition in human pancreatic carcinoma cells. *Cancer Res.* **2006**, *66*, 46–51. [CrossRef] [PubMed]
96. Wang, Y.; Jin, G.; Li, Q.; Wang, Z.; Hu, W.; Li, P.; Li, S.; Wu, H.; Kong, X.; Gao, J.; et al. Hedgehog Signaling non-canonical activated by pro-inflammatory cytokines in pancreatic ductal adenocarcinoma. *J. Cancer* **2016**, *7*, 2067–2076. [CrossRef] [PubMed]
97. Huang, H.; Svoboda, R.A.; Lazenby, A.J.; Saowapa, J.; Chaika, N.; Ding, K.; Wheelock, M.J.; Johnson, K.R. Up-regulation of N-cadherin by collagen i-activated discoidin domain receptor 1 in pancreatic cancer requires the adaptor molecule Shc1. *J. Biol. Chem.* **2016**, *291*, 23208–23223. [CrossRef] [PubMed]
98. Zhu, H.; Qin, H.; Li, D.M.; Liu, J.; Zhao, Q. Effect of PPM1H on malignant phenotype of human pancreatic cancer cells. *Oncol. Rep.* **2016**, *36*, 2926–2934. [CrossRef]
99. Ellenrieder, V.; Hendler, S.F.; Boeck, W.; Activation, S.-R.K.; Seufferlein, T.; Menke, A.; Ruhland, C.; Adler, G.; Gress, T.M. Transforming growth factor β 1 treatment leads to an epithelial-mesenchymal transdifferentiation of pancreatic cancer cells requiring extracellular signal-regulated kinase 2 activation. *Cancer Res.* **2001**, *61*, 4222–4228.
100. Buonato, J.M.; Lan, I.S.; Lazzara, M.J. EGF augments TGFBeta-induced epithelial-mesenchymal transition by promoting SHP2 binding to GAB1. *J. Cell Sci.* **2015**, *128*, 3898–3909. [CrossRef]
101. Maier, H.J.; Schmidt-Strassburger, U.; Huber, M.A.; Wiedemann, E.M.; Beug, H.; Wirth, T. NF-kappaB promotes epithelial-mesenchymal transition, migration and invasion of pancreatic carcinoma cells. *Cancer Lett.* **2010**, *295*, 214–228. [CrossRef]
102. Oyanagi, J.; Kojima, N.; Sato, H.; Higashi, S.; Kikuchi, K.; Sakai, K.; Matsumoto, K.; Miyazaki, K. Inhibition of transforming growth factor-beta signaling potentiates tumor cell invasion into collagen matrix induced by fibroblast-derived hepatocyte growth factor. *Exp. Cell Res.* **2014**, *326*, 267–279. [CrossRef]
103. Wajant, H.; Pfizenmaier, K.; Scheurich, P. Tumor necrosis factor signaling. *Cell Death Differ.* **2003**, *10*, 45–65. [CrossRef]
104. Xu, J.; Lamouille, S.; Derynck, R. TGF-β-induced epithelial to mesenchymal transition. *Cell Res.* **2009**, *19*, 156–172. [CrossRef] [PubMed]
105. Liu, M.; Quek, L.E.; Sultani, G.; Turner, N. Epithelial-mesenchymal transition induction is associated with augmented glucose uptake and lactate production in pancreatic ductal adenocarcinoma. *Cancer Metab.* **2016**, *4*, 19. [CrossRef] [PubMed]
106. Gao, S.; Sun, Y.; Zhang, X.; Hu, L.; Liu, Y.; Chua, C.Y.; Phillips, L.M.; Ren, H.; Fleming, J.B.; Wang, H.; et al. IGFBP2 Activates the NF-kappaB Pathway to Drive Epithelial-Mesenchymal Transition and Invasive Character in Pancreatic Ductal Adenocarcinoma. *Cancer Res* **2016**, *76*, 6543–6554. [CrossRef] [PubMed]
107. Masugi, Y.; Yamazaki, K.; Emoto, K.; Effendi, K.; Tsujikawa, H.; Kitago, M.; Itano, O.; Kitagawa, Y.; Sakamoto, M. Upregulation of integrin beta4 promotes epithelial-mesenchymal transition and is a novel prognostic marker in pancreatic ductal adenocarcinoma. *Lab. Investig. J. Tech. Methods Pathol.* **2015**, *95*, 308–319. [CrossRef]
108. Chen, J.; Li, Q.; An, Y.; Lv, N.; Xue, X.; Wei, J.; Jiang, K.; Wu, J.; Gao, W.; Qian, Z.; et al. CEACAM6 induces epithelial-mesenchymal transition and mediates invasion and metastasis in pancreatic cancer. *Int. J. Oncol.* **2013**, *43*, 877–885. [CrossRef]

109. Ottaviani, S.; Stebbing, J.; Frampton, A.E.; Zagorac, S.; Krell, J.; de Giorgio, A.; Trabulo, S.M.; Nguyen, V.T.M.; Magnani, L.; Feng, H.; et al. TGF-β induces miR-100 and miR-125b but blocks let-7a through LIN28B controlling PDAC progression. *Nat. Commun.* **2018**, *9*. [CrossRef]
110. Wang, Y.; Li, J.; Guo, S.; Ouyang, Y.; Yin, L.; Liu, S.; Zhao, Z.; Yang, J.; Huang, W.; Qin, H.; et al. Lin28B facilitates the progression and metastasis of pancreatic ductal adenocarcinoma. *Oncotarget* **2017**, *8*, 60414–60428. [CrossRef]
111. Guo, Q.; Qin, W. DKK3 blocked translocation of beta-catenin/EMT induced by hypoxia and improved gemcitabine therapeutic effect in pancreatic cancer Bxpc-3 cell. *J. Cell. Mol. Med.* **2015**, *19*, 2832–2841. [CrossRef]
112. Kim, Y.R.; Park, M.K.; Kang, G.J.; Kim, H.J.; Kim, E.J.; Byun, H.J.; Lee, M.Y.; Lee, C.H. Leukotriene B4 induces EMT and vimentin expression in PANC-1 pancreatic cancer cells: Involvement of BLT2 via ERK2 activation. *Prostaglandins Leukotrienes Essential Fatty Acids* **2016**, *115*, 67–76. [CrossRef]
113. Huang, C.; Xiang, Y.; Chen, S.; Yu, H.; Wen, Z.; Ye, T.; Sun, H.; Kong, H.; Li, D.; Yu, D.; et al. DMKN contributes to the epithelial-mesenchymal transition through increased activation of STAT3 in pancreatic cancer. *Cancer Sci.* **2017**, *108*, 2130–2141. [CrossRef]
114. Tang, D.; Zhang, J.; Yuan, Z.; Zhang, H.; Chong, Y.; Huang, Y.; Wang, J.; Xiong, Q.; Wang, S.; Wu, Q.; et al. PSC-derived Galectin-1 inducing epithelial-mesenchymal transition of pancreatic ductal adenocarcinoma cells by activating the NF-kappaB pathway. *Oncotarget* **2017**, *8*, 86488–86502. [CrossRef] [PubMed]
115. Xu, X.; Zhao, Z.; Guo, S.; Li, J.; Liu, S.; You, Y.; Ni, B.; Wang, H.; Bie, P. Increased semaphorin 3c expression promotes tumor growth and metastasis in pancreatic ductal adenocarcinoma by activating the ERK1/2 signaling pathway. *Cancer Lett.* **2017**, *397*, 12–22. [CrossRef] [PubMed]
116. Zhan, L.; Chen, L.; Chen, Z. Knockdown of FUT3 disrupts the proliferation, migration, tumorigenesis and TGF-β induced EMT in pancreatic cancer cells. *Oncol. Lett.* **2018**, *16*, 924–930. [CrossRef]
117. Yang, S.; He, P.; Wang, J.; Schetter, A.; Tang, W.; Funamizu, N.; Yanaga, K.; Uwagawa, T.; Satoskar, A.R.; Gaedcke, J.; et al. A Novel MIF signaling pathway drives the malignant character of pancreatic cancer by targeting NR3C2. *Cancer Res.* **2016**, *76*, 3838–3850. [CrossRef] [PubMed]
118. Bo, H.; Zhang, S.; Gao, L.; Chen, Y.; Zhang, J.; Chang, X.; Zhu, M. Upregulation of Wnt5a promotes epithelial-to-mesenchymal transition and metastasis of pancreatic cancer cells. *BMC Cancer* **2013**, *13*, 496. [CrossRef]
119. Xu, B.; Jin, D.Y.; Lou, W.H.; Wang, D.S. Lipocalin-2 is associated with a good prognosis and reversing epithelial-to-mesenchymal transition in pancreatic cancer. *World J. Surg.* **2013**, *37*, 1892–1900. [CrossRef]
120. Cui, L.; Xie, R.; Dang, S.; Zhang, Q.; Mao, S.; Chen, J.; Qu, J.; Zhang, J. NOV promoted the growth and migration of pancreatic cancer cells. *Tumor Biol.* **2014**, *35*, 3195–3201. [CrossRef]
121. Meng, F.; Li, W.; Li, C.; Gao, Z.; Guo, K.; Song, S. CCL18 promotes epithelial-mesenchymal transition, invasion and migration of pancreatic cancer cells in pancreatic ductal adenocarcinoma. *Int. J. Oncol.* **2015**, *46*, 1109–1120. [CrossRef]
122. Zhou, B.; Zhan, H.; Tin, L.; Liu, S.; Xu, J.; Dong, Y.; Li, X.; Wu, L.; Guo, W. TUFT1 regulates metastasis of pancreatic cancer through HIF1-Snail pathway induced epithelial-mesenchymal transition. *Cancer Lett.* **2016**, *382*, 11–20. [CrossRef]
123. Zhang, J.; Zhang, L.; Li, C.; Yang, C.; Li, L.; Song, S.; Wu, H.; Liu, F.; Wang, L.; Gu, J. LOX-1 is a poor prognostic indicator and induces epithelial-mesenchymal transition and metastasis in pancreatic cancer patients. *Cell. Oncol. (Dordr.)* **2017**, *41*, 73–84. [CrossRef]
124. Park, J.S.; Lee, J.H.; Lee, Y.S.; Kim, J.K.; Dong, S.M.; Yoon, D.S. Emerging role of LOXL2 in the promotion of pancreas cancer metastasis. *Oncotarget* **2016**, *7*, 42539–42552. [CrossRef] [PubMed]
125. Yamaguchi, J.; Yokoyama, Y.; Kokuryo, T.; Ebata, T.; Enomoto, A.; Nagino, M. Trefoil factor 1 inhibits epithelial-mesenchymal transition of pancreatic intraepithelial neoplasm. *J. Clin. Investig.* **2018**, *128*, 3619–3629. [CrossRef] [PubMed]
126. Gurbuz, N.; Ashour, A.A.; Alpay, S.N.; Ozpolat, B. Down-regulation of 5-HT1B and 5-HT1D receptors inhibits proliferation, clonogenicity and invasion of human pancreatic cancer cells. *PLoS ONE* **2014**, *9*, e110067. [CrossRef] [PubMed]

127. Subramani, R.; Lopez-Valdez, R.; Arumugam, A.; Nandy, S.; Boopalan, T.; Lakshmanaswamy, R. Targeting insulin-like growth factor 1 receptor inhibits pancreatic cancer growth and metastasis. *PLoS ONE* **2014**, *9*, e97016. [CrossRef]
128. Wang, F.; Ma, L.; Zhang, Z.; Liu, X.; Gao, H.; Zhuang, Y.; Yang, P.; Kornmann, M.; Tian, X.; Yang, Y. Hedgehog signaling regulates epithelial-mesenchymal transition in pancreatic cancer stem-like cells. *J. Cancer* **2016**, *7*, 408–417. [CrossRef]
129. Liu, C.; Huang, H.; Wang, C.; Kong, Y.; Zhang, H. Involvement of ephrin receptor A4 in pancreatic cancer cell motility and invasion. *Oncol. Lett.* **2014**, *7*, 2165–2169. [CrossRef]
130. Tekin, C.; Shi, K.; Daalhuisen, J.B.; Ten Brink, M.S.; Bijlsma, M.F.; Spek, C.A. PAR1 signaling on tumor cells limits tumor growth by maintaining a mesenchymal phenotype in pancreatic cancer. *Oncotarget* **2018**, *9*, 32010–32023. [CrossRef]
131. Miura, S.; Hamada, S.; Masamune, A.; Satoh, K.; Shimosegawa, T. CUB-domain containing protein 1 represses the epithelial phenotype of pancreatic cancer cells. *Exp. Cell Res.* **2014**, *321*, 209–218. [CrossRef]
132. Muniyan, S.; Haridas, D.; Chugh, S.; Rachagani, S.; Lakshmanan, I.; Gupta, S.; Seshacharyulu, P.; Smith, L.M.; Ponnusamy, M.P.; Batra, S.K. MUC16 contributes to the metastasis of pancreatic ductal adenocarcinoma through focal adhesion mediated signaling mechanism. *Genes Cancer* **2016**, *7*, 110–124. [CrossRef]
133. Belvedere, R.; Bizzarro, V.; Forte, G.; Dal Piaz, F.; Parente, L.; Petrella, A. Annexin A1 contributes to pancreatic cancer cell phenotype, behaviour and metastatic potential independently of Formyl Peptide Receptor pathway. *Sci. Rep.* **2016**, *6*, 29660. [CrossRef]
134. Belvedere, R.; Saggese, P.; Pessolano, E.; Memoli, D.; Bizzarro, V.; Rizzo, F.; Parente, L.; Weisz, A.; Petrella, A. miR-196a Is able to restore the aggressive phenotype of annexin a1 knock-out in pancreatic cancer cells by CRISPR/Cas9 genome editing. *Int. J. Mol. Sci.* **2018**, *19*, 1967. [CrossRef] [PubMed]
135. Zheng, B.; Ohuchida, K.; Cui, L.; Zhao, M.; Shindo, K.; Fujiwara, K.; Manabe, T.; Torata, N.; Moriyama, T.; Miyasaka, Y.; et al. TM4SF1 as a prognostic marker of pancreatic ductal adenocarcinoma is involved in migration and invasion of cancer cells. *Int. J. Oncol.* **2015**, *47*, 490–498. [CrossRef] [PubMed]
136. Ye, C.; Tian, X.; Yue, G.; Yan, L.; Guan, X.; Wang, S.; Hao, C. Suppression of CD26 inhibits growth and metastasis of pancreatic cancer. *Tumour Biol* **2016**, *37*, 15677–15686. [CrossRef] [PubMed]
137. Liu, M.; Yang, J.; Zhang, Y.; Zhou, Z.; Cui, X.; Zhang, L.; Fung, K.M.; Zheng, W.; Allard, F.D.; Yee, E.U.; et al. ZIP4 promotes pancreatic cancer progression by repressing ZO-1 and claudin-1 through a ZEB1-dependent transcriptional mechanism. *Clin. Cancer Res. Off. J. Am. Assoc. Cancer Res.* **2018**, *24*, 3186–3196. [CrossRef]
138. Huang, S. WAVE3 promotes proliferation, migration and invasion via the AKT pathway in pancreatic cancer. *Int. J. Oncol.* **2018**, *53*, 672–684. [CrossRef]
139. Su, H.T.; Weng, C.C.; Hsiao, P.J.; Chen, L.H.; Kuo, T.L.; Chen, Y.W.; Kuo, K.K.; Cheng, K.H. Stem cell marker nestin is critical for TGF-beta1-mediated tumor progression in pancreatic cancer. *Mol. Cancer Res. MCR* **2013**, *11*, 768–779. [CrossRef]
140. Hagio, M.; Matsuda, Y.; Suzuki, T.; Ishiwata, T. Nestin regulates epithelial-mesenchymal transition marker expression in pancreatic ductal adenocarcinoma cell lines. *Mol. Clin. Oncol.* **2013**, *1*, 83–87. [CrossRef]
141. Razidlo, G.L.; Wang, Y.; Chen, J.; Krueger, E.W.; Billadeau, D.D.; McNiven, M.A. Dynamin 2 potentiates invasive migration of pancreatic tumor cells through stabilization of the Rac1 GEF Vav1. *Dev. Cell* **2013**, *24*, 573–585. [CrossRef]
142. Eppinga, R.D.; Krueger, E.W.; Weller, S.G.; Zhang, L.; Cao, H.; McNiven, M.A. Increased expression of the large GTPase dynamin 2 potentiates metastatic migration and invasion of pancreatic ductal carcinoma. *Oncogene* **2012**, *31*, 1228–1241. [CrossRef]
143. Igarashi, T.; Araki, K.; Yokobori, T.; Altan, B.; Yamanaka, T.; Ishii, N.; Tsukagoshi, M.; Watanabe, A.; Kubo, N.; Handa, T.; et al. Association of RAB5 overexpression in pancreatic cancer with cancer progression and poor prognosis via E-cadherin suppression. *Oncotarget* **2017**, *8*, 12290–12300. [CrossRef]
144. Ashour, A.A.; Gurbuz, N.; Alpay, S.N.; Abdel-Aziz, A.A.; Mansour, A.M.; Huo, L.; Ozpolat, B. Elongation factor-2 kinase regulates TG2/beta1 integrin/Src/uPAR pathway and epithelial-mesenchymal transition mediating pancreatic cancer cells invasion. *J. Cell. Mol. Med.* **2014**, *18*, 2235–2251. [CrossRef] [PubMed]
145. Zheng, L.; Zhou, Z.; He, Z. Knockdown of PFTK1 inhibits tumor cell proliferation, invasion and epithelial-to-mesenchymal transition in pancreatic cancer. *Int. J. Clin. Exp. Pathol.* **2015**, *8*, 14005–14012. [PubMed]

146. Tactacan, C.M.; Phua, Y.W.; Liu, L.; Zhang, L.; Humphrey, E.S.; Cowley, M.; Pinese, M.; Biankin, A.V.; Daly, R.J. The pseudokinase SgK223 promotes invasion of pancreatic ductal epithelial cells through JAK1/Stat3 signaling. *Mol. Cancer* **2015**, *14*, 139. [CrossRef] [PubMed]
147. Santoro, R.; Zanotto, M.; Carbone, C.; Piro, G.; Tortora, G.; Melisi, D. MEKK3 sustains EMT and stemness in pancreatic cancer by regulating YAP and TAZ transcriptional activity. *Anticancer Res.* **2018**, *38*, 1937–1946. [CrossRef]
148. Ungefroren, H.; Sebens, S.; Giehl, K.; Helm, O.; Groth, S.; Fandrich, F.; Rocken, C.; Sipos, B.; Lehnert, H.; Gieseler, F. Rac1b negatively regulates TGF-beta1-induced cell motility in pancreatic ductal epithelial cells by suppressing Smad signaling. *Oncotarget* **2014**, *5*, 277–290. [CrossRef]
149. Ning, Z.; Wang, A.; Liang, J.; Xie, Y.; Liu, J.; Yan, Q.; Wang, Z. USP22 promotes epithelial-mesenchymal transition via the FAK pathway in pancreatic cancer cells. *Oncol. Rep.* **2014**, *32*, 1451–1458. [CrossRef]
150. Strnadel, J.; Choi, S.; Fujimura, K.; Wang, H.; Zhang, W.; Wyse, M.; Wright, T.; Croso, E.; Peinado, C.; Park, H.W.; et al. eIF5A-PEAK1 signaling regulates YAP1/TAZ protein expression and pancreatic cancer cell growth. *Cancer Res.* **2017**, *77*, 1997–2007. [CrossRef]
151. Zhu, L.; Zhao, Q. Hypoxia-inducible factor 1alpha participates in hypoxia-induced epithelial-mesenchymal transition via response gene to complement 32. *Exp. Ther. Med.* **2017**, *14*, 1825–1831. [CrossRef]
152. Mody, H.R.; Hung, S.W.; Naidu, K.; Lee, H.; Gilbert, C.A.; Hoang, T.T.; Pathak, R.K.; Manoharan, R.; Muruganandan, S.; Govindarajan, R. SET contributes to the epithelial-mesenchymal transition of pancreatic cancer. *Oncotarget* **2017**, *8*, 67966–67979. [CrossRef]
153. Meng, Q.; Shi, S.; Liang, C.; Liang, D.; Hua, J.; Zhang, B.; Xu, J.; Yu, X. Abrogation of glutathione peroxidase-1 drives EMT and chemoresistance in pancreatic cancer by activating ROS-mediated Akt/GSK3beta/Snail signaling. *Oncogene* **2018**, *37*, 5843. [CrossRef]
154. Shinke, G.; Yamada, D.; Eguchi, H.; Iwagami, Y.; Asaoka, T.; Noda, T.; Wada, H.; Kawamoto, K.; Gotoh, K.; Kobayashi, S.; et al. Role of histone deacetylase 1 in distant metastasis of pancreatic ductal cancer. *Cancer Sci.* **2018**, *109*, 2520–2531. [CrossRef] [PubMed]
155. Mishra, V.K. Histone deacetylase class-I inhibition promotes epithelial gene expression in pancreatic cancer cells in a BRD4- and MYC-dependent manner. *Nucleic Acids Res.* **2017**, *45*, 6334–6349. [CrossRef] [PubMed]
156. Ma, C.; Guo, Y.; Zhang, Y.; Duo, A.; Jia, Y.; Liu, C.; Li, B. PAFAH1B2 is a HIF1a target gene and promotes metastasis in pancreatic cancer. *Biochem. Biophys. Res. Commun.* **2018**, *501*, 654–660. [CrossRef]
157. Li, S.; Wu, L.; Wang, Q.; Li, Y.; Wang, X. KDM4B promotes epithelial-mesenchymal transition through up-regulation of ZEB1 in pancreatic cancer. *Acta Biochim. Biophys. Sin.* **2015**, *47*, 997–1004. [CrossRef] [PubMed]
158. Zhang, W.L.; Zhang, J.H.; Wu, X.Z.; Yan, T.; Lv, W. miR-15b promotes epithelial-mesenchymal transition by inhibiting SMURF2 in pancreatic cancer. *Int. J. Oncol.* **2015**, *47*, 1043–1053. [CrossRef] [PubMed]
159. Zhang, J.Q.; Chen, S.; Gu, J.N.; Zhu, Y.; Zhan, Q.; Cheng, D.F.; Chen, H.; Deng, X.X.; Shen, B.Y.; Peng, C.H. MicroRNA-300 promotes apoptosis and inhibits proliferation, migration, invasion and epithelial-mesenchymal transition via the Wnt/beta-catenin signaling pathway by targeting CUL4B in pancreatic cancer cells. *J. Cell. Biochem.* **2017**, *119*, 1027–1040. [CrossRef] [PubMed]
160. Viotti, M.; Wilson, C.; McCleland, M.; Koeppen, H.; Haley, B.; Jhunjhunwala, S.; Klijn, C.; Modrusan, Z.; Arnott, D.; Classon, M.; et al. SUV420H2 is an epigenetic regulator of epithelial/mesenchymal states in pancreatic cancer. *J. Cell Biol.* **2017**, *217*, 763–777. [CrossRef]
161. Hiraga, R.; Kato, M.; Miyagawa, S.; Kamata, T. Nox4-derived ROS signaling contributes to TGF-beta-induced epithelial-mesenchymal transition in pancreatic cancer cells. *Anticancer Res.* **2013**, *33*, 4431–4438.
162. Tan, J.; You, Y.; Xu, T.; Yu, P.; Wu, D.; Deng, H.; Zhang, Y.; Bie, P. Par-4 downregulation confers cisplatin resistance in pancreatic cancer cells via PI3K/Akt pathway-dependent EMT. *Toxicol. Lett.* **2014**, *224*, 7–15. [CrossRef]
163. Zhao, J.; Wang, Y.; Wu, X. HMGN5 promotes proliferation and invasion via the activation of Wnt/β-catenin signaling pathway in pancreatic ductal adenocarcinoma. *Oncol. Lett.* **2018**, *16*, 4013–4019. [CrossRef]
164. Song, Y.X.; Xu, Z.C.; Li, H.L.; Yang, P.L.; Du, J.K.; Xu, J. Overexpression of GP73 promotes cell invasion, migration and metastasis by inducing epithelial-mesenchymal transition in pancreatic cancer. *Pancreatology* **2018**, *18*, 812–821. [CrossRef] [PubMed]

165. Xu, X.; Su, B.; Xie, C.; Wei, S.; Zhou, Y.; Liu, H.; Dai, W.; Cheng, P.; Wang, F.; Xu, X.; et al. Sonic hedgehog-Gli1 signaling pathway regulates the epithelial mesenchymal transition (EMT) by mediating a new target gene, S100A4, in pancreatic cancer cells. *PLoS ONE* **2014**, *9*, e96441. [CrossRef] [PubMed]
166. Inaguma, S.; Kasai, K.; Ikeda, H. GLI1 facilitates the migration and invasion of pancreatic cancer cells through MUC5AC-mediated attenuation of E-cadherin. *Oncogene* **2011**, *30*, 714–723. [CrossRef] [PubMed]
167. Nagai, S.; Nakamura, M.; Yanai, K.; Wada, J.; Akiyoshi, T.; Nakashima, H.; Ohuchida, K.; Sato, N.; Tanaka, M.; Katano, M. Gli1 contributes to the invasiveness of pancreatic cancer through matrix metalloproteinase-9 activation. *Cancer Sci.* **2008**, *99*, 1377–1384. [CrossRef]
168. Inaguma, S.; Kasai, K.; Hashimoto, M.; Ikeda, H. GLI1 modulates EMT in pancreatic cancer—Letter. *Cancer Res.* **2012**, *72*, 3702–3703. [CrossRef]
169. Huang, C.; Xie, D.; Cui, J.; Li, Q.; Gao, Y.; Xie, K. FOXM1c promotes pancreatic cancer epithelial-to-mesenchymal transition and metastasis via upregulation of expression of the urokinase plasminogen activator system. *Clin. Cancer Res. Off. J. Am. Assoc. Cancer Res.* **2014**, *20*, 1477–1488. [CrossRef]
170. Xie, D.; Cui, J.; Xia, T.; Jia, Z.; Wang, L.; Wei, W.; Zhu, A.; Gao, Y.; Xie, K.; Quan, M. Hippo transducer TAZ promotes epithelial mesenchymal transition and supports pancreatic cancer progression. *Oncotarget* **2015**, *6*, 35949–35963. [CrossRef]
171. Yuan, Y.; Li, D.; Li, H.; Wang, L.; Tian, G.; Dong, Y. YAP overexpression promotes the epithelial-mesenchymal transition and chemoresistance in pancreatic cancer cells. *Mol. Med. Rep.* **2016**, *13*, 237–242. [CrossRef]
172. Chen, K.; Qian, W.; Li, J.; Jiang, Z.; Cheng, L.; Yan, B.; Cao, J.; Sun, L.; Zhou, C.; Lei, M.; et al. Loss of AMPK activation promotes the invasion and metastasis of pancreatic cancer through an HSF1-dependent pathway. *Mol. Oncol.* **2017**, *11*, 1475–1492. [CrossRef]
173. Subramani, R.; Camacho, F.A.; Levin, C.I.; Flores, K.; Clift, A.; Galvez, A.; Terres, M.; Rivera, S.; Kolli, S.N.; Dodderer, J.; et al. FOXC1 plays a crucial role in the growth of pancreatic cancer. *Oncogenesis* **2018**, *7*, 52. [CrossRef]
174. Li, X.; Chen, H.; Liu, Z.; Ye, Z.; Gou, S.; Wang, C. Overexpression of MIST1 reverses the epithelial-mesenchymal transition and reduces the tumorigenicity of pancreatic cancer cells via the Snail/E-cadherin pathway. *Cancer Lett.* **2018**, *431*, 96–104. [CrossRef] [PubMed]
175. Yi, X.; Zai, H.; Long, X.; Wang, X.; Li, W.; Li, Y. Kruppel-like factor 8 induces epithelial-to-mesenchymal transition and promotes invasion of pancreatic cancer cells through transcriptional activation of four and a half LIM-only protein 2. *Oncol. Lett.* **2017**, *14*, 4883–4889. [CrossRef] [PubMed]
176. Thakur, A.K.; Nigri, J.; Lac, S.; Leca, J.; Bressy, C.; Berthezene, P.; Bartholin, L.; Chan, P.; Calvo, E.; Iovanna, J.L.; et al. TAp73 loss favors Smad-independent TGF-β signaling that drives EMT in pancreatic ductal adenocarcinoma. *Cell Death Differ.* **2016**, *23*, 1358–1370. [CrossRef] [PubMed]
177. Takano, S.; Reichert, M.; Bakir, B.; Das, K.K.; Nishida, T.; Miyazaki, M.; Heeg, S.; Collins, M.A.; Marchand, B.; Hicks, P.D.; et al. Prrx1 isoform switching regulates pancreatic cancer invasion and metastatic colonization. *Genes Dev.* **2016**, *30*, 233–247. [CrossRef] [PubMed]
178. Yu, C.; Zhan, L.; Jiang, J.; Pan, Y.; Zhang, H.; Li, X.; Pen, F.; Wang, M.; Qin, R.; Sun, C. KAP-1 is overexpressed and correlates with increased metastatic ability and tumorigenicity in pancreatic cancer. *Med. Oncol. (Northwood Lond. Engl.)* **2014**, *31*, 25. [CrossRef]
179. Li, C.; Wang, Z.; Chen, Y.; Zhou, M.; Zhang, H.; Chen, R.; Shi, F.; Wang, C.; Rui, Z. Transcriptional silencing of ETS-1 abrogates epithelial-mesenchymal transition resulting in reduced motility of pancreatic cancer cells. *Oncol. Rep.* **2015**, *33*, 559–565. [CrossRef]
180. Arfmann-Knubel, S.; Struck, B.; Genrich, G.; Helm, O.; Sipos, B.; Sebens, S.; Schafer, H. The Crosstalk between Nrf2 and TGF-beta1 in the epithelial-mesenchymal transition of pancreatic duct epithelial cells. *PLoS ONE* **2015**, *10*, e0132978. [CrossRef]
181. Roy, N.; Takeuchi, K.K.; Ruggeri, J.M.; Bailey, P.; Chang, D.; Li, J.; Leonhardt, L.; Puri, S.; Hoffman, M.T.; Gao, S.; et al. PDX1 dynamically regulates pancreatic ductal adenocarcinoma initiation and maintenance. *Genes Dev.* **2016**, *30*, 2669–2683. [CrossRef]
182. Sannino, G.; Armbruster, N.; Bodenhofer, M.; Haerle, U.; Behrens, D.; Buchholz, M.; Rothbauer, U.; Sipos, B.; Schmees, C. Role of BCL9L in transforming growth factor-beta (TGF-beta)-induced epithelial-to-mesenchymal-transition (EMT) and metastasis of pancreatic cancer. *Oncotarget* **2016**, *7*, 73725–73738. [CrossRef]

183. Heeg, S.; Das, K.K.; Reichert, M.; Bakir, B.; Takano, S.; Caspers, J.; Aiello, N.M.; Wu, K.; Neesse, A.; Maitra, A.; et al. ETS-Transcription Factor ETV1 Regulates Stromal Expansion and Metastasis in Pancreatic Cancer. *Gastroenterology* **2016**, *151*, 540–553.e14. [CrossRef]
184. Yang, J.; Zhang, X.; Zhang, Y.; Zhu, D.; Zhang, L.; Li, Y.; Zhu, Y.; Li, D.; Zhou, J. HIF-2alpha promotes epithelial-mesenchymal transition through regulating Twist2 binding to the promoter of E-cadherin in pancreatic cancer. *J. Exp. Clin. Cancer Res. CR* **2016**, *35*, 26. [CrossRef] [PubMed]
185. Lerbs, T.; Bisht, S.; Scholch, S.; Pecqueux, M.; Kristiansen, G.; Schneider, M.; Hofmann, B.T.; Welsch, T.; Reissfelder, C.; Rahbari, N.N.; et al. Inhibition of Six1 affects tumour invasion and the expression of cancer stem cell markers in pancreatic cancer. *BMC Cancer* **2017**, *17*, 249. [CrossRef] [PubMed]
186. Nishino, H.; Takano, S.; Yoshitomi, H.; Suzuki, K.; Kagawa, S.; Shimazaki, R.; Shimizu, H.; Furukawa, K.; Miyazaki, M.; Ohtsuka, M. Grainyhead-like 2 (GRHL2) regulates epithelial plasticity in pancreatic cancer progression. *Cancer Med.* **2017**, *6*, 2686–2696. [CrossRef]
187. Martinelli, P.; Carrillo-de Santa Pau, E.; Cox, T.; Sainz, B., Jr.; Dusetti, N.; Greenhalf, W.; Rinaldi, L.; Costello, E.; Ghaneh, P.; Malats, N.; et al. GATA6 regulates EMT and tumour dissemination, and is a marker of response to adjuvant chemotherapy in pancreatic cancer. *Gut* **2017**, *66*, 1665–1676. [CrossRef] [PubMed]
188. Dai, S.; Zhang, J.; Huang, S.; Lou, B.; Fang, B.; Ye, T.; Huang, X.; Chen, B.; Zhou, M. HNRNPA2B1 regulates the epithelial-mesenchymal transition in pancreatic cancer cells through the ERK/snail signaling pathway. *Cancer Cell. Int.* **2017**, *17*, 12. [CrossRef] [PubMed]
189. Chen, J.; Sun, Y.; Xu, X.; Wang, D.; He, J.; Zhou, H.; Lu, Y.; Zeng, J.; Du, F.; Gong, A.; et al. YTH domain family 2 orchestrates epithelial-mesenchymal transition/proliferation dichotomy in pancreatic cancer cells. *Cell Cycle* **2017**, *16*, 2259–2271. [CrossRef]
190. Zhao, L.; Sun, H.; Kong, H.; Chen, Z.; Chen, B.; Zhou, M. The Lncrna-TUG1/EZH2 Axis promotes pancreatic cancer cell proliferation, migration and EMT phenotype formation through sponging Mir-382. *Cell. Physiol. Biochem. Int. J. Exp. Cell. Physiol. Biochem. Pharmacol.* **2017**, *42*, 2145–2158. [CrossRef]
191. Gao, Y.; Zhang, Z.; Li, K.; Gong, L.; Yang, Q.; Huang, X.; Hong, C.; Ding, M.; Yang, H. Linc-DYNC2H1-4 promotes EMT and CSC phenotypes by acting as a sponge of miR-145 in pancreatic cancer cells. *Cell Death Dis.* **2017**, *8*, e2924. [CrossRef]
192. Wu, G.; Li, Z.; Jiang, P.; Zhang, X.; Xu, Y.; Chen, K.; Li, X. MicroRNA-23a promotes pancreatic cancer metastasis by targeting epithelial splicing regulator protein 1. *Oncotarget* **2017**, *8*, 82854–82871. [CrossRef]
193. Li, H.; Wang, X.; Wen, C.; Huo, Z.; Wang, W.; Zhan, Q.; Cheng, D.; Chen, H.; Deng, X.; Peng, C.; et al. Long noncoding RNA NORAD, a novel competing endogenous RNA, enhances the hypoxia-induced epithelial-mesenchymal transition to promote metastasis in pancreatic cancer. *Mol. Cancer* **2017**, *16*, 169. [CrossRef]
194. Ma, C.; Nong, K.; Zhu, H.; Wang, W.; Huang, X.; Yuan, Z.; Ai, K. H19 promotes pancreatic cancer metastasis by derepressing let-7's suppression on its target HMGA2-mediated EMT. *Tumor Biol.* **2014**, *35*, 9163–9169. [CrossRef] [PubMed]
195. Zhan, H.X.; Wang, Y.; Li, C.; Xu, J.W.; Zhou, B.; Zhu, J.K.; Han, H.F.; Wang, L.; Wang, Y.S.; Hu, S.Y. LincRNA-ROR promotes invasion, metastasis and tumor growth in pancreatic cancer through activating ZEB1 pathway. *Cancer Lett.* **2016**, *374*, 261–271. [CrossRef] [PubMed]
196. Hu, J.; Li, L.; Chen, H.; Zhang, G.; Liu, H.; Kong, R.; Chen, H.; Wang, Y.; Li, Y.; Tian, F.; et al. MiR-361-3p regulates ERK1/2-induced EMT via DUSP2 mRNA degradation in pancreatic ductal adenocarcinoma. *Cell Death Dis.* **2018**, *9*, 807. [CrossRef] [PubMed]
197. Li, N.; Wang, C.; Zhang, P.; You, S. Emodin inhibits pancreatic cancer EMT and invasion by up-regulating microRNA-1271. *Mol. Med. Rep.* **2018**, *18*, 3366–3374. [CrossRef] [PubMed]
198. Little, E.C.; Camp, E.R.; Wang, C.; Watson, P.M.; Watson, D.K.; Cole, D.J. The CaSm (LSm1) oncogene promotes transformation, chemoresistance and metastasis of pancreatic cancer cells. *Oncogenesis* **2016**, *5*, e182. [CrossRef] [PubMed]
199. Suzuki, K.; Takano, S.; Yoshitomi, H.; Nishino, H.; Kagawa, S.; Shimizu, H.; Furukawa, K.; Miyazaki, M.; Ohtsuka, M. Metadherin promotes metastasis by supporting putative cancer stem cell properties and epithelial plasticity in pancreatic cancer. *Oncotarget* **2017**, *8*, 66098–66111. [CrossRef] [PubMed]

200. Fabregat, A.; Jupe, S.; Matthews, L.; Sidiropoulos, K.; Gillespie, M.; Garapati, P.; Haw, R.; Jassal, B.; Korninger, F.; May, B.; et al. The Reactome Pathway Knowledgebase. *Nucleic Acids Res.* **2018**, *46*, D649–D655. [CrossRef]
201. Kelder, T.; Pico, A.R.; Hanspers, K.; van Iersel, M.P.; Evelo, C.; Conklin, B.R. Mining biological pathways using WikiPathways web services. *PLoS ONE* **2009**, *4*, e6447. [CrossRef]
202. Szklarczyk, D.; Gable, A.L.; Lyon, D.; Junge, A.; Wyder, S.; Huerta-Cepas, J.; Simonovic, M.; Doncheva, N.T.; Morris, J.H.; Bork, P.; et al. STRING v11: Protein-protein association networks with increased coverage, supporting functional discovery in genome-wide experimental datasets. *Nucleic Acids Res.* **2019**, *47*, D607–D613. [CrossRef]
203. Shannon, P.; Markiel, A.; Ozier, O.; Baliga, N.S.; Wang, J.T.; Ramage, D.; Amin, N.; Schwikowski, B.; Ideker, T. Cytoscape: A software environment for integrated models of biomolecular interaction networks. *Genome Res.* **2003**, *13*, 2498–2504. [CrossRef]
204. Maresch, R.; Mueller, S.; Veltkamp, C.; Ollinger, R.; Friedrich, M.; Heid, I.; Steiger, K.; Weber, J.; Engleitner, T.; Barenboim, M.; et al. Multiplexed pancreatic genome engineering and cancer induction by transfection-based CRISPR/Cas9 delivery in mice. *Nat. Commun.* **2016**, *7*, 10770. [CrossRef] [PubMed]

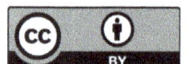

© 2019 by the authors. Licensee MDPI, Basel, Switzerland. This article is an open access article distributed under the terms and conditions of the Creative Commons Attribution (CC BY) license (http://creativecommons.org/licenses/by/4.0/).

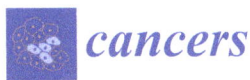

Review

Tumor Endothelial Heterogeneity in Cancer Progression

Nako Maishi [1,2], Dorcas A. Annan [1,2], Hiroshi Kikuchi [2,3], Yasuhiro Hida [4] and Kyoko Hida [1,2,*]

1. Department of Vascular Biology and Molecular Pathology, Hokkaido University Graduate School of Dental Medicine, Sapporo 060-8586, Japan; mnako@den.hokudai.ac.jp (N.M.); annandorcasam@gmail.com (D.A.A.)
2. Vascular Biology, Frontier Research Unit, Institute for Genetic Medicine, Hokkaido University, Sapporo 060-0815, Japan; hiroshikikuchi16@yahoo.co.jp
3. Department of Renal and Genitourinary Surgery, Hokkaido University Graduate School of Medicine, Sapporo 060-8636, Japan
4. Department of Cardiovascular and Thoracic Surgery, Hokkaido University Faculty of Medicine, Sapporo 060-8638, Japan; yhida@med.hokudai.ac.jp
* Correspondence: khida@den.hokudai.ac.jp; Tel.: +81-11-706-4239

Received: 15 September 2019; Accepted: 2 October 2019; Published: 9 October 2019

Abstract: Tumor blood vessels supply nutrients and oxygen to tumor cells for their growth and provide routes for them to enter circulation. Thus, angiogenesis, the formation of new blood vessels, is essential for tumor progression and metastasis. Tumor endothelial cells (TECs) that cover the inner surfaces of tumor blood vessels reportedly show phenotypes distinct from those of their normal counterparts. As examples, TECs show cytogenetic abnormalities, resistance to anticancer drugs, activated proliferation and migration, and specific gene expression patterns. TECs contain stem-like cell populations, which means that the origin of TECs is heterogeneous. In addition, since some abnormal phenotypes in TECs are induced by factors in the tumor microenvironment, such as hypoxia and tumor cell-derived factors, phenotypic diversity in TECs may be caused in part by intratumoral heterogeneity. Recent studies have identified that the interaction of tumor cells and TECs by juxtacrine and paracrine signaling contributes to tumor malignancy. Understanding TEC abnormality and heterogeneity is important for treatment of cancers. This review provides an overview of the diversity of TECs and discusses the interaction between TECs and tumor cells in the tumor microenvironment.

Keywords: tumor endothelial cell; metastasis; heterogeneity; angiocrine factor

---

1. Introduction

Cancer is one of the leading causes of death in most of the advanced countries, and the main cause of cancer death is distant metastasis. Hematogenous metastasis is still incurable, although patient survival has improved. Understanding and overcoming tumor progression and metastasis are crucial in cancer therapy. Tumor tissues require oxygen and nutrients to grow, and these are supplied by blood flow to the tumor. Without neovascularization, most tumors may become dormant at a diameter of 2–3 mm [1]. Blood vessels support tumor cell expansion by providing the routes from intravasation in primary tumors to extravasation in distant organs. Tumor blood vessels play an important role in tumor growth and dissemination.

Antiangiogenic therapy was proposed by Dr. Folkman [1]. Since solid tumors are dependent on neovascularization for their growth, Folkman suggested that the prevention of neovascularization may restrict tumor growth to a very small diameter [1]. Angiogenic inhibitors such as bevacizumab, a humanized anti-vascular endothelial growth factor (VEGF) antibody [2], have been used for the past 15 years. Because VEGF is known as a permeability factor [3–5], antiangiogenic therapy not only suppresses the growth of tumors, it also normalizes blood vessel structures and improves the delivery of oxygen and drugs, which potentially affects both radiotherapy and chemotherapy [6,7]. However, the clinical benefits of antiangiogenic therapies have been limited, resulting in slight improvements in prognosis, such as enhancing progression-free survival [8]. In addition, resistance to antiangiogenic therapy has emerged because of the complex interaction between tumor cells and stromal cells, including endothelial cells (ECs), which allows for tumor cells to escape these targeted therapies [9].

Tumor endothelial cells (TECs) that cover the inner surfaces of tumor blood vessels are the primary targets of antiangiogenic therapy. Several reports have demonstrated that TECs are abnormal, and their abnormality is one of the causes of resistance to antiangiogenic therapy. In addition, TECs show intertumoral and intratumoral heterogeneity in terms of communicating with the surrounding tumor microenvironment. Reviewing how to overcome cancer from a TEC perspective, we focus on the abnormality and diversity of TECs, incorporating a discussion regarding the interaction between TECs and tumor cells in the tumor microenvironment.

2. Abnormalities of TECs

2.1. Tumor Blood Vessels and Normal Blood Vessels

At the organ level, the vasculature in the tumors from which TECs originate has an atypical morphology described as "abnormal" in terms of structure and function. Vasculature in normal nondiseased organs has an organized hierarchical structure that supports the efficient distribution of blood and its components to cells [10]. The order of blood flow in the normal vessels is from arteries to arterioles, and subsequently to capillaries, postcapillary venules, and lastly veins. In terms of function, tumor blood vessels do not support a sequential pattern of blood flow due to the chaotic order of organization.

The formation of tumor blood vessels from existing ones, called angiogenesis, occurs in response to the proangiogenic stimuli, including VEGF, basic fibroblast growth factor (bFGF), placental growth factor, and angiopoietin, among others that are produced by the tumor cells [11,12]. Hypoxia [13] and acidity [14], which are commonly associated with the tumor microenvironment, also can stimulate VEGF production in tumors. The abundance of VEGF and/or the other angiogenic factors in the tumor microenvironment sustains a continuous process of angiogenesis, leading to the formation of tumor blood vessels with various structural defects [12]. These tumor blood vessels are tortuous, highly permeable, and dilated, and show differential coverage and a loose association of perivascular cells along the vessels and weakened EC junctions [15,16].

Another important contribution to the abnormal phenotype of tumor vasculature is the insufficient control of the angiogenesis process. It has been documented that there exists an imbalance in the expression of the angiogenesis stimulators and inhibitors [17,18]. Furthermore, it was recently demonstrated that uncontrolled glycolysis in TECs due to an upregulated expression of glycolysis genes, including the enzyme 6-phosphofructo-2-kinase/fructose-2,6-biphosphatase 3 (PFKFB3), contributes to structural deformities observed in tumor blood vessels [19].

These abnormal structural changes make tumor blood vessels highly permeable compared with normal vessels. Proteins and fluids leak out of the vessels into the extracellular environment and create a high tumor interstitial pressure [20,21]. In addition, the expanding tumor population exerts more pressure on the blood vessels, causing some portions to collapse. Concomitantly, blood flow to certain portions of the tumor is cut off, leading to hypoxia [22], a switch to glycolytic metabolism in some tumors, and an increase in tumor acidosis. Hypoxia in tumors further induces tumor aggressiveness through epithelial-mesenchymal transition, resulting in tumor metastasis [23].

2.2. Differential Characteristics of Tumor and Normal Endothelial Cells

Endothelial cells (ECs) in blood vessels are the primary cells in blood vessel formation, and in a similar way as tumor blood vessels show alterations compared with the normal vessels, the resident endothelial cells in tumor blood vessels are also different. Compared with normal endothelial cells (NECs), TECs differ in their genetic makeup, protein expression, and functional output (Figure 1).

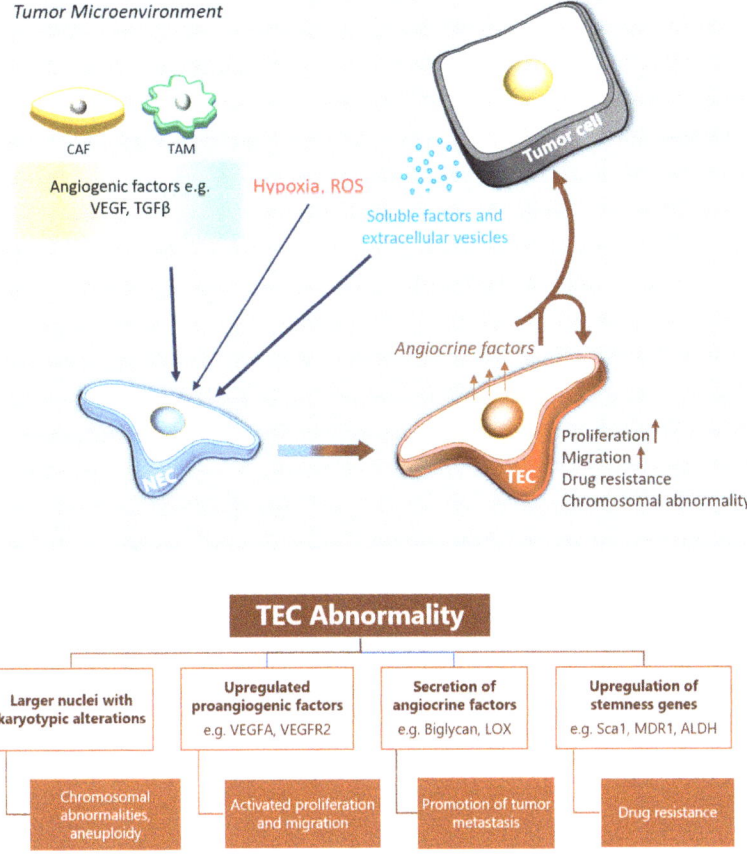

Figure 1. TEC abnormality. Soluble factors and extracellular vesicles released from tumor cells, CAFs and TAMs, induce endothelial cells in pre-existing blood vessels to initiate angiogenesis to form tumor blood vessels. In the process, the NECs are transformed into TECs in the formed tumor vessels. Additionally, hypoxia and ROS in the TME may contribute to the TEC phenotype. TECs have higher proliferative and migration abilities as compared to the NECs. They have an abnormal karyotype characterized by various chromosomal abnormalities and aneuploidy. The genetic changes that occur lead to the upregulated expression of proangiogenic genes e.g., VEGFA and angiocrine factors such as biglycan, which induces angiogenic function in the TECs and may also affect the tumor cells. Furthermore, the upregulation of stemness genes such as MDR1 and ALDH lead to the development of a drug resistant phenotype in the TECs. ROS, reactive oxygen species; TEC tumor endothelial cells; NEC, normal endothelial cell; CAF, cancer-associated fibroblast; TAM, tumor-associated macrophages; TME, tumor microenvironment.

We have previously reported that human renal TECs show various percentages of aneuploidy as compared to NECs [24]. Similarly, in murine TECs the karyotype indicated the presence of larger nuclei and more aneuploidy than in NECs. Within the nuclei in the TECs were chromosomal aberrations, including missing whole or portions of chromosomes, translocations, and abnormal centrosomes characterized by larger sizes and excess numbers than in NECs [25]. These observations indicate that generally TECs have chromosomal instability.

At the molecular level, TECs express angiogenesis-sustaining genes; for example, receptors such as VEGFR-1, VEGFR-2, and VEGFR-3, angiopoietin receptor tie-2, and an upregulated expression of angiopoietin 1 and VEGF-D compared with NECs [26]. With these genes, TECs exhibit a strong response to the respective angiogenic factors for the receptors [27,28]. In addition, we have also previously reported that TECs show an upregulated expression of nonconventional angiogenic factors such as biglycan [29], lysyl oxidase (LOX) [30], and pentraxin 3 (PTX3) [31]. Furthermore, TECs have been described as being "activated" and "chronically inflamed" [32]; they express adhesion molecules ICAM-1, VCAM-1, and E-selectin [27], through which they interact with proinflammatory and tumor cells.

In performing angiogenesis, both human and murine TECs are highly proliferative [28], self-sustaining, and are not dependent on serum for proliferation the way that NECs are [26]. Differentially expressed in FDCP 6 homolog (DEF6) and PTX3 play a role in regulating EC proliferation [31,33], and their expression in TECs could partly account for how TECs regulate and sustain continuous proliferation. The migration ability of TECs is also higher than that for NECs [28,34]. We have demonstrated that some genes upregulated in TECs are important for TEC migration. For example, we showed that interrupting LOX and biglycan, which were upregulated in isolated TECs, decreased migration and tube-forming ability and caused morphological changes in the TEC [29,30]. Pharmacological LOX inhibition in vivo also led to a decrease in tumor metastasis [30]. Moreover, murine TECs maintain their biological characteristics after longer periods of cell culture than do NECs [28].

The exposure of tumor cells to the hypoxic tumor microenvironment induces the expression of stemness genes [35]. Provided that TECs are exposed to a similar microenvironment, some studies have identified the upregulated expression of stemness genes such as stem cell antigen-1 (Sca-1) [28], MDR-1 [36], and ALDH [37] in the TECs. We have shown that the expression of MDR-1 [36] and ALDH in TECs that are derived from highly metastatic melanoma, for example, induces in the TECs a property of drug resistance to the drug paclitaxel [37]. Another study, involving TECs derived from a human hepatocellular carcinoma, showed that the CD105+ TECs acquired resistance to 5-fluorouracil (an anticancer drug) and sorafenib (an antiangiogenic drug) as compared to the CD105+ NECs or human umbilical vein endothelial cells (HUVECs) [38].

3. Heterogeneity of TECs

3.1. Different Roles in ECs during Angiogenesis

Angiogenesis starts in response to cues in injury or pathological condition. VEGF and other proangiogenic factors stimulate quiescent ECs and activate to adopt angiogenic phenotype. Three types of cells, namely tip, stalk, and phalanx cells, are known to coordinate the sprouting of capillaries from pre-existing vessels. Migrating tip cells lead the nascent vessel sprouts at the forefront. Proliferating stalk cells trail the tip cells and elongate blood vessels [39]. Acquiescent phalanx cells form continuous monolayers, forming a tight barrier. These specializations of ECs are transient and reversible by altering the balance between proangiogenic factors, such as VEGF, and suppressors of EC proliferation, such as Dll4-Notch activity [40,41]. Tip cells migrate in response to the VEGF gradient, while stalk cells that proliferate are dependent on the VEGF concentration [42]. Phalanx cells secrete soluble Flt1 (VEGFR-1), which neutralizes VEGF activity to end angiogenesis [43].

These ECs differ in their metabolism [44,45]. Since angiogenic sprouting is metabolically demanding [46], ECs rely on glycolysis [44], which is stimulated by the regulator PFKFB3. ECs can interchange their position depending on their metabolic condition during angiogenesis. Stalk cells overtake the tip cell position when they express higher levels of PFKFB3 [44]. This specialization is one of the heterogeneities of ECs in a tumor microenvironment.

3.2. Origin of TECs

Angiogenesis is the process of sprouting from a pre-existing vessel, while vasculogenesis is mediated by the mobilization of precursor cells, such as endothelial progenitor cells (EPCs) from bone marrow. EPCs were named by Asahara et al., who isolated from adult peripheral blood mononuclear cells showing the same characteristics as the embryonic angioblasts [47–49]. Although the identity and the contribution of EPCs in tumors are controversial and are still under discussion, several studies have shown that EPCs are incorporated into newly formed tumor blood vessels [50–53]. The surface markers of EPCs are classically expected to express CD34, VEGFR-2, and CD133 [49]. Numerous studies have aimed to target EPCs to develop novel therapeutic strategies, since EPCs or circulating endothelial precursor cells contribute to tumor angiogenesis [50,51].

ECs are heterogeneous [54]; for example, the EC structure and function are different depending on vascular size, which is described in terms of the macrovasculature, including arterial and venous, and in terms of microvascular capillaries [55]. Morphology and marker expression in ECs show differences depending on the EC origin [56,57]. Organ-specific or tissue-specific phenotypes in ECs have also been reported [55,58,59]. ECs show heterogeneity in structure and function, and in time and space [60]. TEC heterogeneity can be caused by the surrounding endothelial heterogeneity, with an activating angiogenic switch.

The concept that tumor cells could generate TECs was introduced by some groups of investigators. Streubel et al., demonstrated that chromosomal aberrations were shared by B-cell lymphoma cells and TECs, which means that TECs in B-cell lymphomas are in part tumor related [61]. In glioblastomas, some studies reported that glioblastoma stem cells may give rise to TECs [62–64]. Ricchi-Vitiani et al., showed that various TECs in glioblastoma carry the same genomic alteration as tumor cells, which indicates that some TECs have neoplastic origin [62]. Want et al., also demonstrated that members of a subpopulation of TECs share the same somatic mutations as glioblastoma cells, and that the stem-cell-like CD133+ fraction includes a subset of CD144-expressing cells [63]. Soda et al., demonstrated that tumor cells directly transdifferentiate into CD31+CD34+ ECs, which may play a role in resistance found toward anti-VEGF therapy [64]. On the contrary, another study showed that glioblastoma cells give rise to pericytes rather than to ECs, using lineage tracing with pericyte- or EC-specific promoter-driven fluorescent reporters [65]. The study reported that such an event wherein glioblastoma stem cells give rise to ECs may be very rare because ECs rarely carry the cancer genetic mutations, as other groups of investigators have demonstrated [65–67] Transdifferentiation to ECs in tumors may occur in other cell types. In multiple myeloma, tumor-derived pleiotrophin and macrophage colony-stimulating factor stimulate monocytes to induce the expression of EC markers, and the cells become transdifferentiated into ECs that incorporate into tumor blood vessels [68]. Since Fernandez et al., demonstrated that monocyte-derived immature dendritic cells behave as endothelial-like cells in the presence of specific cytokines such as VEGF [69,70], it has been proposed that dendritic cells may possibly transdifferentiate into TECs in a cytokine-rich tumor microenvironment. These variations could lead to TEC diversity.

3.3. Stem Cell Population in TECs

TEC heterogeneity and diversity have also been reported at functional and molecular levels [71]. TECs upregulate aldehyde dehydrogenase (ALDH) expression. There are two populations in TECs, such that some have high ALDH activity and some have low. ALDH^{high} TECs formed more tubes on Matrigel and sustained the tubular networks longer, with the upregulation of VEGFR2 expression, than ALDH^{low} TECs did [72]. The ALDH^{high} population was resistant to fluorouracil (5-FU) in vitro and in vivo, with upregulation of stem-related genes compared with ALDH^{low} TECs [37]. Naito et al., reported that vascular-resident stem/progenitor-like ECs, which form a minor population in tumors, contribute to tumor angiogenesis. Because of their ability to efflux Hoechst 33342 dye, they are termed side population cells, and cause drug resistance [73]. These reports suggested that the heterogeneity of

ECs in tumor tissues may be a mechanism contributing to resistance to anticancer and antiangiogenic therapy (Figure 2).

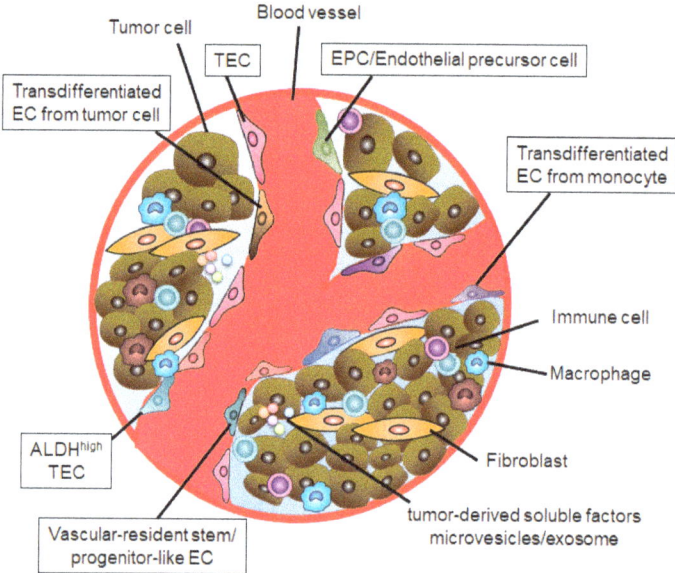

Figure 2. TEC heterogeneity in the tumor microenvironment. TECs are derived from multiple cells. TECs acquire their specific characteristics by several factors in the tumor microenvironment. These variations could lead to TEC diversity.

3.4. The Effect of Tumor Microenvironment on TEC Heterogeneity

The heterogeneity of TECs in highly metastatic tumors and in tumors with low metastasis has been also described [34]. TECs derived from highly metastatic tumors display activated proliferation and migration with the upregulation of proangiogenic factors [34]. TECs in highly metastatic tumors show a stem-like phenotype with an upregulation of stem cell markers, such as CD90 and Sca-1, and a high ability to form spheres [34]. These data suggested that the microenvironment surrounding TECs, including tumor cell phenotype and metastatic potential, affects TEC characteristics and induces heterogeneity among TECs.

TECs acquire their specific characteristics in the tumor microenvironment during tumor angiogenesis. One of the factors in tumor microenvironment is hypoxia. It is well known that tumors are hypoxic [74]. Since the tumor blood vessel pattern is nonhierarchical and disorganized due to the excessive VEGF causing high permeability, which in turn results in an insufficient blood supply, tumor blood vessels are also sometimes exposed to hypoxia. Hypoxia induces the expression of hypoxia-inducible factor-1 alpha and transcribes several molecules, such as VEGF-A. In highly metastatic tumors, TECs are exposed to hypoxia and the expression of VEGF-A is high compared with TECs in tumors with low metastasis [34]. Hypoxia induces the accumulation of reactive oxygen species (ROS). We have previously demonstrated that ROS induces some TEC marker expression in ECs [75]. TECs show chromosomal instability [24,25], and the abnormalities are accumulated in TECs in highly metastatic tumors [34] or ALDH^{high} TECs [72]. One of the causes of cytogenic abnormality in TECs was excessive VEGF [76] and ROS [77]. These factors in the tumor microenvironment induce abnormalities and heterogeneity in ECs.

Tumor-derived soluble factors and microvesicles/exosomes are also among the causes of abnormalities in TECs. TEC marker expression was induced by tumor-derived soluble factors.

For example, the expression of CXCR7 [78], biglycan [79], and MDR1 [36] was upregulated by soluble factors derived from highly metastatic tumors. Tumor-derived microvesicles induce a proangiogenic phenotype in ECs via endocytosis [80]. TECs acquire their specific characteristics by several factors in the tumor microenvironment.

Previous studies have demonstrated that endothelial-to-mesenchymal transition (EndMT) can occur in cancer [81]. EndMT is recognized as a unique source of cancer-associated fibroblasts (CAFs). These CAFs coexpress the EC marker CD31, along with one of the mesenchymal markers, FSP1, or αSMA [81]. Transforming growth factor β (TGFβ) is known to induce EndMT [82]. Conversely, recent studies demonstrated that ECs resist specific conversion to alpha-SMA+ myofibroblast-like cells when the cells are challenged with TGFβ through secretion of bFGF [83]. TGFβ and bFGF could oppose and cooperate with each other during EndMT via Elk1 [84]. These data suggest that EndMT is another mechanism producing TEC heterogeneity.

4. The Role of TECs in Cancer Progression

Tumors often become more malignant and aggressive progressively, step by step. In a primary tumor, tumor cells increase and gain malignant potential, and tumor cells invade the surrounding stroma and extracellular matrix (ECM). At the metastatic phase, tumor cells intravasate into vessels and reach distant organs [85]. Tumor stromal cells such as CAFs or immunosuppressive cells contribute to tumor progression [86], and TECs also play crucial roles at these steps, in addition to supplying oxygen and nutrients by blood flow. The upregulated expression of VEGF receptors may contribute to the rapid response of TECs to VEGF to facilitate disorganized blood vessel formation, through which tumor cells could get into the blood stream. Upregulation of adhesion molecules in TECs gives tumor cells scaffolds to invade between TECs, which lead to extravasation to drive metastatic dissemination [87]. In addition, TECs provide a number of inductive factors named "angiocrine factors" (Table 1), and these factors stimulate tumor growth and tumor cell migration [88]. TECs produce various molecules such as endothelin-1, bFGF, TGFβ, interleukin (IL)-6, and IL-8 as paracrine mediators of prostate cancer progression [89]. Other angiocrine factors, including IL-6, IL-3, granulocyte colony-stimulating factor (G-CSF), granulocyte-macrophage-CSF (GM-CSF), IL-1, and nitric oxide, promote leukemic cell proliferation. In addition, Jag1 derived from TECs activates Notch2 in lymphoma cells to promote tumor invasiveness [90]. CXCR7 on TECs is involved in tumor growth and angiogenesis [78,91,92]. CXCR7 regulates CXCL12-CXCR4-mediated tumor cell transendothelial migration [93]. Platelet-derived growth factor (PDGF) signaling plays a crucial role in inhibitor of differentiation 4 (ID4)-mediated regulation of ECs and Glioma-initiating cells by promoting the PDGF-NOS (nitric oxide synthase)-ID4 signaling axis. These effects maintain cancer stemness and promote tumor angiogenesis [94]. In addition, TECs downregulate tumor-suppressive factors such as Slit2. Slit2 is one of the tumor-suppressive angiocrine factors that is negatively regulated by the EphA2 receptor on ECs [95].

Table 1. Angiocrine factors produced by tumor endothelial cells.

Angiocrine Factors	Functions	Refs
Angiopoietin-2 (Ang2)	Recruit innate immune cells	[96]
Basic fibroblast growth factor (bFGF)	Organogenesis and tumorigenesis	[89,97]
Biglycan	Stimulate tumor cell intravasation	[79]
Bone morphogenetic protein-2, 4 (BMP2, 4)	Tumorigenesis	[98]
Calcineurin	Vascular stabilization and promote metastatic outgrowth	[99]
C-X-C motif chemokine 12 (CXCL12)	Tumorigenesis and tumor progression	[100,101]
Endothelin-1	Promote tumor growth	[102]
Granulocyte colony stimulating factor (G-CSF)	Promote leukemic cell proliferation	[103]
Granulocyte macrophage colony stimulating factor (GM-CSF)	Angiogenesis	[104]
Insulin growth factor binding protein-7 (IGFBP7)	Tumor-suppressive checkpoint	[105]
Insulin growth factor-1 (IGF1)	Stimulate chemoresistance and angiogenesis	[105,106]
Interleukin-3 (IL-3)	Promote leukemic cell proliferation	[103]
Interleukin-6 (IL-6)	Macrophage activation and tumor progression	[107]
Interleukin-8 (IL-8)	Angiogenesis and tumor progression	[108]
Jagged-1 (Jag1)	Promote tumor invasiveness and chemoresistance	[90]
laminin α4 (LAMA4)	Tumorigenesis	[109]
Lysyl oxidase (Lox)	Angiogenesis and stimulate tumor cell intravasation	[30]
Nitric oxide (NO)	Tumorigenesis	[110]
Platelet-derived growth factor (PDGF)	Angiogenesis and tumorigenesis	[94]
Placental growth factor (PGF)	Angiogenesis and tumorigenesis	[111]
Pentraxin 3 (PTX3)	Stimulate TEC proliferation	[31]
Slit2	Tumor suppression	[95]
Suprabasin	Angiogenesis	[112]
Transforming growth factor beta (TGF-β)	Tumorigenesis and tumor progression	[113]
Vascular endothelial growth factor-A (VEGFA)	Angiogenesis and autocrine loop	[114]

Moreover, TECs stimulate tumor cell intravasation and metastasis. Wieland et al., demonstrated that Notch1 in TECs activates the migration of tumor cells and promotes intravasation. Endothelial Notch1 promotes lung metastasis with neutrophil infiltration. In addition, TECs frequently express elevated Notch1 in human tumor tissues, including melanoma, breast carcinoma, lung adenocarcinoma, serous ovarian carcinoma, and colorectal carcinoma, and this expression correlates with poor prognosis [115]. ALK1 in TECs is also involved in tumor metastasis. ALK1 expression in TECs is an independent prognostic factor for metastasis of breast cancer [116]. The oxygen-sensing prolyl hydroxylase domain protein 2 (PHD2) in TECs is involved in vessel shaping. Haplodeficiency of PHD2 did not affect vessel density or lumen size, however, it normalized the endothelial lining and vessel maturation in tumors, which leads to the reduction of tumor cell intravasation and metastasis [43]. We have shown that biglycan, a small leucine-rich repeat proteoglycan, was remarkably upregulated in TECs and facilitated the migration of toll-like receptor-expressing tumor cells, which increased circulating tumor cells and lung metastasis [79]. Endothelial calcineurin have a unique function, which does not affect primary tumor growth, but activates the outgrowth of metastases [99]. These studies suggested that TECs actively promote tumor cell progression and metastasis.

Drugs for anticancer treatment include cytotoxic drugs and molecular targeting drugs. In most cases, these drugs gradually become ineffective in cancer treatment, and this is considered to be caused by tumor cells acquiring drug resistance. It is generally known that tumor cells acquire drug resistance via phenotypic changes, such as increased drug transporter expression [117]. On the contrary, TEC characteristics also cause drug resistance. Renal cell carcinoma-derived TECs are resistant to vincristine [26], and hepatocellular carcinoma-derived TECs are resistant to 5-FU and adriamycin [36,38]. TEC-derived Jag1 confers Notch-dependent chemoresistance in lymphoma cells [90]. TECs have acquired resistance to anticancer drugs via the upregulated expression of ATP-binding cassette transporters, similar to cancer stem cells [36,118]. TECs also play a role as a molecular checkpoint in chemotherapy. IGFBP7 expressed by TECs suppresses IGF1R signaling and the stem-cell-like property of tumor cells. Chemotherapy triggers TECs to suppress IGFBP7, and the upregulation of IGF1 activates the FGF4-FGFR1-ETS2 pathway in TECs and accelerates the conversion of tumor cells to chemoresistant tumor stem-like cells [105]. The drug resistance property of TECs also serves to promote tumor survival. Residual TECs in drug-treated tumors will restore angiogenesis in the more resistant tumor cells that have survived antiangiogenic therapy.

In recent years, tumor immunity has been noted as an important factor for anticancer treatment, and immune checkpoint inhibitors have become key drugs for antitumor immunity [119,120]. ECs play an important role in controlling immune cell entry into tissues with chemokines and adhesion molecules [121]. In tumor tissues, the abnormalities of TECs suppress T-cell trafficking and function and cause an immune-suppressive environment [122]. For example, the high expression of VEGF and other growth factors reduces endothelial ICAM-1 and VCAM-1 expressions in tumor tissues, causing the lymphocyte–endothelial interactions to become inefficient [123]. VEGF and prostaglandins induce CD95 (FasL) expression on TECs, leading to apoptosis of activated anticancer CD8+ T cells. In contrast, regulatory T cells that suppress antitumor immune responses are protected by antiapoptotic genes, such as Bcl2 and Bclxl, and these cells can selectively migrate into tumor tissues [124]. Upregulation of CD73 on TECs reduces effector T-cell homing, whereas anti-CD73 antibodies can restore efficacy of antitumor immunotherapy and decrease tumor angiogenesis [125,126]. In addition, PD-L1, which is a negative regulator of T-cell activation, is expressed in TECs. PD-L1 blockade enhances tumor vascular normalization during anti-VEGF therapy [127]. Macrophage also plays an important role for tumor immunity. TECs are one of the major sources of IL-6 in glioblastoma. Angiocrine IL-6 induces arginase-1 expression and promotes macrophage alternative activation [107]. Thus, vascular normalization is a promising concept in anticancer treatment and can potentially improve the outcome of immunotherapies [128–130].

5. Conclusions

In this review, we addressed the abnormality and heterogeneity of TECs to understand their roles in the tumor microenvironment. The functions of ECs in newly formed blood vessels in tumor tissues are not only to transport nutrients and oxygen for tumor survival and growth, but also to actively promote tumor progression and chemoresistance.

Antiangiogenic therapy has been widely used in many types of tumors; however, since it is now clear that TECs are heterogeneous, to overcome and regulate tumor angiogenesis is a difficult and urgent task. To understand the complex situation in the tumor microenvironment, companion diagnostics to monitor vascularization is required. In addition, both angiogenesis and vasculogenesis need to be targeted to regulate aberrant excessive blood vessels. Targeting multiple growth factors as combination therapy have shown improved outcomes, but the therapeutic effects are sometimes not enough. Another therapy, such as combination with immunotherapy or targeting EC metabolism is expected to normalize tumor microenvironment to cure cancer disease.

Author Contributions: N.M., D.A.A., H.K., Y.H., and K.H. conceived and wrote the review.

Funding: This research was partially funded by JSPS Grants-in-Aid for Scientific Research on Integrated analysis and regulation of cellular diversity Innovative Areas to K.H. (JP18H05092), JSPS Grants-in-Aid for Scientific Research to N.M. (JP18K09715), D.A.A. (JP19K19220), H.K. (JP19K18549), Y.H. (JP18H02891), and K.H. (JP18H02996), Grants from Japan Agency for Medical Research and Development (AMED) to K.H. (JP19ck0106406h0002).

Conflicts of Interest: The authors declare no conflict of interest.

References

1. Folkman, J. Anti-angiogenesis: New concept for therapy of solid tumors. *Ann. Surg.* **1972**, *175*, 409–416. [CrossRef] [PubMed]
2. Culy, C. Bevacizumab: Antiangiogenic cancer therapy. *Drugs Today (Barc)* **2005**, *41*, 23–36. [CrossRef] [PubMed]
3. Leung, D.W.; Cachianes, G.; Kuang, W.J.; Goeddel, D.V.; Ferrara, N. Vascular endothelial growth factor is a secreted angiogenic mitogen. *Science* **1989**, *246*, 1306–1309. [CrossRef] [PubMed]
4. Rosenthal, R.A.; Megyesi, J.F.; Henzel, W.J.; Ferrara, N.; Folkman, J. Conditioned medium from mouse sarcoma 180 cells contains vascular endothelial growth factor. *Growth Factors* **1990**, *4*, 53–59. [CrossRef] [PubMed]
5. Senger, D.R.; Galli, S.J.; Dvorak, A.M.; Perruzzi, C.A.; Harvey, V.S.; Dvorak, H.F. Tumor cells secrete a vascular permeability factor that promotes accumulation of ascites fluid. *Science* **1983**, *219*, 983–985. [CrossRef] [PubMed]
6. Jain, R.K. Normalizing tumor vasculature with anti-angiogenic therapy: A new paradigm for combination therapy. *Nat. Med.* **2001**, *7*, 987–989. [CrossRef] [PubMed]
7. Jain, R.K. Normalization of tumor vasculature: An emerging concept in antiangiogenic therapy. *Science* **2005**, *307*, 58–62. [CrossRef] [PubMed]
8. Ebos, J.M.; Kerbel, R.S. Antiangiogenic therapy: Impact on invasion, disease progression, and metastasis. *Nat. Rev. Clin. Oncol.* **2011**, *8*, 210–221. [CrossRef] [PubMed]
9. van Beijnum, J.R.; Nowak-Sliwinska, P.; Huijbers, E.J.; Thijssen, V.L.; Griffioen, A.W. The great escape; the hallmarks of resistance to antiangiogenic therapy. *Pharmacol. Rev.* **2015**, *67*, 441–461. [CrossRef]
10. Endrich, B.; Reinhold, H.S.; Gross, J.F.; Intaglietta, M. Tissue perfusion inhomogeneity during early tumor growth in rats. *J. Natl. Cancer Inst.* **1979**, *62*, 387–395.
11. Zhang, X.; Nie, D.; Chakrabarty, S. Growth factors in tumor microenvironment. *Front. Biosci. (Landmark Ed)* **2010**, *15*, 151–165. [CrossRef] [PubMed]
12. Dvorak, H.F. Rous-Whipple Award Lecture. How tumors make bad blood vessels and stroma. *Am. J. Pathol.* **2003**, *162*, 1747–1757. [CrossRef]
13. Krock, B.L.; Skuli, N.; Simon, M.C. Hypoxia-induced angiogenesis: Good and evil. *Genes Cancer* **2011**, *2*, 1117–1133. [CrossRef] [PubMed]
14. Xu, L.; Fukumura, D.; Jain, R.K. Acidic extracellular pH induces vascular endothelial growth factor (VEGF) in human glioblastoma cells via ERK1/2 MAPK signaling pathway: Mechanism of low pH-induced VEGF. *J. Biol. Chem.* **2002**, *277*, 11368–11374. [CrossRef] [PubMed]
15. Konerding, M.A.; Malkusch, W.; Klapthor, B.; van Ackern, C.; Fait, E.; Hill, S.A.; Parkins, C.; Chaplin, D.J.; Presta, M.; Denekamp, J. Evidence for characteristic vascular patterns in solid tumours: Quantitative studies using corrosion casts. *Br. J. Cancer* **1999**, *80*, 724–732. [CrossRef] [PubMed]
16. Morikawa, S.; Baluk, P.; Kaidoh, T.; Haskell, A.; Jain, R.K.; McDonald, D.M. Abnormalities in pericytes on blood vessels and endothelial sprouts in tumors. *Am. J. Pathol.* **2002**, *160*, 985–1000. [CrossRef]
17. Folkman, J. Angiogenesis in cancer, vascular, rheumatoid and other disease. *Nat. Med.* **1995**, *1*, 27–31. [CrossRef]
18. Sund, M.; Zeisberg, M.; Kalluri, R. Endogenous Stimulators and Inhibitors of Angiogenesis in Gastrointestinal Cancers: Basic Science to Clinical Application. *Gastroenterology* **2005**, *129*, 2076–2091. [CrossRef]
19. Cantelmo, A.R.; Conradi, L.C.; Brajic, A.; Goveia, J.; Kalucka, J.; Pircher, A.; Chaturvedi, P.; Hol, J.; Thienpont, B.; Teuwen, L.A.; et al. Inhibition of the Glycolytic Activator PFKFB3 in Endothelium Induces Tumor Vessel Normalization, Impairs Metastasis, and Improves Chemotherapy. *Cancer Cell* **2016**, *30*, 968–985. [CrossRef]
20. Hashizume, H.; Baluk, P.; Morikawa, S.; McLean, J.W.; Thurston, G.; Roberge, S.; Jain, R.K.; McDonald, D.M. Openings between defective endothelial cells explain tumor vessel leakiness. *Am. J. Pathol.* **2000**, *156*, 1363–1380. [CrossRef]
21. Heldin, C.-H.; Rubin, K.; Pietras, K.; Östman, A. High interstitial fluid pressure — an obstacle in cancer therapy. *Nat. Rev. Cancer* **2004**, *4*, 806–813. [CrossRef] [PubMed]
22. Chaplin, D.J.; Olive, P.L.; Durand, R.E. Intermittent Blood Flow in a Murine Tumor: Radiobiological Effects. *Cancer Res.* **1987**, *47*, 597–601. [PubMed]

23. Jiang, J.; Tang, Y.L.; Liang, X.H. EMT: A new vision of hypoxia promoting cancer progression. *Cancer Biol. Ther.* **2011**, *11*, 714–723.
24. Akino, T.; Hida, K.; Hida, Y.; Tsuchiya, K.; Freedman, D.; Muraki, C.; Ohga, N.; Matsuda, K.; Akiyama, K.; Harabayashi, T.; et al. Cytogenetic abnormalities of tumor-associated endothelial cells in human malignant tumors. *Am. J. Pathol.* **2009**, *175*, 2657–2667. [CrossRef] [PubMed]
25. Hida, K.; Hida, Y.; Amin, D.N.; Flint, A.F.; Panigrahy, D.; Morton, C.C.; Klagsbrun, M. Tumor-associated endothelial cells with cytogenetic abnormalities. *Cancer Res.* **2004**, *64*, 8249–8255. [CrossRef] [PubMed]
26. Bussolati, B.; Deambrosis, I.; Russo, S.; Deregibus, M.C.; Camussi, G. Altered angiogenesis and survival in human tumor-derived endothelial cells. *FASEB J.* **2003**, *17*, 1159–1161. [CrossRef]
27. Alessandri, G.; Chirivi, R.G.; Fiorentini, S.; Dossi, R.; Bonardelli, S.; Giulini, S.M.; Zanetta, G.; Landoni, F.; Graziotti, P.P.; Turano, A.; et al. Phenotypic and functional characteristics of tumour-derived microvascular endothelial cells. *Clin. Exp. Metastasis* **1999**, *17*, 655–662.
28. Matsuda, K.; Ohga, N.; Hida, Y.; Muraki, C.; Tsuchiya, K.; Kurosu, T.; Akino, T.; Shih, S.C.; Totsuka, Y.; Klagsbrun, M.; et al. Isolated tumor endothelial cells maintain specific character during long-term culture. *Biochem. Biophys. Res. Commun.* **2010**, *394*, 947–954. [CrossRef]
29. Yamamoto, K.; Ohga, N.; Hida, Y.; Maishi, N.; Kawamoto, T.; Kitayama, K.; Akiyama, K.; Osawa, T.; Kondoh, M.; Matsuda, K.; et al. Biglycan is a specific marker and an autocrine angiogenic factor of tumour endothelial cells. *Br. J. Cancer.* **2012**, *106*, 1214–1223. [CrossRef]
30. Osawa, T.; Ohga, N.; Akiyama, K.; Hida, Y.; Kitayama, K.; Kawamoto, T.; Yamamoto, K.; Maishi, N.; Kondoh, M.; Onodera, Y.; et al. Lysyl oxidase secreted by tumour endothelial cells promotes angiogenesis and metastasis. *Br. J. Cancer* **2013**, *109*, 2237–2247. [CrossRef]
31. Hida, K.; Maishi, N.; Kawamoto, T.; Akiyama, K.; Ohga, N.; Hida, Y.; Yamada, K.; Hojo, T.; Kikuchi, H.; Sato, M.; et al. Tumor endothelial cells express high pentraxin 3 levels. *Pathol. Int.* **2016**, *66*, 687–694. [CrossRef] [PubMed]
32. Dudley, A.C. Tumor endothelial cells. *Cold Spring Harb. Perspect. Med.* **2012**, *2*, a006536. [CrossRef] [PubMed]
33. Otsubo, T.; Hida, Y.; Ohga, N.; Sato, H.; Kai, T.; Matsuki, Y.; Takasu, H.; Akiyama, K.; Maishi, N.; Kawamoto, T.; et al. Identification of novel targets for antiangiogenic therapy by comparing the gene expressions of tumor and normal endothelial cells. *Cancer Sci.* **2014**, *105*, 560–567. [CrossRef] [PubMed]
34. Ohga, N.; Ishikawa, S.; Maishi, N.; Akiyama, K.; Hida, Y.; Kawamoto, T.; Sadamoto, Y.; Osawa, T.; Yamamoto, K.; Kondoh, M.; et al. Heterogeneity of tumor endothelial cells: Comparison between tumor endothelial cells isolated from high- and low-metastatic tumors. *Am. J. Pathol.* **2012**, *180*, 1294–1307. [CrossRef] [PubMed]
35. Carnero, A.; Lleonart, M. The hypoxic microenvironment: A determinant of cancer stem cell evolution. *Bioessays* **2016**, *38* (Suppl. 1), S65–S74. [CrossRef] [PubMed]
36. Akiyama, K.; Ohga, N.; Hida, Y.; Kawamoto, T.; Sadamoto, Y.; Ishikawa, S.; Maishi, N.; Akino, T.; Kondoh, M.; Matsuda, A.; et al. Tumor endothelial cells acquire drug resistance by MDR1 up-regulation via VEGF signaling in tumor microenvironment. *Am. J. Pathol.* **2012**, *180*, 1283–1293. [CrossRef]
37. Hida, K.; Maishi, N.; Akiyama, K.; Ohmura-Kakutani, H.; Torii, C.; Ohga, N.; Osawa, T.; Kikuchi, H.; Morimoto, H.; Morimoto, M.; et al. Tumor endothelial cells with high aldehyde dehydrogenase activity show drug resistance. *Cancer Sci.* **2017**, *108*, 2195–2203. [CrossRef]
38. Xiong, Y.Q.; Sun, H.C.; Zhang, W.; Zhu, X.D.; Zhuang, P.Y.; Zhang, J.B.; Wang, L.; Wu, W.Z.; Qin, L.X.; Tang, Z.Y. Human hepatocellular carcinoma tumor-derived endothelial cells manifest increased angiogenesis capability and drug resistance compared with normal endothelial cells. *Clin. Cancer Res.* **2009**, *15*, 4838–4846. [CrossRef]
39. Gerhardt, H.; Betsholtz, C. Endothelial-pericyte interactions in angiogenesis. *Cell Tissue Res.* **2003**, *314*, 15–23. [CrossRef]
40. Eilken, H.M.; Adams, R.H. Dynamics of endothelial cell behavior in sprouting angiogenesis. *Curr. Opin. Cell Biol.* **2010**, *22*, 617–625. [CrossRef]
41. Geudens, I.; Gerhardt, H. Coordinating cell behaviour during blood vessel formation. *Development* **2011**, *138*, 4569–4583. [CrossRef] [PubMed]
42. Gerhardt, H.; Golding, M.; Fruttiger, M.; Ruhrberg, C.; Lundkvist, A.; Abramsson, A.; Jeltsch, M.; Mitchell, C.; Alitalo, K.; Shima, D.; et al. VEGF guides angiogenic sprouting utilizing endothelial tip cell filopodia. *J. Cell Biol.* **2003**, *161*, 1163–1177. [CrossRef] [PubMed]

43. Mazzone, M.; Dettori, D.; de Oliveira, R.L.; Loges, S.; Schmidt, T.; Jonckx, B.; Tian, Y.M.; Lanahan, A.A.; Pollard, P.; de Almodovar, C.R.; et al. Heterozygous deficiency of PHD2 restores tumor oxygenation and inhibits metastasis via endothelial normalization. *Cell* **2009**, *136*, 839–851. [CrossRef] [PubMed]
44. De Bock, K.; Georgiadou, M.; Schoors, S.; Kuchnio, A.; Wong, B.W.; Cantelmo, A.R.; Quaegebeur, A.; Ghesquiere, B.; Cauwenberghs, S.; Eelen, G.; et al. Role of PFKFB3-driven glycolysis in vessel sprouting. *Cell* **2013**, *154*, 651–663. [CrossRef] [PubMed]
45. Schoors, S.; Bruning, U.; Missiaen, R.; Queiroz, K.C.; Borgers, G.; Elia, I.; Zecchin, A.; Cantelmo, A.R.; Christen, S.; Goveia, J.; et al. Fatty acid carbon is essential for dNTP synthesis in endothelial cells. *Nature* **2015**, *520*, 192–197. [CrossRef] [PubMed]
46. Potente, M.; Carmeliet, P. The Link Between Angiogenesis and Endothelial Metabolism. *Annu. Rev. Physiol.* **2017**, *79*, 43–66. [CrossRef] [PubMed]
47. Asahara, T.; Murohara, T.; Sullivan, A.; Silver, M.; van der Zee, R.; Li, T.; Witzenbichler, B.; Schatteman, G.; Isner, J.M. Isolation of putative progenitor endothelial cells for angiogenesis. *Science* **1997**, *275*, 964–967. [CrossRef]
48. Asahara, T.; Masuda, H.; Takahashi, T.; Kalka, C.; Pastore, C.; Silver, M.; Kearne, M.; Magner, M.; Isner, J.M. Bone marrow origin of endothelial progenitor cells responsible for postnatal vasculogenesis in physiological and pathological neovascularization. *Circ. Res.* **1999**, *85*, 221–228. [CrossRef]
49. Asahara, T.; Kawamoto, A. Endothelial progenitor cells for postnatal vasculogenesis. *Am. J. Physiol. Cell Physiol.* **2004**, *287*, C572–C579. [CrossRef]
50. Lyden, D.; Hattori, K.; Dias, S.; Costa, C.; Blaikie, P.; Butros, L.; Chadburn, A.; Heissig, B.; Marks, W.; Witte, L.; et al. Impaired recruitment of bone-marrow-derived endothelial and hematopoietic precursor cells blocks tumor angiogenesis and growth. *Nat. Med.* **2001**, *7*, 1194–1201. [CrossRef]
51. Rafii, S.; Lyden, D.; Benezra, R.; Hattori, K.; Heissig, B. Vascular and haematopoietic stem cells: Novel targets for anti-angiogenesis therapy? *Nat. Rev. Cancer* **2002**, *2*, 826–835. [CrossRef] [PubMed]
52. Nolan, D.J.; Ciarrocchi, A.; Mellick, A.S.; Jaggi, J.S.; Bambino, K.; Gupta, S.; Heikamp, E.; McDevitt, M.R.; Scheinberg, D.A.; Benezra, R.; et al. Bone marrow-derived endothelial progenitor cells are a major determinant of nascent tumor neovascularization. *Genes Dev.* **2007**, *21*, 1546–1558. [CrossRef] [PubMed]
53. Marcola, M.; Rodrigues, C.E. Endothelial progenitor cells in tumor angiogenesis: Another brick in the wall. *Stem Cells Int.* **2015**, *2015*, 832649. [CrossRef] [PubMed]
54. Risau, W. Differentiation of endothelium. *FASEB J.* **1995**, *9*, 926–933. [CrossRef] [PubMed]
55. Aird, W.C. Phenotypic heterogeneity of the endothelium: I. Structure, function, and mechanisms. *Circ. Res.* **2007**, *100*, 158–173. [CrossRef] [PubMed]
56. Kumar, S.; West, D.C.; Ager, A. Heterogeneity in endothelial cells from large vessels and microvessels. *Differentiation* **1987**, *36*, 57–70. [CrossRef]
57. Chi, J.T.; Chang, H.Y.; Haraldsen, G.; Jahnsen, F.L.; Troyanskaya, O.G.; Chang, D.S.; Wang, Z.; Rockson, S.G.; van de Rijn, M.; Botstein, D.; et al. Endothelial cell diversity revealed by global expression profiling. *Proc. Natl. Acad. Sci. USA* **2003**, *100*, 10623–10628. [CrossRef]
58. Nolan, D.J.; Ginsberg, M.; Israely, E.; Palikuqi, B.; Poulos, M.G.; James, D.; Ding, B.S.; Schachterle, W.; Liu, Y.; Rosenwaks, Z.; et al. Molecular signatures of tissue-specific microvascular endothelial cell heterogeneity in organ maintenance and regeneration. *Dev. Cell* **2013**, *26*, 204–219. [CrossRef]
59. Zhao, Q.; Eichten, A.; Parveen, A.; Adler, C.; Huang, Y.; Wang, W.; Ding, Y.; Adler, A.; Nevins, T.; Ni, M.; et al. Single-Cell Transcriptome Analyses Reveal Endothelial Cell Heterogeneity in Tumors and Changes following Antiangiogenic Treatment. *Cancer Res.* **2018**, *78*, 2370–2382. [CrossRef]
60. Aird, W.C. Endothelial cell heterogeneity. *Cold Spring Harb. Perspect. Med.* **2012**, *2*, a006429. [CrossRef]
61. Streubel, B.; Chott, A.; Huber, D.; Exner, M.; Jager, U.; Wagner, O.; Schwarzinger, I. Lymphoma-specific genetic aberrations in microvascular endothelial cells in B-cell lymphomas. *N. Engl. J. Med.* **2004**, *351*, 250–259. [CrossRef] [PubMed]
62. Ricci-Vitiani, L.; Pallini, R.; Biffoni, M.; Todaro, M.; Invernici, G.; Cenci, T.; Maira, G.; Parati, E.A.; Stassi, G.; Larocca, L.M.; et al. Tumour vascularization via endothelial differentiation of glioblastoma stem-like cells. *Nature* **2010**, *468*, 824–828. [CrossRef] [PubMed]
63. Wang, R.; Chadalavada, K.; Wilshire, J.; Kowalik, U.; Hovinga, K.E.; Geber, A.; Fligelman, B.; Leversha, M.; Brennan, C.; Tabar, V. Glioblastoma stem-like cells give rise to tumour endothelium. *Nature* **2010**, *468*, 829–833. [CrossRef] [PubMed]

64. Soda, Y.; Marumoto, T.; Friedmann-Morvinski, D.; Soda, M.; Liu, F.; Michiue, H.; Pastorino, S.; Yang, M.; Hoffman, R.M.; Kesari, S.; et al. Transdifferentiation of glioblastoma cells into vascular endothelial cells. *Proc. Natl. Acad. Sci. USA* **2011**, *108*, 4274–4280. [CrossRef]
65. Cheng, L.; Huang, Z.; Zhou, W.; Wu, Q.; Donnola, S.; Liu, J.K.; Fang, X.; Sloan, A.E.; Mao, Y.; Lathia, J.D.; et al. Glioblastoma stem cells generate vascular pericytes to support vessel function and tumor growth. *Cell* **2013**, *153*, 139–152. [CrossRef]
66. Kulla, A.; Burkhardt, K.; Meyer-Puttlitz, B.; Teesalu, T.; Asser, T.; Wiestler, O.D.; Becker, A.J. Analysis of the TP53 gene in laser-microdissected glioblastoma vasculature. *Acta Neuropathol.* **2003**, *105*, 328–332.
67. Rodriguez, F.J.; Orr, B.A.; Ligon, K.L.; Eberhart, C.G. Neoplastic cells are a rare component in human glioblastoma microvasculature. *Oncotarget* **2012**, *3*, 98–106. [CrossRef]
68. Chen, H.; Campbell, R.A.; Chang, Y.; Li, M.; Wang, C.S.; Li, J.; Sanchez, E.; Share, M.; Steinberg, J.; Berenson, A.; et al. Pleiotrophin produced by multiple myeloma induces transdifferentiation of monocytes into vascular endothelial cells: A novel mechanism of tumor-induced vasculogenesis. *Blood* **2009**, *113*, 1992–2002. [CrossRef]
69. Fernandez Pujol, B.; Lucibello, F.C.; Gehling, U.M.; Lindemann, K.; Weidner, N.; Zuzarte, M.L.; Adamkiewicz, J.; Elsasser, H.P.; Muller, R.; Havemann, K. Endothelial-like cells derived from human CD14 positive monocytes. *Differentiation* **2000**, *65*, 287–300. [CrossRef]
70. Fernandez Pujol, B.; Lucibello, F.C.; Zuzarte, M.; Lutjens, P.; Muller, R.; Havemann, K. Dendritic cells derived from peripheral monocytes express endothelial markers and in the presence of angiogenic growth factors differentiate into endothelial-like cells. *Eur. J. Cell Biol.* **2001**, *80*, 99–110. [CrossRef]
71. Nagy, J.A.; Chang, S.H.; Shih, S.C.; Dvorak, A.M.; Dvorak, H.F. Heterogeneity of the tumor vasculature. *Semin. Thromb. Hemost.* **2010**, *36*, 321–331. [CrossRef] [PubMed]
72. Ohmura-Kakutani, H.; Akiyama, K.; Maishi, N.; Ohga, N.; Hida, Y.; Kawamoto, T.; Iida, J.; Shindoh, M.; Tsuchiya, K.; Shinohara, N.; et al. Identification of tumor endothelial cells with high aldehyde dehydrogenase activity and a highly angiogenic phenotype. *PLoS ONE* **2014**, *9*, e113910. [CrossRef] [PubMed]
73. Naito, H.; Wakabayashi, T.; Kidoya, H.; Muramatsu, F.; Takara, K.; Eino, D.; Yamane, K.; Iba, T.; Takakura, N. Endothelial Side Population Cells Contribute to Tumor Angiogenesis and Antiangiogenic Drug Resistance. *Cancer Res.* **2016**, *76*, 3200–3210. [CrossRef] [PubMed]
74. Moulder, J.E.; Rockwell, S. Tumor hypoxia: Its impact on cancer therapy. *Cancer Metastasis Rev.* **1987**, *5*, 313–341. [CrossRef] [PubMed]
75. Hojo, T.; Maishi, N.; Towfik, A.M.; Akiyama, K.; Ohga, N.; Shindoh, M.; Hida, Y.; Minowa, K.; Fujisawa, T.; Hida, K. ROS enhance angiogenic properties via regulation of NRF2 in tumor endothelial cells. *Oncotarget* **2017**, *8*, 45484–45495. [CrossRef] [PubMed]
76. Taylor, S.M.; Nevis, K.R.; Park, H.L.; Rogers, G.C.; Rogers, S.L.; Cook, J.G.; Bautch, V.L. Angiogenic factor signaling regulates centrosome duplication in endothelial cells of developing blood vessels. *Blood* **2010**, *116*, 3108–3117. [CrossRef] [PubMed]
77. Kondoh, M.; Ohga, N.; Akiyama, K.; Hida, Y.; Maishi, N.; Towfik, A.M.; Inoue, N.; Shindoh, M.; Hida, K. Hypoxia-induced reactive oxygen species cause chromosomal abnormalities in endothelial cells in the tumor microenvironment. *PLoS ONE* **2013**, *8*, e80349. [CrossRef]
78. Maishi, N.; Ohga, N.; Hida, Y.; Akiyama, K.; Kitayama, K.; Osawa, T.; Onodera, Y.; Shinohara, N.; Nonomura, K.; Shindoh, M.; et al. CXCR7: A novel tumor endothelial marker in renal cell carcinoma. *Pathol. Int.* **2012**, *62*, 309–317. [CrossRef]
79. Maishi, N.; Ohba, Y.; Akiyama, K.; Ohga, N.; Hamada, J.; Nagao-Kitamoto, H.; Alam, M.T.; Yamamoto, K.; Kawamoto, T.; Inoue, N.; et al. Tumour endothelial cells in high metastatic tumours promote metastasis via epigenetic dysregulation of biglycan. *Sci. Rep.* **2016**, *6*, 28039. [CrossRef]
80. Kawamoto, T.; Ohga, N.; Akiyama, K.; Hirata, N.; Kitahara, S.; Maishi, N.; Osawa, T.; Yamamoto, K.; Kondoh, M.; Shindoh, M.; et al. Tumor-derived microvesicles induce proangiogenic phenotype in endothelial cells via endocytosis. *PLoS ONE* **2012**, *7*, e34045. [CrossRef]
81. Zeisberg, E.M.; Potenta, S.; Xie, L.; Zeisberg, M.; Kalluri, R. Discovery of endothelial to mesenchymal transition as a source for carcinoma-associated fibroblasts. *Cancer Res.* **2007**, *67*, 10123–10128. [CrossRef] [PubMed]

82. Cooley, B.C.; Nevado, J.; Mellad, J.; Yang, D.; St Hilaire, C.; Negro, A.; Fang, F.; Chen, G.; San, H.; Walts, A.D.; et al. TGF-beta signaling mediates endothelial-to-mesenchymal transition (EndMT) during vein graft remodeling. *Sci. Transl. Med.* **2014**, *6*, 227ra234. [CrossRef]
83. Xiao, L.; Kim, D.J.; Davis, C.L.; McCann, J.V.; Dunleavey, J.M.; Vanderlinden, A.K.; Xu, N.; Pattenden, S.G.; Frye, S.V.; Xu, X.; et al. Tumor Endothelial Cells with Distinct Patterns of TGFbeta-Driven Endothelial-to-Mesenchymal Transition. *Cancer Res.* **2015**, *75*, 1244–1254. [CrossRef] [PubMed]
84. Akatsu, Y.; Takahashi, N.; Yoshimatsu, Y.; Kimuro, S.; Muramatsu, T.; Katsura, A.; Maishi, N.; Suzuki, H.I.; Inazawa, J.; Hida, K.; et al. Fibroblast growth factor signals regulate transforming growth factor-beta-induced endothelial-to-myofibroblast transition of tumor endothelial cells via Elk1. *Mol. Oncol.* **2019**, *13*, 1706–1724. [CrossRef] [PubMed]
85. Fidler, I.J. The pathogenesis of cancer metastasis: The 'seed and soil' hypothesis revisited. *Nat. Rev. Cancer* **2003**, *3*, 453–458. [CrossRef] [PubMed]
86. Quail, D.F.; Joyce, J.A. Microenvironmental regulation of tumor progression and metastasis. *Nat. Med.* **2013**, *19*, 1423–1437. [CrossRef] [PubMed]
87. Sokeland, G.; Schumacher, U. The functional role of integrins during intra- and extravasation within the metastatic cascade. *Mol. Cancer* **2019**, *18*, 12. [CrossRef]
88. Butler, J.M.; Kobayashi, H.; Rafii, S. Instructive role of the vascular niche in promoting tumour growth and tissue repair by angiocrine factors. *Nat. Rev. Cancer* **2010**, *10*, 138–146. [CrossRef]
89. Pirtskhalaishvili, G.; Nelson, J.B. Endothelium-derived factors as paracrine mediators of prostate cancer progression. *Prostate* **2000**, *44*, 77–87. [CrossRef]
90. Cao, Z.; Ding, B.S.; Guo, P.; Lee, S.B.; Butler, J.M.; Casey, S.C.; Simons, M.; Tam, W.; Felsher, D.W.; Shido, K.; et al. Angiocrine factors deployed by tumor vascular niche induce B cell lymphoma invasiveness and chemoresistance. *Cancer Cell* **2014**, *25*, 350–365. [CrossRef]
91. Yamada, K.; Maishi, N.; Akiyama, K.; Towfik Alam, M.; Ohga, N.; Kawamoto, T.; Shindoh, M.; Takahashi, N.; Kamiyama, T.; Hida, Y.; et al. CXCL12-CXCR7 axis is important for tumor endothelial cell angiogenic property. *Int. J. Cancer* **2015**, *137*, 2825–2836. [CrossRef]
92. Miao, Z.; Luker, K.E.; Summers, B.C.; Berahovich, R.; Bhojani, M.S.; Rehemtulla, A.; Kleer, C.G.; Essner, J.J.; Nasevicius, A.; Luker, G.D.; et al. CXCR7 (RDC1) promotes breast and lung tumor growth in vivo and is expressed on tumor-associated vasculature. *Proc. Natl. Acad. Sci. USA* **2007**, *104*, 15735–15740. [CrossRef] [PubMed]
93. Zabel, B.A.; Wang, Y.; Lewen, S.; Berahovich, R.D.; Penfold, M.E.; Zhang, P.; Powers, J.; Summers, B.C.; Miao, Z.; Zhao, B.; et al. Elucidation of CXCR7-mediated signaling events and inhibition of CXCR4-mediated tumor cell transendothelial migration by CXCR7 ligands. *J. Immunol.* **2009**, *183*, 3204–3211. [CrossRef] [PubMed]
94. Jeon, H.M.; Kim, S.H.; Jin, X.; Park, J.B.; Kim, S.H.; Joshi, K.; Nakano, I.; Kim, H. Crosstalk between glioma-initiating cells and endothelial cells drives tumor progression. *Cancer Res.* **2014**, *74*, 4482–4492. [CrossRef] [PubMed]
95. Brantley-Sieders, D.M.; Dunaway, C.M.; Rao, M.; Short, S.; Hwang, Y.; Gao, Y.; Li, D.; Jiang, A.; Shyr, Y.; Wu, J.Y.; et al. Angiocrine factors modulate tumor proliferation and motility through EphA2 repression of Slit2 tumor suppressor function in endothelium. *Cancer Res.* **2011**, *71*, 976–987. [CrossRef] [PubMed]
96. Scholz, A.; Harter, P.N.; Cremer, S.; Yalcin, B.H.; Gurnik, S.; Yamaji, M.; Di Tacchio, M.; Sommer, K.; Baumgarten, P.; Bahr, O.; et al. Endothelial cell-derived angiopoietin-2 is a therapeutic target in treatment-naive and bevacizumab-resistant glioblastoma. *EMBO Mol. Med.* **2016**, *8*, 39–57. [CrossRef] [PubMed]
97. Carmeliet, P.; Jain, R.K. Angiogenesis in cancer and other diseases. *Nature* **2000**, *407*, 249–257. [CrossRef]
98. Mathieu, C.; Sii-Felice, K.; Fouchet, P.; Etienne, O.; Haton, C.; Mabondzo, A.; Boussin, F.D.; Mouthon, M.A. Endothelial cell-derived bone morphogenetic proteins control proliferation of neural stem/progenitor cells. *Mol. Cell Neurosci.* **2008**, *38*, 569–577. [CrossRef]
99. Hendrikx, S.; Coso, S.; Prat-Luri, B.; Wetterwald, L.; Sabine, A.; Franco, C.A.; Nassiri, S.; Zangger, N.; Gerhardt, H.; Delorenzi, M.; et al. Endothelial Calcineurin Signaling Restrains Metastatic Outgrowth by Regulating Bmp2. *Cell Rep.* **2019**, *26*, 1227–1241. [CrossRef]

100. Hayakawa, Y.; Ariyama, H.; Stancikova, J.; Sakitani, K.; Asfaha, S.; Renz, B.W.; Dubeykovskaya, Z.A.; Shibata, W.; Wang, H.; Westphalen, C.B.; et al. Mist1 Expressing Gastric Stem Cells Maintain the Normal and Neoplastic Gastric Epithelium and Are Supported by a Perivascular Stem Cell Niche. *Cancer Cell* **2015**, *28*, 800–814. [CrossRef]
101. Pitt, L.A.; Tikhonova, A.N.; Hu, H.; Trimarchi, T.; King, B.; Gong, Y.; Sanchez-Martin, M.; Tsirigos, A.; Littman, D.R.; Ferrando, A.A.; et al. CXCL12-Producing Vascular Endothelial Niches Control Acute T Cell Leukemia Maintenance. *Cancer Cell* **2015**, *27*, 755–768. [CrossRef] [PubMed]
102. Nelson, J.B.; Chan-Tack, K.; Hedican, S.P.; Magnuson, S.R.; Opgenorth, T.J.; Bova, G.S.; Simons, J.W. Endothelin-1 production and decreased endothelin B receptor expression in advanced prostate cancer. *Cancer Res.* **1996**, *56*, 663–668. [PubMed]
103. Hatfield, K.; Ryningen, A.; Corbascio, M.; Bruserud, O. Microvascular endothelial cells increase proliferation and inhibit apoptosis of native human acute myelogenous leukemia blasts. *Int. J. Cancer* **2006**, *119*, 2313–2321. [CrossRef] [PubMed]
104. Hood, J.L. Melanoma exosome induction of endothelial cell GM-CSF in pre-metastatic lymph nodes may result in different M1 and M2 macrophage mediated angiogenic processes. *Med. Hypotheses* **2016**, *94*, 118–122. [CrossRef] [PubMed]
105. Cao, Z.; Scandura, J.M.; Inghirami, G.G.; Shido, K.; Ding, B.S.; Rafii, S. Molecular Checkpoint Decisions Made by Subverted Vascular Niche Transform Indolent Tumor Cells into Chemoresistant Cancer Stem Cells. *Cancer Cell* **2017**, *31*, 110–126. [CrossRef] [PubMed]
106. De Francesco, E.M.; Sims, A.H.; Maggiolini, M.; Sotgia, F.; Lisanti, M.P.; Clarke, R.B. GPER mediates the angiocrine actions induced by IGF1 through the HIF-1alpha/VEGF pathway in the breast tumor microenvironment. *Breast Cancer Res.* **2017**, *19*, 129. [CrossRef] [PubMed]
107. Wang, Q.; He, Z.; Huang, M.; Liu, T.; Wang, Y.; Xu, H.; Duan, H.; Ma, P.; Zhang, L.; Zamvil, S.S.; et al. Vascular niche IL-6 induces alternative macrophage activation in glioblastoma through HIF-2alpha. *Nat. Commun.* **2018**, *9*, 559. [CrossRef] [PubMed]
108. Ye, B.G.; Sun, H.C.; Zhu, X.D.; Chai, Z.T.; Zhang, Y.Y.; Ao, J.Y.; Cai, H.; Ma, D.N.; Wang, C.H.; Qin, C.D.; et al. Reduced expression of CD109 in tumor-associated endothelial cells promotes tumor progression by paracrine interleukin-8 in hepatocellular carcinoma. *Oncotarget* **2016**, *7*, 29333–29345. [CrossRef] [PubMed]
109. Nikolova, G.; Strilic, B.; Lammert, E. The vascular niche and its basement membrane. *Trends Cell Biol.* **2007**, *17*, 19–25. [CrossRef] [PubMed]
110. Charles, N.; Ozawa, T.; Squatrito, M.; Bleau, A.M.; Brennan, C.W.; Hambardzumyan, D.; Holland, E.C. Perivascular nitric oxide activates notch signaling and promotes stem-like character in PDGF-induced glioma cells. *Cell Stem Cell* **2010**, *6*, 141–152. [CrossRef] [PubMed]
111. Fischer, C.; Mazzone, M.; Jonckx, B.; Carmeliet, P. FLT1 and its ligands VEGFB and PlGF: Drug targets for anti-angiogenic therapy? *Nat. Rev. Cancer* **2008**, *8*, 942–956. [CrossRef] [PubMed]
112. Alam, M.T.; Nagao-Kitamoto, H.; Ohga, N.; Akiyama, K.; Maishi, N.; Kawamoto, T.; Shinohara, N.; Taketomi, A.; Shindoh, M.; Hida, Y.; et al. Suprabasin as a novel tumor endothelial cell marker. *Cancer Sci.* **2014**, *105*, 1533–1540. [CrossRef] [PubMed]
113. Ghiabi, P.; Jiang, J.; Pasquier, J.; Maleki, M.; Abu-Kaoud, N.; Halabi, N.; Guerrouahen, B.S.; Rafii, S.; Rafii, A. Breast cancer cells promote a notch-dependent mesenchymal phenotype in endothelial cells participating to a pro-tumoral niche. *J. Transl. Med.* **2015**, *13*, 27. [CrossRef] [PubMed]
114. Lee, S.; Chen, T.T.; Barber, C.L.; Jordan, M.C.; Murdock, J.; Desai, S.; Ferrara, N.; Nagy, A.; Roos, K.P.; Iruela-Arispe, M.L. Autocrine VEGF signaling is required for vascular homeostasis. *Cell* **2007**, *130*, 691–703. [CrossRef] [PubMed]
115. Wieland, E.; Rodriguez-Vita, J.; Liebler, S.S.; Mogler, C.; Moll, I.; Herberich, S.E.; Espinet, E.; Herpel, E.; Menuchin, A.; Chang-Claude, J.; et al. Endothelial Notch1 Activity Facilitates Metastasis. *Cancer Cell* **2017**, *31*, 355–367. [CrossRef] [PubMed]
116. Cunha, S.I.; Bocci, M.; Lovrot, J.; Eleftheriou, N.; Roswall, P.; Cordero, E.; Lindstrom, L.; Bartoschek, M.; Haller, B.K.; Pearsall, R.S.; et al. Endothelial ALK1 Is a Therapeutic Target to Block Metastatic Dissemination of Breast Cancer. *Cancer Res.* **2015**, *75*, 2445–2456. [CrossRef] [PubMed]
117. Baker, E.K.; Johnstone, R.W.; Zalcberg, J.R.; El-Osta, A. Epigenetic changes to the MDR1 locus in response to chemotherapeutic drugs. *Oncogene* **2005**, *24*, 8061–8075. [CrossRef] [PubMed]

118. Akiyama, K.; Maishi, N.; Ohga, N.; Hida, Y.; Ohba, Y.; Alam, M.T.; Kawamoto, T.; Ohmura, H.; Yamada, K.; Torii, C.; et al. Inhibition of multidrug transporter in tumor endothelial cells enhances antiangiogenic effects of low-dose metronomic paclitaxel. *Am. J. Pathol.* **2015**, *185*, 572–580. [CrossRef] [PubMed]
119. Topalian, S.L.; Hodi, F.S.; Brahmer, J.R.; Gettinger, S.N.; Smith, D.C.; McDermott, D.F.; Powderly, J.D.; Carvajal, R.D.; Sosman, J.A.; Atkins, M.B.; et al. Safety, activity, and immune correlates of anti-PD-1 antibody in cancer. *N. Engl. J. Med.* **2012**, *366*, 2443–2454. [CrossRef]
120. Iwai, Y.; Ishida, M.; Tanaka, Y.; Okazaki, T.; Honjo, T.; Minato, N. Involvement of PD-L1 on tumor cells in the escape from host immune system and tumor immunotherapy by PD-L1 blockade. *Proc. Natl. Acad. Sci. USA* **2002**, *99*, 12293–12297. [CrossRef]
121. Vestweber, D. How leukocytes cross the vascular endothelium. *Nat. Rev. Immunol.* **2015**, *15*, 692–704. [CrossRef] [PubMed]
122. Johansson-Percival, A.; He, B.; Ganss, R. Immunomodulation of Tumor Vessels: It Takes Two to Tango. *Trends Immunol.* **2018**, *39*, 801–814. [CrossRef] [PubMed]
123. Dirkx, A.E.; Oude Egbrink, M.G.; Kuijpers, M.J.; van der Niet, S.T.; Heijnen, V.V.; Bouma-ter Steege, J.C.; Wagstaff, J.; Griffioen, A.W. Tumor angiogenesis modulates leukocyte-vessel wall interactions in vivo by reducing endothelial adhesion molecule expression. *Cancer Res.* **2003**, *63*, 2322–2329. [PubMed]
124. Motz, G.T.; Santoro, S.P.; Wang, L.P.; Garrabrant, T.; Lastra, R.R.; Hagemann, I.S.; Lal, P.; Feldman, M.D.; Benencia, F.; Coukos, G. Tumor endothelium FasL establishes a selective immune barrier promoting tolerance in tumors. *Nat. Med.* **2014**, *20*, 607–615. [CrossRef] [PubMed]
125. Wang, L.; Fan, J.; Thompson, L.F.; Zhang, Y.; Shin, T.; Curiel, T.J.; Zhang, B. CD73 has distinct roles in nonhematopoietic and hematopoietic cells to promote tumor growth in mice. *J. Clin. Investig.* **2011**, *121*, 2371–2382. [CrossRef] [PubMed]
126. Allard, B.; Turcotte, M.; Spring, K.; Pommey, S.; Royal, I.; Stagg, J. Anti-CD73 therapy impairs tumor angiogenesis. *Int. J. Cancer* **2014**, *134*, 1466–1473. [CrossRef]
127. Schmittnaegel, M.; Rigamonti, N.; Kadioglu, E.; Cassara, A.; Wyser Rmili, C.; Kiialainen, A.; Kienast, Y.; Mueller, H.J.; Ooi, C.H.; Laoui, D.; et al. Dual angiopoietin-2 and VEGFA inhibition elicits antitumor immunity that is enhanced by PD-1 checkpoint blockade. *Sci. Transl. Med.* **2017**, *9*. [CrossRef]
128. Huang, Y.; Yuan, J.; Righi, E.; Kamoun, W.S.; Ancukiewicz, M.; Nezivar, J.; Santosuosso, M.; Martin, J.D.; Martin, M.R.; Vianello, F.; et al. Vascular normalizing doses of antiangiogenic treatment reprogram the immunosuppressive tumor microenvironment and enhance immunotherapy. *Proc. Natl. Acad. Sci. USA* **2012**, *109*, 17561–17566. [CrossRef]
129. Johansson, A.; Hamzah, J.; Payne, C.J.; Ganss, R. Tumor-targeted TNFalpha stabilizes tumor vessels and enhances active immunotherapy. *Proc. Natl. Acad. Sci. USA* **2012**, *109*, 7841–7846. [CrossRef]
130. Johansson-Percival, A.; Li, Z.J.; Lakhiani, D.D.; He, B.; Wang, X.; Hamzah, J.; Ganss, R. Intratumoral LIGHT Restores Pericyte Contractile Properties and Vessel Integrity. *Cell Rep.* **2015**, *13*, 2687–2698. [CrossRef]

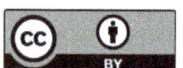

© 2019 by the authors. Licensee MDPI, Basel, Switzerland. This article is an open access article distributed under the terms and conditions of the Creative Commons Attribution (CC BY) license (http://creativecommons.org/licenses/by/4.0/).

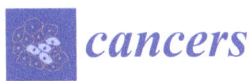

Review

Morphologic and Genomic Heterogeneity in the Evolution and Progression of Breast Cancer

Jamie R. Kutasovic [1,2], Amy E. McCart Reed [1,2], Anna Sokolova [1,3], Sunil R. Lakhani [1,3] and Peter T. Simpson [1,*]

1. UQ Centre for Clinical Research, Faculty of Medicine, The University of Queensland, Herston, Brisbane 4029, Australia; j.kutasovic@uq.edu.au (J.R.K.); amy.reed@uq.edu.au (A.E.M.R.); Anna.Sokolova@health.qld.gov.au (A.S.); s.lakhani@uq.edu.au (S.R.L.)
2. QIMR Berghofer Medical Research Institute, Herston 4006, Australia
3. Pathology Queensland, The Royal Brisbane & Women's Hospital, Herston, Brisbane 4029, Australia
* Correspondence: p.simpson@uq.edu.au

Received: 6 March 2020; Accepted: 26 March 2020; Published: 31 March 2020

Abstract: Breast cancer is a remarkably complex and diverse disease. Subtyping based on morphology, genomics, biomarkers and/or clinical parameters seeks to stratify optimal approaches for management, but it is clear that every breast cancer is fundamentally unique. Intra-tumour heterogeneity adds further complexity and impacts a patient's response to neoadjuvant or adjuvant therapy. Here, we review some established and more recent evidence related to the complex nature of breast cancer evolution. We describe morphologic and genomic diversity as it arises spontaneously during the early stages of tumour evolution, and also in the context of treatment where the changing subclonal architecture of a tumour is driven by the inherent adaptability of tumour cells to evolve and resist the selective pressures of therapy.

Keywords: breast cancer; genomics; intra-tumour heterogeneity; metastasis; subclonal diversity; treatment resistance

1. Introduction

That breast cancer is heterogeneous is beyond all doubt. We now count at least 20 histological subtypes of invasive breast cancer, defined by morphologic growth patterns and cytological appearance [1] and three broad biological subtypes, based on the expression of diagnostic biomarkers (oestrogen (ER) and progesterone (PR) receptor positive; HER2 positive; and triple negative (lacking hormone receptors and HER2). The 'big data' revolution has dramatically enhanced our appreciation of the molecular heterogeneity of breast cancer, further stratifying the disease into biologically and clinically meaningful subtypes, including six or more intrinsic subtypes (normal, claudin-low, luminals A and B, HER2 enriched and basal) [2–5]; four triple negative molecular subtypes (basal-like 1, basal-like 2, mesenchymal and luminal androgen receptor) [6]; and, ten integrative clusters captured by combined transcriptional and DNA copy number profiling [7]. Adding to this, the diversity of extra-tumoral components such as the tumour matrix and immune infiltrate is substantial and so it is easy to imagine that no two breast cancers will respond to therapy, or potentially progress to metastasis in quite the same way.

The recent advances in genomics technology is providing elaborate detail to the somatic architecture of breast tumour genomes, and with it, unprecedented insight into the mechanisms at play driving tumour development, adaptation and progression in response to treatment. Next generation sequencing technology has built on foundational knowledge created by candidate gene sequencing and comparative genomic hybridisation to provide very high depth, targeted gene panel sequencing for identifying targetable mutations and subclonal mutations; whole exome sequencing (WES) for comprehensive mutational analysis of all coding sequences; and whole genome sequencing (WGS) for an unbiased survey of all coding and non-coding sequences to capture the full repertoire of genetic alterations, encompassing single nucleotide variants (SNVs), small insertions and deletions (indels), copy number alterations (CNAs) and structural variants (SVs). Most somatic genetic alterations are perceived to provide little or no advantage to the neoplastic cells in which they arise (passenger mutations), however some enhance or inhibit the activity of cancer genes, and hence are termed driver mutations. One of the great powers of WGS is the ability to use the large numbers of SNVs, indels, CNAs and SVs to call mutational signatures and the analysis of these 'genomic scars' reveal great insight into the causative factors driving an individual cancer [8–12]; i.e., the exogenous carcinogenic processes, defective endogenous cellular processes or germline predisposition that have played a significant role in the aetiology of an individual cancer.

Here we outline how the molecular genetic analysis of tumour genomes has shed light on the inter- and intra-tumour heterogeneity exhibited by breast cancer; we elaborate on the concepts of cancer drivers and clonal evolution linked directly to the diverse morphological characteristics of the disease; and the complex processes of metastasis.

2. Genomic Diversity of Primary Breast Cancer

There are several landmark studies that have characterised the genomic landscape of invasive breast cancers [10,11,13–16]. It is increasingly clear that each breast cancer is genomically distinct, with a high level of diversity in the overall number of individual genetic alterations (SNVs, indels, CNAs, SVs), the cancer genes affected, and the global patterns of mutations captured by mutational signatures.

Most breast cancers have relatively low numbers of SNVs and indels, compared to other cancer types, however, approximately 20% of tumours are associated with defective homologous recombination (HR) double strand break repair (e.g., in particular those arising in *BRCA1*, *BRCA2*, *PALB2*, *RAD51C* germline mutation carriers), and these exhibit high rates of SNVs and indels. Further, a minority of tumours (<10%) exhibit hypermutator phenotypes, for instance in tumours associated with defective base excision repair (e.g., *MUTYH* inactivation), mismatch repair (e.g., *MSH2*, *PMS2*, *MLH1* inactivation) or APOBEC cytidine deaminase activity mutational signatures [8,9,12,14,17–19].

From an architectural point view, some breast cancers have 'simple' genomes (e.g., tumours with the 1q gain and 16q deletion pattern of alterations), whilst other tumours exhibit complex arrays of structural variants involving interchromosomal rearrangements and high level amplification of major oncogenic driver genes (e.g., including *ERBB2*/HER2, *CCND1*, *ZNF703*/FGFR1, *MYC*); and tumours associated with defective HR repair exhibit extremely high levels of chromosomal instability [7,9,13,14,20,21].

A meta-analysis of breast cancer sequencing studies has established that there are at least 147 breast cancer driver genes [22]. Approximately three driver gene mutations are found per tumour [14] and there are a multitude of combinations possible [23]. Some are mutated or altered at high frequency (e.g., *TP53, PIK3CA, MYC, CCND1, ERBB2*) whilst most are affected infrequently, with only 39/147 (26.5%) of these driver genes being altered in 5% or more of the TCGA breast cancer samples (Figure 1A). Further, some genes exhibit a strong genotype/phenotype relationship and so when altered they contribute to the resulting molecular and phenotypic lineage that subsequently develops. For instance, the distribution of driver mutations differs between ER positive and ER negative tumours [14], including the most common driver genes, *PIK3CA* and *TP53*, respectively. This is also evident in familial breast cancer, where the inheritance of a pathogenic germline driver mutation is also strongly related to the resulting tumour phenotype: ER-negative in *BRCA1*-associated tumours (with high frequency of TP53 mutations); ER-positive in *BRCA2*, *ATM* and *CHEK2*-associated tumours; HER2-positive in TP53-carriers; and E-cadherin negative and lobular growth pattern in *CDH1*-carriers [19,24–29].

Some driver mutations manifest more frequently in morphologically distinct tumours and some are pathognomonic for special histological types of the disease (Figure 1B–D). Elegant examples of this occur in rare breast cancer special types; for example secretory carcinomas arise due to the highly recurrent oncogenic driver created by a balanced t(12;15) (p13;q25) translocation creating an *ETV6-NTRK3* fusion gene; similarly the *MYB-NFIB* translocation (t(6;9) (q22–23; p23–24)) is a key driver in the development of adenoid cystic carcinomas of the breast. Both these tumour types are low-grade, typically of a triple negative phenotype and have counterparts in other tissues (e.g., salivary gland) driven by the same translocations [30–34].

Invasive lobular carcinoma (ILC) is the most common special histological type of breast cancer, defined by a characteristic diffuse growth pattern, with discohesive neoplastic cells. The archetypal alteration in ILC involves dysfunction of the epithelial cell adhesion complex involving E-cadherin and its binding partners β-catenin and P120-catenin. E-cadherin is encoded by the gene *CDH1*, which is inactivated in ~65% of ILC by gene mutation and loss of heterozygosity. Building on formative work by others, the recent large TCGA study [15], Desmedt et al. [35] defined the unique genomic features of ILC compared to invasive breast carcinoma of no special type (IBC-NST or IC NST, previously called invasive ductal carcinoma, IDC) through a deep characterisation of the TCGA breast cancer multi-omic data and the targeted mutation profiling of a large cohort of ILC. In addition to *CDH1* mutations, the only other highly recurrent oncogenic driver was *PI3KCA* (43–48%), with a plethora of low frequency (<15% of cases) driver mutations affecting *FOXA1, TBX3, ERBB2, ERBB3* and *PTEN* that were enriched in ILC relative to IC NST, while *GATA3* and *TP53* mutations were enriched in IC NST relative to ILC. TP53 mutations occur at significantly different frequencies between ER+ and ER− tumours, and so the *TP53* mutation finding is likely driven by the presence of ER negative tumours in the IC NST cohort. Metaplastic breast cancers are at the other end of the histological spectrum to ILC; they are a rare and heterogeneous special tumour type, which exhibit metaplastic change to squamous and/or mesenchymal elements; tumours are high grade and are associated with an overall poor outcome. Although generally triple-negative, they have a high frequency of *PIK3CA* mutations [36–38], and indeed have the unusual co-occurrence of *PIK3CA* and *TP53* driver mutations in some instances [36].

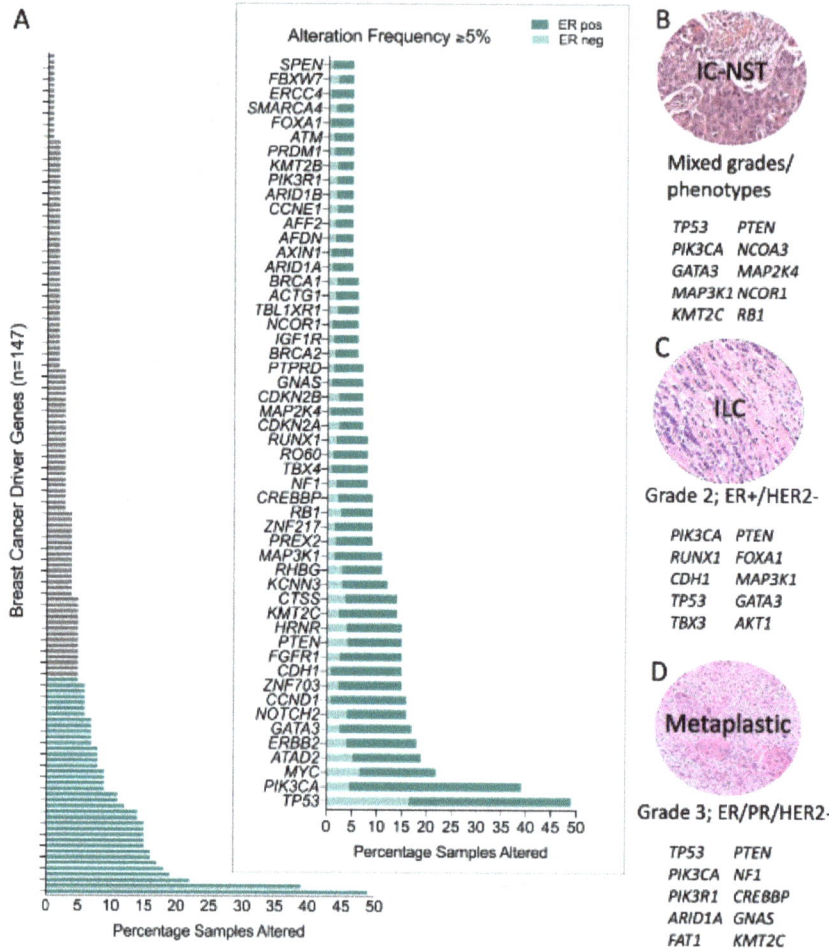

Figure 1. Genomic alterations across breast cancers. (**A**) Frequency of genomic alteration (mutation and copy number variation) in the 147 breast cancer driver genes across the TCGA pancancer breast cancer dataset ($n = 1033$); and stratified by oestrogen receptor (ER) status (in magnified plot): ER positive, $n = 795$; ER negative, $n = 238$. Top ten most frequently mutated genes in (**B**) Invasive Carcinoma-No Special Type (IC-NST) [15]; (**C**) Invasive Lobular Carcinoma (ILC) [15]; and, (**D**) Metaplastic breast cancer [36–38].

3. Subclonal Genomic Diversity in Primary Breast Cancer

Multi-region sequencing of an individual tumour gives intriguing insights into the subclonal nature of the disease (Figure 2A). The level of subclonal heterogeneity identified across a cohort of 50 breast cancers was variable [39]: most cases had a driver mutation that was shared by all regions sequenced (i.e., an early founder driver gene mutation, and indicating an evolutionarily conserved lineage); about half the cancers showed limited variation in the mutations identified across different regions sequenced, whereas for three tumours there was profound subclonal diversity. Sub-clonal driver mutations (e.g., in *TP53, PIK3CA, PTEN, MYC* amplification) were identified in a subset of tumour regions sequenced. Subclonal driver alterations have been previously evident, but not to such detail, through more standard in situ techniques in the diagnostic setting, i.e., breast tumours with heterogenous *ERBB2* amplification. The geographical expansion of mutant subclones was often confined to 1–3 adjacent regions, but interestingly in some cases, mutationally distinct subclones were found to be growing admixed with one another. Cases studied pre- and post- neoadjuvant chemotherapy or targeted therapy revealed evidence that treatment can dramatically alter the clonal make-up of a tumour [39,40].

Eirew and colleagues [41] studied mutations and subclonal dynamics using patient-derived xenograft (PDX) models, and demonstrated that engraftment and subsequent propagation of patient samples led to selective changes in subclonal frequencies. Notably, independent grafts of the same tumour resulted in reproducible expansion of specific subclones that were presumably 'fitter' in this new environment [41]. These striking findings recapitulates the clonal diversity observed in patient samples, but also highlights the idea that human tumour cells in PDX models are dynamic and continually evolve in response to the pressures they are subjected to.

Mixed ductal lobular carcinomas are a unique histological subtype of breast cancer; like metaplastic breast cancers they elicit morphological evidence of intra-tumour heterogeneity, this time showing tumour regions with both ductal and lobular-like differentiation. Multi-region exome sequencing supplemented by copy number profiling of cases exhibiting distinct morphological components demonstrated these were clonally related tumour regions as opposed to being collision tumours [42]. In contrast to the above studies, where topographically defined regions were analysed, here morphologically defined populations of cells representing the different growth patterns (ductal and lobular, including associated pre-invasive lesions) were isolated by microdissection and analysed. In individual cases, all lesions shared precise genetic alterations as likely early events in tumour development; all cases also exhibited private mutations unique to a morphological lineage (e.g., *TBX3*), suggesting they may be important in the separate evolution from a common antecedent [42].

This theory is supported by data from an analysis of multiple invasive tumours from patients with multifocal breast cancer, using targeted gene sequencing analysis, supplemented by low coverage WGS to identify structural and copy number variants [43]. Here, all lesions within an individual case were morphologically identical and expressed the same biomarker profile (same grade, ER and HER2 status). In two thirds of cases, all lesions shared precise genetic alterations, whilst the remaining cases shared no common mutations, from the panel of 360 genes analysed, but they shared structural/copy number variants. Thus, all cases exhibited compelling evidence for the multifocal invasive tumours having a common clonal origin, and for there being subclonal, parallel/branched evolution occurring prior to invasion into the tissue stroma.

4. The Early Clonal Nature of Breast Cancer—Going Back to the Beginning

The early stages of breast neoplasia are defined by a plethora of morphologically characterised lesions which reside within the ductal tree. The frequency with which such morphologically distinct lesions co-existed in the same specimen gave credence to the idea that lesions were evolutionarily related (later supported by molecular evaluation). Ductal carcinoma in situ (DCIS) and lobular carcinoma in situ (LCIS) are genetically advanced lesions and direct precursors to invasive cancer. Columnar cell lesions (CCL), flat epithelial atypia (FEA), atypical ductal hyperplasia (ADH) and atypical lobular hyperplasia/lobular neoplasia (ALH/LN), among others, are considered 'earlier' steps along the multistep pathway to breast cancer development. Each of these lesions harbour genetic alterations and are considered clonal neoplastic proliferations; CCL harbour both DNA copy number alterations and gene mutations, including an usually high rate of *PIK3CA* mutations (54%) [44–46]. Likewise, ADH may be considered a genetically advanced precursor lesion [47].

The role these lesions play in the evolution of ER-positive and ER-negative disease types has been well described [34,48–51] (Figure 2B). Early hypotheses for the evolution of ER-positive breast cancer, in particular, was that of a linear progression from CCL to ADH to DCIS to IDC. Yet the level of intra-tumoural heterogeneity seen within precursor lesions of an individual specimen points to a more complex situation. For instance, within a surgical specimen both DCIS and LCIS can exhibit morphological (e.g., different grades/level of differentiation) and biological (e.g., variable expression of ER, PR, HER2, Ki67) heterogeneity as well as evidence of subclonal genomic diversity [52–54]; these lesions can also co-exist, even admixed within the same duct (Figures 2C and 3). Whilst a linear process of evolution might occur, there is more likely a complex array of parallel/branching clones evolving within the normal ductal structure, and that this probably arises from an underlying bed of genetic instability already present in normal breast epithelium (Figures 2 and 3).

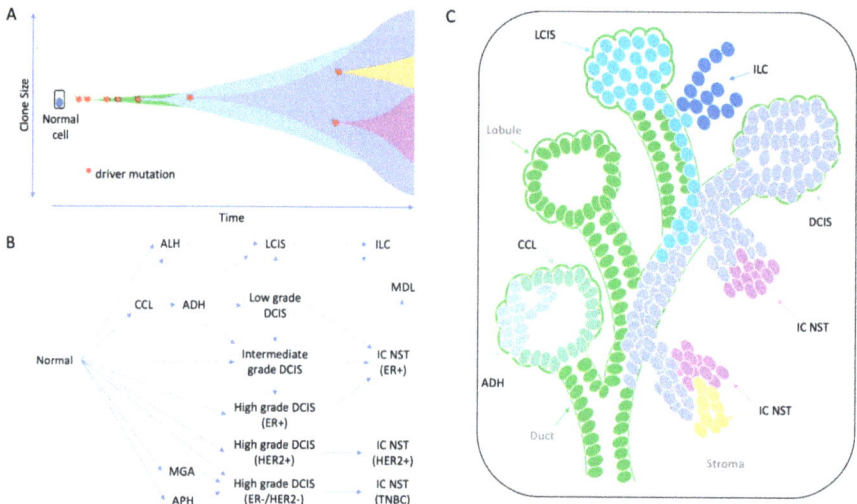

Figure 2. The morphological and molecular evolution of breast cancer. (A) Hypothetical schematic showing how the mutation of cancer genes drives the clonal and subclonal evolution of cancer (adapted from [55]). Key early driver genes impact the subsequent lineage and tumour type that arises, including mutations in *PI3KCA* in ER+ tumours, *CDH1* in lobular lineage, *TP53* in high grade ER- tumours, *ETV6-NTRK3* and *MYB-NFIB* translocations in secretory and adenoid cystic carcinomas respectively. (B) the multistep model of breast cancer showing morphological stages of development from normal epithelium. This simplified model is based on the evolution of ER positive and ER negative breast cancer, as portrayed in more detail elsewhere [49–51]; evidence derived from morphological evaluation and the frequency with which lesions are co-localized, as well as molecular evidence showing co-localized lesions share identical mutations indicating clonal relatedness. (C) Cartoon to illustrate how this might arise in a 'sick lobe', that is a clonal outgrowth of apparently morphologically normal-looking epithelial cells (green), which harbour early genetic changes. In some areas of the lobe, the earliest morphologically abnormal changes may appear in some terminal duct-lobular units (lobule) as columnar cell lesions. These lesions are considered precursors of ADH (light blue cells) and DCIS (purple cells), which arise in lobules and may travel down ducts. The mutation or loss of *CDH1* (E-cadherin) triggers the evolution of the 'lobular lineage' (sky blue cells) as ALH then LCIS (lobular neoplasia); these cells may travel down ducts underneath the normal epithelial lining (pageotoid spread). Both LCIS and DCIS are genetically advanced lesions and so likely exhibit sub-clonal mutations. As these neoplastic cells can travel along ductal structures then this means invasion can occur at multiple sites giving rise to multifocal invasive disease (ILC, IC NST), which continues to undergo subclonal change. CCL: columnar cell lesion; ADH: atypical ductal hyperplasia. ALH: atypical lobular hyperplasia; APH: atypical apocrine hyperplasia; DCIS: ductal carcinoma in situ; LCIS: lobular carcinoma in situ; IC NST: invasive carcinoma no special type; ILC: invasive lobular carcinoma; MDL: mixed ductal lobular carcinoma; MGA: microglandular adenosis.

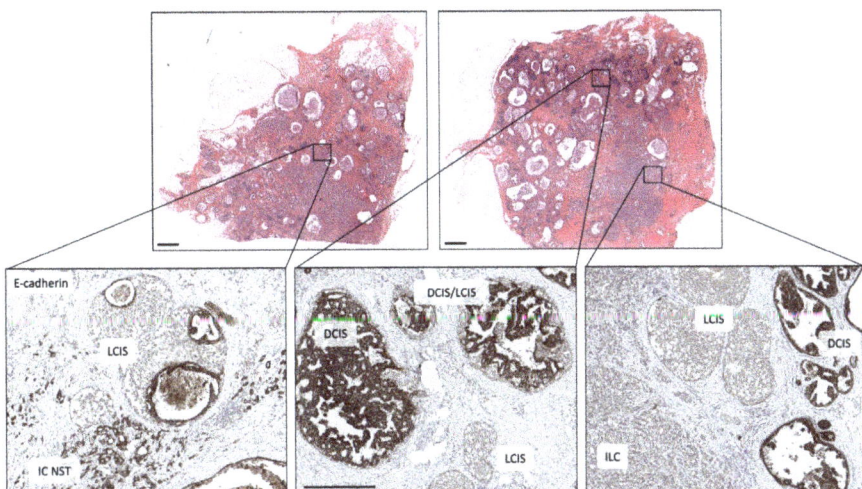

Figure 3. Illustrating morphological and molecular heterogeneity. Low power, haematoxylin and eosin stained sections of two tissue blocks from the same surgical specimen (scale bar = 2 mm). Both blocks are widely affected by breast disease with cystically dilated ducts, in situ carcinoma and invasive carcinoma. The three images in the lower panel are high power views of the same sections stained for E-cadherin (scale bar in middle image = 0.5 mm). Left picture shows cells of LCIS (E-cadherin negative) that have grown and then expanded underneath normal epithelial cells lining a duct (pagetoid spread), adjacent to E-cadherin positive, invasive cells of IC NST. Middle picture shows adjacent ducts in a complex branching network, one duct populated by DCIS (E-cadherin positive), two smaller ducts by LCIS and two other ducts co-involved by cells of DCIS and LCIS (DCIS/LCIS). Right picture showing ducts separately involved by DCIS or LCIS, plus an area of invasive cancer (ILC, E-cadherin negative). The individual components of this case were previously analysed by whole exome sequencing and all lesions were shown to be clonally related with early, common diver mutations identified in *BRCA2* and *TBX3*, 'lobular' lineage-specific mutations including in *CDH1* and 'ductal' lineage-specific mutations including in *NF1* (see [42]). DCIS: ductal carcinoma in situ; LCIS: lobular carcinoma in situ; IC NST: invasive carcinoma no special type; ILC: invasive lobular carcinoma.

Molecular analysis of morphologically complex cases has given great insight into this diversity. Topographically mapped single cell sequencing has elegantly demonstrated that most copy number alterations identified in invasive cancer arise in DCIS; and that clonal diversity observed in invasive cancer is driven in large part by existing clonal diversity present within DCIS, whereby distinct subclones may escape from the ductal tree to seed polyclonal invasive disease (neoplastic cells escaping from different regions of the ductal tree could seed apparently multifocal invasive cancer) [54,56] (Figure 2C). Weng and colleagues [57] also explored these relationships in detail using massively parallel sequencing of normal epithelium, various low-grade proliferative and pre-invasive lesions and associated invasive cancer. Using the somatic mutations to resolve phylogenetic relations between the lesions, the authors revealed a fascinating and complex hierarchy between lesions within individual cases; while IC NST and DCIS were always linked by a shared mutational history; CCLs were either (i) closely related to this DCIS/IC NST lineage with numerous shared somatic mutations, (ii) distantly related to this lineage owing to sharing very early mutations but subsequently evolving down a parallel pathway, or (iii) arose quite independently with no mutations detectable or no mutations in common to higher grade lesions analysed. Interestingly, *PIK3CA* mutations arise frequently but quite heterogeneously within this early stage of disease, including in normal epithelium. Sometimes these mutations are discordant between lesions examined, or are present in CCL but not in synchronous in situ and invasive lesions [45,57], suggesting such early driver events may enhance cellular proliferation, on a background of which other driver mutations may (or may not) arise to trigger progression (or not) to more advanced lesions.

Recent sequencing has revealed an amazing level of genetic instability in 'normal' cells of various tissues, caused by environmental exposure or local pathological processes related to tissue injury [58–61]. There is a growing wealth of evidence suggesting the same is true in breast tissue, acting as a primer for neoplasia. Indeed, morphologically normal epithelium adjacent to tumour harbours a higher level of genetic instability relative to reduction mammoplasty tissue, particularly when normal is within 1 cm of tumour; furthermore normal epithelium from cancer-free patients who carry a pathogenic germline mutation in BRCA1 or BRCA2 also acquire an elevated level of chromosomal instability compared to controls [57,62–66]. In the case of germline mutation carriers, haploinsufficiency for genes with clear roles in DNA damage response (such as BRCA1 and BRCA2) is likely to underpin the predilection to acquire genomic alterations in cells prior to morphological abnormalities being observed [67–69]; in non-carriers the genetic instability may be arising as part of a field cancerisation or 'sick lobe' effect, in which a duct/lobe or a proportion of a lobe is clonally affected by genetic instability and hence the entire lobe is 'at risk' of further genetic instability and oncogenic activation [70]. Indeed, this might explain the observation of multiple atypical proliferations (e.g., CCL, ADH, LCIS, DCIS) co-existing across the same specimen (Figures 2C and 3).

5. Genomics and Clonal Dynamic Changes During Metastatic Progression

Metastatic dissemination is the cause of most cancer-related deaths, therefore, the goal to develop a deep understanding of the mechanisms of metastasis cannot be understated. Large scale sequencing projects of metastatic samples from breast cancer patients, and the analysis of matched cases of the primary tumour and distant metastasis or multiple metastases from an individual have started to reveal important advances in knowledge of clonal progression and treatment resistance.

In many cases the growth pattern (histological type), the expression of phenotypic biomarkers and the molecular subtype of the primary tumour remains quite stable during progression of disease. Genomic data reveal a high concordance in the mutations and in particular copy number alterations between matched primary and metastatic tumours [71–75]. Thus, there is a clear clonal ancestry during progression, and the early molecular drivers of behaviour and phenotype (e.g., mutations in TP53, PIK3CA, CDH1, GATA3, amplification of MYC, CCND1, ERRB2/HER2) remain prevalent drivers in metastatic deposits [71–74,76–80]. Despite this, significant intra-patient heterogeneity develops during progression, even in the absence of systemic therapy; this occurs to a greater extent in progression to distant metastases relative to local lymph nodes and is exacerbated by the selective pressures applied during adjuvant therapy [73,77,81–84]. Changes in tumour phenotype or in the intrinsic molecular subtype during progression occurs in around 30% of patients (most often involving the down regulation of PR, but may also involve ER and less frequently a change in HER2 status) and may occur in a non-random manner at specific metastatic sites (e.g., lung, liver and bone metastases) [85–88]. To further complicate matters, the phenotype of different metastases within a patient can be heterogenous [83,86,89–92].

Compared to early breast cancer, distant metastases tend to harbour a higher mutation burden and more frequent alterations to driver genes that may confer resistance to chemotherapy or targeted therapy, in particular endocrine therapy [74,75,78–80]. Most notably, activating mutations in ESR1 and amplification of the ESR1 gene region (6q25.1) are rarely observed in primary disease, but are prominent and critical drivers of resistance observed in around 20% of metastases arising following endocrine therapy [73,74,78–80,93,94]. Enrichment of mutations in TP53, GATA3, KMT2C, AKT1, NF1, PTEN, ERBB2, FGFR4, or amplification of 7p11.2 (EGFR), 8q24 (MYC), 11q13.3 (CCND1) and 20q13.2 (AURKA) may also underpin endocrine therapy resistance as they are more frequently identified in ER+/HER2− breast cancer metastases compared to ER+/HER2− primary tumours; many of these gene mutations are mutually exclusive to ESR1 mutations, emphasising their potential equivalence in driving resistance [78–80,95].

Mutational signatures found in the primary tumour are also found in metastases; but as with individual gene mutations, the frequencies of individual mutation signatures may also change, with an enrichment in signatures associated with APOBEC enzymatic activity and homologous recombination deficiency being higher in metastases than in primary tumours [75,78,82]. Evidence suggests the acquisition of APOBEC signature maybe a driver of intra tumour heterogeneity and endocrine resistance [17,84,96,97].

The genomic analysis of matched primary and metastatic samples has revealed fascinating insight regarding the evolution of metastatic disease [73,75,82–84,86,90,98–100]. Such efforts reveal, for example, that driver mutations that are enriched in metastasis are indeed rarely found in the matched primary tumour, indicating they arose either in a small subclone not sampled when the primary tumour was sequenced, or they occurred during the metastatic process after cells had disseminated from the breast (i.e., treatment induced mutations) [39,73,79,80,82,101]. Indeed, mutations in *ESR1*, *ERBB2* and *NF1* were significantly enriched in ER+/HER2− tumours post hormone treatment compared to tumours from ER+/HER2− untreated patients [80].

The genetic relationship between multiple metastases within a patient is exceedingly complex but accruing sequencing data and phylogenetic analysis suggests that all metastases within a patient are genetically related, arising from a common ancestral clone. However, subclonal divergence of metastases is invariably observed within patients: driver and non-driver gene mutations are heterogeneously accumulated in different metastases, subsets of metastases may therefore be more closely related to each other than they are to other metastases, and heterogenous tumour phenotypes (ER positive and ER negative) often coincide with this divergent history [75,84,90].

The data supports various models of progression; evidence for both linear and parallel models are evident, in which multiple metastases may arise from a single seeding event from cells disseminating from the primary tumour, or indeed metastases may be seeded from already established metastases in a more linear fashion. The longer the time span between diagnosis of primary tumour and that of the metastases, then the larger the divergence in genetic make-up of the metastases, as expected [98]. Further, in patients with advanced disease at the time of diagnosis, there is evidence of multiple seeding events from the primary tumour, or even from different parts of the same primary tumour [84,98].

An important finding arose through the analysis of the variant allele frequency of shared mutations between metastases or between the primary tumour and resulting metastases: subclonal mutations remained subclonal in the resulting tumour, indicating that metastases were seeded by heterogeneous collections of disseminated cells as opposed to being seeded by a single cell or a single clone (monoclonal origin) [75].

6. Capturing Intra-Tumour Heterogeneity in Tissue or Liquid Biopsy

Predicting the extent of intra-tumour heterogeneity in primary or metastatic disease may provide valuable diagnostic insight into improving the management of patients undergoing neoadjuvant or adjuvant therapy, respectively. This may provide a framework for understanding likely response to chemotherapy or targeted therapy in these settings. As described above, it is clear that tumours may develop and progress on a linear, monoclonal trajectory, with little diversity in phenotype. A single biopsy of the primary tumour or a metastatic deposit may therefore be sufficient to capture the most functionally important alterations to determine therapy.

However, tumours that exhibit intra-tumour heterogeneity and hence with parallel/branching models of progression at play, are more likely to harbour subclones with innate treatment resistance or metastatic capability, or to harbour the capability to evolve in response to treatment to develop resistance. Capturing this level of intra-tumour heterogeneity at diagnosis maybe challenging, but could encompass the recording of a heterogeneity score with regards to morphology and biomarker expression/molecular subtype. Pathologists already record the presence of mixed growth patterns or grades, or the diversity across a tumour for the expression of ER, PR, HER2. Comprehensive sequencing of the entire primary tumour to characterise the subclonal architecture of a mass is not feasible, but evidence suggests that sequencing of two different regions of the tumour provides meaningful information to record clonal heterogeneity and to identify targetable genomic alterations [40].

There has been some reluctance to biopsy metastatic disease in the past, but it has great value in the era of molecular evaluation and the potential offerings for precision medicine. Various studies have demonstrated the feasibility in performing molecular testing on metastatic biopsies [71,79], but this approach is only possible if the metastasis is accessible and may not be appropriate when a patient has multiple organs involved.

Alternative approaches to examine tumour heterogeneity or for capturing important phenotypic or genomic alterations have advanced significantly in recent years. Circulating tumour cells (CTCs) and cell-free tumour DNA (ctDNA) [102–104] are shed into the circulation from both primary and metastatic tumour deposits. Such liquid biopsies are very accessible, and very amenable to repeat sampling while the patient is on treatment to monitor disease. They are, therefore, of great potential benefit in capturing phenotypic heterogeneity or driver mutations acquired or enriched for during treatment; and they are not biased by tumour sampling.

Increased concentration of CTCs in early [105,106] and metastatic [107–110] breast cancer is associated with poor prognosis. The application of single cell analysis technologies to PDX models has shown that CTCs are continuously released by the primary tumour, however only a proportion of clones have the capacity to seed a metastatic deposit, and as such the utility of CTCs in predicting the characteristics of subsequent metastases may be limited [111]. Nevertheless, analysis of CTCs can capture phenotypic heterogeneity of the tumour of origin, for example in the expression of ER, HER2 and androgen receptors [112–114], and also of biological processes driving metastasis such as dynamic changes in epithelial and mesenchymal composition [115,116]. Clusters of CTCs, which may show intermediate epithelial/mesenchymal properties [115,117], demonstrate higher metastatic capacity than single cells [118–121]. Genomic analysis of single CTCs reveals important heterogeneity in the mutation of various driver genes (e.g., *PIK3CA*, *ESR1*, *KRAS*, *PTCH1*, *NOTCH1*) reflecting the presence of discrete subclonal mutations within the tumour of origin and/or the presence of genomic alterations driving resistance/metastasis [122–127].

To illustrate clinical utility of the serial evaluation of molecular heterogeneity within single CTCs, Paoletti and colleagues comprehensively profiled single CTCs in a patient with metastatic lobular carcinoma who progressed following chemotherapy [124]. They demonstrated the presence of four alterations (*CDH1* and *TP53* frameshift mutations; *PIK3CA* and *SOX2* amplifications) in CTC samples at baseline and progression. However, high-level *MYCN* amplifications were only identified in CTCs sampled at progression, likely conferring treatment resistance. Similarly, the development of mutations and splice variants within *ESR1* identified in single CTCs of metastatic patients on endocrine therapy also correlated with the onset of endocrine resistance [124,126,128,129].

ESR1 mutations are also readily detected in ctDNA [130–133], and in fact, ctDNA represents a more sensitive method of detection compared to CTCs [129]. ctDNA is released from tumour cells undergoing apoptosis, necrosis and phagocytosis. Like CTC analysis, ctDNA provides an opportunity for non-invasive molecular testing, akin to the non-invasive prenatal testing (NIPT) in pregnancy, for monitoring patients on therapy. In early breast cancer, the detection of ctDNA in patients undergoing neoadjuvant chemotherapy correlated with tumour grade and stage and a slow (versus rapid) drop of ctDNA levels after one cycle of chemotherapy was associated with a shorter disease-free survival [134]. The detection of minimal residual disease was also demonstrated in patients who continued to have detectable ctDNA *PIK3CA* mutations after surgery [135]. In the metastatic setting, the mutational status is highly concordant between ctDNA and tumour tissue [136,137] with additional private mutations identified in some cases [137].

Serial ctDNA mutation analysis can help characterise the dynamic evolution of subclonal mutations in real time [138–140] and hence represents a powerful approach for the prospective analysis of patients on targeted therapy and the early detection of tumour subclones with resistance capability. This has been demonstrated in the setting of endocrine therapy (various types of *ESR1* alterations, including mutations, rearrangements and amplifications), CDK4/6 inhibition with endocrine therapy (*ESR1*, *RB1* and *PIK3CA* mutations) and anti-HER2 therapy (copy number variations in the *ERBB2* gene as well as increase in *TP53* or PI3K/AKT/mTOR pathway mutations) [131,132,141,142]. Importantly, and reflecting the inter-metastasis molecular heterogeneity described above, *ESR1* mutations identified from either CTC or ctDNA from an individual patient are often heterogenous, suggesting that distinct subclones develop in parallel and utilise overlapping mechanisms of resistance [124,131].

7. Clinical Implications and Utility in Breast Cancer

Many major centres around the world operate routine cancer sequencing programs integrating clinical applications with research, and commonly using targeted panels of cancer genes [143] for triaging patients into clinical trials for targeted therapies. For example; Dana Farbor Cancer Centre/Brigham and Womens' Cancer Centre (BWCC) offers the 'Profile' study wherein cancer gene panel testing may help doctors enrol a patient in a clinical trial or choose the right combination of FDA-approved targeted therapies. Memorial Sloan Kettering Cancer Centre has been pioneering 'basket trials' implementing the use of their in-house MSK-IMPACT panel sequencing assay [144], where trial inclusion is based on mutation status rather than disease origin. UC San Diego Moores Cancer Centre uses the Foundation One panel and has matched 45% of BC patients to a 'personalised' therapy [145,146], however it should be noted that most of these matches were *ERBB2* amplifications to HER2 therapies and the applicability of this panel outside of *ERBB2* in breast cancer is uncertain. Increasing numbers of tools are emerging to facilitate the matching of alterations and therapies, including for example, PanDrugs [147], while the MD Anderson program [148] is feeding back 'sequence-drug' matching data into the public arena through their Precision Cancer Therapy interface.

By the end of 2015, 39 gene targets with matched FDA-approved therapies were noted in an extensive review of precision oncology [149] while the OncoKB resource [150] details 20 genes (42 alterations) as FDA-recognised biomarkers (Level 1 evidence) and 10 genes (22 alterations) as Level 2 (standard of care; predictive of response in breast cancer or another indication). In breast cancer, *ERBB2* amplifications (targeted with anti-HER2 therapies) and *PIK3CA* mutations (targeted with Alpelisib + Fulvestrant) are the only Level 1 biomarkers as noted by OncoKB, while inactivating mutations of *BRCA1* and *BRCA2* are classed as Level 2 biomarkers for intervention with talazoparib and olaparib. Increasing data therefore supports the clinical application of genomics to inform therapeutic intervention in breast cancer. Whole exome and whole genome sequencing will be required to account for the diversity of genes mutated in breast cancer [14,151] as well as larger scale alterations and mutation signatures that may predict treatment response. It is now clear, through mutation signature analysis, that hallmarks of defective DNA damage repair (specifically homologous recombination which BRCA1/2 mediate) are indicative of dysfunctional *BRCA1/2* [8,10]. A weighted model (HRDetect) can detect *BRCA1/BRCA2*-deficient samples using WGS data [9]. The HRDetect algorithm was independently validated, and its association with platinum response in advanced breast cancer demonstrated, where a high HRDetect score was associated with clinical improvement on platinum therapies [152,153]. Recent research has applied a functional HR assay (RECAP) to breast cancer samples and demonstrated that 29% of HR-defective tumours were not *BRCA*-related [154], although the researchers themselves classify this approach as pseudo-diagnostic.

The introduction of immune checkpoint inhibitors (ICI) has revolutionised therapeutics across a number of advanced solid tumours. While a subset of patients displays a durable response, the implementation of a robust biomarker has been challenging. Tumour mutation burden (TMB) is now emerging as a diagnostic biomarker for ICIs such as PD-1/PD-L1 inhibitors [155,156]. It is now possible to calculate TMB from panel sequencing data [157], not just exome or genome sequencing, and with time we expect to see a rationalisation of diagnostic 'cut-offs'. Small molecular inhibitors of the PI3K/AKT/mTOR pathway are fast approaching the clinic. The pan-AKT inhibitor, AZD5363, is potent and sensitivity is predicted by *PIK3CA* mutations [158]. The SOLAR trial [159] investigating the mutant PIK3CA inhibitor, alpelisib, demonstrated that a combination of alpelisib with fulvestrant prolonged progression-free survival among patients with *PIK3CA*-mutated, HR-positive, HER2-negative advanced breast cancer.

The application of these genotype–phenotype relationships in the clinical context of heterogeneity remains to be rationalised. Tumour heterogeneity exclusive of a histological subtype is not standardly reported; for example, ER positivity is recorded in a binary fashion with a low cut-off for positivity. Whether drugs are used sequentially to target residual clones, or in combination for simultaneous targeting will depend on myriad factors including the application of robust biomarkers of sensitivity to the therapy and the extent of intra-tumour heterogeneity.

Author Contributions: J.R.K., A.E.M.R., A.S., S.R.L. and P.T.S. all contributed to the researching, writing and reviewing of this manuscript. All authors have read and agreed to the published version of the manuscript.

Funding: The authors are supported, in part, by Program and Project grant funding from the National Health and Medical Research Council (NHMRC) of Australia (APP1159902, APP1164770, APP1113867).

Acknowledgments: We apologise to authors whose work is relevant to this topic but has not been referenced herein.

Conflicts of Interest: The authors declare no conflict of interest

References

1. WHO Classification of Tumours Editorial Board. *World Health Organisation Classification of Tumours: Breast Tumours*, 5th ed.; International Agency for Research on Cancer (IARC): Lyon, France, 2019.
2. Perou, C.M.; Sorlie, T.; Eisen, M.B.; van de Rijn, M.; Jeffrey, S.S.; Rees, C.A.; Pollack, J.R.; Ross, D.T.; Johnsen, H.; Akslen, L.A.; et al. Molecular portraits of human breast tumours. *Nature* **2000**, *406*, 747–752. [CrossRef] [PubMed]
3. Sorlie, T.; Perou, C.M.; Tibshirani, R.; Aas, T.; Geisler, S.; Johnsen, H.; Hastie, T.; Eisen, M.B.; van de Rijn, M.; Jeffrey, S.S.; et al. Gene expression patterns of breast carcinomas distinguish tumor subclasses with clinical implications. *Proc. Natl. Acad. Sci. USA* **2001**, *98*, 10869–10874. [CrossRef] [PubMed]
4. Prat, A.; Parker, J.S.; Karginova, O.; Fan, C.; Livasy, C.; Herschkowitz, J.I.; He, X.; Perou, C.M. Phenotypic and molecular characterization of the claudin-low intrinsic subtype of breast cancer. *Breast Cancer Res.* **2010**, *12*, R68. [CrossRef] [PubMed]
5. Mathews, J.C.; Nadeem, S.; Levine, A.J.; Pouryahya, M.; Deasy, J.O.; Tannenbaum, A. Robust and interpretable PAM50 reclassification exhibits survival advantage for myoepithelial and immune phenotypes. *NPJ Breast Cancer* **2019**, *5*, 30. [CrossRef] [PubMed]
6. Lehmann, B.D.; Jovanovic, B.; Chen, X.; Estrada, M.V.; Johnson, K.N.; Shyr, Y.; Moses, H.L.; Sanders, M.E.; Pietenpol, J.A. Refinement of Triple-Negative Breast Cancer Molecular Subtypes: Implications for Neoadjuvant Chemotherapy Selection. *PLoS ONE* **2016**, *11*, e0157368. [CrossRef] [PubMed]
7. Curtis, C.; Shah, S.P.; Chin, S.F.; Turashvili, G.; Rueda, O.M.; Dunning, M.J.; Speed, D.; Lynch, A.G.; Samarajiwa, S.; Yuan, Y.; et al. The genomic and transcriptomic architecture of 2000 breast tumours reveals novel subgroups. *Nature* **2012**, *486*, 346–352. [CrossRef]
8. Alexandrov, L.B.; Nik-Zainal, S.; Wedge, D.C.; Aparicio, S.A.; Behjati, S.; Biankin, A.V.; Bignell, G.R.; Bolli, N.; Borg, A.; Borresen-Dale, A.L.; et al. Signatures of mutational processes in human cancer. *Nature* **2013**, *500*, 415–421. [CrossRef]
9. Davies, H.; Glodzik, D.; Morganella, S.; Yates, L.R.; Staaf, J.; Zou, X.; Ramakrishna, M.; Martin, S.; Boyault, S.; Sieuwerts, A.M.; et al. HRDetect is a predictor of BRCA1 and BRCA2 deficiency based on mutational signatures. *Nat. Med.* **2017**, *23*, 517–525. [CrossRef]
10. Nik-Zainal, S.; Alexandrov, L.B.; Wedge, D.C.; Van Loo, P.; Greenman, C.D.; Raine, K.; Jones, D.; Hinton, J.; Marshall, J.; Stebbings, L.A.; et al. Mutational processes molding the genomes of 21 breast cancers. *Cell* **2012**, *149*, 979–993. [CrossRef]
11. Nik-Zainal, S.; Van Loo, P.; Wedge, D.C.; Alexandrov, L.B.; Greenman, C.D.; Lau, K.W.; Raine, K.; Jones, D.; Marshall, J.; Ramakrishna, M.; et al. The life history of 21 breast cancers. *Cell* **2012**, *149*, 994–1007. [CrossRef]
12. Alexandrov, L.B.; Kim, J.; Haradhvala, N.J.; Huang, M.N.; Tian Ng, A.W.; Wu, Y.; Boot, A.; Covington, K.R.; Gordenin, D.A.; Bergstrom, E.N.; et al. The repertoire of mutational signatures in human cancer. *Nature* **2020**, *578*, 94–101. [CrossRef]

13. The Cancer Genome Atlas Network. Comprehensive molecular portraits of human breast tumours. *Nature* **2012**, *490*, 61–70. [CrossRef] [PubMed]
14. Nik-Zainal, S.; Davies, H.; Staaf, J.; Ramakrishna, M.; Glodzik, D.; Zou, X.; Martincorena, I.; Alexandrov, L.B.; Martin, S.; Wedge, D.C.; et al. Landscape of somatic mutations in 560 breast cancer whole-genome sequences. *Nature* **2016**, *534*, 47–54. [CrossRef] [PubMed]
15. Ciriello, G.; Gatza, M.L.; Beck, A.H.; Wilkerson, M.D.; Rhie, S.K.; Pastore, A.; Zhang, H.; McLellan, M.; Yau, C.; Kandoth, C.; et al. Comprehensive Molecular Portraits of Invasive Lobular Breast Cancer. *Cell* **2015**, *163*, 506–519. [CrossRef] [PubMed]
16. Pereira, B.; Chin, S.F.; Rueda, O.M.; Vollan, H.K.; Provenzano, E.; Bardwell, H.A.; Pugh, M.; Jones, L.; Russell, R.; Sammut, S.J.; et al. The somatic mutation profiles of 2433 breast cancers refines their genomic and transcriptomic landscapes. *Nat. Commun.* **2016**, *7*, 11479. [CrossRef]
17. Burns, M.B.; Lackey, L.; Carpenter, M.A.; Rathore, A.; Land, A.M.; Leonard, B.; Refsland, E.W.; Kotandeniya, D.; Tretyakova, N.; Nikas, J.B.; et al. APOBEC3B is an enzymatic source of mutation in breast cancer. *Nature* **2013**, *494*, 366–370. [CrossRef]
18. Davies, H.; Morganella, S.; Purdie, C.A.; Jang, S.J.; Borgen, E.; Russnes, H.; Glodzik, D.; Zou, X.; Viari, A.; Richardson, A.L.; et al. Whole-Genome Sequencing Reveals Breast Cancers with Mismatch Repair Deficiency. *Cancer Res.* **2017**, *77*, 4755–4762. [CrossRef]
19. Nones, K.; Johnson, J.; Newell, F.; Patch, A.M.; Thorne, H.; Kazakoff, S.H.; de Luca, X.M.; Parsons, M.T.; Ferguson, K.; Reid, L.E.; et al. Whole-genome sequencing reveals clinically relevant insights into the aetiology of familial breast cancers. *Ann. Oncol.* **2019**, *30*. [CrossRef]
20. Ferrari, A.; Vincent-Salomon, A.; Pivot, X.; Sertier, A.S.; Thomas, E.; Tonon, L.; Boyault, S.; Mulugeta, E.; Treilleux, I.; MacGrogan, G.; et al. A whole-genome sequence and transcriptome perspective on HER2-positive breast cancers. *Nat. Commun.* **2016**, *7*, 12222. [CrossRef]
21. Hicks, J.; Krasnitz, A.; Lakshmi, B.; Navin, N.E.; Riggs, M.; Leibu, E.; Esposito, D.; Alexander, J.; Troge, J.; Grubor, V.; et al. Novel patterns of genome rearrangement and their association with survival in breast cancer. *Genome Res.* **2006**, *16*, 1465–1479. [CrossRef]
22. Michailidou, K.; Lindstrom, S.; Dennis, J.; Beesley, J.; Hui, S.; Kar, S.; Lemacon, A.; Soucy, P.; Glubb, D.; Rostamianfar, A.; et al. Association analysis identifies 65 new breast cancer risk loci. *Nature* **2017**, *551*, 92–94. [CrossRef] [PubMed]
23. Stephens, P.J.; Tarpey, P.S.; Davies, H.; Van Loo, P.; Greenman, C.; Wedge, D.C.; Nik-Zainal, S.; Martin, S.; Varela, I.; Bignell, G.R.; et al. The landscape of cancer genes and mutational processes in breast cancer. *Nature* **2012**, *486*, 400–404. [CrossRef] [PubMed]
24. Lakhani, S.R.; Reis-Filho, J.S.; Fulford, L.; Penault-Llorca, F.; van der Vijver, M.; Parry, S.; Bishop, T.; Benitez, J.; Rivas, C.; Bignon, Y.J.; et al. Prediction of BRCA1 status in patients with breast cancer using estrogen receptor and basal phenotype. *Clin. Cancer Res.* **2005**, *11*, 5175–5180. [CrossRef] [PubMed]
25. Hu, C.; Polley, E.C.; Yadav, S.; Lilyquist, J.; Shimelis, H.; Na, J.; Hart, S.N.; Goldgar, D.E.; Shah, S.; Pesaran, T.; et al. The contribution of germline predisposition gene mutations to clinical subtypes of invasive breast cancer from a clinical genetic testing cohort. *J. Natl. Cancer Inst.* **2020**, djaa023. [CrossRef] [PubMed]
26. Weigelt, B.; Bi, R.; Kumar, R.; Blecua, P.; Mandelker, D.L.; Geyer, F.C.; Pareja, F.; James, P.A.; kConFab, I.; Couch, F.J.; et al. The Landscape of Somatic Genetic Alterations in Breast Cancers from ATM Germline Mutation Carriers. *J. Natl. Cancer Inst.* **2018**, *110*, 1030–1034. [CrossRef]
27. Mandelker, D.; Kumar, R.; Pei, X.; Selenica, P.; Setton, J.; Arunachalam, S.; Ceyhan-Birsoy, O.; Brown, D.N.; Norton, L.; Robson, M.E.; et al. The Landscape of Somatic Genetic Alterations in Breast Cancers from CHEK2 Germline Mutation Carriers. *JNCI Cancer Spectr.* **2019**, *3*, pkz027. [CrossRef]
28. Wilson, J.R.; Bateman, A.C.; Hanson, H.; An, Q.; Evans, G.; Rahman, N.; Jones, J.L.; Eccles, D.M. A novel HER2-positive breast cancer phenotype arising from germline TP53 mutations. *J. Med. Genet.* **2010**, *47*, 771–774. [CrossRef]
29. Corso, G.; Intra, M.; Trentin, C.; Veronesi, P.; Galimberti, V. CDH1 germline mutations and hereditary lobular breast cancer. *Fam. Cancer* **2016**, *15*, 215–219. [CrossRef]
30. Fusco, N.; Geyer, F.C.; De Filippo, M.R.; Martelotto, L.G.; Ng, C.K.; Piscuoglio, S.; Guerini-Rocco, E.; Schultheis, A.M.; Fuhrmann, L.; Wang, L.; et al. Genetic events in the progression of adenoid cystic carcinoma of the breast to high-grade triple-negative breast cancer. *Mod. Pathol.* **2016**, *29*, 1292–1305. [CrossRef]

31. Miyai, K.; Schwartz, M.R.; Divatia, M.K.; Anton, R.C.; Park, Y.W.; Ayala, A.G.; Ro, J.Y. Adenoid cystic carcinoma of breast: Recent advances. *World J. Clin. Cases* **2014**, *2*, 732–741. [CrossRef]
32. Letessier, A.; Ginestier, C.; Charafe-Jauffret, E.; Cervera, N.; Adelaide, J.; Gelsi-Boyer, V.; Ahomadegbe, J.C.; Benard, J.; Jacquemier, J.; Birnbaum, D.; et al. ETV6 gene rearrangements in invasive breast carcinoma. *Genes Chromosomes Cancer* **2005**, *44*, 103–108. [CrossRef] [PubMed]
33. Tognon, C.; Knezevich, S.R.; Huntsman, D.; Roskelley, C.D.; Melnyk, N.; Mathers, J.A.; Becker, L.; Carneiro, F.; MacPherson, N.; Horsman, D.; et al. Expression of the ETV6-NTRK3 gene fusion as a primary event in human secretory breast carcinoma. *Cancer Cell* **2002**, *2*, 367–376. [CrossRef]
34. Geyer, F.C.; Pareja, F.; Weigelt, B.; Rakha, E.; Ellis, I.O.; Schnitt, S.J.; Reis-Filho, J.S. The Spectrum of Triple-Negative Breast Disease: High- and Low-Grade Lesions. *Am. J. Pathol.* **2017**, *187*, 2139–2151. [PubMed]
35. Desmedt, C.; Zoppoli, G.; Gundem, G.; Pruneri, G.; Larsimont, D.; Fornili, M.; Fumagalli, D.; Brown, D.; Rothe, F.; Vincent, D.; et al. Genomic Characterization of Primary Invasive Lobular Breast Cancer. *J. Clin. Oncol.* **2016**, *34*, 1872–1881. [CrossRef] [PubMed]
36. McCart Reed, A.E.; Kalaw, E.; Nones, K.; Bettington, M.; Lim, M.; Bennett, J.; Johnstone, K.; Kutasovic, J.R.; Saunus, J.M.; Kazakoff, S.; et al. Phenotypic and molecular dissection of Metaplastic Breast Cancer and the prognostic implications. *J. Pathol.* **2019**, *247*, 214–227. [CrossRef]
37. Ng, C.K.Y.; Piscuoglio, S.; Geyer, F.C.; Burke, K.A.; Pareja, F.; Eberle, C.A.; Lim, R.S.; Natrajan, R.; Riaz, N.; Mariani, O.; et al. The Landscape of Somatic Genetic Alterations in Metaplastic Breast Carcinomas. *Clin. Cancer Res.* **2017**, *23*, 3859–3870. [CrossRef]
38. Yates, L.R.; Gerstung, M.; Knappskog, S.; Desmedt, C.; Gundem, G.; Van Loo, P.; Aas, T.; Alexandrov, L.B.; Larsimont, D.; Davies, H.; et al. Genomic and transcriptomic heterogeneity in metaplastic carcinomas of the breast. *NPJ Breast Cancer* **2017**, *3*, 48.
39. Yates, L.R.; Gerstung, M.; Knappskog, S.; Desmedt, C.; Gundem, G.; Van Loo, P.; Aas, T.; Alexandrov, L.B.; Larsimont, D.; Davies, H.; et al. Subclonal diversification of primary breast cancer revealed by multiregion sequencing. *Nat. Med.* **2015**, *21*, 751–759. [CrossRef]
40. Caswell-Jin, J.L.; McNamara, K.; Reiter, J.G.; Sun, R.; Hu, Z.; Ma, Z.; Ding, J.; Suarez, C.J.; Tilk, S.; Raghavendra, A.; et al. Clonal replacement and heterogeneity in breast tumors treated with neoadjuvant HER2-targeted therapy. *Nat. Commun.* **2019**, *10*, 657. [CrossRef]
41. Eirew, P.; Steif, A.; Khattra, J.; Ha, G.; Yap, D.; Farahani, H.; Gelmon, K.; Chia, S.; Mar, C.; Wan, A.; et al. Dynamics of genomic clones in breast cancer patient xenografts at single-cell resolution. *Nature* **2015**, *518*, 422–426. [CrossRef]
42. McCart Reed, A.E.; Kutasovic, J.R.; Nones, K.; Saunus, J.M.; Da Silva, L.; Newell, F.; Kazakoff, S.; Melville, L.; Jayanthan, J.; Vargas, A.C.; et al. Mixed ductal-lobular carcinomas: Evidence for progression from ductal to lobular morphology. *J. Pathol.* **2018**, *244*, 460–468. [CrossRef] [PubMed]
43. Desmedt, C.; Fumagalli, D.; Pietri, E.; Zoppoli, G.; Brown, D.; Nik-Zainal, S.; Gundem, G.; Rothe, F.; Majjaj, S.; Garuti, A.; et al. Uncovering the genomic heterogeneity of multifocal breast cancer. *J. Pathol.* **2015**, *236*, 457–466. [CrossRef] [PubMed]
44. Simpson, P.T.; Gale, T.; Reis-Filho, J.S.; Jones, C.; Parry, S.; Sloane, J.P.; Hanby, A.; Pinder, S.E.; Lee, A.H.; Humphreys, S.; et al. Columnar cell lesions of the breast: The missing link in breast cancer progression? A morphological and molecular analysis. *Am. J. Surg. Pathol.* **2005**, *29*, 734–746. [CrossRef] [PubMed]
45. Troxell, M.L.; Brunner, A.L.; Neff, T.; Warrick, A.; Beadling, C.; Montgomery, K.; Zhu, S.; Corless, C.L.; West, R.B. Phosphatidylinositol-3-kinase pathway mutations are common in breast columnar cell lesions. *Mod. Pathol.* **2012**, *25*, 930–937. [CrossRef] [PubMed]
46. Dabbs, D.J.; Carter, G.; Fudge, M.; Peng, Y.; Swalsky, P.; Finkelstein, S. Molecular alterations in columnar cell lesions of the breast. *Mod. Pathol.* **2006**, *19*, 344–349. [CrossRef] [PubMed]
47. Kader, T.; Hill, P.; Zethoven, M.; Goode, D.L.; Elder, K.; Thio, N.; Doyle, M.; Semple, T.; Sufyan, W.; Byrne, D.J.; et al. Atypical ductal hyperplasia is a multipotent precursor of breast carcinoma. *J. Pathol.* **2019**, *248*, 326–338. [CrossRef]
48. Abdel-Fatah, T.M.; Powe, D.G.; Hodi, Z.; Lee, A.H.; Reis-Filho, J.S.; Ellis, I.O. High frequency of coexistence of columnar cell lesions, lobular neoplasia, and low grade ductal carcinoma in situ with invasive tubular carcinoma and invasive lobular carcinoma. *Am. J. Surg. Pathol.* **2007**, *31*, 417–426. [CrossRef]

49. Simpson, P.T.; Reis-Filho, J.S.; Gale, T.; Lakhani, S.R. Molecular evolution of breast cancer. *J. Pathol.* **2005**, *205*, 248–254. [CrossRef]
50. Lopez-Garcia, M.A.; Geyer, F.C.; Lacroix-Triki, M.; Marchio, C.; Reis-Filho, J.S. Breast cancer precursors revisited: Molecular features and progression pathways. *Histopathology* **2010**, *57*, 171–192. [CrossRef]
51. Bombonati, A.; Sgroi, D.C. The molecular pathology of breast cancer progression. *J. Pathol.* **2011**, *223*, 307–317. [CrossRef]
52. Allred, D.C.; Wu, Y.; Mao, S.; Nagtegaal, I.D.; Lee, S.; Perou, C.M.; Mohsin, S.K.; O'Connell, P.; Tsimelzon, A.; Medina, D. Ductal carcinoma in situ and the emergence of diversity during breast cancer evolution. *Clin. Cancer Res.* **2008**, *14*, 370–378. [CrossRef] [PubMed]
53. Lee, J.Y.; Schizas, M.; Geyer, F.C.; Selenica, P.; Piscuoglio, S.; Sakr, R.A.; Ng, C.K.Y.; Carniello, J.V.S.; Towers, R.; Giri, D.D.; et al. Lobular Carcinomas in Situ Display Intralesion Genetic Heterogeneity and Clonal Evolution in the Progression to Invasive Lobular Carcinoma. *Clin. Cancer Res.* **2019**, *25*, 674–686. [CrossRef] [PubMed]
54. Martelotto, L.G.; Baslan, T.; Kendall, J.; Geyer, F.C.; Burke, K.A.; Spraggon, L.; Piscuoglio, S.; Chadalavada, K.; Nanjangud, G.; Ng, C.K.; et al. Whole-genome single-cell copy number profiling from formalin-fixed paraffin-embedded samples. *Nat. Med.* **2017**, *23*, 376–385. [CrossRef] [PubMed]
55. Yates, L.R.; Campbell, P.J. Evolution of the cancer genome. *Nat. Rev. Genet.* **2012**, *13*, 795–806. [CrossRef] [PubMed]
56. Casasent, A.K.; Schalck, A.; Gao, R.; Sei, E.; Long, A.; Pangburn, W.; Casasent, T.; Meric-Bernstam, F.; Edgerton, M.E.; Navin, N.E. Multiclonal Invasion in Breast Tumors Identified by Topographic Single Cell Sequencing. *Cell* **2018**, *172*, 205–217. [CrossRef]
57. Weng, Z.; Spies, N.; Zhu, S.X.; Newburger, D.E.; Kashef-Haghighi, D.; Batzoglou, S.; Sidow, A.; West, R.B. Cell-lineage heterogeneity and driver mutation recurrence in pre-invasive breast neoplasia. *Genome Med.* **2015**, *7*, 28. [CrossRef]
58. Brunner, S.F.; Roberts, N.D.; Wylie, L.A.; Moore, L.; Aitken, S.J.; Davies, S.E.; Sanders, M.A.; Ellis, P.; Alder, C.; Hooks, Y.; et al. Somatic mutations and clonal dynamics in healthy and cirrhotic human liver. *Nature* **2019**, *574*, 538–542. [CrossRef]
59. Lee-Six, H.; Olafsson, S.; Ellis, P.; Osborne, R.J.; Sanders, M.A.; Moore, L.; Georgakopoulos, N.; Torrente, F.; Noorani, A.; Goddard, M.; et al. The landscape of somatic mutation in normal colorectal epithelial cells. *Nature* **2019**, *574*, 532–537. [CrossRef]
60. Martincorena, I.; Fowler, J.C.; Wabik, A.; Lawson, A.R.J.; Abascal, F.; Hall, M.W.J.; Cagan, A.; Murai, K.; Mahbubani, K.; Stratton, M.R.; et al. Somatic mutant clones colonize the human esophagus with age. *Science* **2018**, *362*, 911–917. [CrossRef]
61. Martincorena, I.; Roshan, A.; Gerstung, M.; Ellis, P.; Van Loo, P.; McLaren, S.; Wedge, D.C.; Fullam, A.; Alexandrov, L.B.; Tubio, J.M.; et al. Tumor evolution. High burden and pervasive positive selection of somatic mutations in normal human skin. *Science* **2015**, *348*, 880–886. [CrossRef]
62. Clarke, C.L.; Sandle, J.; Jones, A.A.; Sofronis, A.; Patani, N.R.; Lakhani, S.R. Mapping loss of heterozygosity in normal human breast cells from BRCA1/2 carriers. *Br. J. Cancer* **2006**, *95*, 515–519. [CrossRef] [PubMed]
63. Deng, G.; Lu, Y.; Zlotnikov, G.; Thor, A.D.; Smith, H.S. Loss of heterozygosity in normal tissue adjacent to breast carcinomas. *Science* **1996**, *274*, 2057–2059. [CrossRef] [PubMed]
64. Ellsworth, D.L.; Ellsworth, R.E.; Love, B.; Deyarmin, B.; Lubert, S.M.; Mittal, V.; Shriver, C.D. Genomic patterns of allelic imbalance in disease free tissue adjacent to primary breast carcinomas. *Breast Cancer Res. Treat.* **2004**, *88*, 131–139. [CrossRef] [PubMed]
65. Heaphy, C.M.; Bisoffi, M.; Fordyce, C.A.; Haaland, C.M.; Hines, W.C.; Joste, N.E.; Griffith, J.K. Telomere DNA content and allelic imbalance demonstrate field cancerization in histologically normal tissue adjacent to breast tumors. *Int. J. Cancer* **2006**, *119*, 108–116. [CrossRef] [PubMed]
66. Larson, P.S.; Schlechter, B.L.; de las Morenas, A.; Garber, J.E.; Cupples, L.A.; Rosenberg, C.L. Allele imbalance, or loss of heterozygosity, in normal breast epithelium of sporadic breast cancer cases and BRCA1 gene mutation carriers is increased compared with reduction mammoplasty tissues. *J. Clin. Oncol.* **2005**, *23*, 8613–8619. [CrossRef] [PubMed]
67. Karaayvaz-Yildirim, M.; Silberman, R.E.; Langenbucher, A.; Saladi, S.V.; Ross, K.N.; Zarcaro, E.; Desmond, A.; Yildirim, M.; Vivekanandan, V.; Ravichandran, H.; et al. Aneuploidy and a deregulated DNA damage response suggest haploinsufficiency in breast tissues of BRCA2 mutation carriers. *Sci. Adv.* **2020**, *6*, eaay2611. [CrossRef]

68. Konishi, H.; Mohseni, M.; Tamaki, A.; Garay, J.P.; Croessmann, S.; Karnan, S.; Ota, A.; Wong, H.Y.; Konishi, Y.; Karakas, B.; et al. Mutation of a single allele of the cancer susceptibility gene BRCA1 leads to genomic instability in human breast epithelial cells. *Proc. Natl. Acad. Sci. USA* **2011**, *108*, 17773–17778. [CrossRef]
69. Sedic, M.; Skibinski, A.; Brown, N.; Gallardo, M.; Mulligan, P.; Martinez, P.; Keller, P.J.; Glover, E.; Richardson, A.L.; Cowan, J.; et al. Haploinsufficiency for BRCA1 leads to cell-type-specific genomic instability and premature senescence. *Nat. Commun.* **2015**, *6*, 7505. [CrossRef]
70. Tan, M.P.; Tot, T. The sick lobe hypothesis, field cancerisation and the new era of precision breast surgery. *Gland Surg.* **2018**, *7*, 611–618. [CrossRef]
71. Zehir, A.; Benayed, R.; Shah, R.H.; Syed, A.; Middha, S.; Kim, H.R.; Srinivasan, P.; Gao, J.; Chakravarty, D.; Devlin, S.M.; et al. Mutational landscape of metastatic cancer revealed from prospective clinical sequencing of 10,000 patients. *Nat. Med.* **2017**, *23*, 703–713. [CrossRef]
72. Reiter, J.G.; Makohon-Moore, A.P.; Gerold, J.M.; Heyde, A.; Attiyeh, M.A.; Kohutek, Z.A.; Tokheim, C.J.; Brown, A.; DeBlasio, R.M.; Niyazov, J.; et al. Minimal functional driver gene heterogeneity among untreated metastases. *Science* **2018**, *361*, 1033–1037. [CrossRef] [PubMed]
73. Siegel, M.B.; He, X.; Hoadley, K.A.; Hoyle, A.; Pearce, J.B.; Garrett, A.L.; Kumar, S.; Moylan, V.J.; Brady, C.M.; Van Swearingen, A.E.; et al. Integrated RNA and DNA sequencing reveals early drivers of metastatic breast cancer. *J. Clin. Investig.* **2018**, *128*, 1371–1383. [CrossRef] [PubMed]
74. Priestley, P.; Baber, J.; Lolkema, M.P.; Steeghs, N.; de Bruijn, E.; Shale, C.; Duyvesteyn, K.; Haidari, S.; van Hoeck, A.; Onstenk, W.; et al. Pan-cancer whole-genome analyses of metastatic solid tumours. *Nature* **2019**, *575*, 210–216. [CrossRef] [PubMed]
75. De Mattos-Arruda, L.; Sammut, S.J.; Ross, E.M.; Bashford-Rogers, R.; Greenstein, E.; Markus, H.; Morganella, S.; Teng, Y.; Maruvka, Y.; Pereira, B.; et al. The Genomic and Immune Landscapes of Lethal Metastatic Breast Cancer. *Cell Rep.* **2019**, *27*, 2690–2708. [CrossRef]
76. Hoadley, K.A.; Siegel, M.B.; Kanchi, K.L.; Miller, C.A.; Ding, L.; Zhao, W.; He, X.; Parker, J.S.; Wendl, M.C.; Fulton, R.S.; et al. Tumor Evolution in Two Patients with Basal-like Breast Cancer: A Retrospective Genomics Study of Multiple Metastases. *PLoS Med.* **2016**, *13*, e1002174. [CrossRef]
77. Brastianos, P.K.; Carter, S.L.; Santagata, S.; Cahill, D.P.; Taylor-Weiner, A.; Jones, R.T.; Van Allen, E.M.; Lawrence, M.S.; Horowitz, P.M.; Cibulskis, K.; et al. Genomic Characterization of Brain Metastases Reveals Branched Evolution and Potential Therapeutic Targets. *Cancer Discov.* **2015**, *5*, 1164–1177. [CrossRef]
78. Angus, L.; Smid, M.; Wilting, S.M.; van Riet, J.; Van Hoeck, A.; Nguyen, L.; Nik-Zainal, S.; Steenbruggen, T.G.; Tjan-Heijnen, V.C.G.; Labots, M.; et al. The genomic landscape of metastatic breast cancer highlights changes in mutation and signature frequencies. *Nat. Genet.* **2019**, *51*, 1450–1458. [CrossRef]
79. Bertucci, F.; Ng, C.K.Y.; Patsouris, A.; Droin, N.; Piscuoglio, S.; Carbuccia, N.; Soria, J.C.; Dien, A.T.; Adnani, Y.; Kamal, M.; et al. Genomic characterization of metastatic breast cancers. *Nature* **2019**, *569*, 560–564. [CrossRef]
80. Razavi, P.; Chang, M.T.; Xu, G.; Bandlamudi, C.; Ross, D.S.; Vasan, N.; Cai, Y.; Bielski, C.M.; Donoghue, M.T.A.; Jonsson, P.; et al. The Genomic Landscape of Endocrine-Resistant Advanced Breast Cancers. *Cancer Cell* **2018**, *34*, 427–438. [CrossRef]
81. Ng, C.K.Y.; Bidard, F.C.; Piscuoglio, S.; Geyer, F.C.; Lim, R.S.; de Bruijn, I.; Shen, R.; Pareja, F.; Berman, S.H.; Wang, L.; et al. Genetic Heterogeneity in Therapy-Naive Synchronous Primary Breast Cancers and Their Metastases. *Clin. Cancer Res.* **2017**, *23*, 4402–4415. [CrossRef]
82. Yates, L.R.; Knappskog, S.; Wedge, D.; Farmery, J.H.R.; Gonzalez, S.; Martincorena, I.; Alexandrov, L.B.; Van Loo, P.; Haugland, H.K.; Lilleng, P.K.; et al. Genomic Evolution of Breast Cancer Metastasis and Relapse. *Cancer Cell* **2017**, *32*, 169–184. [CrossRef] [PubMed]
83. Kutasovic, J.R.; McCart Reed, A.E.; Males, R.; Sim, S.; Saunus, J.M.; Dalley, A.; McEvoy, C.R.; Dedina, L.; Miller, G.; Peyton, S.; et al. Breast cancer metastasis to gynaecological organs: A clinico-pathological and molecular profiling study. *J. Pathol. Clin. Res.* **2019**, *5*, 25–39. [CrossRef] [PubMed]
84. Ullah, I.; Karthik, G.M.; Alkodsi, A.; Kjallquist, U.; Stalhammar, G.; Lovrot, J.; Martinez, N.F.; Lagergren, J.; Hautaniemi, S.; Hartman, J.; et al. Evolutionary history of metastatic breast cancer reveals minimal seeding from axillary lymph nodes. *J. Clin. Investig.* **2018**, *128*, 1355–1370. [CrossRef] [PubMed]
85. Aurilio, G.; Disalvatore, D.; Pruneri, G.; Bagnardi, V.; Viale, G.; Curigliano, G.; Adamoli, L.; Munzone, E.; Sciandivasci, A.; De Vita, F.; et al. A meta-analysis of oestrogen receptor, progesterone receptor and human epidermal growth factor receptor 2 discordance between primary breast cancer and metastases. *Eur. J. Cancer* **2014**, *50*, 277–289. [CrossRef]

86. Cummings, M.C.; Simpson, P.T.; Reid, L.E.; Jayanthan, J.; Skerman, J.; Song, S.; McCart Reed, A.E.; Kutasovic, J.R.; Morey, A.L.; Marquart, L.; et al. Metastatic progression of breast cancer: Insights from 50 years of autopsies. *J. Pathol.* **2014**, *232*, 23–31. [CrossRef]
87. De Duenas, E.M.; Hernandez, A.L.; Zotano, A.G.; Carrion, R.M.; Lopez-Muniz, J.I.; Novoa, S.A.; Rodriguez, A.L.; Fidalgo, J.A.; Lozano, J.F.; Gasion, O.B.; et al. Prospective evaluation of the conversion rate in the receptor status between primary breast cancer and metastasis: Results from the GEICAM 2009-03 ConvertHER study. *Breast Cancer Res. Treat.* **2014**, *143*, 507–515. [CrossRef]
88. Niikura, N.; Liu, J.; Hayashi, N.; Mittendorf, E.A.; Gong, Y.; Palla, S.L.; Tokuda, Y.; Gonzalez-Angulo, A.M.; Hortobagyi, G.N.; Ueno, N.T. Loss of human epidermal growth factor receptor 2 (HER2) expression in metastatic sites of HER2-overexpressing primary breast tumors. *J. Clin. Oncol.* **2012**, *30*, 593–599. [CrossRef]
89. Lindstrom, L.S.; Karlsson, E.; Wilking, U.M.; Johansson, U.; Hartman, J.; Lidbrink, E.K.; Hatschek, T.; Skoog, L.; Bergh, J. Clinically used breast cancer markers such as estrogen receptor, progesterone receptor, and human epidermal growth factor receptor 2 are unstable throughout tumor progression. *J. Clin. Oncol.* **2012**, *30*, 2601–2608. [CrossRef]
90. Lluch, A.; Gonzalez-Angulo, A.M.; Casadevall, D.; Eterovic, A.K.; Martinez de Duenas, E.; Zheng, X.; Guerrero-Zotano, A.; Liu, S.; Perez, R.; Chen, K.; et al. Dynamic clonal remodelling in breast cancer metastases is associated with subtype conversion. *Eur. J. Cancer* **2019**, *120*, 54–64. [CrossRef]
91. Saunus, J.M.; Quinn, M.C.; Patch, A.M.; Pearson, J.V.; Bailey, P.J.; Nones, K.; McCart Reed, A.E.; Miller, D.; Wilson, P.J.; Al-Ejeh, F.; et al. Integrated genomic and transcriptomic analysis of human brain metastases identifies alterations of potential clinical significance. *J. Pathol.* **2015**, *237*, 363–378. [CrossRef]
92. Wu, J.M.; Fackler, M.J.; Halushka, M.K.; Molavi, D.W.; Taylor, M.E.; Teo, W.W.; Griffin, C.; Fetting, J.; Davidson, N.E.; De Marzo, A.M.; et al. Heterogeneity of breast cancer metastases: Comparison of therapeutic target expression and promoter methylation between primary tumors and their multifocal metastases. *Clin. Cancer Res.* **2008**, *14*, 1938–1946. [CrossRef] [PubMed]
93. Jeselsohn, R.; Yelensky, R.; Buchwalter, G.; Frampton, G.; Meric-Bernstam, F.; Gonzalez-Angulo, A.M.; Ferrer-Lozano, J.; Perez-Fidalgo, J.A.; Cristofanilli, M.; Gomez, H.; et al. Emergence of constitutively active estrogen receptor-alpha mutations in pretreated advanced estrogen receptor-positive breast cancer. *Clin. Cancer Res.* **2014**, *20*, 1757–1767. [CrossRef] [PubMed]
94. Robinson, D.R.; Wu, Y.M.; Vats, P.; Su, F.; Lonigro, R.J.; Cao, X.; Kalyana-Sundaram, S.; Wang, R.; Ning, Y.; Hodges, L.; et al. Activating ESR1 mutations in hormone-resistant metastatic breast cancer. *Nat. Genet.* **2013**, *45*, 1446–1451. [CrossRef] [PubMed]
95. Levine, K.M.; Priedigkeit, N.; Basudan, A.; Tasdemir, N.; Sikora, M.J.; Sokol, E.S.; Hartmaier, R.J.; Ding, K.; Ahmad, N.Z.; Watters, R.J.; et al. FGFR4 overexpression and hotspot mutations in metastatic ER+ breast cancer are enriched in the lobular subtype. *NPJ Breast Cancer* **2019**, *5*, 19. [CrossRef]
96. Law, E.K.; Sieuwerts, A.M.; LaPara, K.; Leonard, B.; Starrett, G.J.; Molan, A.M.; Temiz, N.A.; Vogel, R.I.; Meijer-van Gelder, M.E.; Sweep, F.C.; et al. The DNA cytosine deaminase APOBEC3B promotes tamoxifen resistance in ER-positive breast cancer. *Sci. Adv.* **2016**, *2*, e1601737. [CrossRef]
97. Swanton, C.; McGranahan, N.; Starrett, G.J.; Harris, R.S. APOBEC Enzymes: Mutagenic Fuel for Cancer Evolution and Heterogeneity. *Cancer Discov.* **2015**, *5*, 704–712. [CrossRef]
98. Brown, D.; Smeets, D.; Szekely, B.; Larsimont, D.; Szasz, A.M.; Adnet, P.Y.; Rothe, F.; Rouas, G.; Nagy, Z.I.; Farago, Z.; et al. Phylogenetic analysis of metastatic progression in breast cancer using somatic mutations and copy number aberrations. *Nat. Commun.* **2017**, *8*, 14944. [CrossRef]
99. Echeverria, G.V.; Powell, E.; Seth, S.; Ge, Z.; Carugo, A.; Bristow, C.; Peoples, M.; Robinson, F.; Qiu, H.; Shao, J.; et al. High-resolution clonal mapping of multi-organ metastasis in triple negative breast cancer. *Nat. Commun.* **2018**, *9*, 5079. [CrossRef]
100. Savas, P.; Teo, Z.L.; Lefevre, C.; Flensburg, C.; Caramia, F.; Alsop, K.; Mansour, M.; Francis, P.A.; Thorne, H.A.; Silva, M.J.; et al. The Subclonal Architecture of Metastatic Breast Cancer: Results from a Prospective Community-Based Rapid Autopsy Program "CASCADE". *PLoS Med.* **2016**, *13*, e1002204. [CrossRef]
101. Robinson, D.R.; Wu, Y.M.; Lonigro, R.J.; Vats, P.; Cobain, E.; Everett, J.; Cao, X.; Rabban, E.; Kumar-Sinha, C.; Raymond, V.; et al. Integrative clinical genomics of metastatic cancer. *Nature* **2017**, *548*, 297–303. [CrossRef]
102. Keller, L.; Pantel, K. Unravelling tumour heterogeneity by single-cell profiling of circulating tumour cells. *Nat. Rev. Cancer* **2019**, *19*, 553–567. [CrossRef] [PubMed]

103. Cappelletti, V.; Appierto, V.; Tiberio, P.; Fina, E.; Callari, M.; Daidone, M.G. Circulating Biomarkers for Prediction of Treatment Response. *J. Natl. Cancer Inst. Monogr.* **2015**, *2015*, 60–63. [CrossRef] [PubMed]
104. Dawson, S.J.; Tsui, D.W.; Murtaza, M.; Biggs, H.; Rueda, O.M.; Chin, S.F.; Dunning, M.J.; Gale, D.; Forshew, T.; Mahler-Araujo, B.; et al. Analysis of circulating tumor DNA to monitor metastatic breast cancer. *N. Engl. J. Med.* **2013**, *368*, 1199–1209. [CrossRef] [PubMed]
105. Janni, W.J.; Rack, B.; Terstappen, L.W.; Pierga, J.Y.; Taran, F.A.; Fehm, T.; Hall, C.; de Groot, M.R.; Bidard, F.C.; Friedl, T.W.; et al. Pooled Analysis of the Prognostic Relevance of Circulating Tumor Cells in Primary Breast Cancer. *Clin. Cancer Res.* **2016**, *22*, 2583–2593. [CrossRef]
106. Rack, B.; Schindlbeck, C.; Juckstock, J.; Andergassen, U.; Hepp, P.; Zwingers, T.; Friedl, T.W.; Lorenz, R.; Tesch, H.; Fasching, P.A.; et al. Circulating tumor cells predict survival in early average-to-high risk breast cancer patients. *J. Natl. Cancer Inst.* **2014**, *106*, dju066. [CrossRef]
107. Cristofanilli, M.; Budd, G.T.; Ellis, M.J.; Stopeck, A.; Matera, J.; Miller, M.C.; Reuben, J.M.; Doyle, G.V.; Allard, W.J.; Terstappen, L.W.; et al. Circulating tumor cells, disease progression, and survival in metastatic breast cancer. *N. Engl. J. Med.* **2004**, *351*, 781–791. [CrossRef]
108. Bidard, F.C.; Peeters, D.J.; Fehm, T.; Nole, F.; Gisbert-Criado, R.; Mavroudis, D.; Grisanti, S.; Generali, D.; Garcia-Saenz, J.A.; Stebbing, J.; et al. Clinical validity of circulating tumour cells in patients with metastatic breast cancer: A pooled analysis of individual patient data. *Lancet Oncol.* **2014**, *15*, 406–414. [CrossRef]
109. Cristofanilli, M.; Pierga, J.Y.; Reuben, J.; Rademaker, A.; Davis, A.A.; Peeters, D.J.; Fehm, T.; Nole, F.; Gisbert-Criado, R.; Mavroudis, D.; et al. The clinical use of circulating tumor cells (CTCs) enumeration for staging of metastatic breast cancer (MBC): International expert consensus paper. *Crit. Rev. Oncol. Hematol.* **2019**, *134*, 39–45. [CrossRef]
110. Ye, Z.; Wang, C.; Wan, S.; Mu, Z.; Zhang, Z.; Abu-Khalaf, M.M.; Fellin, F.M.; Silver, D.P.; Neupane, M.; Jaslow, R.J.; et al. Association of clinical outcomes in metastatic breast cancer patients with circulating tumour cell and circulating cell-free DNA. *Eur. J. Cancer* **2019**, *106*, 133–143. [CrossRef]
111. Merino, D.; Weber, T.S.; Serrano, A.; Vaillant, F.; Liu, K.; Pal, B.; Di Stefano, L.; Schreuder, J.; Lin, D.; Chen, Y.; et al. Barcoding reveals complex clonal behavior in patient-derived xenografts of metastatic triple negative breast cancer. *Nat. Commun.* **2019**, *10*, 766. [CrossRef]
112. Wallwiener, M.; Hartkopf, A.D.; Riethdorf, S.; Nees, J.; Sprick, M.R.; Schonfisch, B.; Taran, F.A.; Heil, J.; Sohn, C.; Pantel, K.; et al. The impact of HER2 phenotype of circulating tumor cells in metastatic breast cancer: A retrospective study in 107 patients. *BMC Cancer* **2015**, *15*, 403. [CrossRef] [PubMed]
113. Fehm, T.; Muller, V.; Aktas, B.; Janni, W.; Schneeweiss, A.; Stickeler, E.; Lattrich, C.; Lohberg, C.R.; Solomayer, E.; Rack, B.; et al. HER2 status of circulating tumor cells in patients with metastatic breast cancer: A prospective, multicenter trial. *Breast Cancer Res. Treat.* **2010**, *124*, 403–412. [CrossRef] [PubMed]
114. De Kruijff, I.E.; Sieuwerts, A.M.; Onstenk, W.; Jager, A.; Hamberg, P.; de Jongh, F.E.; Smid, M.; Kraan, J.; Timmermans, M.A.; Martens, J.W.M.; et al. Androgen receptor expression in circulating tumor cells of patients with metastatic breast cancer. *Int. J. Cancer* **2019**, *145*, 1083–1089. [CrossRef] [PubMed]
115. Yu, M.; Bardia, A.; Wittner, B.S.; Stott, S.L.; Smas, M.E.; Ting, D.T.; Isakoff, S.J.; Ciciliano, J.C.; Wells, M.N.; Shah, A.M.; et al. Circulating breast tumor cells exhibit dynamic changes in epithelial and mesenchymal composition. *Science* **2013**, *339*, 580–584. [CrossRef]
116. Markiewicz, A.; Topa, J.; Nagel, A.; Skokowski, J.; Seroczynska, B.; Stokowy, T.; Welnicka-Jaskiewicz, M.; Zaczek, A.J. Spectrum of Epithelial-Mesenchymal Transition Phenotypes in Circulating Tumour Cells from Early Breast Cancer Patients. *Cancers* **2019**, *11*, 59. [CrossRef]
117. Pastushenko, I.; Brisebarre, A.; Sifrim, A.; Fioramonti, M.; Revenco, T.; Boumahdi, S.; Van Keymeulen, A.; Brown, D.; Moers, V.; Lemaire, S.; et al. Identification of the tumour transition states occurring during EMT. *Nature* **2018**, *556*, 463–468. [CrossRef]
118. Mu, Z.; Wang, C.; Ye, Z.; Austin, L.; Civan, J.; Hyslop, T.; Palazzo, J.P.; Jaslow, R.; Li, B.; Myers, R.E.; et al. Prospective assessment of the prognostic value of circulating tumor cells and their clusters in patients with advanced-stage breast cancer. *Breast Cancer Res. Treat.* **2015**, *154*, 563–571. [CrossRef]
119. Aceto, N.; Bardia, A.; Miyamoto, D.T.; Donaldson, M.C.; Wittner, B.S.; Spencer, J.A.; Yu, M.; Pely, A.; Engstrom, A.; Zhu, H.; et al. Circulating tumor cell clusters are oligoclonal precursors of breast cancer metastasis. *Cell* **2014**, *158*, 1110–1122. [CrossRef]

120. Wang, C.; Mu, Z.; Chervoneva, I.; Austin, L.; Ye, Z.; Rossi, G.; Palazzo, J.P.; Sun, C.; Abu-Khalaf, M.; Myers, R.E.; et al. Longitudinally collected CTCs and CTC-clusters and clinical outcomes of metastatic breast cancer. *Breast Cancer Res. Treat.* **2017**, *161*, 83–94. [CrossRef]
121. Giuliano, M.; Shaikh, A.; Lo, H.C.; Arpino, G.; De Placido, S.; Zhang, X.H.; Cristofanilli, M.; Schiff, R.; Trivedi, M.V. Perspective on Circulating Tumor Cell Clusters: Why It Takes a Village to Metastasize. *Cancer Res.* **2018**, *78*, 845–852. [CrossRef]
122. Appierto, V.; Di Cosimo, S.; Reduzzi, C.; Pala, V.; Cappelletti, V.; Daidone, M.G. How to study and overcome tumor heterogeneity with circulating biomarkers: The breast cancer case. *Semin. Cancer Biol.* **2017**, *44*, 106–116. [CrossRef] [PubMed]
123. Pestrin, M.; Salvianti, F.; Galardi, F.; De Luca, F.; Turner, N.; Malorni, L.; Pazzagli, M.; Di Leo, A.; Pinzani, P. Heterogeneity of PIK3CA mutational status at the single cell level in circulating tumor cells from metastatic breast cancer patients. *Mol. Oncol.* **2015**, *9*, 749–757. [CrossRef] [PubMed]
124. Paoletti, C.; Cani, A.K.; Larios, J.M.; Hovelson, D.H.; Aung, K.; Darga, E.P.; Cannell, E.M.; Baratta, P.J.; Liu, C.J.; Chu, D.; et al. Comprehensive Mutation and Copy Number Profiling in Archived Circulating Breast Cancer Tumor Cells Documents Heterogeneous Resistance Mechanisms. *Cancer Res.* **2018**, *78*, 1110–1122. [CrossRef] [PubMed]
125. Polzer, B.; Medoro, G.; Pasch, S.; Fontana, F.; Zorzino, L.; Pestka, A.; Andergassen, U.; Meier-Stiegen, F.; Czyz, Z.T.; Alberter, B.; et al. Molecular profiling of single circulating tumor cells with diagnostic intention. *EMBO Mol. Med.* **2014**, *6*, 1371–1386. [CrossRef] [PubMed]
126. De Luca, F.; Rotunno, G.; Salvianti, F.; Galardi, F.; Pestrin, M.; Gabellini, S.; Simi, L.; Mancini, I.; Vannucchi, A.M.; Pazzagli, M.; et al. Mutational analysis of single circulating tumor cells by next generation sequencing in metastatic breast cancer. *Oncotarget* **2016**, *7*, 26107–26119. [PubMed]
127. Shaw, J.A.; Guttery, D.S.; Hills, A.; Fernandez-Garcia, D.; Page, K.; Rosales, B.M.; Goddard, K.S.; Hastings, R.K.; Luo, J.; Ogle, O.; et al. Mutation Analysis of Cell-Free DNA and Single Circulating Tumor Cells in Metastatic Breast Cancer Patients with High Circulating Tumor Cell Counts. *Clin. Cancer Res.* **2017**, *23*, 88–96. [CrossRef]
128. Paolillo, C.; Mu, Z.; Rossi, G.; Schiewer, M.J.; Nguyen, T.; Austin, L.; Capoluongo, E.; Knudsen, K.; Cristofanilli, M.; Fortina, P. Detection of Activating Estrogen Receptor Gene (ESR1) Mutations in Single Circulating Tumor Cells. *Clin. Cancer Res.* **2017**, *23*, 6086–6093. [CrossRef]
129. Beije, N.; Sieuwerts, A.M.; Kraan, J.; Van, N.M.; Onstenk, W.; Vitale, S.R.; van der Vlugt-Daane, M.; Dirix, L.Y.; Brouwer, A.; Hamberg, P.; et al. Estrogen receptor mutations and splice variants determined in liquid biopsies from metastatic breast cancer patients. *Mol. Oncol.* **2018**, *12*, 48–57. [CrossRef]
130. Desmedt, C.; Pingitore, J.; Rothe, F.; Marchio, C.; Clatot, F.; Rouas, G.; Richard, F.; Bertucci, F.; Mariani, O.; Galant, C.; et al. ESR1 mutations in metastatic lobular breast cancer patients. *NPJ Breast Cancer* **2019**, *5*, 9. [CrossRef]
131. Chung, J.H.; Pavlick, D.; Hartmaier, R.; Schrock, A.B.; Young, L.; Forcier, B.; Ye, P.; Levin, M.K.; Goldberg, M.; Burris, H.; et al. Hybrid capture-based genomic profiling of circulating tumor DNA from patients with estrogen receptor-positive metastatic breast cancer. *Ann. Oncol.* **2017**, *28*, 2866–2873. [CrossRef]
132. O'Leary, B.; Cutts, R.J.; Liu, Y.; Hrebien, S.; Huang, X.; Fenwick, K.; Andre, F.; Loibl, S.; Loi, S.; Garcia-Murillas, I.; et al. The Genetic Landscape and Clonal Evolution of Breast Cancer Resistance to Palbociclib plus Fulvestrant in the PALOMA-3 Trial. *Cancer Discov.* **2018**, *8*, 1390–1403. [CrossRef] [PubMed]
133. Kuang, Y.; Siddiqui, B.; Hu, J.; Pun, M.; Cornwell, M.; Buchwalter, G.; Hughes, M.E.; Wagle, N.; Kirschmeier, P.; Janne, P.A.; et al. Unraveling the clinicopathological features driving the emergence of ESR1 mutations in metastatic breast cancer. *NPJ Breast Cancer* **2018**, *4*, 22. [CrossRef] [PubMed]
134. Riva, F.; Bidard, F.C.; Houy, A.; Saliou, A.; Madic, J.; Rampanou, A.; Hego, C.; Milder, M.; Cottu, P.; Sablin, M.P.; et al. Patient-Specific Circulating Tumor DNA Detection during Neoadjuvant Chemotherapy in Triple-Negative Breast Cancer. *Clin. Chem.* **2017**, *63*, 691–699. [CrossRef] [PubMed]
135. Beaver, J.A.; Jelovac, D.; Balukrishna, S.; Cochran, R.; Croessmann, S.; Zabransky, D.J.; Wong, H.Y.; Toro, P.V.; Cidado, J.; Blair, B.G.; et al. Detection of cancer DNA in plasma of patients with early-stage breast cancer. *Clin. Cancer Res.* **2014**, *20*, 2643–2650. [CrossRef] [PubMed]
136. Madic, J.; Kiialainen, A.; Bidard, F.C.; Birzele, F.; Ramey, G.; Leroy, Q.; Rio Frio, T.; Vaucher, I.; Raynal, V.; Bernard, V.; et al. Circulating tumor DNA and circulating tumor cells in metastatic triple negative breast cancer patients. *Int. J. Cancer* **2015**, *136*, 2158–2165. [CrossRef]

137. Rothe, F.; Laes, J.F.; Lambrechts, D.; Smeets, D.; Vincent, D.; Maetens, M.; Fumagalli, D.; Michiels, S.; Drisis, S.; Moerman, C.; et al. Plasma circulating tumor DNA as an alternative to metastatic biopsies for mutational analysis in breast cancer. *Ann. Oncol.* **2014**, *25*, 1959–1965. [CrossRef]

138. Murtaza, M.; Dawson, S.J.; Pogrebniak, K.; Rueda, O.M.; Provenzano, E.; Grant, J.; Chin, S.F.; Tsui, D.W.Y.; Marass, F.; Gale, D.; et al. Multifocal clonal evolution characterized using circulating tumour DNA in a case of metastatic breast cancer. *Nat. Commun.* **2015**, *6*, 8760. [CrossRef]

139. Takeshita, T.; Yamamoto, Y.; Yamamoto-Ibusuki, M.; Inao, T.; Sueta, A.; Fujiwara, S.; Omoto, Y.; Iwase, H. Clinical significance of monitoring ESR1 mutations in circulating cell-free DNA in estrogen receptor positive breast cancer patients. *Oncotarget* **2016**, *7*, 32504–32518. [CrossRef]

140. Parikh, A.R.; Leshchiner, I.; Elagina, L.; Goyal, L.; Levovitz, C.; Siravegna, G.; Livitz, D.; Rhrissorrakrai, K.; Martin, E.E.; Van Seventer, E.E.; et al. Liquid versus tissue biopsy for detecting acquired resistance and tumor heterogeneity in gastrointestinal cancers. *Nat. Med.* **2019**, *25*, 1415–1421. [CrossRef]

141. Ma, F.; Zhu, W.; Guan, Y.; Yang, L.; Xia, X.; Chen, S.; Li, Q.; Guan, X.; Yi, Z.; Qian, H.; et al. ctDNA dynamics: A novel indicator to track resistance in metastatic breast cancer treated with anti-HER2 therapy. *Oncotarget* **2016**, *7*, 66020–66031. [CrossRef]

142. Rothe, F.; Silva, M.J.; Venet, D.; Campbell, C.; Bradburry, I.; Rouas, G.; de Azambuja, E.; Maetens, M.; Fumagalli, D.; Rodrik-Outmezguine, V.; et al. Circulating Tumor DNA in HER2-Amplified Breast Cancer: A Translational Research Substudy of the NeoALTTO Phase III Trial. *Clin. Cancer Res.* **2019**, *25*, 3581–3588. [CrossRef] [PubMed]

143. Schuh, A.; Dreau, H.; Knight, S.J.L.; Ridout, K.; Mizani, T.; Vavoulis, D.; Colling, R.; Antoniou, P.; Kvikstad, E.M.; Pentony, M.M.; et al. Clinically actionable mutation profiles in patients with cancer identified by whole-genome sequencing. *Cold Spring Harb. Mol. Case Stud.* **2018**, *4*, a002279. [CrossRef] [PubMed]

144. Cheng, D.T.; Mitchell, T.N.; Zehir, A.; Shah, R.H.; Benayed, R.; Syed, A.; Chandramohan, R.; Liu, Z.Y.; Won, H.H.; Scott, S.N.; et al. Memorial Sloan Kettering-Integrated Mutation Profiling of Actionable Cancer Targets (MSK-IMPACT): A Hybridization Capture-Based Next-Generation Sequencing Clinical Assay for Solid Tumor Molecular Oncology. *J. Mol. Diagn.* **2015**, *17*, 251–264. [CrossRef] [PubMed]

145. Schwaederle, M.; Parker, B.A.; Schwab, R.B.; Daniels, G.A.; Piccioni, D.E.; Kesari, S.; Helsten, T.L.; Bazhenova, L.A.; Romero, J.; Fanta, P.T.; et al. Precision Oncology: The UC San Diego Moores Cancer Center PREDICT Experience. *Mol. Cancer Ther.* **2016**, *15*, 743–752. [CrossRef] [PubMed]

146. Wheler, J.J.; Janku, F.; Naing, A.; Li, Y.; Stephen, B.; Zinner, R.; Subbiah, V.; Fu, S.; Karp, D.; Falchook, G.S.; et al. Cancer Therapy Directed by Comprehensive Genomic Profiling: A Single Center Study. *Cancer Res.* **2016**, *76*, 3690–3701. [CrossRef]

147. Pineiro-Yanez, E.; Reboiro-Jato, M.; Gomez-Lopez, G.; Perales-Paton, J.; Troule, K.; Rodriguez, J.M.; Tejero, H.; Shimamura, T.; Lopez-Casas, P.P.; Carretero, J.; et al. PanDrugs: A novel method to prioritize anticancer drug treatments according to individual genomic data. *Genome Med.* **2018**, *10*, 41. [CrossRef]

148. Dumbrava, E.I.; Meric-Bernstam, F. Personalized cancer therapy-leveraging a knowledge base for clinical decision-making. *Cold Spring Harb. Mol. Case Stud.* **2018**, *4*, a001578. [CrossRef]

149. Meric-Bernstam, F.; Johnson, A.; Holla, V.; Bailey, A.M.; Brusco, L.; Chen, K.; Routbort, M.; Patel, K.P.; Zeng, J.; Kopetz, S.; et al. A decision support framework for genomically informed investigational cancer therapy. *J. Natl. Cancer Inst.* **2015**, djv098. [CrossRef]

150. Chakravarty, D.; Gao, J.; Phillips, S.M.; Kundra, R.; Zhang, H.; Wang, J.; Rudolph, J.E.; Yaeger, R.; Soumerai, T.; Nissan, M.H.; et al. OncoKB: A Precision Oncology Knowledge Base. *JCO Precis. Oncol.* **2017**, *2017*. [CrossRef]

151. Yates, L.R.; Desmedt, C. Translational Genomics: Practical Applications of the Genomic Revolution in Breast Cancer. *Clin. Cancer Res.* **2017**, *23*, 2630–2639. [CrossRef]

152. Zhao, E.Y.; Shen, Y.; Pleasance, E.; Kasaian, K.; Leelakumari, S.; Jones, M.; Bose, P.; Ch'ng, C.; Reisle, C.; Eirew, P.; et al. Homologous Recombination Deficiency and Platinum-Based Therapy Outcomes in Advanced Breast Cancer. *Clin. Cancer Res.* **2017**, *23*, 7521–7530. [CrossRef] [PubMed]

153. Staaf, J.; Glodzik, D.; Bosch, A.; Vallon-Christersson, J.; Reutersward, C.; Hakkinen, J.; Degasperi, A.; Amarante, T.D.; Saal, L.H.; Hegardt, C.; et al. Whole-genome sequencing of triple-negative breast cancers in a population-based clinical study. *Nat. Med.* **2019**, *25*, 1526–1533. [CrossRef] [PubMed]

154. Meijer, T.G.; Verkaik, N.S.; Sieuwerts, A.M.; van Riet, J.; Naipal, K.A.T.; van Deurzen, C.H.M.; den Bakker, M.A.; Sleddens, H.; Dubbink, H.J.; den Toom, T.D.; et al. Correction: Functional Ex Vivo Assay Reveals Homologous Recombination Deficiency in Breast Cancer Beyond BRCA Gene Defects. *Clin. Cancer Res.* **2019**, *25*, 2935. [CrossRef] [PubMed]
155. Chan, T.A.; Yarchoan, M.; Jaffee, E.; Swanton, C.; Quezada, S.A.; Stenzinger, A.; Peters, S. Development of tumor mutation burden as an immunotherapy biomarker: Utility for the oncology clinic. *Ann. Oncol.* **2019**, *30*, 44–56. [CrossRef] [PubMed]
156. Goodman, A.M.; Kato, S.; Bazhenova, L.; Patel, S.P.; Frampton, G.M.; Miller, V.; Stephens, P.J.; Daniels, G.A.; Kurzrock, R. Tumor Mutational Burden as an Independent Predictor of Response to Immunotherapy in Diverse Cancers. *Mol. Cancer Ther.* **2017**, *16*, 2598–2608. [CrossRef]
157. Samstein, R.M.; Lee, C.H.; Shoushtari, A.N.; Hellmann, M.D.; Shen, R.; Janjigian, Y.Y.; Barron, D.A.; Zehir, A.; Jordan, E.J.; Omuro, A.; et al. Tumor mutational load predicts survival after immunotherapy across multiple cancer types. *Nat. Genet.* **2019**, *51*, 202–206. [CrossRef]
158. Banerji, U.; Dean, E.J.; Perez-Fidalgo, J.A.; Batist, G.; Bedard, P.L.; You, B.; Westin, S.N.; Kabos, P.; Garrett, M.D.; Tall, M.; et al. A Phase I Open-Label Study to Identify a Dosing Regimen of the Pan-AKT Inhibitor AZD5363 for Evaluation in Solid Tumors and in PIK3CA-Mutated Breast and Gynecologic Cancers. *Clin. Cancer Res.* **2018**, *24*, 2050–2059. [CrossRef]
159. Andre, F.; Ciruelos, E.; Rubovszky, G.; Campone, M.; Loibl, S.; Rugo, H.S.; Iwata, H.; Conte, P.; Mayer, I.A.; Kaufman, B.; et al. Alpelisib for PIK3CA-Mutated, Hormone Receptor-Positive Advanced Breast Cancer. *N. Engl. J. Med.* **2019**, *380*, 1929–1940. [CrossRef]

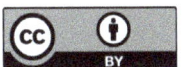

© 2020 by the authors. Licensee MDPI, Basel, Switzerland. This article is an open access article distributed under the terms and conditions of the Creative Commons Attribution (CC BY) license (http://creativecommons.org/licenses/by/4.0/).

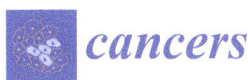

Review

Single-Cell Analysis of Circulating Tumor Cells: Why Heterogeneity Matters

Su Bin Lim [1,2], Chwee Teck Lim [1,2,3,4] and Wan-Teck Lim [5,6,7,*]

1. NUS Graduate School for Integrative Sciences & Engineering, National University of Singapore, Singapore 117456, Singapore; sblim@u.nus.edu (S.B.L.); ctlim@nus.edu.sg (C.T.L.)
2. Department of Biomedical Engineering, National University of Singapore, Singapore 117583, Singapore
3. Mechanobiology Institute, National University of Singapore, Singapore 117411, Singapore
4. Institute for Health Innovation and Technology (iHealthtech), National University of Singapore, Singapore 117599, Singapore
5. Division of Medical Oncology, National Cancer Centre Singapore, Singapore 169610, Singapore
6. Office of Academic and Clinical Development, Duke-NUS Medical School, Singapore 169857, Singapore
7. IMCB NCC MPI Singapore Oncogenome Laboratory, Institute of Molecular and Cell Biology (IMCB), Agency for Science, Technology and Research (A*STAR), Singapore 138673, Singapore
* Correspondence: darren.lim.w.t@singhealth.com.sg; Tel.: +65-6436-8000

Received: 30 September 2019; Accepted: 16 October 2019; Published: 19 October 2019

Abstract: Unlike bulk-cell analysis, single-cell approaches have the advantage of assessing cellular heterogeneity that governs key aspects of tumor biology. Yet, their applications to circulating tumor cells (CTCs) are relatively limited, due mainly to the technical challenges resulting from extreme rarity of CTCs. Nevertheless, recent advances in microfluidics and immunoaffinity enrichment technologies along with sequencing platforms have fueled studies aiming to enrich, isolate, and sequence whole genomes of CTCs with high fidelity across various malignancies. Here, we review recent single-cell CTC (scCTC) sequencing efforts, and the integrated workflows, that have successfully characterized patient-derived CTCs. We examine how these studies uncover DNA alterations occurring at multiple molecular levels ranging from point mutations to chromosomal rearrangements from a single CTC, and discuss their cellular heterogeneity and clinical consequences. Finally, we highlight emerging strategies to address key challenges currently limiting the translation of these findings to clinical practice.

Keywords: single-cell analysis; cellular heterogeneity; circulating tumor cells

---

1. Introduction

The concept of intratumoral heterogeneity (ITH), first described in 1982 by Fidler and Hart [1], has been expanded to include genetic, phenotypic and functional heterogeneity within tumors comprising diverse malignant and non-malignant subpopulations. With accumulations of mutations in DNA damage checkpoint control genes and DNA repair genes, divergent cancer clones may evolve and propagate over time through selection processes driven by constantly changing microenvironment and by the use of therapy [2,3]. In addition to genetic heterogeneity in clonal mutations and subclonal de novo mutations, functional heterogeneity related to developmental pathways and epigenetic programs and spatial variability in tumor microenvironment contribute to ITH, which governs key aspects of tumor biology, including tumor invasion, metastasis, and drug resistance [2].

Recent years have also seen the contribution of non-malignant cells, such as stromal fibroblasts, immune cells, bone-marrow-derived cells, mesenchymal stem cells, and endothelial cells, to ITH within a tumor. Malignant and benign cells interact locally through a complex network of extracellular matrix (ECM) and the related components, collectively termed as matrisome, which has been linked to tumor progression, response to adjuvant therapy, and immune system [4–7], driving tumor phenotypes supporting their metastatic competence. The tumor cells can be shed passively (through corrupted blood vessel) and/or actively (through epithelial–mesenchymal transition (EMT)) from tumors into the circulation, referred to as circulating tumor cells (CTCs), in which only a minority of cell populations survive under the physiological blood flow and succeed in early colonization phases [8]. Despite the low frequency of occurrence, CTCs allow for repeated sampling, which is not clinically practical for tissue biopsy, and may thus be an excellent tool for assessing tumor heterogeneity and for revealing clonal diversity underlying resistance to treatment [9].

The prevalence of phenotypic plasticity involving programmed death-ligand 1 (PD-L1) [10], stemness [11], drug resistance [12], and EMT [13], within CTC populations has fueled investigation of cellular heterogeneity using single-cell high-throughput enrichment and sequencing platforms over the past five years. Emerging single-cell RNA sequencing (scRNA-seq) data further suggest that CTCs may interact with hematopoietic cells or platelets in blood through direct and/or indirect routes, adding another layer of heterogeneity [14]. Bulk-cell approaches traditionally deployed in existing CTC literature, however, have provided insights into cellular processes averaged throughout the enriched blood sample, which largely comprises leukocytes, or white blood cells (WBCs). The leukocyte contamination is inevitable in any given primarily enriched sample due in part to extremely rare CTCs occurring at a frequency of ~1 in 10^7 WBCs in blood from a cancer patient [15] and the relatively low cell capture efficiency of existing cell sorting technologies, which are further limited to isolating only certain CTC subpopulations (refer to the Section 2.1 for further details). It is therefore essential to reach single-cell resolution to precisely characterize CTCs at the genomic level and further to investigate the clinical impact of cellular heterogeneity present within CTC populations.

2. Methods and Technologies

Despite technical challenges, single-cell CTC (scCTC) analyses have so far revealed genomic variations specific to each CTC, including mutations that are not yet present in the Catalogue of Somatic Mutations in Cancer (COSMIC) database [16–20] or subclonal alterations that are not easily discernible from tissue biopsies [16,17], cells of origin of cancer (e.g., bone marrow-derived multiple myeloma) [21], or with bulk-cell approaches [22], providing comprehensive landscape of evolving tumor cells. Such private genomic variations shared by CTCs may represent "CTC phenotypes", including intravasation competency, increased migration/motility, enhanced cell–cell interactions, variation in energy metabolism, interaction with platelet and blood immune cells, resistance to anoikis, and resistance to therapy [19,23]. Single nucleotide variations (SNVs) and/or copy number variations (CNVs) in these putative precursors of metastasis present early in clonal evolution or in tumor progression may be excellent targets for therapeutic intervention. Examined below are scCTC DNA sequencing studies that have successfully assessed DNA alterations in patient-derived CTCs across various cancer types (Table 1).

Table 1. Summary of single-cell circulating tumor cells (scCTC) sequencing studies that analyzed DNA alterations in patient-derived CTCs.

CTC Enrichment	Single-Cell Isolation	CTC Criteria	WGA	Profiling	Investigated Genes	Genomic Analysis	Number of Single CTCs (Patients)[1]	Ref.
Prostate cancer								
MagSweeper	CellCelector	DAPI− CD45− EpCAM+	MDA	NGS	All	SNVs	42 (5)	[24]
Epic Sciences CTC Platform	Micromanipulation	CD45− CK+/−	DOP-PCR	NGS	All	CNVs, LSTs	67 (7)	[25]
NanoVelcro CTC Chip	LCM	CD45− CK+	MDA	NGS, Sanger, aCGH	All	SNVs, SVs, CNVs	12 (1)	[26]
HD-CTC Assay	Micromanipulation	DAPI+ CK+ CD45−	LA-PCR	NGS	All	CNVs	41 (1)	[27]
CellSearch, Spectra Optia Apheresis System	FACS	DAPI+ CK+ CD45−	LA-PCR	aCGH	All	CNVs	205 (14)	[17]
Breast cancer								
MagSweeper	Micromanipulation	DAPI+ CK+ CD45−	No WGA	Sanger	PIK3CA	SNVs	185 (11)	[28]
CellSearch	DEPArray	DAPI+ CK+ CD45−	LA-PCR	Sanger	TP53	SNVs	11 (2)	[29]
				Sanger	PIK3CA	SNVs	241 (43)	
CellSearch	DEPArray	DAPI+ CK+ CD45−	LA-PCR	qPCR	HER2	CNVs	192 (42)	[30]
				aCGH	All	CNVs	37 (15)	
CellSearch	DEPArray	DAPI+ CK+ CD45− CD34−	LA-PCR	Sanger	PIK3CA	SNVs	115 (18)	[18]
CellSearch	DEPArray	DAPI+ CK+ CD45−	LA-PCR	Targeted NGS	50 cancer-related genes	SNVs	14 (4)	[31]
Leukapheresis, CellSearch	Micromanipulation	CK+ CD45−	DOP-PCR	CGH	All	CNVs	65 (19)	[32]
				aCGH	All	CNVs		
CellSearch	MoFlo XDP flow-sorting	DAPI+ CK+ CD45−	LA-PCR	qPCR	CCND1 locus	CNVs	26 (12)	[33]
				Sanger	PIK3CA, TP53	SNVs		
FACS	DEPArray	DAPI− CD45− EpCAM− CD44+ CD24− uPAR+/− intβ1+/−	LA-PCR	MassARRAY	>200 hallmark cancer genes	SNVs	7 (-)	[34]
CellSearch	Micromanipulation	DAPI+ CK+ CD45−	MDA, LA-PCR	Sanger	PIK3CA	SNVs	114 (33)	[35]
CellSearch	DEPArray	DAPI+ CK+ CD45−	LA-PCR	Targeted NGS, ddPCR	50 COSMIC genes	SNVs	40 (5)	[36]
CellSearch	CellCelector	DAPI+ CK+ CD45−	LA-PCR	Targeted NGS	50 COSMIC genes	SNVs	7 (2)	[37]
CellSearch	DEPArray	DAPI+ CK+ CD45−	LA-PCR	Sanger	TP53, HER2, PIK3CA, RB1	SNVs	24 (6)	[38]
Ficoll Separation	Micromanipulation	DAPI+ CK+ CD45−	LA-PCR	Sanger	ESR1	SNVs	8 (4)	[39]
AutoMACS Classic Separator	LCM	CK+ CD45−	LA-PCR	SNP Array	All	CNVs	17 (17)	[23]
CellSearch, Oncoquick	CellCelector	EpCAM+ CD45−	MDA	aCGH, targeted NGS	All	SNVs, CNVs	31 (1)	[40]
oHSV-hTERT-GFP method	FACS	CD45− hTERT+	MALBAC	NGS	All	SNVs, CNVs	11 (8)	[19]
ScreenCell	DEPArray	DAPI+ CK+ CD45−	LA-PCR	Sanger	TP53, ESR1	SNVs	7 (1)	[41]
ClearCell FX System	Manipulation	DAPI+ CK+ CD45−	MALBAC	NGS	All	SNVs	3 (1)	[20]

135

Table 1. *Cont.*

CTC Enrichment	Single-Cell Isolation	CTC Criteria	WGA	Profiling	Investigated Genes	Genomic Analysis	Number of Single CTCs (Patients) [1]	Ref.
Lung cancer								
CellSearch	DEPArray	DAPI+ CK+ CD45−	LA-PCR	NGS	All	CNVs	72 (13)	[42]
CellSearch	Micromanipulation	DAPI+ CK+ CD45−	MALBAC	NGS, digital PCR, Sanger	All	SNVs, INDELs	24 (4)	[43]
ClearCell FX System	Microfluidic chip	DAPI+ CK+ CD45−	No WGA	Sanger	EGFR	CNVs	61 (11)	[44]
CellSearch	Micromanipulation	DAPI+ CK+ CD45−	MALBAC	NGS	All	SNVs	26 (7)	[45]
CellSearch	Micromanipulation	DAPI+ CK+ CD45−	MALBAC	NGS	All	SNVs, INDELs, CNVs, SVs	97 (23)	[46]
MagSifter	Single-Nanowell Assay	DAPI+ CK+ CD45− TERT+ MET+	No WGA	Multiplex PCR	EGFR	SNVs, INDELs, CNVs, SVs	91 (10)	[22]
						SNVs	202 (7)	
Colorectal cancer								
CellSearch	Micromanipulation	EpCAM+ CD45− CK+	LA-PCR	aCGH Sanger Multiplex PCR	All KRAS, BRAF, TP53 NCI/ICG-HNPCC marker panel	CNVs SNVs MSI	8 (8) 126 (31) 122 (30)	[47]
CellSearch	Micromanipulation	DAPI+ CK+ CD45−	LA-PCR, MDA	aCGH Targeted NGS	All 68 colorectal cancer-associated genes	CNVs SNVs	37 (6) 8 (2)	[16]
CellSearch	Micromanipulation	DAPI+ CK+ CD45−	LA-PCR, MDA	qPCR Sanger	EGFR KRAS, BRAF, PIK3CA	CNVs SNVs	26 (3) 69 (5)	[48]
Oncoquick	DEPArray	HOECHST+ CK+ CD45−	LA-PCR	Sanger, pyrosequencing	KRAS	SNVs	- (16)	[49]
Melanoma								
Dynabeads	LCM	HMW− MAA+ CD45− MART-1/gp100+	No WGA	Sanger	BRAF KIT	SNVs SNVs	14 (9) 4 (4)	[50]
Dielectrophoretic microwell array	Micromanipulation	CD45− MART-1/gp101/gp100+	No WGA	Sanger	BRAF	SNVs	33 (1)	[51]
Multiple myeloma								
MACS beads	Micromanipulation	CD45−CD138+	MDA	Targeted NGS	35 most commonly mutated loci	SNVs	203 (10)	[21]
Epic Sciences CTC Platform	Micromanipulation	CK+/− CD45−	DOP-PCR	NGS	All	CNVs	9 (1)	[52]
Pancreatic cancer								
NanoVelcro Chip	LCM	HOECHST+ CD45− CK/CEA+	MDA	Sanger	KRAS	SNVs	60 (12)	[53]

[1] QC-passed CTCs that have been included in the final analysis.

2.1. CTC Enrichment

Once collected, blood samples are subjected to CTC enrichment using density gradient centrifugation, 2D/3D microfiltration, microfluidic devices, or immunoaffinity-based technologies (Figure 1; refer to Ref. [14] for detailed summary and comparison of existing CTC enrichment technologies). While CellSearch® remains the choice of primary enrichment tool in scCTC sequencing studies, such immunoaffinity-based enrichment technology relying on epithelial cell surface markers (e.g., EpCAM or CKs) have varying capture efficiency depending on the degree of EMT, stemness, and the resulting differentiation cell state. EpCAM$^+$CK$^+$ cells have also been detected by CellSearch® in patients with benign diseases, but in lower frequency compared to the cancer group [54]. Clinical data supporting the metastatic competence of EpCAM$^-$ CTCs in numerous studies [34,55] have further fueled the transition in the field to the development of label-free approaches leveraging on biophysical properties of CTCs (e.g., size, density, stiffness).

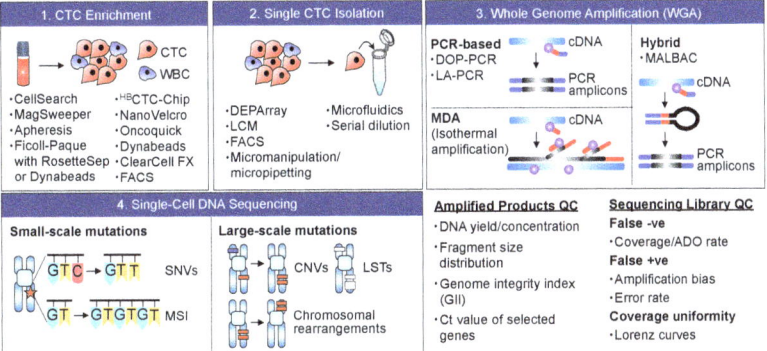

Figure 1. The standard workflow and existing technologies for scCTC sequencing. CTCs are primarily enriched from a whole blood sample, and are isolated as single cells for subsequent downstream molecular analyses. For genomic analysis of whole genome/exome, whole-genome amplification (WGA) is performed and amplified DNA products are QC-checked prior to sequencing.

One of our pioneering efforts in developing such marker-independent technology was the application of inertial microfluidics using spiral microchannels, in which depth and width of each channel can be designed to control the positioning of cells or microparticles in suspension via Dean flow fractionation (DFF). Our technology, so-called ClearCell® FX, enriches intact and viable CTCs from the peripheral blood of cancer patients in a fully automated and high-throughput fashion, with a reported >80% sensitivity and specificity in detecting CTCs from clinical samples (refer to [56] for further details on the system). Mechanobiologically inspired enrichment platforms achieve high sensitivity and are not limited to certain CTC subpopulations, yet the purity of enriched samples may be compromised due to their size distribution overlapping with leukocytes, as observed in breast, colorectal, and prostate cancer [57]. To best interrogate CTCs and their cellular heterogeneity, cell enrichment technology should thus be carefully selected for unbiased capture and recovery of different CTC subpopulations.

2.2. Single-Cell Isolation

CTC enrichment technologies are used in conjunction with microscopic micromanipulators (e.g., Eppendorf Transfer Man NK2/4 micromanipulator, CellCelector^{TM}), laser capture microdissection (LCM) [26], microfluidic devices [44], or DEPArray^{TM} to recover putative CTCs as single cells. Enriched cells are often fixed and stained with the nucleic acid dye DAPI and monoclonal antibodies specific to epithelial cell surface marker cytokeratin (CK) and leukocyte marker CD45, and manually selected by the trained and skilled operator based on DAPI and CK positivity and CD45 negativity. Morphology of the captured cells (e.g., cell shape, size) are concurrently assessed to identify cells having 4 to 40 µm diameter, round or oval shape, and/or high nuclear/cytoplasm ratio [37,39,49].

Even though dozens of CTCs might have been captured in CTC enrichment step, only very few single CTCs (<10 CTCs) have been isolated and transferred successfully to a PCR tube per sample [4,19,49]. Such low recovery rate could be attributed to apoptotic CTCs, which are often excluded from the isolation in most scCTC sequencing studies. Consistent with the classic definition of apoptosis, these cells are defined as CK^+CD45^- CTCs with non-intact nuclei having DAPI pattern of chromosomal condensation and/or nuclear fragmentation and blebbing [52]. Given that low burden of apoptotic CTCs has been associated with poor prognosis and aggressive phenotypes across several cancer types [52,58], characterization of CTC apoptosis in situ may facilitate the development of new platform for real-time monitoring of antitumor drug efficacy.

2.3. Whole-Genome Amplification (WGA)

WGA is an active area of development with wide applications to study rare tumor cells or single-celled organisms, such as bacteria and archaea. There exist different WGA approaches based on specific, degenerate, and/or hybrid primers: Linker-adapter PCR (LA-PCR), interspersed repetitive sequence PCR (IRS-PCR), primer extension preamplification (PEP-PCR), degenerate oligonucleotide primed PCR (DOP-PCR), displacement degenerate oligonucleotide primed PCR (D-DOP-PCR), multiple displacement amplification (MDA), single primer isothermal amplification (SPIA), and multiple annealing and looping-based amplification cycles (MALBAC; refer to ref. [59] for a comprehensive summary on working principles and characteristics of each WGA method).

Briefly, LA-PCR and IRS-PCR methods utilize specific primers, each amplifying digested DNA litigated to adapter fragments and repeating sequence elements, respectively, while the rest of the methods, such as PEP-PCR, DOP-PCR, and D-DOP-PCR, are based on the use of degenerated primers. MDA has been commonly applied to single-cell sequencing of microorganisms as well as patient-derived CTCs. It employs a unique polymerase with strong strand displacement activity (e.g., phi29 DNA polymerase), which can amplify fragments of up to 100 kb with high replication fidelity compared to purely PCR-based (e.g., Taq polymerase) methods [59]. MALBAC has been proposed as a hybrid PCR/MDA method, relying on two relatively error-prone DNA polymerases, *Bst* DNA polymerase and Taq DNA polymerase, for isothermal strand displacement and PCR, respectively. Each WGA technique has its own advantages and limitations in terms of sensitivity, specificity, uniformity, and amplification bias. For example, while LA-PCR, DOP-PCR, and MALBAC may be the choice of method for detection of CNVs but not SNVs, MDA (REPLI-g^{TM}) has proven to be most sensitive in detecting mutations at a single-base resolution compared to LA-PCR methods (GenomePlex^{TM}, Ampli1^{TM}) [60].

The challenge is that the yield of amplified DNA varies significantly across CTCs, where the success rate of amplification ranges from 11% to 100% [24,61], and WGA step itself is subjected to coverage biases and errors, such as preferential allelic amplification, GC bias, dropout events, and nucleotide copy errors [60]. To account for such variability, studies have established an additional QC step prior to in-depth sequencing to probe only CTCs with yields of DNA greater than negative controls [24] or a fixed concentration level [27] or those showing specific bands corresponding to targets of interest on the Agilent 2100 Bioanalyzer [19,29]. The author-defined QC assays have also been developed to identify CTCs suited for single-cell targeted sequencing and analysis. For example, genome integrity index (GII), which is determined from detectable PCR bands corresponding to three Mse fragments and KRAS fragment, has been proven to be predictive of successful analysis of sequence-based molecular changes, including point mutations, gene amplifications, and CNVs [30,36,42].

2.4. Sequencing and Profiling

Amplified DNA samples are subjected to library preparation and quantification. To date, scCTC studies have most commonly employed next-generation sequencing (NGS), Sanger sequencing, single nucleotide polymorphism (SNP), and array comparative genomic hybridization (aCGH) platforms, and conventional PCR technologies to analyze somatic SNVs, structural variations, (SVs), CNVs, and chromosomal breakpoints and rearrangements for whole exome/genome or selected cancer-associated genes, often comparatively with matched primary tumors and/or metastatic tissues or disseminated tumor cells (DTCs).

In the library QC step, the sequencing depth, percentage of area covered, homogeneity of coverage, and/or SNP densities are assessed to only select high-quality CTC libraries based on author-defined assessment techniques, such as autocorrelation analysis [24] and Lorenz curves [26]. Fluorimetric assays (e.g., Fluorometer) and analytical tool provided by the sequencing platform (e.g., Torrent Suite) may also be used to quantify DNA samples and to assess the performance of sequencing runs and the quality of generated data, respectively [19,31,37]. In some cases, the variants identified by NGS were specifically selected and further validated by Sanger sequencing [31,45] or digital droplet PCR (ddPCR) [36] using the same samples.

The sequence queried in single CTCs in prior studies vary from small-scale mutations (<1 kb) to large-scale mutations (1 kb–100 Mb). Targeting larger regions may come with the trade-off of increased number of false variant calls and sequencing costs and reduced number of individual cells to be sequenced [62]. Nevertheless, whole-genome sequencing (WGS) allows new discoveries of genomic variations occurring even in non-coding regions that may add significant values to the analysis of rare tumor cells.

3. CTC Heterogeneity and Clinical Impact

While resolving cellular heterogeneity, single-cell approaches may link specific CTC subpopulation programs to cancer cell phenotypes, metastasis, patient outcomes, and drug resistance, as demonstrated by recent studies. Examined below are genomic aberrations commonly analyzed in CTCs and their clinical impact (Figure 2). Clinical data derived from scCTC transcriptomic analyses are discussed elsewhere [14].

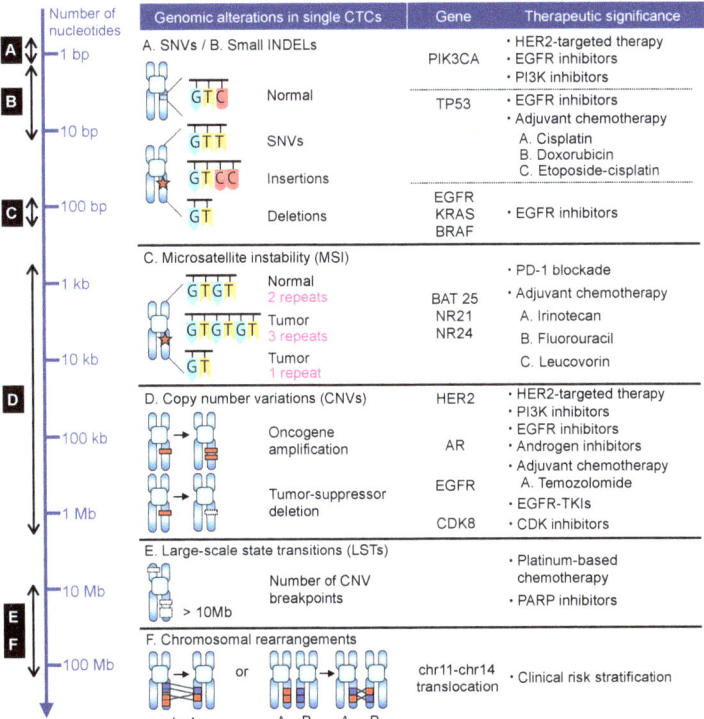

Figure 2. Summary of genomic alterations found in scCTC sequencing studies.

3.1. Single Nucleotide Variation (SNV)

3.1.1. PIK3CA

PIK3CA is a gene harboring major driver mutations in many cancer types [63,64]. Its mutational status has increasingly been recognized as a promising predictor of resistance to targeted therapies [65]. In breast cancer, tumors harboring PIK3CA mutations are often resistant to HER2-based therapy [66–68], and are less likely to achieve pathologic complete response to anti-HER2 treatments [69,70]. Though limited to the analysis of EpCAM-expressing CTCs, scCTC studies have applied targeted sequencing approaches to examine mutational hotspots, most commonly in exon 9 and 20 [16,18,28,30,35,37,48,71]. The assessment of pre-existing resistant clones through scCTC analysis prior to the administration of HER2-based therapies has been suggested to be of clinical significance for patients harboring CTCs with HER2 amplification and double-mutant PIK3CA/HER2 [30]. Longitudinal monitoring of therapy response through HER2 mutational analysis of CTCs in this subset of patients will be of particular clinical interest, given the known drug efficacy of PIK3CA pathway inhibitors in patients with HER2$^+$ primary tumors [72].

PIK3CA mutational status in CTCs indicative of resistance against HER2-targeted therapy has been demonstrated for HER2$^-$ metastatic breast cancer patients screened for German multicentric phase III trial (i.e., DETECT III study) harboring HER2$^+$ CTCs [35]. Further, studies have noted a high degree of intrapatient cellular heterogeneity and discordant PIK3CA status between CTCs and matched primary tumors [18,28,35,36], of which PIK3CA was one of two genes (among >2200 COSMIC mutations analyzed) frequently mutated in CTCs, cfDNA, and matched primary tumor in HER2$^-$ breast cancer [36]. PIK3CA mutation has also been implicated in drug resistance of EGFR tyrosine kinase inhibitor (TKI) treatment. Notably, a lung cancer patient harboring PIK3CA mutation in almost all CTCs (7/8 CTCs) but not in primary tumor (low abundance) had progressive disease and presented distant metastasis after one month of treatment with erlotinib. Early detection of such resistant cells in such a less invasive way may thus be tremendously useful in drug selection.

3.1.2. TP53

TP53 is a tumor suppressor gene frequently mutated in most human cancers [73]. TP53 mutations have functional implications in key molecular events in tumor progression, such as EMT [74], stemness [75], cancer prognosis, and survival outcomes [76]. Highly heterogeneous TP53 mutational status was observed across individual CTCs in prostate [24], lung [43], colorectal [16], and breast cancer [29,31,36,38,41]. In metastatic prostate cancer, ubiquitous TP53 mutations were found among multiple foci of the primary tumor and metastases, suggesting divergent cancer evolution from a single ancestor cancer [24].

In breast cancer, TP53 harbored the highest number of mutations across CTCs [31]. Mutant TP53 p.R273C has been associated with cisplatin chemotherapy resistance [77]. Concurrent mutations of RB1 and TP53 genes were also found in the majority of CTCs from a lung cancer patient who experienced a phenotypic transition from adenocarcinoma to small-cell lung cancer (SCLC) [43]. Notably, dramatic clinical response was observed in this patient upon etoposide-cisplatin treatment, which is a standard chemotherapy for SCLC patients [78,79]. These studies altogether highlight how scCTC profiling may provide an early signal of phenotypic transition in tumor to guide new therapeutic regimen.

3.1.3. EGFR

Despite promising efficacy of EGFR in multiple cancer types [80], prediction of response against EGFR inhibition still remains ambiguous. The mere assessment of EGFR expression at the DNA or protein level using bulk primary tumor samples has not been an ideal indicator for predicting the response to anti-EGFR drugs [81,82]. Whole-exome sequencing of lung CTCs revealed specific INDEL in the EGFR gene (p.Lys746_Ala750del) shared by primary tumors and metastases, which could be targeted with TKIs [43]. In our earlier work, we reported highly sensitive detection of EGFR mutations

(T790M and L868R) in microfluidically enriched CTCs, which showed a complete concordance of mutation status with matched primary tumors in non-small-cell lung cancer (NSCLC) patients [44]. Similarly, an integrated method using a magnetic sifter (MagSifter) and nanowell system has been described for accurate detection of EGFR (del19, T790M, and L868R) mutations in CTCs from lung cancer patients [22]. Notably, RT-qPCR readings of bulk blood samples did not reach detectable level to be analyzed for same mutations in this study [22].

3.1.4. KRAS

KRAS, one of the genes involved in the EGFR signaling pathway, may have predictive value of clinical response to anti-EGFR therapies, such as cetuximab [83], panitumumab [84], and gefitinib [85]. Patients exhibited mutational disparity between CTCs and matched primary tumors and/or across individual CTCs in breast [36], colorectal [47–49], and multiple myeloma [24], and breast cancer [36]. This may explain the variable response to anti-EGFR treatment in these cancer patients. Similarly, a highly varying degree of concordance in KRAS mutational status between CTCs and primary/metastatic lesions was observed, reflecting intratumoral heterogeneity of point mutations in KRAS occurring in 48–76% of various cancers [86].

3.1.5. BRAF

Another mutation predictive of response to EGFR-inhibiting therapy is BRAF, which is associated with a very poor prognosis particularly in colorectal cancer and melanoma [87]. Further, the predictive values of V600E and V601E mutations have been demonstrated for the use of RAF kinase inhibitor (vemurafenib) and MEK inhibitor (trametinib), respectively, in BRAF-mutated melanomas [50,88]. Somatic missense mutations in BRAF have been found in approximately 10% and 60% of colorectal tumors and melanoma lesions, respectively [50,89]. Single-cell genomic characterization of CTCs across these cancer types have revealed highly heterogeneous BRAF status across CTCs [47,48,50,51], with disparities in BRAF mutations to the corresponding primary tumor [47,50]. While such considerable heterogeneity observed in these selected genes might be the result of newly acquired mutations in CTCs, it is likely that these mutations were missed by single sector-based tissue biopsies. Through the additional deep sequencing of tissue samples, other groups indeed found mutations that were initially unique to CTCs in the primary tumors and metastases at subclonal level [16].

3.2. Microsatellite Instability (MSI)

Defective DNA mismatch repair (MMR) machinery leads to hypermutation and instability in nucleotide repeat sequences [90]. MSI is an established prognostic [91–93] and predictive marker [94,95] in many cancer types. In colorectal cancer (CRC), tumors with high-level MSI, or MSI-H phenotype account for ~15% of metastatic disease [96], and have distinct pathologic and clinical features [97]. MSI typing may serve as a predictor of benefit from adjuvant 5-fluorouracil chemotherapy for non-MSI-H CRC patients [95,98]. The standard MSI assessment recommended by the National Cancer Institute/International Collaborative Group/HNPCC (NCI/ICG-HNPCC) involves the examination of two mononucleotide repeats and three dinucleotide repeats in tumor and non-tumor adjacent normal tissues [99].

A comprehensive genomic study of CRC identified microsatellite stable (MSS) tumor harboring MSI CTCs, through aCGH, mutational profiling, and MSI analyses at the single-cell level [47]. Of note, immunohistochemical (IHC) expression analysis of DNA MMR proteins (i.e., MLH1, MSH2, MSH6, and PMS2) in multiple sectors obtained from matched primary tumor and metastatic lesions did not indicate MSI-H status in this patient. Such discordance was also found in mutational profiles, where mutations in key genes such as KRAS and TP53 were detectable only in CTCs but not in the tumor. Given that contaminating stromal cells or surrounding non-tumor cells in the tissue may obscure MSI, single-cell approaches will be essential for MSI typing.

3.3. Copy-Number Variation (CNV)

With the advent of SNP/aCGH arrays and NGS technologies, identification and characterization of CNVs in primary and metastatic tumors have provided insight into the role of CNVs in cellular functions and cancer pathogenesis [100–102]. Gain of oncogenes and loss of tumor suppressors are frequent drivers of tumor progression, and are closely associated with therapeutic responses [103]. In CTCs, genome-wide CNVs were found to be highly reproducible from cell to cell within the same individual and across different lung cancer patients with same pathological subtypes [43,45]. This is consistent with homogeneity found in CTCs from SCLC [42,46] and colorectal cancer patients [45].

While harboring a substantial number of genomic aberrations, CTCs exhibit concordant changes in chromosomes observed in matched primary and/or metastatic tumors, supporting their malignant origin, but to different extents across individual CTC, as demonstrated in colorectal [45,47], breast [40], and bladder [52] cancers. For example, phylogenetic analysis of CNV profiles identified homozygous deletion of a chromosomal region containing the tumor suppressor gene, PTEN, in CTCs and lymph node metastases, but not in primary tumor, suggesting that such CTC subsets might have metastasized in colorectal cancer [45].

A unique signature of recurrent CNVs specific to CTCs was also found in breast cancer, consisting of genes and miRNAs related to CTC phenotypes, such as resistance to anoikis, TGFβ signaling, and metastasis [23]. This copy number signature clustered patients into two groups, independent of subtype, revealing distinct functional or metastatic features in different populations. Gain of a chromosomal region harboring the HER2 gene was further consistently observed across CTCs regardless of HER2 status of matched primary tumors in this study, suggesting a potential role of HER2 amplification in CTC biology. Notably, HER2 amplification associated with the degree of chromosomal changes was identified in another multi-scale scCTC study, where a significantly higher number of genomic rearrangements was observed in breast CTCs with HER2 amplification than those without amplification, whereas no such change was seen for PIK3CA mutations [30].

CNV profiling of CTCs could potentially be used as a tool for risk stratification. CNV-based classifiers that can assign SCLC patients as chemosensitive or chemorefractory have been developed [42,46], one of which have been validated in an independent patient cohort [42]. The two patient groups stratified by these classifiers were found to have significant different progression-free survival (PFS) and/or overall survival (OS), demonstrating prognostic and predictive value of CTC CNV profiles [42,46]. Further, apheresis-acquired, CK^+ CTCs harboring >10 chromosomal alterations were associated with risk of early metastasis [32]. Better therapeutic strategies may also be inferred from sequential single-cell characterization of CNV changes in CTCs over the course of treatment; MYC amplification occurred along with AR protein expression and AR amplification in a prostate cancer patient progressing through targeted therapy [27]. While direct targeting of MYC proves to be difficult, scCTC data suggest that co-targeting of c-Myc in conjunction with AR may serve as an alternative path to prevent the emergence of drug-resistant subclones.

3.4. Chromosomal Breakpoints

In addition to focal CNV analyses, whole genome-wide CNV profiles have been extensively analyzed in bulk primary tumors. They are often associated with therapeutic resistance against platinum-based chemotherapy and PARP inhibitors [104]. Large-scale state transition (LST), which is defined as the number of chromosomal breaks between adjacent regions of at least 10Mb, is one of surrogates of such large-scale genomic instability. Significantly higher and heterogeneous LST scores were observed in CTCs from metastatic castration resistant prostate cancer (mCRPC) patients compared to cancer cell lines and WBCs from healthy donors, implying unstable CTC genomes at the single-cell level [25]. The ability to assess genomic instability with LST scoring could potentially improve risk stratification for therapeutic strategies.

3.5. Chromosomal Rearrangement

Two SVs common in all CTCs and both primary and metastatic tumors were found in prostate cancer [26]: TMEM207 in chr3, which facilitates tumor invasion, migration, and metastasis [105,106], and chr13-chr15 translocation. An extensive assessment further revealed heterogeneous status of SVs involving tumor suppressor genes, such as BRCA2, RB1, and PTEN, which are common in prostate cancer [107]. Heterogeneous status of PTEN SVs in single CTCs may suggest the acquirement of variations at different time-points, as PTEN point mutations emerges as a late event during cancer evolution [108]. Parallel transcriptomic profiling for detecting such SVs encoding oncogenes or tumor suppressors that carry founder mutation will further allow discovery of novel fusion products.

4. Longitudinal Studies

While it has long been recognized that CTC count could serve as a robust predictor of patient outcomes in breast, prostate, and colorectal cancers [36,39,109–112], CTC enumeration at a single time point alone may not provide sufficient information in terms of treatment regimen. Alternatively, phenotyping of CTCs with morphometric parameters and protein expression has been shown to be better correlated with therapy response [27,113]. Another major advantage of CTC profiling is the feasibility to analyze longitudinal samples to study mechanisms related to acquired resistance to therapy (Figure 3). Yet, such analyses may be challenging in the absence of evident de novo global chromosomal changes upon relapse and progression, requiring larger patient cohorts [42].

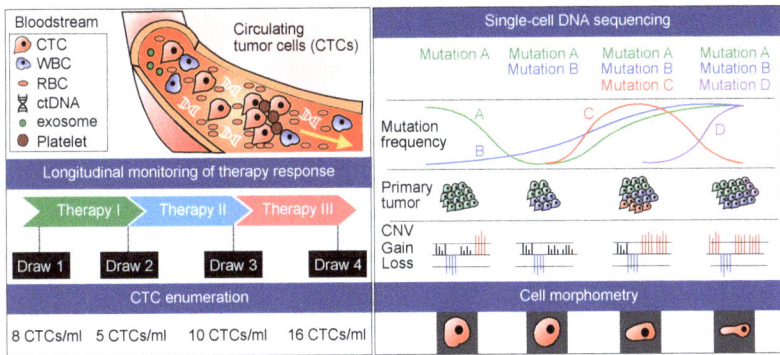

Figure 3. scCTC DNA sequencing for longitudinal monitoring of therapy response.

Selection of patients for targeted therapy has been based on the IHC detection of protein of interest and/or fluorescence in situ hybridization-based analysis of gene-level alterations, typically in known oncogenes, using primary tumor tissues. An underlying assumption is that only marker-positive patients will respond to mutant oncogene-targeted therapy. These treatments may include vemurafenib (BRAF inhibitor) for melanoma patients with V600E/V600K mutation in the BRAF gene [114], Neratinib (HER2 TKI) [115], trastuzumab (HER2 antibody) [116] and pertuzumab (HER2 antibody) [117] for breast cancer patients with amplification and/or overexpression of the HER2 gene, and erlotinib (EGFR TKI) for non-small cell lung cancer patients with exon 19 deletion or L858R mutation in the EGFR gene [118].

Such oncogene-targeted therapies, however, should carefully be applied in the clinical settings. IHC detection of EGFR expression in bulk tumor tissue alone, for example, may not be an ideal tool for prediction of response to gefitinib [119]. Discordance in genomic profiles between primary and recurring/metastatic tumors [120–122] attributed to clonal changes, sampling error in clonal selection, and/or technical flaws in the assay has complicated the decision-making process in treatment selection. Repeat biopsy for marker reassessment does not guarantee improved accuracy, nor is it without false-negative readings [123].

Varying genomic status of oncogenes has thus been re-evaluated with CTC pools over the course of therapy. Studies have examined the feasibility of detection of HER2$^+$ CTCs in patients with HER2$^-$ primary tumors [124,125] and that of KRAS-mutated CTCs in patients with nonmutated colorectal primary tumor and mutated metastases [89]. Notably, it was found that treatment with trastuzumab, an anti-HER2 antibody traditionally prescribed for patients with HER2$^+$ primary tumor, was shown to be effective in improving survival outcomes of patients with HER2$^-$ tumor by eliminating CK$^+$HER2$^+$ CTCs [126]. This was the first study that clearly demonstrated the potential of CTCs to effectively monitor evolving mutational landscape reflecting time-varying changes in drug susceptibility. Since then, several prospectively conducted studies have been carried out to facilitate the phenotyping and genetic characterization of CTCs as targeted-therapeutic intervention in metastatic cancer [127].

Longitudinal genomic data on SNVs and CNVs have so far been obtained in scCTC studies where CTCs were collected in a sequential manner during the course of treatment in lung [42,43] and prostate cancer [17]. A unique set of somatic CNV variations distinct from those observed in response to standard chemotherapy, was identified in single prostate CTCs at the time of targeted therapy failure, inferring rapidly evolving genomic organization and the emergent putative-resistant clones [27]. In another study where single-cell characterization was done before and during treatment for a breast cancer patient, while CTCs revealed distinct mutational profiles at different time points, all CTCs harbored mutation in the HER2 gene (p.V777L), regardless of sampling time, indicating resistance to HER2-targeted treatment in this patient. Interestingly, the best treatment response to chemotherapy with capecitabine and vinerolbine was observed in a patient who had the highest number of mutated genes and sequence variants in single breast CTCs [31].

Not all longitudinal studies, however, have demonstrated a clear association between CTCs and metastatic status. PIK3CA mutational status in majority of breast CTCs (7 out of 9 blood draws) sequentially sampled over time was not reflective of bone and lung metastases while DTCs achieved 100% concordance in a patient with progressive metastatic breast cancer [28]. Such highly discordant results, however, may be attributed to EpCAM-based approach employed in this study for CTC enrichment, missing out de-differentiated EpCAM$^-$ or mesenchymally shifted CTCs, all of which may be major constituents of putative metastatic founders [4].

5. Challenges and Emerging Technologies

Clearly, recent CTC studies have uncovered new perspectives in tumor biology and cancer management, through the application of rare cell sorting and single-cell sequencing technologies. Practically, however, there are challenges and technical errors associated with the developed workflows presented in this work.

5.1. Fresh-Frozen Versus Formalin-Fixed

Immunoaffinity-based enrichment technologies, including CellSearch®, involve a fixation step, which makes use of fixatives to stabilize whole blood for up to 96 h. Yet, fixed CTCs may be not suitable for RNA-based measurements, ex vivo culture and expansion, drug screening, and xenograft model-based functional studies, for compromised cell viability and degraded RNAs. Alternatively, multiparametric flow cytometry or FACS can be used to keep viable CTCs, which can further be expanded ex vivo to generate patient-derived 3D-spheroids, as demonstrated in prostate and breast cancers [17,34]. DEPArray^{TM} and microfluidic technologies can also be used to isolate viable CTCs for subsequent molecular screening on a cell-per-cell basis.

To preserve cell viability, peripheral blood sample should be delivered on ice immediately to the laboratory once collected from a cancer patient. RNA degradation occurs within 2–4 h, and sample processing >5 h after the blood draw may result in >60% loss in CTC yield [128]. Similar to tissue acquisition of solid lesions, these requirements impose practical challenges in hospitals and labs, particularly for longitudinal cohort studies. Nevertheless, emerging technologies may be applied to CTCs to circumvent such issues, through the use of nuclear RNA or preservation protocol that retains cell viability and RNA quality for up to 72 h for single-cell transcriptomic profiling. Studies have demonstrated high concordance between nuclear RNA and whole cell RNA in the expression of cell-type specific and metabolic modeling genes [129], and that between fresh and preserved blood in detecting cancer-specific transcripts [128]. Alternatively, frozen-optimized scRNA-seq protocols (e.g., Nuc-seq) may be applied to CTC profiling, which will be particularly useful for serial monitoring of previously inaccessible tissues [2].

5.2. Increasing Number of CTC Libraries

Among all the steps, WGA was found to be the most error-prone step in performing scCTC sequencing, with allele dropout (ADO) being a significant source of failure for scCTC sequencing [53]. Such prevalent limitations may be overcome if the amount of DNA template is increased. For example, it has been suggested that at least 10 CTCs are required to reliably detect point mutations in KRAS from pancreatic CTCs [53]. Similarly, sequencing multiple independent libraries of CTCs has been proposed to improve sensitivity in determining variants and to better represent bulk library from a matched primary tumor in prostate cancer [24]. The development of WGA methods providing improved uniformity in genome-wide coverage of the amplified DNA may further facilitate reproducible and accurate sequencing for clinical use.

Alternatively, highly sensitive CTC enrichment technologies may be applied to scCTC sequencing studies to capture, assumedly, all CTCs present in blood so as to generate more DNA templates. Recently, methods of performing single-cell CNV analysis of CTCs acquired by apheresis was described in prostate and breast cancers [17], where CTCs harvested from an apheresis (mean volume = 59.5 mL) achieved approximately 90-fold increased yield (CTC count = 12,546) [17]. Extrapolation analysis further indicated that CTCs might be concentrated along with the mononuclear cell populations during diagnostic leukapheresis (DLA), thereby enhancing CTC detection frequency even in nonmetastatic cancer patients, as compared to standard CTC blood tests processing a volume of 1–10 mL of peripheral blood [32].

In recent years, scRNA-seq technologies coupled with massively parallel microfluidics have enabled high-throughput analysis of mouse retinal cells [130], human macrophages [131], embryonic stem cells [132], and peripheral blood mononuclear cells (PBMCs) [133]. Their application to CTCs, however, has been relatively limited due to the inefficiency of bead-cell pairing and the inevitable contamination of blood cells even in primarily enriched samples [134]. To overcome these limitations, Cheng et al. have recently developed Hydro-seq, which enable high-throughput contamination-free scRNA-seq of CTCs from breast cancer patients, uncovering cellular heterogeneity in metastasis and therapy related genes [134]. Having the scale-up capability while achieving high cell-capture efficiency and high-fidelity single-cell sequencing results, these technologies will play an increasingly important role in future studies aiming to generate more accurate and reproducible data at high throughput with low cost.

5.3. Multidimensional Measurements

While others have attributed the appearance of CK^+CD45^+ cells to false-positive CK^+ staining of WBCs [32], such "double-positive" cells may have functional roles or clinical implication within circulation given their occurrence at a much lower frequency in healthy blood samples [135]. Similarly, the exact role of apoptotic CTCs (e.g., CK^+CD45^- cells with abnormal chromosomal patterns and/or nuclear fragmentation), $PD-L1^+CD45^-$ cells, and CK^-CD45^- cells in metastasis is not yet fully clear. Technologies enabling joint profiling of multiple modalities from the same individual cell may provide accurate means to understand clinical implication on the occurrence of these specific CTC subpopulations in circulation.

The high definition-CTC (HD-CTC) is an exemplary technology that facilitates real-time single-cell characterization of morphometric (i.e., cell roundness, cell area, AR subcellular localization) and protein expression changes in AR for prostate cancer [27]. Similarly, the functional EPISPOT assay, which is now named EPIDROP, allows simultaneous single-cell analysis of proteome and secretome of viable CTCs or of CTC clusters [136]. Such functional assays or microfluidic technologies, which have been successfully applied to patient-derived CTCs for analysis of genome [44], transcriptome [4], proteome [137], metabolome [138], and secretome [139] at the single-cell level, may further be integrated into the framework for deriving multidimensional data. Along with the increasingly available genomic data derived from tissue biopsies spanning diverse cancer types [140,141], the combined analysis of tissue and liquid biopsies may further uncover new insights into tumor heterogeneity and provide additional clinical information, as recently shown in lung cancer [4].

6. Conclusions

Recent scCTC studies have focused on how best to (1) identify and isolate extremely heterogeneous, fragile, and rare CTCs in a highly specific and unbiased manner, (2) discriminate false negatives and detect actionable mutations, and (3) relate the findings to clinically meaningful outcomes that could not have been caught by a tissue biopsy. Emerging data pointing towards the prevalence of CTC subpopulations and their differing metastatic potential have further stimulated studies aiming to identify and genetically/phenotypically characterize such premetastatic subsets of CTC populations that are favored to be liberated from primary tumors, survive in the bloodstream, and succeed in the early colonization phases.

While past efforts in deconvoluting the complex nature of CTCs have been largely ineffective with bulk-cell analysis, single-cell approaches are beginning to unmask cellular heterogeneity of CTCs and their clinical significance, providing a foundation for liquid biopsy in the clinic. As we continue to develop sensitive CTC enrichment technologies and generate more sequencing data from patient-derived CTCs, clinicians will continue to find a better way to apply liquid biopsies, possibly (1) at initial diagnosis, for prognostication, (2) after tumor resection, for assessment of residual disease, and (3) after adjuvant therapies, for prediction of early recurrence or relapse. With mounting molecular evidence suggesting prognostic value of CTC-derived biomarkers predictive of response to chemotherapy, targeted therapy, and immune checkpoint inhibitors, we anticipate that, in the near future, liquid biopsies will become a routine screening and monitoring of cancer patients.

Author Contributions: Conceptualization, S.B.L., C.T.L., and W.-T.L.; writing—original draft preparation, S.B.L.; writing—review and editing, S.B.L., C.T.L., and W.-T.L.; visualization, S.B.L.; supervision, C.T.L. and W.-T.L.; project administration, W.-T.L.; funding acquisition, W.-T.L.

Funding: This research was funded by the National Medical Research Council (NMRC), NMRC/CSA/040/2012 and NMRC/CSA-INV/0025/2017.

Acknowledgments: This work was carried out at the MechanoBioengineering Laboratory at the Department of Biomedical Engineering, National University of Singapore (NUS). The authors thank support provided by the Institute for Health Innovation and Technology (iHealthtech) at NUS. S.B.L. acknowledges support provided by NUS Graduate School for Integrative Sciences and Engineering (NGS), Mogam Science Scholarship Foundation, and Daewoong Foundation.

Conflicts of Interest: C.T.L. serves as an advisor of Biolidics. C.T.L. and W.-T.L. are shareholders of Biolidics. The remaining author declares no competing interest.

References

1. Fidler, I.J.; Hart, I.R. Biological diversity in metastatic neoplasms: Origins and implications. *Science* **1982**, *217*, 998–1003. [CrossRef] [PubMed]
2. Tirosh, I.; Suvà, M.L. Deciphering Human Tumor Biology by Single-Cell Expression Profiling. *Annu. Rev. Cancer Biol.* **2019**, *3*, 151–166. [CrossRef]
3. Shi, X.; Chakraborty, P.; Chaudhuri, A. Unmasking tumor heterogeneity and clonal evolution by single-cell analysis. *J. Cancer Metastasis Treat.* **2018**, *4*, 47. [CrossRef]
4. Lim, S.B.; Yeo, T.; Lee, W.D.; Bhagat, A.A.S.; Tan, S.J.; Tan, D.S.W.; Lim, W.T.; Lim, C.T. Addressing cellular heterogeneity in tumor and circulation for refined prognostication. *Proc. Natl. Acad. Sci. USA* **2019**, *116*, 17957–17962. [CrossRef]

5. Lim, S.B.; Tan, S.J.; Lim, W.T.; Lim, C.T. An extracellular matrix-related prognostic and predictive indicator for early-stage non-small cell lung cancer. *Nat. Commun.* 2017, *8*, 1734. [CrossRef]
6. Lim, S.B.; Lim, C.T.; Lim, D.W.-T. MO2-6-3Matrisomal abnormality: A predictive biomarker for cancer immunotherapy. *Ann. Oncol.* 2019, *30*. [CrossRef]
7. Lim, S.B.; Chua, M.L.K.; Yeong, J.P.S.; Tan, S.J.; Lim, W.-T.; Lim, C.T. Pan-cancer analysis connects tumor matrisome to immune response. *NPJ Precis. Oncol.* 2019, *3*, 15. [CrossRef]
8. Francart, M.E.; Lambert, J.; Vanwynsberghe, A.M.; Thompson, E.W.; Bourcy, M.; Polette, M.; Gilles, C. Epithelial-mesenchymal plasticity and circulating tumor cells: Travel companions to metastases. *Dev. Dyn.* 2018, *247*, 432–450. [CrossRef]
9. Menon, N.V.; Lim, S.B.; Lim, C.T. Microfluidics for personalized drug screening of cancer. *Curr. Opin. Pharmacol.* 2019, *48*, 155–161. [CrossRef]
10. Koh, Y.; Yagi, S.; Akamatsu, H.; Kanai, K.; Hayata, A.; Tokudome, N.; Akamatsu, K.; Higuchi, M.; Kanbara, H.; Nakanishi, M.; et al. Heterogeneous Expression of Programmed Death Receptor-ligand 1 on Circulating Tumor Cells in Patients with Lung Cancer. *Clin. Lung Cancer* 2019, *20*, 270–277.e271. [CrossRef]
11. Grillet, F.; Bayet, E.; Villeronce, O.; Zappia, L.; Lagerqvist, E.L.; Lunke, S.; Charafe-Jauffret, E.; Pham, K.; Molck, C.; Rolland, N.; et al. Circulating tumour cells from patients with colorectal cancer have cancer stem cell hallmarks in ex vivo culture. *Gut* 2017, *66*, 1802. [CrossRef] [PubMed]
12. Jordan, N.V.; Bardia, A.; Wittner, B.S.; Benes, C.; Ligorio, M.; Zheng, Y.; Yu, M.; Sundaresan, T.K.; Licausi, J.A.; Desai, R.; et al. HER2 expression identifies dynamic functional states within circulating breast cancer cells. *Nature* 2016, *537*, 102–106. [CrossRef] [PubMed]
13. Agnoletto, C.; Corra, F.; Minotti, L.; Baldassari, F.; Crudele, F.; Cook, W.J.J.; Di Leva, G.; d'Adamo, A.P.; Gasparini, P.; Volinia, S. Heterogeneity in Circulating Tumor Cells: The Relevance of the Stem-Cell Subset. *Cancers* 2019, *11*, 483. [CrossRef] [PubMed]
14. Lim, S.B.; Di Lee, W.; Vasudevan, J.; Lim, W.-T.; Lim, C.T. Liquid biopsy: One cell at a time. *NPJ Precis. Oncol.* 2019, *3*, 23. [CrossRef]
15. Racila, E.; Euhus, D.; Weiss, A.J.; Rao, C.; McConnell, J.; Terstappen, L.W.M.M.; Uhr, J.W. Detection and characterization of carcinoma cells in the blood. *Proc. Natl. Acad. Sci. USA* 1998, *95*, 4589. [CrossRef]
16. Heitzer, E.; Auer, M.; Gasch, C.; Pichler, M.; Ulz, P.; Hoffmann, E.M.; Lax, S.; Waldispuehl-Geigl, J.; Mauermann, O.; Lackner, C.; et al. Complex tumor genomes inferred from single circulating tumor cells by array-CGH and next-generation sequencing. *Cancer Res.* 2013, *73*, 2965–2975. [CrossRef]
17. Lambros, M.B.; Seed, G.; Sumanasuriya, S.; Gil, V.; Crespo, M.; Fontes, M.; Chandler, R.; Mehra, N.; Fowler, G.; Ebbs, B.; et al. Single-Cell Analyses of Prostate Cancer Liquid Biopsies Acquired by Apheresis. *Clin. Cancer Res.* 2018, *24*, 5635–5644. [CrossRef]
18. Pestrin, M.; Salvianti, F.; Galardi, F.; De Luca, F.; Turner, N.; Malorni, L.; Pazzagli, M.; Di Leo, A.; Pinzani, P. Heterogeneity of PIK3CA mutational status at the single cell level in circulating tumor cells from metastatic breast cancer patients. *Mol. Oncol.* 2015, *9*, 749–757. [CrossRef]
19. Wang, Y.; Guo, L.; Feng, L.; Zhang, W.; Xiao, T.; Di, X.; Chen, G.; Zhang, K. Single nucleotide variant profiles of viable single circulating tumour cells reveal CTC behaviours in breast cancer. *Oncol. Rep.* 2018, *39*, 2147–2159. [CrossRef]
20. Yin, J.; Wang, Z.; Li, G.; Lin, F.; Shao, K.; Cao, B.; Hou, Y. Characterization of circulating tumor cells in breast cancer patients by spiral microfluidics. *Cell Biol. Toxicol.* 2019, *35*, 59–66. [CrossRef]
21. Lohr, J.G.; Kim, S.; Gould, J.; Knoechel, B.; Drier, Y.; Cotton, M.J.; Gray, D.; Birrer, N.; Wong, B.; Ha, G.; et al. Genetic interrogation of circulating multiple myeloma cells at single-cell resolution. *Sci. Transl. Med.* 2016, *8*, 363ra147. [CrossRef] [PubMed]
22. Park, S.M.; Wong, D.J.; Ooi, C.C.; Kurtz, D.M.; Vermesh, O.; Aalipour, A.; Suh, S.; Pian, K.L.; Chabon, J.J.; Lee, S.H.; et al. Molecular profiling of single circulating tumor cells from lung cancer patients. *Proc. Natl. Acad. Sci. USA* 2016, *113*, E8379–E8386. [CrossRef] [PubMed]
23. Kanwar, N.; Hu, P.; Bedard, P.; Clemons, M.; McCready, D.; Done, S.J. Identification of genomic signatures in circulating tumor cells from breast cancer. *Int. J. Cancer* 2015, *137*, 332–344. [CrossRef] [PubMed]
24. Lohr, J.G.; Adalsteinsson, V.A.; Cibulskis, K.; Choudhury, A.D.; Rosenberg, M.; Cruz-Gordillo, P.; Francis, J.M.; Zhang, C.-Z.; Shalek, A.K.; Satija, R.; et al. Whole-exome sequencing of circulating tumor cells provides a window into metastatic prostate cancer. *Nat. Biotechnol.* 2014, *32*, 479–484. [CrossRef]

25. Greene, S.B.; Dago, A.E.; Leitz, L.J.; Wang, Y.; Lee, J.; Werner, S.L.; Gendreau, S.; Patel, P.; Jia, S.; Zhang, L.; et al. Chromosomal Instability Estimation Based on Next Generation Sequencing and Single Cell Genome Wide Copy Number Variation Analysis. *PLoS ONE* **2016**, *11*, e0165089. [CrossRef] [PubMed]
26. Jiang, R.; Lu, Y.-T.; Ho, H.; Li, B.; Chen, J.-F.; Lin, M.; Li, F.; Wu, K.; Wu, H.; Lichterman, J.; et al. A comparison of isolated circulating tumor cells and tissue biopsies using whole-genome sequencing in prostate cancer. *Oncotarget* **2015**, *6*, 44781–44793. [CrossRef]
27. Dago, A.E.; Stepansky, A.; Carlsson, A.; Luttgen, M.; Kendall, J.; Baslan, T.; Kolatkar, A.; Wigler, M.; Bethel, K.; Gross, M.E.; et al. Rapid phenotypic and genomic change in response to therapeutic pressure in prostate cancer inferred by high content analysis of single circulating tumor cells. *PLoS ONE* **2014**, *9*, e101777. [CrossRef]
28. Deng, G.; Krishnakumar, S.; Powell, A.A.; Zhang, H.; Mindrinos, M.N.; Telli, M.L.; Davis, R.W.; Jeffrey, S.S. Single cell mutational analysis of PIK3CA in circulating tumor cells and metastases in breast cancer reveals heterogeneity, discordance, and mutation persistence in cultured disseminated tumor cells from bone marrow. *BMC Cancer* **2014**, *14*, 456. [CrossRef]
29. Fernandez, S.V.; Bingham, C.; Fittipaldi, P.; Austin, L.; Palazzo, J.; Palmer, G.; Alpaugh, K.; Cristofanilli, M. TP53 mutations detected in circulating tumor cells present in the blood of metastatic triple negative breast cancer patients. *Breast Cancer Res.* **2014**, *16*, 445. [CrossRef]
30. Polzer, B.; Medoro, G.; Pasch, S.; Fontana, F.; Zorzino, L.; Pestka, A.; Andergassen, U.; Meier-Stiegen, F.; Czyz, Z.T.; Alberter, B.; et al. Molecular profiling of single circulating tumor cells with diagnostic intention. *EMBO Mol. Med.* **2014**, *6*, 1371–1386. [CrossRef]
31. De Luca, F.; Rotunno, G.; Salvianti, F.; Galardi, F.; Pestrin, M.; Gabellini, S.; Simi, L.; Mancini, I.; Vannucchi, A.M.; Pazzagli, M.; et al. Mutational analysis of single circulating tumor cells by next generation sequencing in metastatic breast cancer. *Oncotarget* **2016**, *7*, 26107–26119. [CrossRef] [PubMed]
32. Fischer, J.C.; Niederacher, D.; Topp, S.A.; Honisch, E.; Schumacher, S.; Schmitz, N.; Zacarias Fohrding, L.; Vay, C.; Hoffmann, I.; Kasprowicz, N.S.; et al. Diagnostic leukapheresis enables reliable detection of circulating tumor cells of nonmetastatic cancer patients. *Proc. Natl. Acad. Sci. USA* **2013**, *110*, 16580–16585. [CrossRef] [PubMed]
33. Neves, R.P.; Raba, K.; Schmidt, O.; Honisch, E.; Meier-Stiegen, F.; Behrens, B.; Mohlendick, B.; Fehm, T.; Neubauer, H.; Klein, C.A.; et al. Genomic high-resolution profiling of single CKpos/CD45neg flow-sorting purified circulating tumor cells from patients with metastatic breast cancer. *Clin. Chem.* **2014**, *60*, 1290–1297. [CrossRef] [PubMed]
34. Vishnoi, M.; Peddibhotla, S.; Yin, W.; Scamardo, A.T.; George, G.C.; Hong, D.S.; Marchetti, D. The isolation and characterization of CTC subsets related to breast cancer dormancy. *Sci. Rep.* **2015**, *5*, 17533. [CrossRef] [PubMed]
35. Gasch, C.; Oldopp, T.; Mauermann, O.; Gorges, T.M.; Andreas, A.; Coith, C.; Muller, V.; Fehm, T.; Janni, W.; Pantel, K.; et al. Frequent detection of PIK3CA mutations in single circulating tumor cells of patients suffering from HER2-negative metastatic breast cancer. *Mol. Oncol.* **2016**, *10*, 1330–1343. [CrossRef] [PubMed]
36. Shaw, J.A.; Guttery, D.S.; Hills, A.; Fernandez-Garcia, D.; Page, K.; Rosales, B.M.; Goddard, K.S.; Hastings, R.K.; Luo, J.; Ogle, O.; et al. Mutation Analysis of Cell-Free DNA and Single Circulating Tumor Cells in Metastatic Breast Cancer Patients with High Circulating Tumor Cell Counts. *Clin. Cancer Res.* **2017**, *23*, 88–96. [CrossRef] [PubMed]
37. Neumann, M.H.D.; Schneck, H.; Decker, Y.; Schömer, S.; Franken, A.; Endris, V.; Pfarr, N.; Weichert, W.; Niederacher, D.; Fehm, T.; et al. Isolation and characterization of circulating tumor cells using a novel workflow combining the CellSearch®system and the CellCelector™. *Biotechnol. Prog.* **2017**, *33*, 125–132. [CrossRef]
38. Bingham, C.; Fernandez, S.V.; Fittipaldi, P.; Dempsey, P.W.; Ruth, K.J.; Cristofanilli, M.; Katherine Alpaugh, R. Mutational studies on single circulating tumor cells isolated from the blood of inflammatory breast cancer patients. *Breast Cancer Res. Treat.* **2017**, *163*, 219–230. [CrossRef]
39. Babayan, A.; Hannemann, J.; Spotter, J.; Muller, V.; Pantel, K.; Joosse, S.A. Heterogeneity of estrogen receptor expression in circulating tumor cells from metastatic breast cancer patients. *PLoS ONE* **2013**, *8*, e75038. [CrossRef]

40. Heidary, M.; Auer, M.; Ulz, P.; Heitzer, E.; Petru, E.; Gasch, C.; Riethdorf, S.; Mauermann, O.; Lafer, I.; Pristauz, G.; et al. The dynamic range of circulating tumor DNA in metastatic breast cancer. *Breast Cancer Res.* **2014**, *16*, 421. [CrossRef]
41. Mu, Z.; Benali-Furet, N.; Uzan, G.; Znaty, A.; Ye, Z.; Paolillo, C.; Wang, C.; Austin, L.; Rossi, G.; Fortina, P.; et al. Detection and Characterization of Circulating Tumor Associated Cells in Metastatic Breast Cancer. *Int. J. Mol. Sci.* **2016**, *17*, 1665. [CrossRef] [PubMed]
42. Carter, L.; Rothwell, D.G.; Mesquita, B.; Smowton, C.; Leong, H.S.; Fernandez-Gutierrez, F.; Li, Y.; Burt, D.J.; Antonello, J.; Morrow, C.J.; et al. Molecular analysis of circulating tumor cells identifies distinct copy-number profiles in patients with chemosensitive and chemorefractory small-cell lung cancer. *Nat. Med.* **2017**, *23*, 114–119. [CrossRef] [PubMed]
43. Ni, X.; Zhuo, M.; Su, Z.; Duan, J.; Gao, Y.; Wang, Z.; Zong, C.; Bai, H.; Chapman, A.R.; Zhao, J.; et al. Reproducible copy number variation patterns among single circulating tumor cells of lung cancer patients. *Proc. Natl. Acad. Sci. USA* **2013**, *110*, 21083–21088. [CrossRef] [PubMed]
44. Yeo, T.; Tan, S.J.; Lim, C.L.; Lau, D.P.; Chua, Y.W.; Krisna, S.S.; Iyer, G.; Tan, G.S.; Lim, T.K.; Tan, D.S.; et al. Microfluidic enrichment for the single cell analysis of circulating tumor cells. *Sci. Rep.* **2016**, *6*, 22076. [CrossRef]
45. Gao, Y.; Ni, X.; Guo, H.; Su, Z.; Ba, Y.; Tong, Z.; Guo, Z.; Yao, X.; Chen, X.; Yin, J.; et al. Single-cell sequencing deciphers a convergent evolution of copy number alterations from primary to circulating tumor cells. *Genome Res.* **2017**, *27*, 1312–1322. [CrossRef]
46. Su, Z.; Wang, Z.; Ni, X.; Duan, J.; Gao, Y.; Zhuo, M.; Li, R.; Zhao, J.; Ma, Q.; Bai, H.; et al. Inferring the Evolution and Progression of Small-Cell Lung Cancer by Single-Cell Sequencing of Circulating Tumor Cells. *Clin. Cancer Res.* **2019**, *25*, 5049–5060. [CrossRef]
47. Steinert, G.; Schölch, S.; Niemietz, T.; Iwata, N.; García, S.A.; Behrens, B.; Voigt, A.; Kloor, M.; Benner, A.; Bork, U.; et al. Immune Escape and Survival Mechanisms in Circulating Tumor Cells of Colorectal Cancer. *Cancer Res.* **2014**, *74*, 1694–1704. [CrossRef]
48. Gasch, C.; Bauernhofer, T.; Pichler, M.; Langer-Freitag, S.; Reeh, M.; Seifert, A.M.; Mauermann, O.; Izbicki, J.R.; Pantel, K.; Riethdorf, S. Heterogeneity of epidermal growth factor receptor status and mutations of KRAS/PIK3CA in circulating tumor cells of patients with colorectal cancer. *Clin. Chem.* **2013**, *59*, 252–260. [CrossRef]
49. Fabbri, F.; Carloni, S.; Zoli, W.; Ulivi, P.; Gallerani, G.; Fici, P.; Chiadini, E.; Passardi, A.; Frassineti, G.L.; Ragazzini, A.; et al. Detection and recovery of circulating colon cancer cells using a dielectrophoresis-based device: KRAS mutation status in pure CTCs. *Cancer Lett.* **2013**, *335*, 225–231. [CrossRef]
50. Sakaizawa, K.; Goto, Y.; Kiniwa, Y.; Uchiyama, A.; Harada, K.; Shimada, S.; Saida, T.; Ferrone, S.; Takata, M.; Uhara, H.; et al. Mutation analysis of BRAF and KIT in circulating melanoma cells at the single cell level. *Br. J. Cancer* **2012**, *106*, 939–946. [CrossRef]
51. Kiniwa, Y.; Nakamura, K.; Mikoshiba, A.; Akiyama, Y.; Morimoto, A.; Okuyama, R. Diversity of circulating tumor cells in peripheral blood: Detection of heterogeneous BRAF mutations in a patient with advanced melanoma by single-cell analysis. *J. Derm. Sci.* **2018**, *90*, 211–213. [CrossRef] [PubMed]
52. Anantharaman, A.; Friedlander, T.; Lu, D.; Krupa, R.; Premasekharan, G.; Hough, J.; Edwards, M.; Paz, R.; Lindquist, K.; Graf, R.; et al. Programmed death-ligand 1 (PD-L1) characterization of circulating tumor cells (CTCs) in muscle invasive and metastatic bladder cancer patients. *BMC Cancer* **2016**, *16*, 744. [CrossRef] [PubMed]
53. Court, C.M.; Ankeny, J.S.; Sho, S.; Hou, S.; Li, Q.; Hsieh, C.; Song, M.; Liao, X.; Rochefort, M.M.; Wainberg, Z.A.; et al. Reality of Single Circulating Tumor Cell Sequencing for Molecular Diagnostics in Pancreatic Cancer. *J. Mol. Diagn.* **2016**, *18*, 688–696. [CrossRef] [PubMed]
54. Pantel, K.; Deneve, E.; Nocca, D.; Coffy, A.; Vendrell, J.P.; Maudelonde, T.; Riethdorf, S.; Alix-Panabieres, C. Circulating epithelial cells in patients with benign colon diseases. *Clin. Chem.* **2012**, *58*, 936–940. [CrossRef]
55. Zhang, L.; Ridgway, L.D.; Wetzel, M.D.; Ngo, J.; Yin, W.; Kumar, D.; Goodman, J.C.; Groves, M.D.; Marchetti, D. The identification and characterization of breast cancer CTCs competent for brain metastasis. *Sci. Transl. Med.* **2013**, *5*, 180ra148. [CrossRef]
56. Lee, Y.; Guan, G.; Bhagat, A.A. ClearCell®FX, a label-free microfluidics technology for enrichment of viable circulating tumor cells. *Cytom. Part. A* **2018**, *93*, 1251–1254. [CrossRef]

57. Ligthart, S.T.; Coumans, F.A.; Bidard, F.C.; Simkens, L.H.; Punt, C.J.; de Groot, M.R.; Attard, G.; de Bono, J.S.; Pierga, J.Y.; Terstappen, L.W. Circulating Tumor Cells Count and Morphological Features in Breast, Colorectal and Prostate Cancer. *PLoS ONE* **2013**, *8*, e67148. [CrossRef]
58. Kallergi, G.; Konstantinidis, G.; Markomanolaki, H.; Papadaki, M.A.; Mavroudis, D.; Stournaras, C.; Georgoulias, V.; Agelaki, S. Apoptotic circulating tumor cells in early and metastatic breast cancer patients. *Mol. Cancer Ther.* **2013**, *12*, 1886–1895. [CrossRef]
59. Blainey, P.C. The future is now: Single-cell genomics of bacteria and archaea. *FEMS Microbiol. Rev.* **2013**, *37*, 407–427. [CrossRef]
60. Salvianti, F.; Pazzagli, M.; Pinzani, P. Single circulating tumor cell sequencing as an advanced tool in cancer management. *Expert Rev. Mol. Diagn.* **2016**, *16*, 51–63. [CrossRef]
61. Swennenhuis, J.F.; Reumers, J.; Thys, K.; Aerssens, J.; Terstappen, L.W. Efficiency of whole genome amplification of single circulating tumor cells enriched by CellSearch and sorted by FACS. *Genome Med.* **2013**, *5*, 106. [CrossRef] [PubMed]
62. Gawad, C.; Koh, W.; Quake, S.R. Single-cell genome sequencing: Current state of the science. *Nat. Rev. Genet.* **2016**, *17*, 175–188. [CrossRef] [PubMed]
63. Pao, W.; Girard, N. New driver mutations in non-small-cell lung cancer. *Lancet Oncol.* **2011**, *12*, 175–180. [CrossRef]
64. Stephens, P.J.; Tarpey, P.S.; Davies, H.; Van Loo, P.; Greenman, C.; Wedge, D.C.; Nik-Zainal, S.; Martin, S.; Varela, I.; Bignell, G.R.; et al. The landscape of cancer genes and mutational processes in breast cancer. *Nature* **2012**, *486*, 400–404. [CrossRef] [PubMed]
65. Jhawer, M.; Goel, S.; Wilson, A.J.; Montagna, C.; Ling, Y.H.; Byun, D.S.; Nasser, S.; Arango, D.; Shin, J.; Klampfer, L.; et al. PIK3CA mutation/PTEN expression status predicts response of colon cancer cells to the epidermal growth factor receptor inhibitor cetuximab. *Cancer Res.* **2008**, *68*, 1953–1961. [CrossRef] [PubMed]
66. Berns, K.; Horlings, H.M.; Hennessy, B.T.; Madiredjo, M.; Hijmans, E.M.; Beelen, K.; Linn, S.C.; Gonzalez-Angulo, A.M.; Stemke-Hale, K.; Hauptmann, M.; et al. A Functional Genetic Approach Identifies the PI3K Pathway as a Major Determinant of Trastuzumab Resistance in Breast Cancer. *Cancer Cell* **2007**, *12*, 395–402. [CrossRef] [PubMed]
67. Chandarlapaty, S.; Sakr, R.A.; Giri, D.; Patil, S.; Heguy, A.; Morrow, M.; Modi, S.; Norton, L.; Rosen, N.; Hudis, C.; et al. Frequent mutational activation of the PI3K-AKT pathway in trastuzumab-resistant breast cancer. *Clin. Cancer Res.* **2012**, *18*, 6784–6791. [CrossRef]
68. Mukohara, T. Mechanisms of resistance to anti-human epidermal growth factor receptor 2 agents in breast cancer. *Cancer Sci.* **2011**, *102*, 1–8. [CrossRef]
69. Ibrahim, E.M.; Kazkaz, G.A.; Al-Mansour, M.M.; Al-Foheidi, M.E. The predictive and prognostic role of phosphatase phosphoinositol-3 (PI3) kinase (PIK3CA) mutation in HER2-positive breast cancer receiving HER2-targeted therapy: A meta-analysis. *Breast Cancer Res. Treat.* **2015**, *152*, 463–476. [CrossRef]
70. Loibl, S.; von Minckwitz, G.; Schneeweiss, A.; Paepke, S.; Lehmann, A.; Rezai, M.; Zahm, D.M.; Sinn, P.; Khandan, F.; Eidtmann, H.; et al. PIK3CA mutations are associated with lower rates of pathologic complete response to anti-human epidermal growth factor receptor 2 (her2) therapy in primary HER2-overexpressing breast cancer. *J. Clin. Oncol.* **2014**, *32*, 3212–3220. [CrossRef]
71. Neumann, M.; Decker, Y.; Franken, A.; Schömer, S.; Schneck, H.; Fehm, T.; Weichert, W.; Endriss, V.; Neubauer, H.; Niederacher, D. Sequential analysis of circulating tumor cells on genome and protein level: Potential regulation of the invasion marker CapG by PIK3CA. *Senologie Zeitschrift für Mammadiagnostik und Herapie* **2016**, *13*, A95. [CrossRef]
72. Janku, F.; Wheler, J.J.; Westin, S.N.; Moulder, S.L.; Naing, A.; Tsimberidou, A.M.; Fu, S.; Falchook, G.S.; Hong, D.S.; Garrido-Laguna, I.; et al. PI3K/AKT/mTOR inhibitors in patients with breast and gynecologic malignancies harboring PIK3CA mutations. *J. Clin. Oncol.* **2012**, *30*, 777–782. [CrossRef] [PubMed]
73. Olivier, M.; Eeles, R.; Hollstein, M.; Khan, M.A.; Harris, C.C.; Hainaut, P. The IARC TP53 database: New online mutation analysis and recommendations to users. *Hum. Mutat.* **2002**, *19*, 607–614. [CrossRef] [PubMed]
74. Kim, T.; Veronese, A.; Pichiorri, F.; Lee, T.J.; Jeon, Y.-J.; Volinia, S.; Pineau, P.; Marchio, A.; Palatini, J.; Suh, S.-S.; et al. p53 regulates epithelial–mesenchymal transition through microRNAs targeting ZEB1 and ZEB2. *J. Exp. Med.* **2011**, *208*, 875. [CrossRef]

75. Chang, C.-J.; Chao, C.-H.; Xia, W.; Yang, J.-Y.; Xiong, Y.; Li, C.-W.; Yu, W.-H.; Rehman, S.K.; Hsu, J.L.; Lee, H.-H.; et al. p53 regulates epithelial-mesenchymal transition and stem cell properties through modulating miRNAs. *Nat. Cell Biol.* **2011**, *13*, 317–323. [CrossRef]
76. Petitjean, A.; Achatz, M.I.; Borresen-Dale, A.L.; Hainaut, P.; Olivier, M. TP53 mutations in human cancers: Functional selection and impact on cancer prognosis and outcomes. *Oncogene* **2007**, *26*, 2157–2165. [CrossRef]
77. Li, J.; Yang, L.; Gaur, S.; Zhang, K.; Wu, X.; Yuan, Y.-C.; Li, H.; Hu, S.; Weng, Y.; Yen, Y. Mutants TP53 p.R273H and p.R273C but not p.R273G Enhance Cancer Cell Malignancy. *Hum. Mutat.* **2014**, *35*, 575–584. [CrossRef]
78. Kalemkerian, G.P. Chemotherapy for small-cell lung cancer. *Lancet Oncol.* **2014**, *15*, 13–14. [CrossRef]
79. Sutherland, K.D.; Proost, N.; Brouns, I.; Adriaensen, D.; Song, J.Y.; Berns, A. Cell of origin of small cell lung cancer: Inactivation of Trp53 and Rb1 in distinct cell types of adult mouse lung. *Cancer Cell* **2011**, *19*, 754–764. [CrossRef]
80. Nicholson, R.I.; Gee, J.M.; Harper, M.E. EGFR and cancer prognosis. *Eur. J. Cancer* **2001**, *37* (Suppl. S4), S9–S15. [CrossRef]
81. Ciardiello, F.; Tortora, G. Epidermal growth factor receptor (EGFR) as a target in cancer therapy: Understanding the role of receptor expression and other molecular determinants that could influence the response to anti-EGFR drugs. *Eur. J. Cancer* **2003**, *39*, 1348–1354. [CrossRef]
82. Moroni, M.; Veronese, S.; Benvenuti, S.; Marrapese, G.; Sartore-Bianchi, A.; Di Nicolantonio, F.; Gambacorta, M.; Siena, S.; Bardelli, A. Gene copy number for epidermal growth factor receptor (EGFR) and clinical response to antiEGFR treatment in colorectal cancer: A cohort study. *Lancet Oncol.* **2005**, *6*, 279–286. [CrossRef]
83. Lièvre, A.; Bachet, J.-B.; Le Corre, D.; Boige, V.; Landi, B.; Emile, J.-F.; Côté, J.-F.; Tomasic, G.; Penna, C.; Ducreux, M.; et al. KRAS Mutation Status Is Predictive of Response to Cetuximab Therapy in Colorectal Cancer. *Cancer Res.* **2006**, *66*, 3992. [CrossRef]
84. Amado, R.G.; Wolf, M.; Peeters, M.; Van Cutsem, E.; Siena, S.; Freeman, D.J.; Juan, T.; Sikorski, R.; Suggs, S.; Radinsky, R.; et al. Wild-Type KRAS Is Required for Panitumumab Efficacy in Patients with Metastatic Colorectal Cancer. *J. Clin. Oncol.* **2008**, *26*, 1626–1634. [CrossRef]
85. Zhu, C.-Q.; da Cunha Santos, G.; Ding, K.; Sakurada, A.; Cutz, J.-C.; Liu, N.; Zhang, T.; Marrano, P.; Whitehead, M.; Squire, J.A.; et al. Role of KRAS and EGFR as Biomarkers of Response to Erlotinib in National Cancer Institute of Canada Clinical Trials Group Study BR.21. *J. Clin. Oncol.* **2008**, *26*, 4268–4275. [CrossRef]
86. Watanabe, T.; Kobunai, T.; Yamamoto, Y.; Matsuda, K.; Ishihara, S.; Nozawa, K.; Iinuma, H.; Shibuya, H.; Eshima, K. Heterogeneity of KRAS Status May Explain the Subset of Discordant KRAS Status Between Primary and Metastatic Colorectal Cancer. *Dis. Colon Rectum* **2011**, *54*, 1170–1178. [CrossRef]
87. Ducreux, M.; Chamseddine, A.; Laurent-Puig, P.; Smolenschi, C.; Hollebecque, A.; Dartigues, P.; Samallin, E.; Boige, V.; Malka, D.; Gelli, M. Molecular targeted therapy of BRAF-mutant colorectal cancer. *Ther. Adv. Med. Oncol.* **2019**, *11*. [CrossRef]
88. Marconcini, R.; Galli, L.; Antonuzzo, A.; Bursi, S.; Roncella, C.; Fontanini, G.; Sensi, E.; Falcone, A. Metastatic BRAF K601E-mutated melanoma reaches complete response to MEK inhibitor trametinib administered for over 36 months. *Exp. Hematol. Oncol.* **2017**, *6*, 6. [CrossRef]
89. Mostert, B.; Jiang, Y.; Sieuwerts, A.M.; Wang, H.; Bolt-de Vries, J.; Biermann, K.; Kraan, J.; Lalmahomed, Z.; van Galen, A.; de Weerd, V.; et al. KRAS and BRAF mutation status in circulating colorectal tumor cells and their correlation with primary and metastatic tumor tissue. *Int. J. Cancer* **2013**, *133*, 130–141. [CrossRef]
90. Wheeler, J.M.; Bodmer, W.F.; Mortensen, N.J. DNA mismatch repair genes and colorectal cancer. *Gut* **2000**, *47*, 148–153. [CrossRef]
91. Mackay, H.J.; Gallinger, S.; Tsao, M.S.; McLachlin, C.M.; Tu, D.; Keiser, K.; Eisenhauer, E.A.; Oza, A.M. Prognostic value of microsatellite instability (MSI) and PTEN expression in women with endometrial cancer: Results from studies of the NCIC Clinical Trials Group (NCIC CTG). *Eur. J. Cancer* **2010**, *46*, 1365–1373. [CrossRef] [PubMed]
92. Popat, S.; Hubner, R.; Houlston, R.S. Systematic Review of Microsatellite Instability and Colorectal Cancer Prognosis. *J. Clin. Oncol.* **2005**, *23*, 609–618. [CrossRef] [PubMed]
93. Thibodeau, S.N.; Bren, G.; Schaid, D. Microsatellite instability in cancer of the proximal colon. *Science* **1993**, *260*, 816–819. [CrossRef] [PubMed]

94. Kim, G.P.; Colangelo, L.H.; Wieand, H.S.; Paik, S.; Kirsch, I.R.; Wolmark, N.; Allegra, C.J.; National Cancer, I. Prognostic and predictive roles of high-degree microsatellite instability in colon cancer: A National Cancer Institute-National Surgical Adjuvant Breast and Bowel Project Collaborative Study. *J. Clin. Oncol.* **2007**, *25*, 767–772. [CrossRef] [PubMed]
95. Ribic, C.M.; Sargent, D.J.; Moore, M.J.; Thibodeau, S.N.; French, A.J.; Goldberg, R.M.; Hamilton, S.R.; Laurent-Puig, P.; Gryfe, R.; Shepherd, L.E.; et al. Tumor Microsatellite-Instability Status as a Predictor of Benefit from Fluorouracil-Based Adjuvant Chemotherapy for Colon Cancer. *N. Engl. J. Med.* **2003**, *349*, 247–257. [CrossRef]
96. Goldstein, J.; Tran, B.; Ensor, J.; Gibbs, P.; Wong, H.L.; Wong, S.F.; Vilar, E.; Tie, J.; Broaddus, R.; Kopetz, S.; et al. Multicenter retrospective analysis of metastatic colorectal cancer (CRC) with high-level microsatellite instability (MSI-H). *Ann. Oncol.* **2014**, *25*, 1032–1038. [CrossRef] [PubMed]
97. Findeisen, P.; Kloor, M.; Merx, S.; Sutter, C.; Woerner, S.M.; Dostmann, N.; Benner, A.; Dondog, B.; Pawlita, M.; Dippold, W.; et al. T25 repeat in the 3′ untranslated region of the CASP2 gene: A sensitive and specific marker for microsatellite instability in colorectal cancer. *Cancer Res.* **2005**, *65*, 8072–8078. [CrossRef]
98. Carethers, J.M.; Smith, E.J.; Behling, C.A.; Nguyen, L.; Tajima, A.; Doctolero, R.T.; Cabrera, B.L.; Goel, A.; Arnold, C.A.; Miyai, K.; et al. Use of 5-fluorouracil and survival in patients with microsatellite-unstable colorectal cancer. *Gastroenterology* **2004**, *126*, 394–401. [CrossRef]
99. Boland, C.R.; Thibodeau, S.N.; Hamilton, S.R.; Sidransky, D.; Eshleman, J.R.; Burt, R.W.; Meltzer, S.J.; Rodriguez-Bigas, M.A.; Fodde, R.; Ranzani, G.N.; et al. A National Cancer Institute Workshop on Microsatellite Instability for cancer detection and familial predisposition: Development of international criteria for the determination of microsatellite instability in colorectal cancer. *Cancer Res.* **1998**, *58*, 5248–5257.
100. Bergamaschi, A.; Kim, Y.H.; Wang, P.; Sorlie, T.; Hernandez-Boussard, T.; Lonning, P.E.; Tibshirani, R.; Borresen-Dale, A.L.; Pollack, J.R. Distinct patterns of DNA copy number alteration are associated with different clinicopathological features and gene-expression subtypes of breast cancer. *Genes Chromosomes Cancer* **2006**, *45*, 1033–1040. [CrossRef]
101. Chin, K.; DeVries, S.; Fridlyand, J.; Spellman, P.T.; Roydasgupta, R.; Kuo, W.L.; Lapuk, A.; Neve, R.M.; Qian, Z.; Ryder, T.; et al. Genomic and transcriptional aberrations linked to breast cancer pathophysiologies. *Cancer Cell* **2006**, *10*, 529–541. [CrossRef] [PubMed]
102. Zhao, X.; Li, C.; Paez, J.G.; Chin, K.; Jänne, P.A.; Chen, T.-H.; Girard, L.; Minna, J.; Christiani, D.; Leo, C.; et al. An Integrated View of Copy Number and Allelic Alterations in the Cancer Genome Using Single Nucleotide Polymorphism Arrays. *Cancer Res.* **2004**, *64*, 3060. [CrossRef] [PubMed]
103. Cappuzzo, F.; Varella-Garcia, M.; Shigematsu, H.; Domenichini, I.; Bartolini, S.; Ceresoli, G.L.; Rossi, E.; Ludovini, V.; Gregorc, V.; Toschi, L.; et al. Increased HER2 Gene Copy Number Is Associated with Response to Gefitinib Therapy in Epidermal Growth Factor Receptor–Positive Non–Small-Cell Lung Cancer Patients. *J. Clin. Oncol.* **2005**, *23*, 5007–5018. [CrossRef]
104. Watkins, J.A.; Irshad, S.; Grigoriadis, A.; Tutt, A.N. Genomic scars as biomarkers of homologous recombination deficiency and drug response in breast and ovarian cancers. *Breast Cancer Res.* **2014**, *16*, 211. [CrossRef]
105. Humar, B.; Blair, V.; Charlton, A.; More, H.; Martin, I.; Guilford, P. E-cadherin deficiency initiates gastric signet-ring cell carcinoma in mice and man. *Cancer Res.* **2009**, *69*, 2050–2056. [CrossRef]
106. Takeuchi, T.; Adachi, Y.; Nagayama, T. A WWOX-binding molecule, transmembrane protein 207, is related to the invasiveness of gastric signet-ring cell carcinoma. *Carcinogenesis* **2012**, *33*, 548–554. [CrossRef]
107. Berger, M.F.; Lawrence, M.S.; Demichelis, F.; Drier, Y.; Cibulskis, K.; Sivachenko, A.Y.; Sboner, A.; Esgueva, R.; Pflueger, D.; Sougnez, C.; et al. The genomic complexity of primary human prostate cancer. *Nature* **2011**, *470*, 214–220. [CrossRef]
108. Baca, S.C.; Prandi, D.; Lawrence, M.S.; Mosquera, J.M.; Romanel, A.; Drier, Y.; Park, K.; Kitabayashi, N.; MacDonald, T.Y.; Ghandi, M.; et al. Punctuated Evolution of Prostate Cancer Genomes. *Cell* **2013**, *153*, 666–677. [CrossRef]
109. Budd, G.T.; Cristofanilli, M.; Ellis, M.J.; Stopeck, A.; Borden, E.; Miller, M.C.; Matera, J.; Repollet, M.; Doyle, G.V.; Terstappen, L.W.M.M.; et al. Circulating Tumor Cells versus Imaging—Predicting Overall Survival in Metastatic Breast Cancer. *Clin. Cancer Res.* **2006**, *12*, 6403. [CrossRef]

110. Cohen, S.J.; Punt, C.J.A.; Iannotti, N.; Saidman, B.H.; Sabbath, K.D.; Gabrail, N.Y.; Picus, J.; Morse, M.; Mitchell, E.; Miller, M.C.; et al. Relationship of Circulating Tumor Cells to Tumor Response, Progression-Free Survival, and Overall Survival in Patients with Metastatic Colorectal Cancer. *J. Clin. Oncol.* **2008**, *26*, 3213–3221. [CrossRef]
111. De Bono, J.S.; Scher, H.I.; Montgomery, R.B.; Parker, C.; Miller, M.C.; Tissing, H.; Doyle, G.V.; Terstappen, L.W.; Pienta, K.J.; Raghavan, D. Circulating tumor cells predict survival benefit from treatment in metastatic castration-resistant prostate cancer. *Clin. Cancer Res.* **2008**, *14*, 6302–6309. [CrossRef] [PubMed]
112. Hayes, D.F.; Cristofanilli, M.; Budd, G.T.; Ellis, M.J.; Stopeck, A.; Miller, M.C.; Matera, J.; Allard, W.J.; Doyle, G.V.; Terstappen, L.W.W.M. Circulating Tumor Cells at Each Follow-up Time Point during Therapy of Metastatic Breast Cancer Patients Predict Progression-Free and Overall Survival. *Clin. Cancer Res.* **2006**, *12*, 4218. [CrossRef] [PubMed]
113. Miyamoto, D.T.; Lee, R.J.; Stott, S.L.; Ting, D.T.; Wittner, B.S.; Ulman, M.; Smas, M.E.; Lord, J.B.; Brannigan, B.W.; Trautwein, J.; et al. Androgen Receptor Signaling in Circulating Tumor Cells as a Marker of Hormonally Responsive Prostate Cancer. *Cancer Discov.* **2012**, *2*, 995. [CrossRef] [PubMed]
114. McArthur, G.A.; Chapman, P.B.; Robert, C.; Larkin, J.; Haanen, J.B.; Dummer, R.; Ribas, A.; Hogg, D.; Hamid, O.; Ascierto, P.A.; et al. Safety and efficacy of vemurafenib in BRAFV600E and BRAFV600K mutation-positive melanoma (BRIM-3): Extended follow-up of a phase 3, randomised, open-label study. *Lancet Oncol.* **2014**, *15*, 323–332. [CrossRef]
115. Cortés-Funes, H.; Mendiola, C.; Manso, L.; Ciruelos, E. Neratinib, an irreversible pan erB receptor tyrosine kinase inhibitor active for advanced HER2+breast cancer. *Breast Cancer Res.* **2009**, *11*, S19. [CrossRef]
116. Slamon, D.J.; Leyland-Jones, B.; Shak, S.; Fuchs, H.; Paton, V.; Bajamonde, A.; Fleming, T.; Eiermann, W.; Wolter, J.; Pegram, M.; et al. Use of Chemotherapy plus a Monoclonal Antibody against HER2 for Metastatic Breast Cancer That Overexpresses HER2. *N. Engl. J. Med.* **2001**, *344*, 783–792. [CrossRef]
117. Baselga, J.; Gelmon, K.A.; Verma, S.; Wardley, A.; Conte, P.; Miles, D.; Bianchi, G.; Cortes, J.; McNally, V.A.; Ross, G.A.; et al. Phase II Trial of Pertuzumab and Trastuzumab in Patients with Human Epidermal Growth Factor Receptor 2–Positive Metastatic Breast Cancer That Progressed During Prior Trastuzumab Therapy. *J. Clin. Oncol.* **2010**, *28*, 1138–1144. [CrossRef]
118. Zhou, C.; Wu, Y.-L.; Chen, G.; Feng, J.; Liu, X.-Q.; Wang, C.; Zhang, S.; Wang, J.; Zhou, S.; Ren, S.; et al. Erlotinib versus chemotherapy as first-line treatment for patients with advanced EGFR mutation-positive non-small-cell lung cancer (OPTIMAL, CTONG-0802): A multicentre, open-label, randomised, phase 3 study. *Lancet Oncol.* **2011**, *12*, 735–742. [CrossRef]
119. Bailey, R.; Kris, M.; Wolf, M.; Kay, A.; Averbuch, S.; Askaa, J.; Janas, M.; Schmidt, K.; Fukuoka, M. O-242 Gefitinib ('Iressa', ZD1839) monotherapy for pretreated advanced non-small-cell lung cancer in IDEAL 1 and 2: Tumor response is not clinically relevantly predictable from tumor EGFR membrane staining alone. *Lung Cancer* **2003**, *41*, S71. [CrossRef]
120. Amir, E.; Miller, N.; Geddie, W.; Freedman, O.; Kassam, F.; Simmons, C.; Oldfield, M.; Dranitsaris, G.; Tomlinson, G.; Laupacis, A.; et al. Prospective study evaluating the impact of tissue confirmation of metastatic disease in patients with breast cancer. *J. Clin. Oncol.* **2012**, *30*, 587–592. [CrossRef]
121. Lindström, L.S.; Karlsson, E.; Wilking, U.M.; Johansson, U.; Hartman, J.; Lidbrink, E.K.; Hatschek, T.; Skoog, L.; Bergh, J. Clinically Used Breast Cancer Markers Such as Estrogen Receptor, Progesterone Receptor, and Human Epidermal Growth Factor Receptor 2 Are Unstable Throughout Tumor Progression. *J. Clin. Oncol.* **2012**, *30*, 2601–2608. [CrossRef] [PubMed]
122. Turner, N.H.; Di Leo, A. HER2 discordance between primary and metastatic breast cancer: Assessing the clinical impact. *Cancer Treat. Rev.* **2013**, *39*, 947–957. [CrossRef]
123. Pusztai, L.; Viale, G.; Kelly, C.M.; Hudis, C.A. Estrogen and HER-2 Receptor Discordance Between Primary Breast Cancer and Metastasis. *Oncologist* **2010**, *15*, 1164–1168. [CrossRef] [PubMed]
124. Fehm, T.; Muller, V.; Aktas, B.; Janni, W.; Schneeweiss, A.; Stickeler, E.; Lattrich, C.; Lohberg, C.R.; Solomayer, E.; Rack, B.; et al. HER2 status of circulating tumor cells in patients with metastatic breast cancer: A prospective, multicenter trial. *Breast Cancer Res. Treat.* **2010**, *124*, 403–412. [CrossRef] [PubMed]
125. Wallwiener, M.; Hartkopf, A.D.; Riethdorf, S.; Nees, J.; Sprick, M.R.; Schonfisch, B.; Taran, F.A.; Heil, J.; Sohn, C.; Pantel, K.; et al. The impact of HER2 phenotype of circulating tumor cells in metastatic breast cancer: A retrospective study in 107 patients. *BMC Cancer* **2015**, *15*, 403. [CrossRef]

126. Georgoulias, V.; Bozionelou, V.; Agelaki, S.; Perraki, M.; Apostolaki, S.; Kallergi, G.; Kalbakis, K.; Xyrafas, A.; Mavroudis, D. Trastuzumab decreases the incidence of clinical relapses in patients with early breast cancer presenting chemotherapy-resistant CK-19mRNA-positive circulating tumor cells: Results of a randomized phase II study. *Ann. Oncol.* **2012**, *23*, 1744–1750. [CrossRef]
127. Schramm, A.; Friedl, T.W.P.; Schochter, F.; Scholz, C.; de Gregorio, N.; Huober, J.; Rack, B.; Trapp, E.; Alunni-Fabbroni, M.; Müller, V.; et al. Therapeutic intervention based on circulating tumor cell phenotype in metastatic breast cancer: Concept of the DETECT study program. *Arch. Gynecol. Obstet.* **2016**, *293*, 271–281. [CrossRef]
128. Wong, K.H.K.; Tessier, S.N.; Miyamoto, D.T.; Miller, K.L.; Bookstaver, L.D.; Carey, T.R.; Stannard, C.J.; Thapar, V.; Tai, E.C.; Vo, K.D.; et al. Whole blood stabilization for the microfluidic isolation and molecular characterization of circulating tumor cells. *Nat. Commun.* **2017**, *8*, 1733. [CrossRef]
129. Lake, B.B.; Codeluppi, S.; Yung, Y.C.; Gao, D.; Chun, J.; Kharchenko, P.V.; Linnarsson, S.; Zhang, K. A comparative strategy for single-nucleus and single-cell transcriptomes confirms accuracy in predicted cell-type expression from nuclear RNA. *Sci. Rep.* **2017**, *7*, 6031. [CrossRef]
130. Macosko, E.Z.; Basu, A.; Satija, R.; Nemesh, J.; Shekhar, K.; Goldman, M.; Tirosh, I.; Bialas, A.R.; Kamitaki, N.; Martersteck, E.M.; et al. Highly Parallel Genome-wide Expression Profiling of Individual Cells Using Nanoliter Droplets. *Cell* **2015**, *161*, 1202–1214. [CrossRef]
131. Gierahn, T.M.; Wadsworth, M.H., 2nd; Hughes, T.K.; Bryson, B.D.; Butler, A.; Satija, R.; Fortune, S.; Love, J.C.; Shalek, A.K. Seq-Well: Portable, low-cost RNA sequencing of single cells at high throughput. *Nat. Methods* **2017**, *14*, 395–398. [CrossRef] [PubMed]
132. Klein, A.M.; Mazutis, L.; Akartuna, I.; Tallapragada, N.; Veres, A.; Li, V.; Peshkin, L.; Weitz, D.A.; Kirschner, M.W. Droplet barcoding for single-cell transcriptomics applied to embryonic stem cells. *Cell* **2015**, *161*, 1187–1201. [CrossRef] [PubMed]
133. Fan, H.C.; Fu, G.K.; Fodor, S.P. Expression profiling. Combinatorial labeling of single cells for gene expression cytometry. *Science* **2015**, *347*, 1258367. [CrossRef]
134. Cheng, Y.H.; Chen, Y.C.; Lin, E.; Brien, R.; Jung, S.; Chen, Y.T.; Lee, W.; Hao, Z.; Sahoo, S.; Min Kang, H.; et al. Hydro-Seq enables contamination-free high-throughput single-cell RNA-sequencing for circulating tumor cells. *Nat. Commun.* **2019**, *10*, 2163. [CrossRef] [PubMed]
135. Stott, S.L.; Hsu, C.H.; Tsukrov, D.I.; Yu, M.; Miyamoto, D.T.; Waltman, B.A.; Rothenberg, S.M.; Shah, A.M.; Smas, M.E.; Korir, G.K.; et al. Isolation of circulating tumor cells using a microvortex-generating herringbone-chip. *Proc. Natl. Acad. Sci. USA* **2010**, *107*, 18392–18397. [CrossRef]
136. Pantel, K.; Alix-Panabières, C. Liquid biopsy and minimal residual disease—Latest advances and implications for cure. *Nat. Rev. Clin. Oncol.* **2019**, *16*, 409–424. [CrossRef] [PubMed]
137. Sinkala, E.; Sollier-Christen, E.; Renier, C.; Rosàs-Canyelles, E.; Che, J.; Heirich, K.; Duncombe, T.A.; Vlassakis, J.; Yamauchi, K.A.; Huang, H.; et al. Profiling protein expression in circulating tumour cells using microfluidic western blotting. *Nat. Commun.* **2017**, *8*, 14622. [CrossRef]
138. Abouleila, Y.; Onidani, K.; Ali, A.; Shoji, H.; Kawai, T.; Lim, C.T.; Kumar, V.; Okaya, S.; Kato, K.; Hiyama, E.; et al. Live single cell mass spectrometry reveals cancer-specific metabolic profiles of circulating tumor cells. *Cancer Sci.* **2019**, *110*, 697–706. [CrossRef]
139. Deng, Y.; Zhang, Y.; Sun, S.; Wang, Z.; Wang, M.; Yu, B.; Czajkowsky, D.M.; Liu, B.; Li, Y.; Wei, W.; et al. An Integrated Microfluidic Chip System for Single-Cell Secretion Profiling of Rare Circulating Tumor Cells. *Sci. Rep.* **2014**, *4*, 7499. [CrossRef]
140. Lim, S.B.; Tan, S.J.; Lim, W.-T.; Lim, C.T. Compendiums of cancer transcriptomes for machine learning applications. *Sci. Data* **2019**, *6*, 194. [CrossRef]
141. Lim, S.B.; Tan, S.J.; Lim, W.-T.; Lim, C.T. A merged lung cancer transcriptome dataset for clinical predictive modeling. *Sci. Data* **2018**, *5*, 180136. [CrossRef] [PubMed]

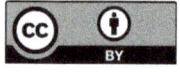

© 2019 by the authors. Licensee MDPI, Basel, Switzerland. This article is an open access article distributed under the terms and conditions of the Creative Commons Attribution (CC BY) license (http://creativecommons.org/licenses/by/4.0/).

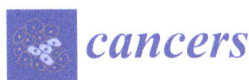

Review

Impact of Tumor and Immunological Heterogeneity on the Anti-Cancer Immune Response

Carolyn Shembrey [1,2], Nicholas D. Huntington [3] and Frédéric Hollande [1,2,*]

1. Department of Clinical Pathology, Victorian Comprehensive Cancer Centre, The University of Melbourne, Melbourne, VIC 3000, Australia
2. Centre for Cancer Research, The University of Melbourne, Melbourne, VIC 3000, Australia
3. Department of Biochemistry and Molecular Biology, Biomedicine Discovery Institute, Monash University, Clayton, VIC 3800, Australia
* Correspondence: frederic.hollande@unimelb.edu.au

Received: 17 July 2019; Accepted: 16 August 2019; Published: 21 August 2019

Abstract: Metastatic tumors are the primary cause of cancer-related mortality. In recent years, interest in the immunologic control of malignancy has helped establish escape from immunosurveillance as a critical requirement for incipient metastases. Our improved understanding of the immune system's interactions with cancer cells has led to major therapeutic advances but has also unraveled a previously unsuspected level of complexity. This review will discuss the vast spatial and functional heterogeneity in the tumor-infiltrating immune system, with particular focus on natural killer (NK) cells, as well as the impact of tumor cell-specific factors, such as secretome composition, receptor–ligand repertoire, and neoantigen diversity, which can further drive immunological heterogeneity. We emphasize how tumor and immunological heterogeneity may undermine the efficacy of T-cell directed immunotherapies and explore the potential of NK cells to be harnessed to circumvent these limitations.

Keywords: tumor heterogeneity; natural killer cells; tumor mutation burden; immunotherapy

1. Introduction

Recent advances in our understanding of cancer, driven by the development of sophisticated biochemical and molecular techniques, have highlighted the complex and heterogenous nature of this disease. Within individual tumors, significant differences in the molecular and phenotypic profiles may arise from tumor cell-intrinsic or extrinsic factors. Genomics has provided the most extensive insights to date about tumor-intrinsic variations, with sequencing studies revealing a large extent of clinically-relevant intra-tumor heterogeneity [1–3]. Thus, next generation sequencing of multiple tumor types identifying the association between increased clonal heterogeneity and higher pathological stage and/or worse prognosis [4]. Moreover, genetic heterogeneity has also been identified across patients, and the incidence of clinically actionable mutations differs significantly between tumors arising from different tissue or cell types, amongst patients with the same class of tumor, and between matched primary and metastatic tumors within the same patient [5–8]. Non-genetic determinants of heterogeneity have also garnered significant interest, as even genetically identical cells may harbor unique chemosensitivity profiles [9]. This points towards the role epigenetic modifications [10–12] and metabolic reprogramming [13], in dictating the functional variation observed within individual populations.

Tumor cell extrinsic factors, such as the cellular and structural elements of the tumor microenvironment (TME), are also known to influence tumor heterogeneity. For instance, the spatial arrangement of cells with receptor tyrosine kinase amplifications in glioblastoma has been shown to correspond with degree of vascularization in the local TME [14]. Similarly, in melanoma patients, the extent of subclonal divergence from the mutational profile of the primary tumor is dependent on the metastatic site [15], suggesting an influence of the local microenvironment. Perhaps the most important component of the TME are the immune cells. Whilst the tumor-sculpting role of the anti-cancer immune response has long been recognised, conflicting reports exist on the impact of this immunoediting on tumor heterogeneity. The selective pressure of the immune response has been shown to profoundly reduce sub-clonal diversity via the targeted elimination of immunogenic cell variants [16], recent evidence indicates that the adaptive immune response may in fact potentiate genomic instability [17], thus promoting the rise of novel subclones thereby increasing tumor heterogeneity. As heterogeneity within the immune or tumor cell compartments could conceivably impact the efficacy of immunotherapies, there is a vital need to improve our understanding of the relationship between the two.

2. Spatial, Functional, and Temporal Heterogeneity of Immune Cell Infiltrates

Tumor cells develop in a dynamic niche; individual tumor cell subpopulations not only compete and cooperate with each other, but also with the surrounding TME and its constituent immune cells. Single-cell sequencing studies have confirmed that tumors may be populated by a vast and diverse array of immune components: innate leukocytes, such as natural killer (NK) cells and mast cells; phagocytes, such as macrophages, neutrophils, and dendritic cells; and adaptive effectors, including naïve, memory, and effector B- and T-lymphocytes [18]. It is clear that the degree of immune infiltration and the composition of this infiltrate can vary markedly across tumor types [19] and stages [18], as well as between patients with the same tumor type [20,21]. Similarly, whether synchronous metastases within a single patient regress or progress has been associated with their distinct immune profile [22]. Within a tumor, complexity is further compounded by the differing spatial distribution of immune effectors between the core and invasive fronts, as well as within the adjacent tertiary lymphoid structures [23,24].

However, as increased infiltration of CD8+ T-cells is prognostic for better outcome in numerous tumor types [25–28], traditional scoring of tumor immunogenicity has been based upon the degree of T-cell inflammation alone. Immunologically 'hot' tumors, such as melanoma and non-small cell lung cancer (NSCLC), present with a high degree of T-cell permeation, whereas tumor-infiltrating lymphocytes (TILs) are scarcely observed in 'cold' tumors, such as ovarian, prostate, and pancreatic cancers. More recently, a third immunologically 'altered' phenotype has been proposed, denoting cases where peri-tumoral sites are densely inflamed with immune cells which lack the ability to infiltrate into the tumor [29]. As the T-cell inflamed gene expression profiles of 'hot' tumors have been strongly linked with positive response to checkpoint blockade therapies [30,31], significant attention has been focused on developing therapeutic strategies which can convert immunologically 'cold' or 'altered' phenotypes into 'hot' environments [32–34]. Yet, as the immune contexture may vary across non-adjacent tumor regions, it should be emphasized that many tumors may not be universally 'hot' nor 'cold'.

To address this disparity, the Immunoscore method proposed by the Galon group incorporates spatial context into its immunological quantitation metric, computed by the ratio of memory CD3+ and cytotoxic CD8+ TILs at the tumor centre and invasive margins. In colorectal cancer (CRC), this index has been validated as an independent prognostic marker which performs better than both Tumor-Node-Metastasis (TNM) staging and microsatellite instability (MSI) status [35–37] and an in vitro diagnostic assay has been made clinically available for assessing relapse risk in Stage II and III CRC. Yet, there is substantial evidence that quantification varies between non-adjacent areas of tumor biopsies [38–40], suggesting that single biopsies may not be representative of the broader infiltrating immune landscape. Pertinently, a phenomenon termed Immunoskew has been documented, whereby a minority of tumor regions are densely infiltrated with TILs despite an otherwise barren TME [41]. Determining whether Immunoskew extends to other immune cell populations, and identifying the specific intra-tumor differences which drive this differential infiltration pattern, are worthy areas for future study.

Beyond TILs, the contribution of other cell types to tumor immunogenicity should not be overlooked. NK cells are inversely correlated with cancer incidence [42,43] and intra-tumoral NK cell infiltrates have been identified as a positive prognostic marker in multiple solid cancers [44–48] and haematological malignancies [49]. Additionally, NK cells are supremely important in the control of metastasis. A wealth of in vivo studies have demonstrated that mice depleted of NK cells via pharmacological inhibition [50–52] or genetic knockout [53] are more vulnerable to metastasis than their NK cell-proficient counterparts. The same is true for mice reconstituted with NK cells deficient in cytotoxic molecules, such as perforin and interferon-γ (IFNγ) [54,55] or activating receptors [56–59]. This notion has been confirmed in a clinical study of CRC liver metastases, where increased frequency of intra-tumoral NK cells was the variable most significantly ($p = 0.01$) associated with better overall survival, performing better than other clinical parameters including TNM stage, number/size of metastases, and frequency of infiltrating CD3+ lymphocytes [60]. Additionally, there is strong evidence supporting the role of NK cells in the clearance of putative cancer stem cells [61–64], suggesting that NKs may promote long-term recurrence-free survival.

The discordance in immune infiltrate between primary and metastatic tumors is more pronounced in metachronous than synchronous tumors [24,65,66] indicating that temporal changes also contribute to tumor heterogeneity. The composition of immune infiltrates is also known to change as tumors progress, with one study in CRC reporting an increased prevalence of innate immune cells and decreased number of most T-cell lineages in more advanced tumor stages [18]. The latter may be particularly important when considering the age-associated decline in lymphocyte number and function [67], particularly given that the majority of new cancer diagnoses are made in those over the age of 65.

Above all, a limitation of current techniques that quantify immune infiltrates is that they frequently do not assess functionality. Recent evidence suggests that infiltration alone may not be sufficient to elicit anti-tumor responses, as effector cells can be relegated to the peritumoral stroma and therefore lack the direct cell contact required for target cell destruction [68–70]. Similarly, the efficacy of each immune cell population may be influenced by the immunoregulatory cytokines produced by neighboring cell types. For example, infiltrating cytotoxic lymphocytes may be restrained by various immunosuppressive cell types, including myeloid-derived suppressor cells [71], Tregs [33,72–74], and tumor-associated (TA) fibroblasts [68,75–77], which are diversely distributed across cancer types. Conversely, traditionally immunosuppressive cells can act beneficially depending on the surrounding tumor context [78,79].

3. Tumor Cell-Driven Immunological Heterogeneity

The observation that increased TIL fractions have positive prognostic value in numerous tumor types has culminated in the harnessing of this subset for immunotherapy, primarily in the form of immune checkpoint inhibitors. Whilst strikingly effective in tumor types, such as melanoma, renal cell carcinoma (RCC), and NSCLC, the efficacy of immune checkpoint therapies is highly variable across solid malignancies. For example, in CRC, positive therapeutic responses to T-cell directed checkpoint inhibitors are limited to approximately 30% of patients with MSI, which represents 5% of all patients [80]. Whilst the exact molecular mechanisms which underpin this resistance remain elusive, emerging evidence suggests that broad spectrum of clinical responses could be partially attributable to immunological heterogeneity. As well as differences in immune infiltration and interaction of immune cell types, there are multiple tumor cell intrinsic factors, such as the secretome, receptor–ligand profile, and neoantigen repertoire, which can drive immunological heterogeneity (Figure 1).

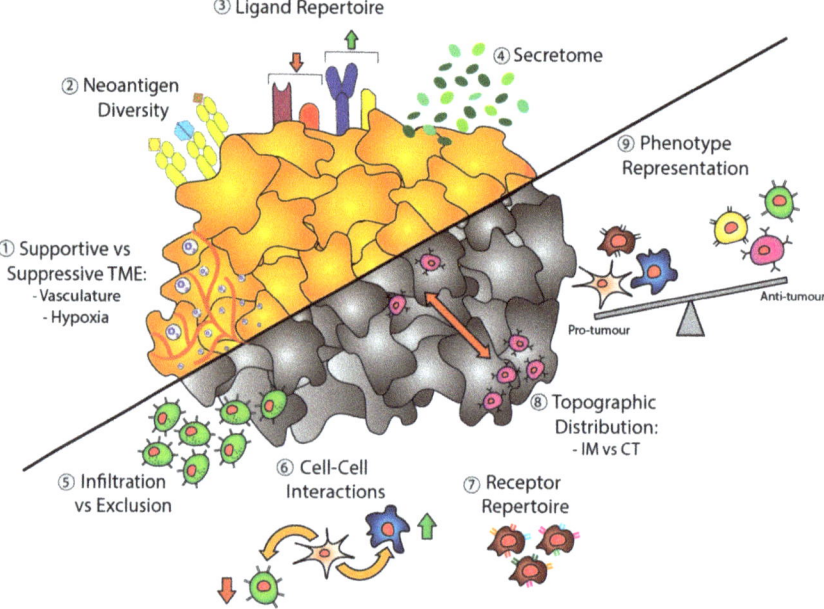

Figure 1. Tumor and immunological heterogeneity. Tumor-intrinsic drivers of heterogeneity (upper left) include diversity in: the degree of tumor vascularization or hypoxia (**1**), which determines whether the local tumor microenvironment (TME) will support or suppress anti-tumor immune cells; the variable expression of neoantigens (**2**) and ligands (**3**), which facilitate interaction with various immune cell types; and the secretion of soluble factors (**4**) (which may also be produced by the immune cells themselves) that may promote or restrain the action of nearby immune cells. Immune cell contributions to heterogeneity (bottom right) include: the type and density of infiltrating versus excluded immune cells (**5**); modulatory interactions between co-localised immune cell types (**6**); the balance of activating versus inhibitory receptors (**7**); effector cell distribution between the invasive margin (IM) and central tumor (CT) (**8**); and the overall balance between pro- and anti-tumor effectors (**9**).

3.1. Secretome Heterogeneity

Infiltrating immune cells can be conditioned by the soluble factors secreted by nearby tumor cells. Tumor cells can directly foster an immunosuppressive TME via the production of enzymes and metabolites including indolamine 2, 3-dioxygenase (IDO) [81,82], lactic acid [83] and prostaglandin E_2 [68,84]. As metabolically heterogeneous regions are detectable within discrete tumors [13], it is conceivable that these immunosuppressive metabolites may be irregularly distributed. Although such mediators are directly implicated in the dampening of T- and NK cell activity, their immunomodulatory effects are not reflected in routine clinical immunohistochemistry, where the focus is on assessing the presence or absence of lymphocytes, not their activation state.

There are multiple reports of tumor-derived cytokines, such as transforming growth factor-β1 (TGF-β1) suppressing cytotoxic effector functions [85–87], frequently acting via the downregulation of activating receptors [88–90]. As TGF-β1 production is exacerbated in hypoxic conditions, it follows that hypoxic tumor cells show heightened resistance to NK cell-mediated killing [91–93]. In response to hypoxia, accumulation of immunosuppressive adenosine and subsequent signaling via the A2A adenosine receptor has been shown to potently inhibit T- and NK cells [94,95]. This tumor-protective effect is abrogated in hyperoxic conditions [96,97], suggesting that supplemental oxygen could be a useful co-adjuvant for immunotherapy. Due to the disorganized vascularization of growing tumors, tumor cells may be irregularly exposed to hypoxia [98]. Interestingly, this intermittent hypoxic conditioning has been shown to enhance inflammatory responses as compared with chronic hypoxia [99–101]. However, this phenomenon has also been shown to enhance tumor growth and promote radiotherapy resistance in in vitro and in vivo models [102]. Thus, more research interrogating the role of intermittent hypoxia in the context of the TME would be valuable.

Additionally, there is mounting evidence that different immune cell subtypes, particularly NK cells, may exhibit tropisms for different tumor types. Human NK cells develop from $CD34^+$ hematopoietic progenitors in the bone marrow and critically rely on interleukin-15 (IL-15) transpresentation for maturation into two functionally distinct mature NK cell subsets in the periphery [103,104], divided based on CD56 expression. Approximately 90% of circulating NK cells exhibit the $CD56^{dim}$ phenotype, which primarily function as cytolytic effectors via production of perforin and granzyme B. Conversely, the immunoregulatory $CD56^{bright}$ subset is charged with production of type I pro-inflammatory cytokines (IFNγ, Tumor necrosis factor (TNF)α, GM-CSF, IL-10, IL-13) and preferentially reside in the secondary lymphoid organs. In breast cancer [105] and gastrointestinal stromal tumours (GIST) [44], tumor-infiltrating NK cells are primarily of the poorly cytotoxic $CD56^{bright}$ subtype, whereas glioblastomas are preferentially infiltrated by $CD56^{dim}$ NK cells [106], and conflicting tropisms have been reported in NSCLC [107,108]. Such differences in NK cell homing may also be associated with the extent of hypoxia in the TME, as hypoxia-induced upregulation of chemokines C-X-C chemokine receptor type 4 (CXCR4) and CCR7 has been shown to favor migration of the $CD56^{bright}$ subset [109]. Intriguingly, this is unlikely to be explained by chemokine profile alone, as NK cell infiltration in CRC is scarce despite elevated expression of chemokines that attract $CD56^{bright}$ (CXCL9, CXCL10, CCL3, CCL4) and $CD56^{dim}$ (CXCL8, CXCL1, CXCL5, and CXCL12) subsets in tumor tissue as compared with adjacent normal mucosa [69].

3.2. Receptor–Ligand Heterogeneity

Through somatic recombination, the adaptive immune system is able to generate immunoglobulin and T-cell receptor (TCR) repertoires which span millions of antigens. Disparate receptor repertoires also exist within the NK cell compartment and underpin their functional heterogeneity. NK cell effector functions are tightly controlled by a complex network of activating and inhibitory receptors, and the ability of NK cells to eliminate target cells and produce cytokines relies upon the integration of signals from both types. Activating receptors, such as the natural cytotoxicity receptors (NKp30, NKp44, and NKp46) and NKG2D, recognise stress-induced ligands which are upregulated in response to DNA damage or viral transformation ("induced-self" recognition) [110,111]. Conversely, inhibitory receptors comprising the highly polymorphic killer cell immunoglobulin-like receptor (KIR) family work to prevent the aberrant targeting of healthy host cells by engaging "self" molecules, such as major histocompatibility complex class I (MHC-I), glycoproteins, and cadherins, and accordingly targeting those that have lost expression of these molecules ("missing-self" recognition).

Whilst NK cell receptors are preformed and, therefore, do not undergo the rearrangements characteristic of B- and T-cell receptors, a remarkable degree of NK cell diversity is conferred by the combinatorial expression of different NK receptors. Utilising a mass cytometry panel of 28 NK cell receptors, Horowitz et al. successfully detected up to 30,000 distinct NK cell phenotypes within a healthy individual. Such heterogeneity may in part be explained by the multiple factors which can regulate NK cell receptor repertoires, including host-genetics [112,113], epigenetic regulation [114] and previous viral infection [115–117].

The KIRs are the most heterogeneously expressed family of receptors. KIRs are encoded by 15 highly polymorphic genes clustered in the leukocyte receptor complex on chromosome 19q13.4 [118]. $CD56^{dim}$ NK cells express between 7 and 11 KIR family members; the presence or absence of individual KIR genes in each haplotype generates considerable genotypic diversity, which is compounded by differing allelic frequencies within each gene. Such heterogeneity is of clinical importance, as KIR-mismatch is a prerequisite for the graft-versus-leukaemia effect of allogenic NK cell transfer [119–121] and specific KIR genotypes have been associated with better responses to combination immunotherapies in neuroblastoma patients [122,123]. Similarly, three splice variants of the activating receptor NKp30 have been identified and the relative abundance of activating versus inhibitory isoforms has been associated with clinical outcome in neuroblastoma [124] and gastrointestinal sarcoma [44]. In the latter study, expression of inhibitory NKp30c as the most abundant isoform was the only independent prognostic factor for overall survival, whose overexpression was traced to a single nucleotide polymorphism in the natural cytotoxicity receptor-3 (NCR3) gene [44].

Importantly, numerous in vitro studies have demonstrated the ability of tumor cell lines to differentially regulate the receptor repertoires of NK cells [62,63,125]. Coordinated patterns of receptor dysregulation have similarly been documented in tumor-infiltrating as compared with peripheral NK cells. Reduced expression of activating receptors (including NKp30, NKp46, NKp80, CD16, DNAX accessory molecule-1 (DNAM-1) and NKG2D) has been documented in lung carcinoma [108], breast cancer [105] and acute myeloid leukaemia [126]. In each case, functional analysis of these patient-derived NK cells revealed that tumor-associated NK cells are poor producers of IFNγ and have an impaired ability to degranulate, although these studies did not investigate whether these defects impacted clinical outcome. Conversely, upregulation of the CD96/NKG2A inhibitory receptor complex has been observed in renal cell [127] and associated with poor prognosis in hepatocellular [128] carcinomas.

Immune cell responsiveness is not only determined by the balance of receptors present on a given cell, but also by the various ligands expressed by the target cell. For instance, a recognised mechanism of tumor escape in is the shedding of soluble 'decoy' ligands for NK cell activating receptors, including BCL2-associated athanogene 6 (BAG-6) [129,130] and B7-H6 [131]. Interestingly, a genome-wide knockout screen performed by Klein and colleagues [132] identified loss of B7-H6 as the sole event which increased resistance of the chronic myeloid leukaemia cells to NK cell killing. Yet, recent studies investigating the functional consequences of NKG2D ligand shedding have challenged the idea that soluble ligands are exclusively immunosuppressive; in human cancers, shedding of MHC class I polypeptide related sequence A (MIC-A), a low-affinity NKG2D ligand, facilitates immune evasion [133,134]; however, shedding of the high-affinity murine analogue, MULT-1, enhances NK cell activation and tumor rejection [135].

Another major mechanism by which tumors evade immune destruction is up-regulation of immune checkpoint ligands, such as CD80/86, 4-1BBL, and OX40-L. Immune checkpoints are a broad group of inhibitory pathways and co-receptors with the primary purpose to restrict the duration and amplitude of an immune response, thereby minimizing collateral damage to healthy tissues [136]. Immune checkpoints primarily regulate T-cell responses, although checkpoint expression has been documented in B cells, NK cells and professional antigen-presenting cells (APCs) [136]. In the context of cancer, chronic antigen exposure coupled with engagement of inhibitory immune checkpoint ligands on tumor cells results in effector T-cell exhaustion, wherein T-cells undergo profound impairment of proliferation, cytokine production and cytotoxicity. Even in hostile immune environments densely infiltrated with cytotoxic T-lymphocytes, checkpoint ligand expression impinges upon tumor clearance [137]. Programmed Death Ligand 1 (PD-L1) has attracted particular attention in that its expression is associated with poor prognosis in multiple cancers [138–141]. Indeed, six of the seven FDA-approved immune checkpoint inhibitors target the PD-1/PD-L1 inhibitory axis [142]. PD-L1 expression by tumor cells is a strong predictive biomarker for response to PD-L1 blockade [143], although positive therapeutic responses to have been reported PD-L1-knockout mice [144] PD-L1-negative patients [145]. This suggests that whilst PD-L1 positivity enriches for responders, combining PD-L1 expression with other predictive factors, such as MSI status, may increase our confidence in patient selection. Indeed, even in tumors classed as PD-L1-positive, individual tumor cells vary widely in terms of PD-L1 expression [66,146]. Individual research groups set thresholds for ligand positivity ranging from 1–50% [147] and in tumors classed as checkpoint-positive, negative-staining cells may be ignored during clinical decision making despite their likely influence on treatment efficacy. Likewise, ligand profiles are labile in response to therapy; conventional chemotherapeutics increase expression ligands for the NK cell activating receptors NKG2D and DNAM-1 in multiple myeloma [148] and ovarian cancer [149] cells.

There is also some degree of binding promiscuity involved in receptor–ligand interactions. An array of NK cell receptors with opposing functional roles compete for binding of CD155 (PVR) ligand, including activating DNAX accessory molecule-1 (DNAM-1) and inhibitory T-cell immunoreceptor with Ig and ITIM domains (TIGIT) [150]. CD96-CD155 ligation is primarily considered an inhibitory checkpoint in the NK-mediated control of metastasis [151], however an activating role for CD96 has also been reported via promoting target adhesion [152]. Such complexity demonstrates how the interplay between immune cell receptors and ligands should be assessed as a network rather than at the single molecule level, and how such assessment should take into account spatial heterogeneity rather than focus on limited areas.

3.3. Neoantigenic Heterogeneity; A Challenge for T-cell Directed Immunotherapies

Just as the ability of the immune system to recognise and destroy invading pathogens or foreign particles relies on the ability to distinguish self from non- or altered-self, the genetic marks carried by tumor cells provide a diverse set of antigens that the immune system can use to detect malignant cells amongst their normal counterparts. Accordingly, T-cell directed immunotherapies have currently proven most efficacious in cancer types with high average tumor mutation burden (TMB) [153,154]. Whilst clinical responses to immune checkpoint blockade in cancer types with traditionally low TMB have been reported, these are generally restricted to virally-induced cancers, such as Merkel cell carcinoma and human papilloma virus-positive head and neck squamous cell carcinoma (HPV+ HNSCC), which show enhanced T-cell infiltration due to the presence of viral antigen [155,156]. Similarly, MSI has been identified as a pan-cancer predictive marker for checkpoint inhibitors [157,158], as MSI tumors harbour DNA mismatch-repair defects and thus present with 10–100 fold greater TMB than genomically stable tumors [159]. MSI tumors also have higher TIL density as compared with their microsatellite stable (MSS) counterparts, due primarily to their increased frequency of mutated neo-epitopes recognisable as non-self [160]. Neoepitope load is predictive of clinical outcome in bladder cancer [161], multiple myeloma [162], melanoma [163], and ovarian cancer [163,164], and there several reports of cytotoxic T-cells recognising epitopes derived from single point mutations [165–167]. Accordingly, heightened TMB is associated with more diversified expansion of T-cells [168] and greater infiltration of neoantigen-specific clonotypes [169].

Neoepitope targeting is an appealing therapeutic avenue in that the lack of neoepitope expression in healthy cells ensures that neoepitope-specific T-cells are not impinged by central tolerance, thereby conferring greater specificity and less toxicity. To this end, multiple studies are currently investigating the possibility of targeting neoepitopes with for personalised immunotherapy (see Türeci et al. [170] 2016 for a complete list of completed and ongoing trials). Yet, a barrier to the clinical applicability of these strategies inheres in the tremendously diverse range of antigenome landscapes observed between patients. In a recent pan-cancer analysis where almost one million unique neoantigens were identified, only 24 were conserved in at least 5% of patients in one or more cancer types [171]. Similar results have been reported in analyses of individual cancer types [172,173]; of note, a cohort study from The Cancer Genome Atlas (TCGA) in CRC (n = 598) revealed that only 4% of predicted neoepitopes were shared by at least two patients [174]. This complexity is compounded by the substantial diversity across patients with respect to human leukocyte antigen (HLA) haplotypes required for antigen presentation. This may be particularly important as, unlike membrane-associated checkpoint molecules, the majority of tumorigenic mutations affect genes which encode for intracellular proteins [175] and are therefore only recognizable by CD8+ T-cells following antigen processing and presentation in the context of MHC-I.

There is also strong evidence supporting the existence of neoantigenic heterogeneity within individual tumors. In lung adenocarcinoma, post-surgical recurrence has been associated with an increased proportion of branched neoantigens, defined as those not homogenously detected throughout the tumor [21]. Importantly, TCR sequencing of 45 tumor regions in these patients demonstrated that the majority of T-cell clones were topographically restricted, and that intra-tumor heterogeneity in TCR repertoires positively correlated with predicted neoantigen variety. Together, these findings suggest that regional differences in T-cell infiltration may be driven by spatially distinct neoantigen profiles, which may have important consequences for the development of therapies which target single neoantigens. There is also accumulating data suggesting that neoantigens are not equally 'potent' in their ability to elicit T-cell effector functions, highlighting that assessing neoantigen quality may be more important than their quantity. Recent work has demonstrated that qualitative neoantigen prediction models, where fitness is conferred by a higher probability of TCR-recognition, have surpassed quantitative models in their ability to stratify for survival [176,177].

4. Neoantigen-Independent Strategies for Immunotherapy

Evidently, neoantigenic heterogeneity presents a formidable challenge in the development of T-cell based immunotherapies. To circumvent this striking degree of variability, clinical attention has been directed towards targeting non-mutated antigens that show heightened tumor specificity, including cancer germline antigens (CGAs). Unlike patient-specific neoepitopes, non-mutated antigens arise from comparatively well-defined mechanisms and are thus more likely to be conserved across patients. CG antigens are proteins that are exclusively expressed by germ cells which can be aberrantly re-expressed in multiple cancers, including the archetypal melanoma antigen (MAGE), synovial sarcoma X-chromosome breakpoint (SSX), and oesophageal squamous cell carcinoma (ESO) families. Expression of CG antigens is epigenetically modulated, being frequently induced following hypomethylation of CpG islands and covalent histone modifications [178]. Due to their absence on healthy somatic cells, CGAs have garnered substantial interest as therapeutic targets. However, development of CGA-directed therapies has been hampered by their low prevalence. Indeed, Kerkar et al. [179] report that only 2–3% of common epithelial cancers uniformly express New York-ESO-1 (NY-ESO-1).

An alternate strategy has been to target TA antigens that, despite basal expression in healthy cells, are preferentially expressed by transformed cells. One class of TA antigens are the differentiation antigens, which are homogenously expressed by cells of a given tissue type or cell lineage and consequently, by all malignant cells arising therefrom. Given that these antigens are concomitantly expressed in healthy tissues, therapeutic efficacy is generally accompanied by 'on-target' toxicity. For example, adoptive cell transfer directed against the metastatic melanoma differentiation antigens gp1000 and melanoma-associated antigen recognised by T cells (MART-1) resulted in regression in 30% of patients, though these individuals frequently experienced uveitis and hearing loss due to destruction of melanocytes in the eye and ear [180]. Similarly, targeting carcinoembryonic antigen (CEA) overexpression in metastatic CRC induced regression but also severe inflammatory colitis [181].

Harnessing NK Cells for Innate Immunotherapy

In recent years, NK cells have emerged as alternative candidates for immunotherapeutic development. Certainly, the MHC-I unrestricted manner of NK cell responses may render this subset a more promising candidate for immunotherapy, as they may overcome the restricted benefit of antigen-specific T-cells in tumors with high mutational diversity. NK-based therapies may prove a new frontier in the treatment of immunologically 'cold' or refractory tumors, given that the one of the most common mechanisms of immune escape employed by tumor cells is downregulation of MHC-I machinery [182]. Similarly, defects in genes implicated in antigen processing and presentation have recently been identified as key drivers of acquired resistance to immune checkpoint therapies [183]. Additionally, NK cell cytotoxicity may be triggered following engagement of ligands upregulated by transformed cells in response to epithelial-mesenchymal transition, such as MIC-A/B and ULBP1-3 [184].

The latter renders NK cells particularly apt in the eradication of early metastatic cells. Importantly, NK cell receptors are preformed and thus do not require prior sensitisation, clonal expansion and co-stimulatory signalling required for T-cell responsiveness, thus allowing for more rapid cytotoxic responses. Whilst adoptive transfer of HLA-mismatched NK cells induces graft-versus-tumor effects, these cells do not contribute to dose-limiting graft-versus-host disease (GvHD) and may even play a protective role by dampening alloreactive T-cell responses [185,186].

Although no therapies directed specifically at NK cells have been approved in the clinic to date, such promising data suggests that a next wave of therapeutic advances could come from targeting this cell type (Table 1). In phase I/II clinical trials, monoclonal antibodies targeting NK cell inhibitory receptors, such as NKG2A [187] and the KIR family [188], have been shown to bolster NK cell-mediated cytotoxicity. Chimeric antigen receptor (CAR) NK cells directed against CD19 [189,190], CD2 subset-1 (CS-1) [191] and epidermal growth factor receptor (EGFR) [192,193] have also shown efficacy in xenograft models. To improve specificity, Bi-Specific Killer cell Engagers (BiKEs) have been developed which co-target the CD16 low affinity IgG receptor (FcγRIII) and epitopes expressed by malignant cells, such as CD33 [194] and EpCAM [195]. BiKEs have been shown to mediate NK cell cytotoxicity, which is markedly enhanced following the incorporation of a modified human IL-15 crosslinker to generate a tri-specific moity (TriKE; [196]. Yet, these approaches all still rely on tumor cell expression of the selected target and may therefore show limited success in eliminating heterogenous tumor cell populations. Addressing this challenge, CAR T-cells have been engineered to co-express members of the natural cytotoxicity receptor (NCR) family of NK cell activating receptors (including NKp46 [197], NKp44 [198], and NKp30 [199]. These 'hybrid' CARs avoid the obstacle of MHC-restriction but retain the long-term persistence of adoptively transferred T-cells, endowing cytotoxic T-cells with an NK cell-like pattern of recognition. It is through such innovations, which consider the complexity of tumor cell heterogeneity and acknowledge that immunotherapy may not be a 'one size fits all' approach, that we may draw the greatest clinical benefit.

Table 1. Completed and currently active clinical trials of NK cell-based immunotherapies.

Approach	Target	Indication	Phase	Clinical Trial ID(s)
Adoptive cell transfer:	Allogenic PBMCs (non-targeted)	Leukemias and lymphomas	Phase I/II	NCT00569283; NCT00799799; NCT00823524; NCT00303667; NCT00187096; NCT00274846; NCT01106950; NCT005626292; NCT01390402; NCT02395822; NCT00586690; NCT00586703; NCT00145626; NCT01386619; NCT00945126; NCT00354172; NCT01313897; NCT01181258
		Solid cancers	Phase I/II	NCT01287104; NCT01212341; NCT01105650; UMIN000013378; NCT01147380; 2005-005125-58
	Autologous PBMCs (non-targeted)	Multiple myeloma	Phase I	NCT02481934
		Advanced digestive cancer	Phase I	UMIN000007527
		Advanced melanoma or kidney cancer	Phase II	NCT00328861
		Advanced renal cell cancer or melanoma	Phase I	N/A [200]
	NK-92 (NK cell line; non-targeted)	End-stage chemotherapy resistant cancer	Phase I	N/A [201]
		Hematologic malignancies	Phase I	NCT00990717
		Relapsed acute myeloid leukemia	Phase I	NCT00900809
		Stage IIIB or Stage IV Merkel cell carcinoma	Phase II	NCT02465957
Chimeric Antigen Receptors	CD19	Solid and hematological malignancies	Phase I/II	NCT03690310; NCT03679927; NCT03056339; NCT01974479; NCT00995137; NCT02892695
	ROBO1	Solid tumors	Phase I/II	NCT03940820
	BCMA	Relapsed and refractory multiple myeloma	Phase I/II	NCT03940833
	PSMA	Castration-resistant prostate cancer	Phase I	NCT03692663
	NKG2D	Metastatic solid tumors	Phase I	NCT03415100
	Mesothelin	Epithelial ovarian cancer	Not yet recruiting	NCT03692637
	CD33 CAR NK-92	Acute myeloid leukemia	Phase I/II	NCT02944162
	CD7	Lymphoma and leukemia	Phase I/II	NCT02742727
	MUC1	Solid tumors	Phase I/II	NCT02839954
	HER2	Glioblastoma	Phase I/II	NCT03383978
	NKG2D ligands	Solid tumors	Phase I	NCT03415100

Table 1. Cont.

Approach	Target	Indication	Phase	Clinical Trial ID(s)
Bi- and Tri- specific Killer cell Engagers (BiKe/TriKes)	CD16 × CD33	Myelodysplastic syndromes	Pre-clinical	N/A [94]
	AFM13 (CD30 × CD16A) BiKe	Hodgkin lymphoma	Phase I	NCT01221571
	AFM13 (CD30 × CD16A) BiKe	Relapsed/refractory cutaneous lymphomas	Phase I/II	NCT03192202
	CD16 × IL-15 × CD33 TriKe	AML & high-risk myelodysplastic syndromes	Phase I/II	NCT03214666
Anti-NKG2A	Monalizumab (anti-NKG2A) + cetuximab	Squamous cell carcinoma of the head and neck	Phase II	NCT02643550
	Monalizumab (anti-NKG2A) + durvalumab	Advanced or metastatic solid cancers	Phase I/II	
Anti-KIR	KIR3DL2			
	IPH4102	Cutaneous T-cell lymphoma	Phase I	NCT02593045
	IPH4102 +/− gemcitabine +/− oxaliplatin	Advanced T-cell lymphoma	Phase II	NCT03902184
	KIR2DL1-2-3-:			
	Lirilumab (IPH2102/BMS-986015)	Smoldering multiple myeloma	Phase II	NCT01222286
	Lirilumab (IPH2102/BMS-986015)	Acute myeloid leukemia	Phase II	NCT01687387
	Lirilumab (IPH2102/BMS-986015) + ipilimumab (anti-PD-1)	Advanced solid tumors	Phase I/II	NCT01714739 & NCT03203876
	Lirilumab (IPH2102/BMS-986015) + ipilimumab (anti-CTLA-4)	NSCLC, Castration Resistant Prostate Cancer, Melanoma	Phase I	NCT01750580
	Lirilumab (IPH2102/BMS-986015) + ipilimumab (anti-CD20)	Chronic lymphocytic leukemia	Phase II	NCT02481297
	1-7F9 (IPH2101)	Multiple myeloma	Phase I	NCT00055296 & NCT00999830
	1-7F9 (IPH2101)	Acute myeloid leukemia	Phase I	NCT01256073

5. Concluding Remarks

Whether driven by immune cell-intrinsic or tumor-induced factors, it is clear that a vast scope of immunological heterogeneity exists across human cancers. Incorporating our understanding of this heterogeneity into clinical studies may improve our ability to further stratify patients who are candidates for immunotherapy and aid in the design of rational combination therapies directed against heterogeneously expressed targets thereby complementing existing therapeutic strategies, such as those targeting PD-L1. Additionally, further research exploring the influence of TMB on the infiltration and effector functions of non-antigen restricted mediators, specifically NK cells, could inform new therapeutic strategies harnessing the innate immune compartment.

Author Contributions: Writing—original draft preparation, C.S.; Writing—review and editing, F.H. and N.D.H.

Funding: This research was funded by the National Health and Medical Research Council of Australia, grants GNT1069024 and GNT1164081 to FH.

Conflicts of Interest: N.D.H. has ownership interest (including patents) in oNKo-innate Pty Ltd and receives research funding from Servier and Paranta Biosciences.

Abbreviations

Common cell types and acronyms used throughout this manuscript.

$CD56^{bright}$ natural killer (NK) cell	Immunoregulatory subset (~10%) of NK cells producing type I pro-inflammatory cytokines
$CD56^{dim}$ NK cell	Cytotoxic subset (~90%) of NK cells characterized by high production of perforin and granzyme B.
Chimeric antigen receptor (CAR)	Chimeric proteins that fuse an extracellular tumor antigen-targeting domain with a lymphocyte (T- or NK cell)-activating intracellular moiety.
Bi-/Tri-specific killer cell engager (Bi-/TriKE)	Advanced biologicals engineered to express antibody domains capable of binding multiple unique antigens (e.g., 2 antigens /Bi- or 3 antigens/Tri on NK cells and tumor cells to promote NK cell activation and binding to tumor cells)
Killer cell immunoglobulin-like receptor (KIR)	Large family of highly polymorphic NK cell receptors (also expressed in a subset of T-cells) which regulate cytotoxicity by engaging "self" molecules, such as MHC-I.
Major histocompatibility complex class I (MHC-I)	Multi-protein complex expressed by all nucleated cells in mammals. MHC-I presents peptide fragments (derived from self, non-self and neo-antigens) to cytotoxic T-cells.
Natural cytotoxicity receptor (NCR)	Family of type I transmembrane proteins which, when stimulated, trigger NK cell degranulation and cytotoxicity; most tumor-associated NCR ligands are unknown.
Neoantigen-dependent killing	Peptides arising from tumor mutations are presented to T-cells in the context of MHC-I, triggering clonal expansion of cytotoxic T-cells which specifically target tumor cells expressing the cognate neoantigen.
Neoantigen-independent killing	Cytotoxicity which does not require priming by a specific antigen; NK cell cytotoxicity is antigen-independent and therefore not restricted to tumor cells that express the cognate neoantigen.
Microsatellite instability (MSI)	Type of genetic instability arising from defective DNA mismatch repair, resulting in a hypermutated phenotype.
Tumor-infiltrating lymphocyte (TIL)	Lymphocyte which has migrated from the peripheral blood into a solid tumor; This term often refers to tumor-infiltrating cytotoxic CD8+ T-cells.
Tumor mutation burden (TMB)	Number of mutations per coding area of a tumor genome; high TMB is associated with better responses to checkpoint immunotherapy.

References

1. Eirew, P.; Steif, A.; Khattra, J.; Ha, G.; Yap, D.; Farahani, H.; Gelmon, K.; Chia, S.; Mar, C.; Wan, A.; et al. Dynamics of genomic clones in breast cancer patient xenografts at single-cell resolution. *Nature* **2015**, *518*, 422–426. [CrossRef] [PubMed]
2. Kim, T.M.; Jung, S.H.; An, C.H.; Lee, S.H.; Baek, I.P.; Kim, M.S.; Park, S.W.; Rhee, J.K.; Lee, S.H.; Chung, Y.J. Subclonal Genomic Architectures of Primary and Metastatic Colorectal Cancer Based on Intratumoral Genetic Heterogeneity. *Clin. Cancer Res.* **2015**, *21*, 4461–4472. [CrossRef]

3. Khalique, L.; Ayhan, A.; Weale, M.E.; Jacobs, I.J.; Ramus, S.J.; Gayther, S.A. Genetic intra-tumor heterogeneity in epithelial ovarian cancer and its implications for molecular diagnosis of tumors. *J. Pathol.* **2007**, *211*, 286–295. [CrossRef] [PubMed]
4. Oh, B.Y.; Shin, H.T.; Yun, J.W.; Kim, K.T.; Kim, J.; Bae, J.S.; Cho, Y.B.; Lee, W.Y.; Yun, S.H.; Park, Y.A.; et al. Intratumor heterogeneity inferred from targeted deep sequencing as a prognostic indicator. *Sci. Rep.* **2019**, *9*, 4542. [CrossRef] [PubMed]
5. Liu, G.; Zhan, X.; Dong, C.; Liu, L. Genomics alterations of metastatic and primary tissues across 15 cancer types. *Sci. Rep.* **2017**, *7*, 13262. [CrossRef] [PubMed]
6. Yang, J.; Luo, H.; Li, Y.; Li, J.; Cai, Z.; Su, X.; Dai, D.; Du, W.; Chen, T.; Chen, M. Intratumoral Heterogeneity Determines Discordant Results of Diagnostic Tests for Human Epidermal Growth Factor Receptor (HER) 2 in Gastric Cancer Specimens. *Cell Biochem. Biophys.* **2012**, *62*, 221–228. [CrossRef] [PubMed]
7. Kalikaki, A.; Voutsinaa, A.; Koutsopoulosb, A.; Pallis, A.; Trypaki, M.; Souglakos, J.; Stathopoulos, E.; Mavroudis, D.; Georgoulias, V. P3-157: Correlation of EGFR mutation status between primary tumor and metastases in NSCLC. *J. Thorac. Oncol.* **2008**, *2*, S746. [CrossRef]
8. Echeverria, G.V.; Powell, E.; Seth, S.; Ge, Z.; Carugo, A.; Bristow, C.; Peoples, M.; Robinson, F.; Qiu, H.; Shao, J.; et al. High-resolution clonal mapping of multi-organ metastasis in triple negative breast cancer. *Nat. Commun.* **2018**, *9*, 5079. [PubMed]
9. Kreso, A.; O'Brien, C.A.; Van Galen, P.; Gan, O.I.; Notta, F.; Brown, A.M.K.; Ng, K.; Jing, M.; Wienholds, E.; Dunant, C.; et al. Variable clonal repopulation dynamics influence chemotherapy response in colorectal cancer. *Science* **2013**, *339*, 543–548. [CrossRef] [PubMed]
10. Cheow, L.F.; Courtois, E.T.; Tan, Y.; Viswanathan, R.; Xing, Q.; Tan, R.Z.; Tan, D.S.W.; Robson, P.; Loh, Y.H.; Quake, S.R.; et al. Single-cell multimodal profiling reveals cellular epigenetic heterogeneity. *Nat. Methods* **2016**, *13*, 833–836. [CrossRef]
11. Henrique, R. Epigenetic Heterogeneity of High-Grade Prostatic Intraepithelial Neoplasia: Clues for Clonal Progression in Prostate Carcinogenesis. *Mol. Cancer Res.* **2006**, *4*, 1–8. [CrossRef]
12. Sigalotti, L.; Fratta, E.; Coral, S.; Tanzarella, S.; Danielli, R.; Colizzi, F.; Fonsatti, E.; Traversari, C.; Altomonte, M.; Maio, M. Intratumor Heterogeneity of Cancer/Testis Antigens Expression in Human Cutaneous Melanoma Is Methylation-Regulated and Functionally Reverted by 5-Aza-2'-deoxycytidine. *Cancer Res.* **2004**, *64*, 9167–9171. [CrossRef]
13. Hensley, C.T.; Faubert, B.; Yuan, Q.; Jin, E.; Kim, J.; Jiang, L.; Ko, B.; Skelton, R.; Loudat, L.; Wodzak, M.; et al. Metabolic Heterogeneity in Human Lung Tumors. *Cell* **2016**, *164*, 681–694. [CrossRef] [PubMed]
14. Little, S.E.; Popov, S.; Jury, A.; Bax, D.A.; Doey, L.; Al-Sarraj, S.; Jurgensmeier, J.M.; Jones, C. Receptor Tyrosine Kinase Genes Amplified in Glioblastoma Exhibit a Mutual Exclusivity in Variable Proportions Reflective of Individual Tumor Heterogeneity. *Cancer Res.* **2012**, *72*, 1614–1620. [CrossRef]
15. Colombino, M.; Capone, M.; Lissia, A.; Cossu, A.; Rubino, C.; De Giorgi, V.; Massi, D.; Fonsatti, E.; Staibano, S.; Nappi, O.; et al. BRAF/NRAS Mutation Frequencies Among Primary Tumors and Metastases in Patients with Melanoma. *J. Clin. Oncol.* **2012**, *30*, 2522–2529. [CrossRef]
16. Milo, I.; Bedora-Faure, M.; Garcia, Z.; Thibaut, R.; Périé, L.; Shakhar, G.; Deriano, L.; Bousso, P. The immune system profoundly restricts intratumor genetic heterogeneity. *Sci. Immunol.* **2018**, *3*, 29. [CrossRef] [PubMed]
17. Takeda, K.; Nakayama, M.; Hayakawa, Y.; Kojima, Y.; Ikeda, H.; Imai, N.; Ogasawara, K.; Okumura, K.; Thomas, D.M.; Smyth, M.J. IFN-γ is required for cytotoxic T cell-dependent cancer genome immunoediting. *Nat. Commun.* **2017**, *8*, 14607. [CrossRef] [PubMed]
18. Bindea, G.; Mlecnik, B.; Tosolini, M.; Kirilovsky, A.; Waldner, M.; Obenauf, A.C.; Angell, H.; Fredriksen, T.; Lafontaine, L.; Berger, A.; et al. Spatiotemporal dynamics of intratumoral immune cells reveal the immune landscape in human cancer. *Immunity* **2013**, *39*, 782–795. [CrossRef] [PubMed]
19. Gentles, A.J.; Newman, A.M.; Liu, C.L.; Bratman, S.V.; Feng, W.; Kim, D.; Nair, V.S.; Xu, Y.; Khuong, A.; Hoang, C.D.; et al. The prognostic landscape of genes and infiltrating immune cells across human cancers. *Nat. Med.* **2015**, *21*, 938–945. [CrossRef] [PubMed]
20. Doucette, T.; Rao, G.; Rao, A.; Shen, L.; Aldape, K.; Wei, J.; Dziurzynski, K.; Gilbert, M.; Heimberger, A.B. Immune Heterogeneity of Glioblastoma Subtypes: Extrapolation from the Cancer Genome Atlas. *Cancer Immunol. Res.* **2013**, *1*, 112–122. [CrossRef] [PubMed]

21. Reuben, A.; Gittelman, R.; Gao, J.; Zhang, J.; Yusko, E.C.; Wu, C.J.; Emerson, R.; Zhang, J.; Tipton, C.; Li, J.; et al. TCR Repertoire Intratumor Heterogeneity in Localized Lung Adenocarcinomas: An Association with Predicted Neoantigen Heterogeneity and Postsurgical Recurrence. *Cancer Discov.* **2017**, *7*, 12–17. [CrossRef]
22. Jiménez-Sánchez, A.; Memon, D.; Pourpe, S.; Veeraraghavan, H.; Li, Y.; Vargas, H.A.; Gill, M.B.; Park, K.J.; Zivanovic, O.; Konner, J.; et al. Heterogeneous Tumor-Immune Microenvironments among Differentially Growing Metastases in an Ovarian Cancer Patient. *Cell* **2017**, *170*, 927–938. [CrossRef] [PubMed]
23. Hu, Z.; Sun, R.; Curtis, C. A population genetics perspective on the determinants of intra-tumor heterogeneity. *Biochim. Biophys. Acta Rev. Cancer* **2017**, *1867*, 109–126. [CrossRef] [PubMed]
24. Obeid, J.M.; Hu, Y.; Erdag, G.; Leick, K.M.; Slingluff, C.L. The heterogeneity of tumor-infiltrating CD8+ T cells in metastatic melanoma distorts their quantification. *Melanoma Res.* **2017**, *27*, 211–217. [CrossRef] [PubMed]
25. Gao, Y.; Souza-Fonseca-Guimaraes, F.; Bald, T.; Ng, S.S.; Young, A.; Ngiow, S.F.; Rautela, J.; Straube, J.; Waddell, N.; Blake, S.J.; et al. Tumor immunoevasion by the conversion of effector NK cells into type 1 innate lymphoid cells. *Nat. Immunol.* **2017**, *18*, 1004–1015. [CrossRef] [PubMed]
26. Hiraoka, K.; Miyamoto, M.; Cho, Y.; Suzuoki, M.; Oshikiri, T.; Nakakubo, Y.; Itoh, T.; Ohbuchi, T.; Kondo, S.; Katoh, H. Concurrent infiltration by CD8 + T cells and CD4 + T cells is a favourable prognostic factor in non-small-cell lung carcinoma. *Br. J. Cancer* **2006**, *94*, 275–280. [CrossRef] [PubMed]
27. Leffers, N.; Gooden, M.J.M.; De Jong, R.A.; Hoogeboom, B.N.; Ten Hoor, K.A.; Hollema, H.; Boezen, H.M.; Van Der Zee, A.G.J.; Daemen, T.; Nijman, H.W. Prognostic significance of tumor-infiltrating T-lymphocytes in primary and metastatic lesions of advanced stage ovarian cancer. *Cancer Immunol. Immunother.* **2009**, *58*, 449–459. [CrossRef]
28. Naito, Y.; Saito, K.; Shiiba, K.; Ohuchi, A.; Saigenji, K.; Nagura, H.; Ohtani, H. CD8+ T cells infiltrated within cancer cell nests as a prognostic factor in human colorectal cancer. *Cancer Res.* **1998**, *58*, 3491–3494. [PubMed]
29. Camus, M.; Tosolini, M.; Mlecnik, B.; Pagè, F.; Kirilovsky, A.; Berger, A.; Costes, A.; Bindea, G.; Charoentong, P.; Bruneval, P.; et al. Coordination of Intratumoral Immune Reaction and Human Colorectal Cancer Recurrence. *Cancer Res* **2009**, *69*, 2685–2693. [CrossRef]
30. Ott, P.A.; Bang, Y.J.; Piha-Paul, S.A.; Abdul Razak, A.R.; Bennouna, J.; Soria, J.C.; Rugo, H.S.; Cohen, R.B.; O'Neil, B.H.; Mehnert, J.M.; et al. T-cell–inflamed gene-expression profile, programmed death ligand 1 expression, and tumor mutational burden predict efficacy in patients treated with pembrolizumab across 20 cancers: KEYNOTE-028. *J. Clin. Oncol.* **2019**, *37*, 318–327. [CrossRef]
31. Ji, R.R.; Chasalow, S.D.; Wang, L.; Hamid, O.; Schmidt, H.; Cogswell, J.; Alaparthy, S.; Berman, D.; Jure-Kunkel, M.; Siemers, N.O.; et al. An immune-active tumor microenvironment favors clinical response to ipilimumab. *Cancer Immunol. Immunother.* **2012**, *61*, 1019–1031. [CrossRef] [PubMed]
32. Prendergast, G.C.; Mondal, A.; Dey, S.; Laury-Kleintop, L.D.; Muller, A.J. Inflammatory Reprogramming with IDO1 Inhibitors: Turning Immunologically Unresponsive 'Cold' Tumors 'Hot'. *Trends Cancer* **2018**, *4*, 38–58. [CrossRef] [PubMed]
33. Ghiringhelli, F.; Ménard, C.; Terme, M.; Flament, C.; Taieb, J.; Chaput, N.; Puig, P.E.; Novault, S.; Escudier, B.; Vivier, E.; et al. CD4 + CD25 + regulatory T cells inhibit natural killer cell functions in a transforming growth factor–β–dependent manner. *J. Exp. Med.* **2005**, *202*, 1075–1085. [CrossRef] [PubMed]
34. Galluzzi, L.; Buqué, A.; Kepp, O.; Zitvogel, L.; Kroemer, G. Immunological Effects of Conventional Chemotherapy and Targeted Anticancer Agents. *Cancer Cell* **2015**, *28*, 690–714. [CrossRef] [PubMed]
35. Mlecnik, B.; Tosolini, M.; Kirilovsky, A.; Berger, A.; Bindea, G.; Meatchi, T.; Bruneval, P.; Trajanoski, Z.; Fridman, W.H.; Pagès, F.; et al. Histopathologic-based prognostic factors of colorectal cancers are associated with the state of the local immune reaction. *J. Clin. Oncol.* **2011**, *29*, 610–618. [CrossRef] [PubMed]
36. Mlecnik, B.; Bindea, G.; Angell, H.K.; Valge-Archer, V.; Latouche, J.B.; Maby, P.; Angelova, M.; Tougeron, D.; Church, S.E.; Lafontaine, L.; et al. Integrative Analyses of Colorectal Cancer Show Immunoscore Is a Stronger Predictor of Patient Survival Than Microsatellite Instability. *Immunity* **2016**, *44*, 698–711. [CrossRef] [PubMed]
37. Pagès, F.; Mlecnik, B.; Marliot, F.; Bindea, G.; Ou, F.S.; Bifulco, C.; Lugli, A.; Zlobec, I.; Rau, T.T.; Berger, M.D.; et al. International validation of the consensus Immunoscore for the classification of colon cancer: A prognostic and accuracy study. *Lancet* **2018**, *391*, 2128–2139. [CrossRef]
38. Gong, C.; Anders, R.A.; Zhu, Q.; Taube, J.M.; Green, B.; Cheng, W.; Bartelink, I.H.; Vicini, P.; Wang, B.; Popel, A.S. Quantitative Characterization of CD8+ T Cell Clustering and Spatial Heterogeneity in Solid Tumors. *Front. Oncol.* **2019**, *8*, 649. [CrossRef]

39. Shi, L.; Zhang, Y.; Feng, L.; Wang, L.; Rong, W.; Wu, F.; Wu, J.; Zhang, K.; Cheng, S.; Shi, L.; et al. Multi-omics study revealing the complexity and spatial heterogeneity of tumor-infiltrating lymphocytes in primary liver carcinoma. *Oncotarget* **2017**, *8*, 34844–34857. [CrossRef]
40. Heindl, A.; Sestak, I.; Naidoo, K.; Cuzick, J.; Dowsett, M.; Yuan, Y. Relevance of Spatial Heterogeneity of Immune Infiltration for Predicting Risk of Recurrence After Endocrine Therapy of ER+ Breast Cancer. *Jnci J. Natl. Cancer Inst.* **2018**, *110*, 166–175. [CrossRef]
41. Khan, A.M.; Yuan, Y. Biopsy variability of lymphocytic infiltration in breast cancer subtypes and the ImmunoSkew score. *Sci. Rep.* **2016**, *6*, 36231. [CrossRef] [PubMed]
42. Orange, J.S. Natural Killer Cell Deficiency. *Stiehm's Immune Defic.* **2014**, *132*, 765–774.
43. Miyake, S.; Suga, K.; Matsuyama, S.; Nakachi, K.; Imai, K. Natural cytotoxic activity of peripheral-blood lymphocytes and cancer incidence: An 11-year follow-up study of a general population. *Lancet* **2002**, *356*, 1795–1799.
44. Delahaye, N.F.; Rusakiewicz, S.; Martins, I.; Ménard, C.; Roux, S.; Lyonnet, L.; Paul, P.; Sarabi, M.; Chaput, N.; Semeraro, M.; et al. Alternatively spliced NKp30 isoforms affect the prognosis of gastrointestinal stromal tumors. *Nat. Med.* **2011**, *17*, 700–707. [CrossRef]
45. Gannon, P.O.; Poisson, A.O.; Delvoye, N.; Lapointe, R.; Mes-Masson, A.-M.; Saad, F. Characterization of the intra-prostatic immune cell infiltration in androgen-deprived prostate cancer patients. *J. Immunol. Methods* **2009**, *348*, 9–17. [CrossRef] [PubMed]
46. Donskov, F.; von der Maase, H. Impact of immune parameters on long-term survival in metastatic renal cell carcinoma. *J. Clin. Oncol.* **2006**, *24*, 1997–2005. [CrossRef] [PubMed]
47. Coca, S.; Perez-Piqueras, J.; Martinez, D.; Colmenarejo, A.; Saez, M.A.; Vallejo, C.; Martos, J.A.; Moreno, M. The prognostic significance of intratumoral natural killer cells in patients with colorectal carcinoma. *Cancer* **1997**, *79*, 2320–2328. [CrossRef]
48. Cursons, J.; Souza-Fonseca Guimaraes, F.; Foroutan, M.; Anderson, A.; Hollande, F.; Hediyeh-Zadeh, S.; Behren, A.; Huntington, N.D.; Davis, M.J. A gene signature predicting natural killer cell infiltration and improved survival in melanoma patients. *Cancer Immunol. Res.* **2018**, 2019. [CrossRef]
49. Ilander, M.; Olsson-Strömberg, U.; Schlums, H.; Guilhot, J.; Brück, O.; Lähteenmäki, H.; Kasanen, T.; Koskenvesa, P.; Söderlund, S.; Höglund, M.; et al. Increased proportion of mature NK cells is associated with successful imatinib discontinuation in chronic myeloid leukemia. *Leukemia* **2017**, *31*, 1108–1116. [CrossRef]
50. Saijo, N.; Ozaki, A.; Beppu, Y.; Takahashi, K.; Fujita, J.; Sasaki, Y.; Nomori, H.; Kimata, M.; Shimizu, E.; Hoshi, A. Analysis of metastatic spread and growth of tumor cells in mice with depressed natural killer activity by anti-asialo GMl antibody or anticancer agents. *J. Cancer Res. Clin. Oncol.* **1984**, *107*, 157–163. [CrossRef]
51. Yano, S.; Nishioka, Y.; Izumi, K.; Tsuruo, T.; Tanaka, T.; Miyasaka, M.; Sone, S. Novel metastasis model of human lung cancer in SCID mice depleted of NK cells. *Int. J. Cancer* **1996**, *67*, 211–217. [CrossRef]
52. Kasai, M.; Yoneda, T.; Habu, S.; Maruyama, Y.; Okumura, K.; Tokunaga, T. Okumura; Tokunaga, T. In vivo effect of anti-asialo GM1 antibody on natural killer activity. *Nature* **1981**, *291*, 334–335. [CrossRef]
53. Sathe, P.; Delconte, R.B.; Souza-Fonseca-Guimaraes, F.; Seillet, C.; Chopin, M.; Vandenberg, C.J.; Rankin, L.C.; Mielke, L.A.; Vikstrom, I.; Kolesnik, T.B.; et al. Innate immunodeficiency following genetic ablation of Mcl1 in natural killer cells. *Nat. Commun.* **2014**, *5*, 4539. [CrossRef] [PubMed]
54. Smyth, M.J.; Thia, K.Y.T.; Cretney, E.; Kelly, J.M.; Snook, M.B.; Forbes, C.A.; Scalzo, A.A. Perforin Is a Major Contributor to NK Cell Control of Tumor Metastasis. *J. Immunol.* **1999**, *162*, 6658–6662.
55. Street, S.E.A.; Cretney, E.; Smyth, M.J. Perforin and interferon-activities independently control tumor initiation, growth, and metastasis. *Blood* **2001**, *97*, 192–197. [CrossRef] [PubMed]
56. Glasner, A.; Ghadially, H.; Gur, C.; Stanietsky, N.; Tsukerman, P.; Enk, J.; Mandelboim, O. Recognition and Prevention of Tumor Metastasis by the NK Receptor NKp46/NCR1. *J. Immunol.* **2012**, *188*, 2509–2515. [CrossRef]
57. Iguchi-Manaka, A.; Kai, H.; Yamashita, Y.; Shibata, K.; Tahara-Hanaoka, S.; Honda, S.; Yasui, T.; Kikutani, H.; Shibuya, K.; Shibuya, A. Accelerated tumor growth in mice deficient in DNAM-1 receptor. *J. Exp. Med.* **2008**, *205*, 2959–2964. [CrossRef]
58. Chan, C.J.; Andrews, D.M.; McLaughlin, N.M.; Yagita, H.; Gilfillan, S.; Colonna, M.; Smyth, M.J. DNAM-1/CD155 Interactions Promote Cytokine and NK Cell-Mediated Suppression of Poorly Immunogenic Melanoma Metastases. *J. Immunol.* **2010**, *184*, 902–911. [CrossRef]

59. Takeda, K.; Hayakawa, Y.; Smyth, M.; Kayagaki, N.; Yamaguchi, N.; Kakuta, S.; Iwakura, Y.; Yagita, H.; Okumura, K. Involvement of tumor necrosis factor-related apoptosis-inducing ligand in surveillance of tumor metastasis by liver natural killer cells. *Nat. Med.* **2001**, *7*, 94–100. [CrossRef] [PubMed]
60. Donadon, M.; Hudspeth, K.; Cimino, M.; Di Tommaso, L.; Preti, M.; Tentorio, P.; Roncalli, M.; Mavilio, D.; Torzilli, G. Increased Infiltration of Natural Killer and T Cells in Colorectal Liver Metastases Improves Patient Overall Survival. *J. Gastrointest. Surg.* **2017**, *21*, 1–11. [CrossRef] [PubMed]
61. Tallerico, R.; Todaro, M.; Di Franco, S.; Maccalli, C.; Garofalo, C.; Sottile, R.; Palmieri, C.; Tirinato, L.; Pangigadde, P.N.; La Rocca, R.; et al. Human NK cells selective targeting of colon cancer-initiating cells: A role for natural cytotoxicity receptors and MHC class I molecules. *J. Immunol.* **2013**, *190*, 2381–2390. [CrossRef] [PubMed]
62. Pietra, G.; Manzini, C.; Vitale, M.; Balsamo, M.; Ognio, E.; Boitano, M.; Queirolo, P.; Moretta, L.; Mingari, M.C. Natural killer cells kill human melanoma cells with characteristics of cancer stem cells. *Int. Immunol.* **2009**, *21*, 793–801. [CrossRef] [PubMed]
63. Castriconi, R.; Daga, A.; Dondero, A.; Zona, G.; Poliani, P.L.; Melotti, A.; Griffero, F.; Marubbi, D.; Spaziante, R.; Bellora, F.; et al. NK Cells Recognize and Kill Human Glioblastoma Cells with Stem Cell-Like Properties. *J. Immunol.* **2009**, *182*, 3530–3539. [CrossRef] [PubMed]
64. Ames, E.; Canter, R.J.; Grossenbacher, S.K.; Mac, S.; Chen, M.; Smith, R.C.; Hagino, T.; Perez-Cunningham, J.; Sckisel, G.D.; Urayama, S.; et al. NK Cells Preferentially Target Tumor Cells with a Cancer Stem Cell Phenotype. *J. Immunol.* **2015**, *195*, 4010–4019. [CrossRef] [PubMed]
65. Mansfield, A.S.; Aubry, M.C.; Moser, J.C.; Harrington, S.M.; Dronca, R.S.; Park, S.S.; Dong, H. Temporal and spatial discordance of programmed cell death-ligand 1 expression and lymphocyte tumor infiltration between paired primary lesions and brain metastases in lung cancer. *Ann. Oncol.* **2016**, *27*, 1953–1958. [CrossRef]
66. Li, M.; Li, A.; Zhou, S.; Xu, Y.; Xiao, Y.; Bi, R.; Yang, W. Heterogeneity of PD-L1 expression in primary tumors and paired lymph node metastases of triple negative breast cancer. *BMC Cancer* **2018**, *18*. [CrossRef] [PubMed]
67. Linton, P.J.; Dorshkind, K. Age-related changes in lymphocyte development and function. *Nat. Immunol.* **2004**, *5*, 133–139. [CrossRef]
68. Li, T.; Yang, Y.; Hua, X.; Wang, G.; Liu, W.; Jia, C.; Tai, Y.; Zhang, Q.; Chen, G. Hepatocellular carcinoma-associated fibroblasts trigger NK cell dysfunction via PGE2 and IDO. *Cancer Lett.* **2012**, *318*, 154–161. [CrossRef]
69. Halama, N.; Braun, M.; Kahlert, C.; Spille, A.; Quack, C.; Rahbari, N.; Koch, M.; Weitz, J.; Kloor, M.; Zoernig, I.; et al. Natural Killer Cells are Scarce in Colorectal Carcinoma Tissue Despite High Levels of Chemokines and Cytokines. *Clin. Cancer Res.* **2011**, *17*, 678–689. [CrossRef]
70. Rosenberg, S.A.; Sherry, R.M.; Morton, K.E.; Scharfman, W.J.; Yang, J.C.; Topalian, S.L.; Royal, R.E.; Kammula, U.; Restifo, N.P.; Hughes, M.S.; et al. Tumor progression can occur despite the induction of very high levels of self/tumor antigen-specific CD8+ T cells in patients with melanoma. *J. Immunol.* **2005**, *175*, 6169–6176. [CrossRef]
71. Hoechst, B.; Voigtlaender, T.; Ormandy, L.; Gamrekelashvili, J.; Zhao, F.; Wedemeyer, H.; Lehner, F.; Manns, M.P.; Greten, T.F.; Korangy, F. Myeloid derived suppressor cells inhibit natural killer cells in patients with hepatocellular carcinoma via the NKp30 receptor. *Hepatology* **2009**, *50*, 799–807. [CrossRef] [PubMed]
72. Hanke, T.; Melling, N.; Simon, R.; Sauter, G.; Bokemeyer, C.; Lebok, P.; Terracciano, L.M.; Izbicki, J.R.; Marx, A.H. High intratumoral FOXP3+ T regulatory cell (Tregs) density is an independent good prognosticator in nodal negative colorectal cancer. *Int. J. Clin. Exp. Pathol.* **2015**, *8*, 8227–8235.
73. Heimberger, A.B.; Abou-Ghazal, M.; Reina-Ortiz, C.; Yang, D.S.; Sun, W.; Qiao, W.; Hiraoka, N.; Fuller, G.N. Incidence and prognostic impact of FoxP3+ regulatory T cells in human gliomas. *Clin. Cancer Res.* **2008**, *14*, 5166–5172. [CrossRef]
74. Shen, Z.; Zhou, S.; Wang, Y.; Li, R.L.; Zhong, C.; Liang, C.; Sun, Y. Higher intratumoral infiltrated Foxp3+ Treg numbers and Foxp3+/CD8+ ratio are associated with adverse prognosis in resectable gastric cancer. *J. Cancer Res. Clin. Oncol.* **2010**, *136*, 1585–1595. [CrossRef] [PubMed]
75. Li, T.; Yi, S.; Liu, W.; Jia, C.; Wang, G.; Hua, X.; Tai, Y.; Zhang, Q.; Chen, G. Colorectal carcinoma-derived fibroblasts modulate natural killer cell phenotype and antitumor cytotoxicity. *Med. Oncol.* **2013**, *30*, 663. [CrossRef] [PubMed]

76. Zhang, R.; Qi, F.; Zhao, F.; Li, G.; Shao, S.; Zhang, X.; Yuan, L.; Feng, Y. Cancer-associated fibroblasts enhance tumor-associated macrophages enrichment and suppress NK cells function in colorectal cancer. *Cell Death Dis.* **2019**, *10*, 273. [CrossRef]
77. Balsamo, M.; Scordamaglia, F.; Pietra, G.; Manzini, C.; Cantoni, C.; Boitano, M.; Queirolo, P.; Vermi, W.; Facchetti, F.; Moretta, A.; et al. Melanoma-associated fibroblasts modulate NK cell phenotype and antitumor cytotoxicity. *Proc. Natl. Acad. Sci.* **2009**, *106*, 20847–20852. [CrossRef] [PubMed]
78. West, N.R.; Kost, S.E.; Martin, S.D.; Milne, K.; Deleeuw, R.J.; Nelson, B.H.; Watson, P.H. Tumor-infiltrating FOXP3 + lymphocytes are associated with cytotoxic immune responses and good clinical outcome in oestrogen receptor-negative breast cancer. *Br. J. Cancer* **2013**, *108*, 155–162. [CrossRef] [PubMed]
79. Salama, P.; Phillips, M.; Grieu, F.; Morris, M.; Zeps, N.; Joseph, D.; Platell, C.; Iacopetta, B. Tumor-infiltrating FOXP3+ T regulatory cells show strong prognostic significance in colorectal cancer. *J. Clin. Oncol.* **2009**, *27*, 186–192. [CrossRef] [PubMed]
80. Birenda, K.; Hwang, J.J. Advances in Immunotherapy in the treatment of Colorectal Cancer. *Am. J. Hematol. Oncol.* **2017**, *13*, 4–8.
81. Peng, Y.P.; Zhang, J.J.; Liang, W.; Tu, Z.P.; Lu, Z.P.; Wei, J.S.; Jiang, K.R.; Gao, W.T.; Wu, J.L.; Xu, Z.K.; et al. Elevation of MMP-9 and IDO induced by pancreatic cancer cells mediates natural killer cell dysfunction. *Bmc Cancer* **2014**, *14*, 738. [CrossRef]
82. Song, H.; Park, H.; Kim, J.; Park, G.; Kim, Y.S.; Kim, S.M.; Kim, D.; Seo, S.K.; Lee, H.K.; Cho, D.; et al. IDO metabolite produced by EBV-transformed B cells inhibits surface expression of NKG2D in NK cells via the c-Jun N-terminal kinase (JNK) pathway. *Immunol. Lett.* **2011**, *136*, 187–193. [CrossRef]
83. Brand, A.; Singer, K.; Koehl, G.E.; Kolitzus, M.; Schoenhammer, G.; Thiel, A.; Matos, C.; Bruss, C.; Klobuch, S.; Peter, K.; et al. LDHA-Associated Lactic Acid Production Blunts Tumor Immunosurveillance by T and NK Cells. *Cell Metab.* **2016**, *24*, 657–671. [CrossRef] [PubMed]
84. Holt, D.; Ma, X.; Kundu, N.; Fulton, A. Prostaglandin E2 (PGE2) suppresses natural killer cell function primarily through the PGE2 receptor EP4. *Cancer Immunol. Immunother.* **2011**, *60*, 1577–1586. [CrossRef] [PubMed]
85. Lee, J.C.; Lee, K.; Kim, D.; Heo, D.S. Elevated TGF- 1 Secretion and Down-Modulation of NKG2D Underlies Impaired NK Cytotoxicity in Cancer Patients. *J. Immunol.* **2004**, *172*, 7335–7340. [CrossRef]
86. Laouar, Y.; Sutterwala, F.S.; Gorelik, L.; Flavell, R.A. Transforming growth factor-β controls T helper type 1 cell development through regulation of natural killer cell interferon-γ. *Nat. Immunol.* **2005**, *6*, 600–607. [CrossRef]
87. Jun, E.; Song, A.Y.; Choi, J.W.; Ko, D.H.; Kang, H.J.; Kim, S.W.; Bryceson, Y.; Kim, S.C.; Kim, H.S. Progressive impairment of NK cell cytotoxic degranulation is associated with TGF-b1 deregulation and disease progression in pancreatic cancer. *Front. Immunol.* **2019**, *10*, 1354. [CrossRef]
88. Crane, C.A.; Han, S.J.; Barry, J.J.; Ahn, B.J.; Lanier, L.L.; Parsa, A.T. TGF-β downregulates the activating receptor NKG2D on NK cells and CD8+ T cells in glioma patients. *Neuro. Oncol.* **2010**, *12*, 7–13. [CrossRef]
89. Castriconi, R.; Dondero, A.; Bellora, F.; Moretta, L.; Castellano, A.; Locatelli, F.; Corrias, M.V.; Moretta, A.; Bottino, C. Transforming growth factor 1 inhibits expression of NKp30 and NKG2D receptors: Consequences for the NK-mediated killing of dendritic cells. *Proc. Natl. Acad. Sci.* **2003**, *100*, 4120–4125. [CrossRef]
90. Balsamo, M.; Manzini, C.; Pietra, G.; Raggi, F.; Blengio, F.; Mingari, M.C.; Varesio, L.; Moretta, L.; Bosco, M.C.; Vitale, M. Hypoxia downregulates the expression of activating receptors involved in NK-cell-mediated target cell killing without affecting ADCC. *Eur. J. Immunol.* **2013**, *43*, 2756–2764. [CrossRef] [PubMed]
91. Baginska, J.; Viry, E.; Berchem, G.; Poli, A.; Noman, M.Z.; van Moer, K.; Medves, S.; Zimmer, J.; Oudin, A.; Niclou, S.P.; et al. Granzyme B degradation by autophagy decreases tumor cell susceptibility to natural killer-mediated lysis under hypoxia. *Proc. Natl. Acad. Sci.* **2013**, *110*, 17450–17455. [CrossRef] [PubMed]
92. Sceneay, J.; Chow, M.T.; Chen, A.; Halse, H.M.; Wong, C.S.F.; Andrews, D.M.; Sloan, E.K.; Parker, B.S.; Bowtell, D.D.; Smyth, M.J.; et al. Primary Tumor Hypoxia Recruits CD11b þ /Ly6C med /Ly6G þ Immune Suppressor Cells and Compromises NK Cell Cytotoxicity in the Premetastatic Niche. *Cancer Res.* **2012**, *72*, 3906–3911. [CrossRef] [PubMed]
93. Berchem, G.; Noman, M.Z.; Bosseler, M.; Paggetti, J.; Baconnais, S.; Le cam, E.; Nanbakhsh, A.; Moussay, E.; Mami-Chouaib, F.; Janji, B.; et al. Hypoxic tumor-derived microvesicles negatively regulate NK cell function by a mechanism involving TGF-β and miR23a transfer. *Oncoimmunology* **2015**, *24*, e1062968. [CrossRef] [PubMed]

94. Häusler, S.F.M.; Montalbán Del Barrio, I.; Strohschein, J.; Anoop Chandran, P.; Engel, J.B.; Hönig, A.; Ossadnik, M.; Horn, E.; Fischer, B.; Krockenberger, M.; et al. Ectonucleotidases CD39 and CD73 on OvCA cells are potent adenosine-generating enzymes responsible for adenosine receptor 2A-dependent suppression of T cell function and NK cell cytotoxicity. *Cancer Immunol. Immunother.* **2011**, *60*, 1405–1418. [CrossRef] [PubMed]
95. Young, A.; Foong Ngiow, S.; Gao, Y.; Patch, A.M.; Barkauskas, D.S.; Messaoudene, M.; Lin, G.; Coudert, J.D.; Stannard, K.A.; Zitvogel, L.; et al. Tumor Biology and Immunology A2AR Adenosine Signaling Suppresses Natural Killer Cell Maturation in the Tumor Microenvironment. *Cancer Res.* **2018**, *78*, 1003–1016. [CrossRef] [PubMed]
96. Hatfield, S.M.; Kjaergaard, J.; Lukashev, D.; Belikoff, B.; Schreiber, T.H.; Sethumadhavan, S.; Abbott, R.; Philbrook, P.; Thayer, M.; Shujia, D.; et al. Systemic oxygenation weakens the hypoxia and hypoxia inducible factor 1α-dependent and extracellular adenosine-mediated tumor protection. *J. Mol. Med.* **2014**, *92*, 1283–1292. [CrossRef] [PubMed]
97. Hatfield, S.M.; Kjaergaard, J.; Lukashev, D.; Schreiber, T.H.; Belikoff, B.; Abbott, R.; Sethumadhavan, S.; Philbrook, P.; Ko, K.; Cannici, R.; et al. Immunological mechanisms of the antitumor effects of supplemental oxygenation. *Sci. Transl. Med.* **2015**, *7*. [CrossRef] [PubMed]
98. Michiels, C.; Tellier, C.; Feron, O. Cycling hypoxia: A key feature of the tumor microenvironment. *Biochim. Biophys. Acta - Rev. Cancer* **2016**, *1866*, 76–86. [CrossRef] [PubMed]
99. Serebrovskaya, T.V.; Nikolsky, I.S.; Nikolska, V.V.; Mallet, R.T.; Ishchuk, V.A. Intermittent Hypoxia Mobilizes Hematopoietic Progenitors and Augments Cellular and Humoral Elements of Innate Immunity in Adult Men. *High Alt. Med. Biol.* **2011**, *1*, 243–252. [CrossRef]
100. Ryan, S.; Taylor, C.T.; McNicholas, W.T. Selective Activation of Inflammatory Pathways by Intermittent Hypoxia in Obstructive Sleep Apnea Syndrome. *Circulation* **2005**, *112*, 2660–2667. [CrossRef]
101. Taylor, C.T.; Kent, B.D.; Crinion, S.J.; McNicholas, W.T.; Ryan, S. Human adipocytes are highly sensitive to intermittent hypoxia induced NF-kappaB activity and subsequent inflammatory gene expression. *Biochem. Biophys. Res. Commun.* **2014**, *447*, 660–665. [CrossRef] [PubMed]
102. Martinive, P.; Defresne, F.; Bouzin, C.; Saliez, J.; Lair, F.; Grégoire, V.; Michiels, C.; Dessy, C.; Feron, O. Preconditioning of the tumor vasculature and tumor cells by intermittent hypoxia: Implications for anticancer therapies. *Cancer Res.* **2006**, *66*, 11736–11744. [CrossRef] [PubMed]
103. Ranson, T.; Vosshenrich, C.A.J.; Corcuff, E.; Richard, O.; Müller, W.; di Santo, J.P. IL-15 is an essential mediator of peripheral NK-cell homeostasis. *Blood* **2003**, *101*, 4887–4893. [CrossRef] [PubMed]
104. Huntington, N.D.; Legrand, N.; Alves, N.L.; Jaron, B.; Weijer, K.; Plet, A.; Corcuff, E.; Mortier, E.; Jacques, Y.; Spits, H.; et al. IL-15 trans-presentation promotes human NK cell development and differentiation in vivo. *J. Exp. Med.* **2008**, *206*, 25–34. [CrossRef] [PubMed]
105. Mamessier, E.; Sylvain, A.; Thibult, M.L.; Houvenaeghel, G.; Jacquemier, J.; Castellano, R.; Gonçalves, A.; André, P.; Romagné, F.; Thibault, G.; et al. Human breast cancer cells enhance self tolerance by promoting evasion from NK cell antitumor immunity. *J. Clin. Invest.* **2011**, *121*, 3609–3622. [CrossRef] [PubMed]
106. Kmiecik, J.; Poli, A.; Brons, N.H.C.; Waha, A.; Eide, G.E.; Enger, P.Ø.; Zimmer, J.; Chekenya, M. Elevated CD3+ and CD8+ tumor-infiltrating immune cells correlate with prolonged survival in glioblastoma patients despite integrated immunosuppressive mechanisms in the tumor microenvironment and at the systemic level. *J. Neuroimmunol.* **2013**, *264*, 71–83. [CrossRef]
107. Carrega, P.; Bonaccorsi, I.; Di Carlo, E.; Morandi, B.; Paul, P.; Rizzello, V.; Cipollone, G.; Navarra, G.; Mingari, M.C.; Moretta, L.; et al. CD56brightPerforinlow Noncytotoxic Human NK Cells Are Abundant in Both Healthy and Neoplastic Solid Tissues and Recirculate to Secondary Lymphoid Organs via Afferent Lymph. *J. Immunol.* **2014**, *192*, 3805–3815. [CrossRef] [PubMed]
108. Platonova, S.; Cherfils-Vicini, J.; Damotte, D.; Crozet, L.; Vieillard, V.; Validire, P.; André, P.; Dieu-Nosjean, M.C.; Alifano, M.; Régnard, J.F.; et al. Profound coordinated alterations of intratumoral NK cell phenotype and function in lung carcinoma. *Cancer Res.* **2011**, *71*, 5412–5422. [CrossRef]
109. Parodi, M.; Raggi, F.; Cangelosi, D.; Manzini, C.; Balsamo, M.; Blengio, F.; Eva, A.; Varesio, L.; Pietra, G.; Moretta, L.; et al. Hypoxia modifies the transcriptome of human NK cells, modulates their immunoregulatory profile, and influences NK cell subset migration. *Front. Immunol.* **2018**, *9*, 2358. [CrossRef]
110. Kärre, K.; Ljunggren, H.G.; Piontek, G.; Kiessling, R. Selective rejection of H-2-deficient lymphoma variants suggests alternative immune defence strategy. *Nature* **1986**, *319*, 675–678. [CrossRef]

111. Karlhofer, F.M.; Ribaudo, R.K.; Yokoyama, W.M. MHC class I alloantigen specificity of Ly-49+ IL-2-activated natural killer cells. *Nature* **1992**, *358*, 66–70. [CrossRef]
112. Horowitz, A.; Strauss-Albee, D.M.; Leipold, M.; Kubo, J.; Nemat-Gorgani, N.; Dogan, O.C.; Dekker, C.L.; Mackey, S.; Maecker, H.; Swan, G.E.; et al. Genetic and environmental determinants of human NK cell diversity revealed by mass cytometry. *Sci. Transl. Med.* **2013**, *5*. [CrossRef]
113. Martin, A.M.; Freitas, E.M.; Witt, C.S.; Christiansen, F.T. The genomic organization and evolution of the natural killer immunoglobulin-like receptor (KIR) gene cluster. *Immunogenetics* **2000**, *51*, 268–280. [CrossRef] [PubMed]
114. Cichocki, F.; Miller, J.S.; Anderson, S.K.; Bryceson, Y.T. Epigenetic regulation of NK cell differentiation and effector functions. *Front. Immunol.* **2013**, *4*, 55. [CrossRef]
115. Béziat, V.; Liu, L.L.; Malmberg, J.A.; Ivarsson, M.A.; Sohlberg, E.; Björklund, A.T.; Retière, C.; Sverremark-Ekström, E.; Traherne, J.; Ljungman, P.; et al. NK cell responses to cytomegalovirus infection lead to stable imprints in the human KIR repertoire and involve activating KIRs. *Blood* **2013**, *121*, 2678–2688. [CrossRef] [PubMed]
116. Debre, P.; Petitdemange, C.; Becquart, P.; Wauquier, N.; Be, V.; Leroy, E.M.; Vieillard, V.; Béziat, V.; Debré, P.; Leroy, E.M.; et al. Unconventional repertoire profile is imprinted during acute chikungunya infection for natural killer cells polarization toward cytotoxicity. *PLoS Pathog.* **2011**, *7*, e1002268.
117. Charoudeh, H.N.; Terszowski, G.; Czaja, K.; Gonzalez, A.; Schmitter, K.; Stern, M. Modulation of the natural killer cell KIR repertoire by cytomegalovirus infection. *Eur. J. Immunol.* **2013**, *43*, 480–487. [CrossRef] [PubMed]
118. Middleton, D.; Gonzelez, F. The extensive polymorphism of KIR genes. *Immunology* **2010**, *129*, 8–19. [CrossRef]
119. Ruggeri, L.; Capanni, M.; Casucci, M.; Volpi, I.; Tosti, A.; Perruccio, K.; Urbani, E.; Negrin, R.S.; Martelli, M.F.; Velardi, A. Role of natural killer cell alloreactivity in HLA-mismatched hematopoietic stem cell transplantation. *Blood* **1999**, *94*, 333–339.
120. Giebel, S.; Locatelli, F.; Lamparelli, T.; Velardi, A.; Davies, S.; Frumento, G.; Maccario, R.; Bonetti, F.; Wojnar, J.; Martinetti, M.; et al. Survival advantage with KIR ligand incompatibility in hematopoietic stem cell transplantation from unrelated donors. *Blood* **2003**, *2*, 814–819. [CrossRef]
121. Pfeiffer, M.; Schumm, M.; Feuchtinger, T.; Dietz, K.; Handgretinger, R.; Lang, P. Intensity of HLA class I expression and KIR-mismatch determine NK-cell mediated lysis of leukaemic blasts from children with acute lymphatic leukaemia. *Br. J. Haematol.* **2007**, *138*, 97–100. [CrossRef] [PubMed]
122. Delgado, D.C.; Hank, J.A.; Kolesar, J.; Lorentzen, D.; Gan, J.; Seo, S.; Kim, K.; Shusterman, S.; Gillies, S.D.; Reisfeld, R.A.; et al. Genotypes of NK Cell KIR Receptors, Their Ligands, and Fc Receptors in the Response of Neuroblastoma Patients to Hu14.18-IL2 Immunotherapy. *Cancer Res.* **2010**, *70*, 9554–9561. [CrossRef] [PubMed]
123. Erbe, A.K.; Wang, W.; Carmichael, L.; Kim, K.M.; Mendonca, E.A.; Song, Y.; Hess, D.; Reville, P.K.; London, W.B.; Naranjo, A.; et al. Neuroblastoma patients' KIR and KIR-ligand genotypes influence clinical outcome for dinutuximab-based immunotherapy: A report from the children's oncology group. *Clin. Cancer Res.* **2018**, *24*, 189–196. [CrossRef] [PubMed]
124. Semeraro, M.; Rusakiewicz, S.; Minard-Colin, V.; Delahaye, N.F.; Enot, D.; Vély, F.; Marabelle, A.; Papoular, B.; Piperoglou, C.; Ponzoni, M.; et al. Clinical impact of the NKp30/B7-H6 axis in high-risk neuroblastoma patients. *Sci. Transl. Med.* **2015**, *7*, ra55–ra283. [CrossRef] [PubMed]
125. Rocca, Y.S.; Roberti, M.P.; Arriaga, J.M.; Amat, M.; Bruno, L.; Pampena, M.B.; Huertas, E.; Loria, F.S.; Pairola, A.; Bianchini, M.; et al. Altered phenotype in peripheral blood and tumor-associated NK cells from colorectal cancer patients. *Innate Immun.* **2013**, *19*, 76–85. [CrossRef] [PubMed]
126. Costello, R.T.; Sivori, S.; Marcenaro, E.; Lafage-Pochitaloff, M.; Mozziconacci, M.J.; Reviron, D.; Gastaut, J.A.; Pende, D.; Olive, D.; Moretta, A. Defective expression and function of natural killer cell-triggering receptors in patients with acute myeloid leukemia. *Blood* **2002**, *99*, 3661–3667. [CrossRef] [PubMed]
127. Schleypen, J.S.; Von Geldern, M.; Weiß, E.H.; Kotzias, N.; Rohrmann, K.; Schendel, D.J.; Falk, C.S.; Pohla, H. Renal cell carcinoma-infiltrating natural killer cells express differential repertoires of activating and inhibitory receptors and are inhibited by specific HLA class I allotypes. *Int. J. Cancer* **2003**, *106*, 905–912. [CrossRef]

128. Sun, C.; Xu, J.; Huang, Q.; Huang, M.; Wen, H.; Zhang, C.; Wang, J.; Song, J.; Zheng, M.; Sun, H.; et al. High NKG2A expression contributes to NK cell exhaustion and predicts a poor prognosis of patients with liver cancer. *Oncoimmunology* **2017**, *6*. [CrossRef]
129. Reiners, K.S.; Topolar, D.; Henke, A.; Simhadri, V.R.; Kessler, J.; Sauer, M.; Bessler, M.; Hansen, H.P.; Tawadros, S.; Herling, M.; et al. Soluble ligands for NK cell receptors promote evasion of chronic lymphocytic leukemia cells from NK cell anti-tumor activity. *Blood* **2013**, *121*, 3658–3665. [CrossRef]
130. Binici, J.; Hartmann, J.; Herrmann, J.; Schreiber, C.; Beyer, S.; Güler, G.; Vogel, V.; Tumulka, F.; Abele, R.; Mäntele, W.; et al. A soluble fragment of the tumor antigen BCL2-associated athanogene 6 (BAG-6) is essential and sufficient for inhibition of NKp30 receptor-dependent cytotoxicity of natural killer cells. *J. Biol. Chem.* **2013**, *288*, 34295–34303. [CrossRef]
131. Schlecker, E.; Fiegler, N.; Arnold, A.; Altevogt, P.; Rose-John, S.; Moldenhauer, G.; Sucker, A.; Paschen, A.; Von Strandmann, E.P.; Textor, S.; et al. Metalloprotease-mediated tumor cell shedding of B7-H6, the ligand of the natural killer cell-activating receptor NKp30. *Cancer Res.* **2014**, *74*, 3429–3440. [CrossRef] [PubMed]
132. Klein, K.; Wang, T.; Lander, E.S.; Altfeld, M.; Garcia-Beltran, W.F. Applying CRISPR-based genetic screens to identify drivers of tumor-cell sensitivity towards NK-cell attack. *bioRxiv* **2019**. [CrossRef]
133. Groh, V.; Wu, J.; Yee, C.; Spies, T. Tumor-derived soluble MIC ligands impair expression of NKG2D and T-cell activation. *Nature* **2002**, *419*, 734–738. [CrossRef] [PubMed]
134. Steinle, A.; Wu, J.D.; Higgins, L.M.; Cosman, D.; Plymate, S.R.; Haugk, K. Prevalent expression of the immunostimulatory MHC class I chain–related molecule is counteracted by shedding in prostate cancer. *J. Clin. Invest.* **2008**, *114*, 560–568.
135. Deng, W.; Gowen, B.G.; Zhang, L.; Wang, L.; Lau, S.; Iannello, A.; Xu, J.; Rovis, T.L.; Xiong, N.; Raulet, D.H. A shed NKG2D ligand that promotes natural killer cell activation and tumor rejection. *Science* **2015**, *348*, 136–139. [CrossRef] [PubMed]
136. Pardoll, D.M. The blockade of immune checkpoints in cancer immunotherapy. *Nat. Rev. Cancer* **2012**, *12*, 252–264. [CrossRef] [PubMed]
137. Llosa, N.J.; Cruise, M.; Tam, A.; Wicks, E.C.; Hechenbleikner, E.M.; Taube, J.M.; Blosser, R.L.; Fan, H.; Wang, H.; Luber, B.S.; et al. The vigorous immune microenvironment of microsatellite instable colon cancer is balanced by multiple counter-inhibitory checkpoints. *Cancer Discov.* **2015**, *5*, 43–51. [CrossRef] [PubMed]
138. Shi, S.J.; Wang, L.J.; Wang, G.D.; Guo, Z.Y.; Wei, M.; Meng, Y.L.; Yang, A.G.; Wen, W.H. B7-H1 Expression Is Associated with Poor Prognosis in Colorectal Carcinoma and Regulates the Proliferation and Invasion of HCT116 Colorectal Cancer Cells. *PLoS ONE* **2013**, *8*, e76012. [CrossRef] [PubMed]
139. Mu, C.Y.; Huang, J.A.; Chen, Y.; Chen, C.; Zhang, X.G. High expression of PD-L1 in lung cancer may contribute to poor prognosis and tumor cells immune escape through suppressing tumor infiltrating dendritic cells maturation. *Med. Oncol.* **2011**, *28*, 682–688. [CrossRef] [PubMed]
140. Muenst, S.; Schaerli, A.R.; Gao, F.; Däster, S.; Trella, E.; Droeser, R.A.; Muraro, M.G.; Zajac, P.; Zanetti, R.; Gillanders, W.E.; et al. Expression of programmed death ligand 1 (PD-L1) is associated with poor prognosis in human breast cancer. *Breast Cancer Res. Treat.* **2014**, *146*, 15–24. [CrossRef] [PubMed]
141. Nakanishi, J.; Wada, Y.; Matsumoto, K.; Azuma, M.; Kikuchi, K.; Ueda, S. Overexpression of B7-H1 (PD-L1) significantly associates with tumor grade and postoperative prognosis in human urothelial cancers. *Cancer Immunol. Immunother.* **2007**, *56*, 1173–1182. [CrossRef] [PubMed]
142. Hargadon, K.M.; Johnson, C.E.; Williams, C.J. Immune checkpoint blockade therapy for cancer: An overview of FDA-approved immune checkpoint inhibitors. *Int. Immunopharmacol.* **2018**, *62*, 29–39. [CrossRef]
143. Patel, S.P.; Kurzrock, R. PD-L1 Expression as a Predictive Biomarker in Cancer Immunotherapy. *Mol. Cancer Ther.* **2015**, *14*, 847–856. [CrossRef]
144. Kleinovink, J.W.; Marijt, K.A.; Schoonderwoerd, M.J.A.; van Hall, T.; Ossendorp, F.; Fransen, M.F. PD-L1 expression on malignant cells is no prerequisite for checkpoint therapy. *Oncoimmunology* **2017**, *6*. [CrossRef] [PubMed]
145. Shen, X.; Zhao, B. Efficacy of PD-1 or PD-L1 inhibitors and PD-L1 expression status in cancer: Meta-analysis. *BMJ* **2018**. [CrossRef] [PubMed]
146. McLaughlin, J.; Han, G.; Schalper, K.A.; Carvajal-Hausdorf, D.; Pelekanou, V.; Rehman, J.; Velcheti, V.; Herbst, R.; LoRusso, P.; Rimm, D.L. Quantitative assessment of the heterogeneity of PD-L1 expression in non-small-cell lung cancer. *JAMA Oncol* **2016**, *2*, 46–54. [CrossRef]

147. Ilie, M.; Long-Mira, E.; Bence, C.; Butori, C.; Lassalle, S.; Bouhlel, L.; Fazzalari, L.; Zahaf, K.; Lalvée, S.; Washetine, K.; et al. Comparative study of the PD-L1 status between surgically resected specimens and matched biopsies of NSCLC patients reveal major discordances: A potential issue for anti-PD-L1 therapeutic strategies. *Ann. Oncol.* **2016**, *27*, 147–153. [CrossRef]
148. Soriani, A.; Zingoni, A.; Cerboni, C.; Iannitto, M.L.; Ricciardi, M.R.; Di Gialleonardo, V.; Cippitelli, M.; Fionda, C.; Petrucci, M.T.; Guarini, A.; et al. ATM-ATR dependent up-regulation of DNAM-1 and NKG2D ligands on multiple myeloma cells by therapeutic agents results in enhanced NK cell susceptibility and is associated with a senescent phenotype. *Blood* **2009**, *113*, 3503–3511. [CrossRef]
149. Siew, Y.Y.; Neo, S.Y.; Yew, H.C.; Lim, S.W.; Ng, Y.C.; Lew, S.M.; Seetoh, W.G.; Seow, S.V.; Koh, H.L. Oxaliplatin regulates expression of stress ligands in ovarian cancer cells and modulates their susceptibility to natural killer cell-mediated cytotoxicity. *Int. Immunol.* **2015**, *27*, 621–632. [CrossRef] [PubMed]
150. Guillerey, C.; Huntington, N.D.; Smyth, M.J. Targeting natural killer cells in cancer immunotherapy. *Nat. Immunol.* **2016**, *17*, 1025–1036. [CrossRef]
151. Blake, S.J.; Stannard, K.; Liu, J.; Allen, S.; Yong, M.C.R.; Mittal, D.; Aguilera, A.R.; Miles, J.J.; Lutzky, V.P.; de Andrade, L.F.; et al. Suppression of metastases using a new lymphocyte checkpoint target for cancer immunotherapy. *Cancer Discov.* **2016**, *4*, 446–459. [CrossRef] [PubMed]
152. Fuchs, A.; Cella, M.; Giurisato, E.; Shaw, A.S.; Colonna, M. Cutting edge: CD96 (tactile) promotes NK cell-target cell adhesion by interacting with the poliovirus receptor (CD155). *J. Immunol.* **2004**, *172*, 3994–3998. [CrossRef] [PubMed]
153. Goodman, A.M.; Kato, S.; Bazhenova, L.; Patel, S.P.; Frampton, G.M.; Miller, V.; Stephens, P.J.; Daniels, G.A.; Kurzrock, R. Tumor Mutational Burden as an Independent Predictor of Response to Immunotherapy in Diverse Cancers. *Mol. Cancer* **2017**, *16*, 2598–2608. [CrossRef] [PubMed]
154. Rizvi, N.A.; Hellmann, M.D.; Snyder, A.; Kvistborg, P.; Makarov, V.; Havel, J.J.; Lee, W.; Yuan, J.; Wong, P.; Ho, T.S.; et al. Cancer immunology. Mutational landscape determines sensitivity to PD-1 blockade in non-small cell lung cancer. *Science* **2015**, *348*, 124–128. [CrossRef] [PubMed]
155. Yarchoan, M.; Hopkins, A.; Jaffee, E.M. Tumor Mutational Burden and Response Rate to PD-1 Inhibition. *N. Engl. J. Med.* **2017**, *377*, 2500–2501. [CrossRef] [PubMed]
156. Kaufman, H.L.; Russell, J.S.; Hamid, O.; Bhatia, S.; Terheyden, P.; D'Angelo, S.P.; Shih, K.C.; Lebbé, C.; Milella, M.; Brownell, I.; et al. Updated efficacy of avelumab in patients with previously treated metastatic Merkel cell carcinoma after ≥1 year of follow-up: JAVELIN Merkel 200, a phase 2 clinical trial. *J. Immunother. Cancer* **2018**, *6*. [CrossRef] [PubMed]
157. Dudley, J.C.; Lin, M.T.; Le, D.T.; Eshleman, J.R. Microsatellite Instability as a Biomarker for PD-1 Blockade. *Clin. Cancer Res.* **2016**, *22*, 813–820. [CrossRef]
158. Le, D.T.; Durham, J.N.; Smith, K.N.; Wang, H.; Bartlett, B.R.; Aulakh, L.K.; Lu, S.; Kemberling, H.; Wilt, C.; Luber, B.S.; et al. Mismatch repair deficiency predicts response of solid tumors to PD-1 blockade. *Science* **2017**, *357*, 409–413. [CrossRef]
159. Timmermann, B.; Kerick, M.; Roehr, C.; Fischer, A.; Isau, M.; Boerno, S.T.; Wunderlich, A.; Barmeyer, C.; Seemann, P.; Koenig, J.; et al. Somatic Mutation Profiles of MSI and MSS Colorectal Cancer Identified by Whole Exome Next Generation Sequencing and Bioinformatics Analysis. *PLoS ONE* **2010**, *5*. [CrossRef]
160. Germano, G.; Lamba, S.; Rospo, G.; Barault, L.; Magri, A.; Maione, F.; Russo, M.; Crisafulli, G.; Bartolini, A.; Lerda, G.; et al. Inactivation of DNA repair triggers neoantigen generation and impairs tumor growth. *Nature* **2017**, *552*, 1–5. [CrossRef]
161. Choudhury, N.J.; Kiyotani, K.; Yap, K.L.; Campanile, A.; Antic, T.; Yew, P.Y.; Steinberg, G.; Park, J.H.; Nakamura, Y.; O'Donnell, P.H. Low T-cell Receptor Diversity, High Somatic Mutation Burden, and High Neoantigen Load as Predictors of Clinical Outcome in Muscle-invasive Bladder Cancer. *Eur. Urol. Focus* **2016**, *2*, 445–452. [CrossRef] [PubMed]
162. Miller, A.; Asmann, Y.; Cattaneo, L.; Braggio, E.; Keats, J.; Auclair, D.; Lonial, S.; Russell, S.J.; Stewart, A.K. High somatic mutation and neoantigen burden are correlated with decreased progression-free survival in multiple myeloma. *Blood Cancer J.* **2017**, *7*. [CrossRef] [PubMed]
163. Lauss, M.; Donia, M.; Harbst, K.; Andersen, R.; Mitra, S.; Rosengren, F.; Salim, M.; Vallon-Christersson, J.; Törngren, T.; Kvist, A.; et al. Mutational and putative neoantigen load predict clinical benefit of adoptive T cell therapy in melanoma. *Nat. Commun.* **2017**, *8*. [CrossRef] [PubMed]

164. Strickland, K.C.; Howitt, B.E.; Shukla, S.A.; Rodig, S.; Ritterhouse, L.L.; Liu, J.F.; Garber, J.E.; Chowdhury, D.; Wu, C.J.; D'Andrea, A.D.; et al. Association and prognostic significance of BRCA1/2-mutation status with neoantigen load, number of tumor-infiltrating lymphocytes and expression of PD-1/PD-L1 in high grade serous ovarian cancer. *Oncotarget* **2016**, *7*, 13587–13598. [CrossRef] [PubMed]
165. Coulie, P.G.; Lehmann, F.; Lethe, B.; Herman, J.; Lurquin, C.; Andrawiss, M.; Boon, T. A mutated intron sequence codes for an antigenic peptide recognized by cytolytic T lymphocytes on a human melanoma. *Proc. Natl. Acad. Sci.* **2006**, *92*, 7976–7980. [CrossRef]
166. Takenoyama, M.; Baurain, J.F.; Yasuda, M.; So, T.; Sugaya, M.; Hanagiri, T.; Sugio, K.; Yasumoto, K.; Boon, T.; Coulie, P.G. A point mutation in the NFYC gene generates an antigenic peptide recognized by autologous cytolytic T lymphocytes on a human squamous cell lung carcinoma. *Int. J. Cancer* **2006**, *118*, 1992–1997. [CrossRef] [PubMed]
167. Lennerz, V.; Fatho, M.; Gentilini, C.; Frye, R.A.; Lifke, A.; Ferel, D.; Wolfel, C.; Huber, C.; Wolfel, T. The response of autologous T cells to a human melanoma is dominated by mutated neoantigens. *Proc. Natl. Acad. Sci. USA* **2005**, *102*, 16013–16018. [CrossRef]
168. Jia, Q.; Wu, W.; Wang, Y.; Alexander, P.B.; Sun, C.; Gong, Z.; Cheng, J.N.; Sun, H.; Guan, Y.; Xia, X.; et al. Local mutational diversity drives intratumoral immune heterogeneity in non-small cell lung cancer. *Nat. Commun.* **2018**, *9*, 5361. [CrossRef]
169. McGranahan, N.; Furness, A.J.S.; Rosenthal, R.; Ramskov, S.; Lyngaa, R.; Saini, S.K.; Jamal-Hanjani, M.; Wilson, G.A.; Birkbak, N.J.; Hiley, C.T.; et al. Clonal neoantigens elicit T cell immunoreactivity and sensitivity to immune checkpoint blockade. *Science* **2016**, *351*, 1463–1469. [CrossRef] [PubMed]
170. Türeci, Ö.; Vormehr, M.; Diken, M.; Kreiter, S.; Huber, C.; Sahin, U. Targeting the heterogeneity of cancer with individualized neoepitope vaccines. *Clin. Cancer Res.* **2016**, *22*, 1885–1896. [CrossRef] [PubMed]
171. Charoentong, P.; Finotello, F.; Angelova, M.; Mayer, C.; Efremova, M.; Rieder, D.; Hackl, H.; Trajanoski, Z. Pan-cancer Immunogenomic Analyses Reveal Genotype-Immunophenotype Relationships and Predictors of Response to Checkpoint Blockade. *Cell Rep.* **2017**, *18*, 248–262. [CrossRef] [PubMed]
172. Tran, E.; Robbins, P.F.; Rosenberg, S.A.; Author, N.I. Final common pathway' of human cancer immunotherapy: Targeting random somatic mutations A brief survey of non-mutant tumor antigens HHS Public Access Author manuscript. *Nat Immunol.* **2017**, *18*, 255–262. [CrossRef] [PubMed]
173. Mcgranahan, N.; Swanton, C. Review Clonal Heterogeneity and Tumor Evolution: Past, Present, and the Future. *Cell* **2017**, *168*, 613–628. [CrossRef] [PubMed]
174. Angelova, M.; Charoentong, P.; Hackl, H.; Fischer, M.L.; Snajder, R.; Krogsdam, A.M.; Waldner, M.J.; Bindea, G.; Mlecnik, B.; Galon, J.; et al. Characterization of the immunophenotypes and antigenomes of colorectal cancers reveals distinct tumor escape mechanisms and novel targets for immunotherapy. *Genome Biol.* **2015**, *16*, 64. [CrossRef] [PubMed]
175. Brown, S.D.; Warren, R.L.; Gibb, E.A.; Martin, S.D.; Spinelli, J.J.; Nelson, B.H.; Holt, R.A. Neo-antigens predicted by tumor genome meta-analysis correlate with increased patient survival. *Genome Res.* **2014**, *24*, 743–750. [CrossRef] [PubMed]
176. Łuksza, M.; Riaz, N.; Makarov, V.; Balachandran, V.P.; Hellmann, M.D.; Solovyov, A.; Rizvi, N.A.; Merghoub, T.; Levine, A.J.; Chan, T.A.; et al. A neoantigen fitness model predicts tumor response to checkpoint blockade immunotherapy. *Nature* **2017**, *551*, 517–520. [CrossRef] [PubMed]
177. Balachandran, V.P.; Luksza, M.; Zhao, J.N.; Makarov, V.; Moral, J.A.; Remark, R.; Herbst, B.; Askan, G.; Bhanot, U.; Senbabaoglu, Y.; et al. Identification of unique neoantigen qualities in long-term survivors of pancreatic cancer. *Nature* **2017**, *551*, S12–S16. [CrossRef] [PubMed]
178. Akers, S.N.; Odunsi, K.; Karpf, A.R. Regulation of cancer germline antigen gene expression: Implications for cancer immunotherapy. *Future Oncol.* **2010**, *6*, 717–732. [CrossRef] [PubMed]
179. Kerkar, S.P.; Wang, Z.F.; Lasota, J.; Park, T.; Patel, K.; Groh, E.; Rosenberg, S.A.; Miettinen, M.M. MAGE-A is more highly expressed than NY-ESO-1 in a systematic immunohistochemical analysis of 3668 cases. *J. Immunother.* **2016**, *39*, 181–187. [CrossRef] [PubMed]
180. Johnson, L.A.; Morgan, R.A.; Dudley, M.E.; Cassard, L.; Yang, J.C.; Hughes, M.S.; Kammula, U.S.; Royal, R.E.; Sherry, R.M.; Wunderlich, J.R.; et al. Gene therapy with human and mouse T-cell receptors mediates cancer regression and targets normal tissues expressing cognate antigen. *Blood* **2009**, *114*, 535–546. [CrossRef] [PubMed]

181. Parkhurst, M.R.; Yang, J.C.; Langan, R.C.; Dudley, M.E.; Nathan, D.A.N.; Feldman, S.A.; Davis, J.L.; Morgan, R.A.; Merino, M.J.; Sherry, R.M.; et al. T cells targeting carcinoembryonic antigen can mediate regression of metastatic colorectal cancer but induce severe transient colitis. *Mol. Ther.* **2011**, *19*, 620–626. [CrossRef] [PubMed]

182. Garrido, F.; Algarra, I. MHC antigens and tumor escape from immune surveillance. *Adv. Cancer Res.* **2001**, *83*, 117–158. [PubMed]

183. Patel, S.J.; Sanjana, N.E.; Kishton, R.J.; Eidizadeh, A.; Vodnala, S.K.; Cam, M.; Gartner, J.J.; Jia, L.; Steinberg, S.M.; Yamamoto, T.N.; et al. Identification of essential genes for cancer immunotherapy. *Nature* **2017**, *548*, 537–542. [CrossRef] [PubMed]

184. Lopez-Soto, A.; Huergo-Zapico, L.; Galvan, J.A.; Rodrigo, L.; de Herreros, A.G.; Astudillo, A.; Gonzalez, S. Epithelial-Mesenchymal Transition Induces an Antitumor Immune Response Mediated by NKG2D Receptor. *J. Immunol.* **2013**, *190*, 4408–4419. [CrossRef] [PubMed]

185. Ruggeri, L. Effectiveness of Donor Natural Killer Cell Alloreactivity in Mismatched Hematopoietic Transplants. *Science* **2002**, *295*, 2097–2100. [CrossRef] [PubMed]

186. Ruggeri, L.; Mancusi, A.; Burchielli, E.; Capanni, M.; Carotti, A.; Aloisi, T.; Aversa, F.; Martelli, M.F.; Velardi, A. NK cell alloreactivity and allogeneic hematopoietic stem cell transplantation. *Blood Cells Mol. Dis.* **2008**, *40*, 84–90. [CrossRef] [PubMed]

187. André, P.; Denis, C.; Soulas, C.; Bourbon-Caillet, C.; Lopez, J.; Arnoux, T.; Bléry, M.; Bonnafous, C.; Gauthier, L.; Morel, A.; et al. Anti-NKG2A mAb Is a Checkpoint Inhibitor that Promotes Anti-Tumor Immunity by Unleashing Both T and NK Cells. *Cell* **2018**, *175*, 1731–1743. [CrossRef]

188. Vey, N.; Karlin, L.; Sadot-Lebouvier, S.; Broussais, F.; Berton-Rigaud, D.; Rey, J.; Charbonnier, A.; Marie, D.; André, P.; Paturel, C.; et al. A phase 1 study of lirilumab (antibody against killer immunoglobulin-like receptor antibody KIR2D; IPH2102) in patients with solid tumors and hematologic malignancies. *Oncotarget* **2018**, *9*, 17675–17688. [CrossRef]

189. Romanski, A.; Uherek, C.; Bug, G.; Seifried, E.; Klingemann, H.; Wels, W.S.; Ottmann, O.G.; Tonn, T. CD19-CAR engineered NK-92 cells are sufficient to overcome NK cell resistance in B-cell malignancies. *J. Cell. Mol. Med.* **2016**, *20*, 1287–1294. [CrossRef]

190. Liu, E.; Tong, Y.; Dotti, G.; Shaim, H.; Savoldo, B.; Mukherjee, M.; Orange, J.; Wan, X.; Lu, X.; Reynolds, A.; et al. Cord blood NK cells engineered to express IL-15 and a CD19-targeted CAR show long-term persistence and potent antitumor activity. *Leukemia* **2018**, *32*, 520–531. [CrossRef]

191. Chu, J.; Deng, Y.; Benson, D.M.; He, S.; Hughes, T.; Zhang, J.; Peng, Y.; Mao, H.; Yi, L.; Ghoshal, K.; et al. CS1-specific chimeric antigen receptor (CAR)-engineered natural killer cells enhance in vitro and in vivo antitumor activity against human multiple myeloma. *Leukemia* **2014**, *28*, 917–927. [CrossRef] [PubMed]

192. Chen, X.; Han, J.; Chu, J.; Zhang, L.; Zhang, J.; Chen, C.; Chen, L.; Wang, Y.; Wang, H.; Yi, L.; et al. A combinational therapy of EGFR-CAR NK cells and oncolytic herpes simplex virus 1 for breast cancer brain metastases. *Oncotarget* **2006**, *7*, 27764–27777. [CrossRef] [PubMed]

193. Han, J.; Chu, J.; Keung Chan, W.; Zhang, J.; Wang, Y.; Cohen, J.B.; Victor, A.; Meisen, W.H.; Kim, S.H.; Grandi, P.; et al. CAR-engineered NK cells targeting wild-type EGFR and EGFRvIII enhance killing of glioblastoma and patient-derived glioblastoma stem cells. *Sci. Rep.* **2015**, *5*. [CrossRef] [PubMed]

194. Gleason, M.K.; Ross, J.A.; Warlick, E.D.; Lund, T.C.; Verneris, M.R.; Wiernik, A.; Spellman, S.; Haagenson, M.D.; Lenvik, A.J.; Litzow, M.R.; et al. CD16xCD33 bispecific killer cell engager (BiKE) activates NK cells against primary MDS and MDSC CD33+ targets. *Blood* **2014**, *123*, 3016–3026. [CrossRef] [PubMed]

195. Vallera, D.A.; Zhang, B.; Gleason, M.K.; Oh, S.; Weiner, L.M.; Kaufman, D.S.; McCullar, V.; Miller, J.S.; Verneris, M.R. Heterodimeric bispecific single-chain variable-fragment antibodies against EpCAM and CD16 induce effective antibody-dependent cellular cytotoxicity against human carcinoma cells. *Cancer Biother. Radiopharm.* **2013**, *28*, 274–282. [CrossRef]

196. Vallera, D.A.; Felices, M.; McElmurry, R.; McCullar, V.; Zhou, X.; Schmohl, J.U.; Zhang, B.; Lenvik, A.J.; Panoskaltsis-Mortari, A.; Verneris, M.R.; et al. IL15 Trispecific Killer Engagers (TriKE) Make Natural Killer Cells Specific to CD33+Targets while Also Inducing Persistence, in Vivo Expansion, and Enhanced Function. *Clin. Cancer Res.* **2016**, *22*, 3440–3450. [CrossRef]

197. Tal, Y.; Yaakobi, S.; Horovitz-Fried, M.; Safyon, E.; Rosental, B.; Porgador, A.; Cohen, C.J. An NCR1-based chimeric receptor endows T-cells with multiple anti-tumor specificities. *Oncotarget* **2014**, *5*, 10949–10958. [CrossRef]

198. Eisenberg, V.; Shamalov, K.; Meir, S.; Hoogi, S.; Sarkar, R.; Pinker, S.; Markel, G.; Porgador, A.; Cohen, C.J. Targeting Multiple Tumors Using T-Cells Engineered to Express a Natural Cytotoxicity Receptor 2-Based Chimeric Receptor. *Front. Immunol.* **2017**, *29*. [CrossRef]
199. Zhang, T.; Wu, M.; Sentman, C.L. An NKp30-Based Chimeric Antigen Receptor Promotes T Cell Effector Functions and Antitumor Efficacy In Vivo. *J. Immunol.* **2012**, *189*, 2290–2299. [CrossRef]
200. Arai, S.; Meagher, R.; Swearingen, M.; Myint, H.; Rich, E.; Martinson, J.; Klingemann, H. Infusion of the allogeneic cell line NK-92 in patients with advanced renal cell cancer or melanoma: A phase I trial. *Cytotherapy* **2008**, *10*, 625–632. [CrossRef]
201. Tonn, T.; Schwabe, D.; Klingemann, HG.; Becker, S.; Esser, R.; Koehl, U.; Suttorp, M.; Seifried, E.; Ottmann, OG.; Bug, G. Treatment of patients with advanced cancer with the natural killer cell line NK-92. *Cytotherapy* **2013**, *15*, 1563–1570. [CrossRef]

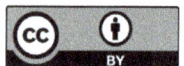

© 2019 by the authors. Licensee MDPI, Basel, Switzerland. This article is an open access article distributed under the terms and conditions of the Creative Commons Attribution (CC BY) license (http://creativecommons.org/licenses/by/4.0/).

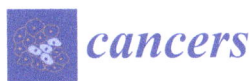

Review

The Immune Microenvironment of Breast Cancer Progression

Helen Tower [1], Meagan Ruppert [1] and Kara Britt [1,2,*]

1. Breast Cancer Risk and Prevention, Peter MacCallum Cancer Centre, 305 Grattan St, Melbourne, Victoria, VIC 3000, Australia; helen.m.tower@gmail.com (H.T.); Meagan.Ruppert@petermac.org (M.R.)
2. The Sir Peter MacCallum Department of Oncology, University of Melbourne, Parkville, Victoria, VIC 3000, Australia
* Correspondence: Kara.Britt@petermac.org

Received: 5 July 2019; Accepted: 4 September 2019; Published: 16 September 2019

Abstract: Inflammation is now recognized as a hallmark of cancer. Genetic changes in the cancer cell are accepted as the match that lights the fire, whilst inflammation is seen as the fuel that feeds the fire. Once inside the tumour, the immune cells secrete cytokines that kick-start angiogenesis to ferry in much-needed oxygen and nutrients that encourage the growth of tumours. There is now irrefutable data demonstrating that the immune contexture of breast tumours can influence growth and metastasis. A higher immune cell count in invasive breast cancer predicts prognosis and response to chemotherapy. We are beginning now to define the specific innate and adaptive immune cells present in breast cancer and their role not just in the progression of invasive disease, but also in the development of pre-invasive lesions and their transition to malignant tumours. This review article focusses on the immune cells present in early stage breast cancer and their relationship with the immunoediting process involved in tumour advancement.

Keywords: breast cancer; immune microenvironment; DCIS; ADH

1. Introduction

The immune system protects the host from pathogens and toxic, allergenic or foreign substances. It is broadly classified into two lines of defence: innate immunity and adaptive immunity. Innate immunity is comprised of the initial immune response, occurring within hours of encountering a foreign antigen, and is antigen-independent (non-specific). On the other hand, adaptive immunity is antigen-dependent and pathogen-specific, but requires approximately 4-7 days to mount a full active response. It is well accepted that the immune system has an integral role in shaping the evolution of cancer through the process of immunoediting. Testament to this, immunotherapy now forms part of some cancer treatments, rallying the body's immune system to fight cancer. Checkpoint inhibitors, for example, have been developed to target and block the immune checkpoint proteins CTLA-4, PD-1 and PD-L1, which are upregulated on tumour cells and immune cells and restrict the immune system from attacking the tumour. The checkpoint inhibitor therapies reactivate the T cells, leading to durable responses and long-term survival in lung cancer and melanoma. Here we discuss the role of the immune system in breast cancer (BCa), including invasive cancers and the pre-invasive in-situ lesions, where recent work shows the innate and adaptive cells are already activated.

2. Lesions of the Breast

Carcinoma of the breast can arise from either the lobular or the ductal epithelium. Lobular carcinomas are less prevalent than ductal, accounting for 4–10% of diagnoses from breast biopsies [1]. Before BCa reaches the invasive stage at which point it can spread to the rest of the body, it is referred to as a pre-invasive lesion (Figure 1). In pre-invasive lesions, the cancerous cells are confined to the ducts or lobules from which they originate and have not yet broken the basement membrane [2]. The pre-invasive lesions in ductal carcinoma are categorized as either atypical ductal hyperplasia (ADH) or ductal carcinoma in situ (DCIS). It can be difficult to histologically distinguish ADH lesions from that of low-grade DCIS, as the lesions look similar and ADH is mostly identified through failing to meeting the diagnostic criteria for DCIS [3,4]. Ducts exhibiting abnormal proliferation that receive a diagnosis of ADH are partially or completely filled with uniform and polarized cells. These cells are hyperchromatic, and the extent of proliferation is greater than that found in usual ductal hyperplasia [4]. Ducts affected by ADH are small, typically defined as less than or equal to 2 millimetres (mm) in size, and are usually found alone or in small, clustered foci [3]. Not all ADH lesions will progress to carcinoma [5], however women with a diagnosis of ADH are four times more likely to develop BCa [6].

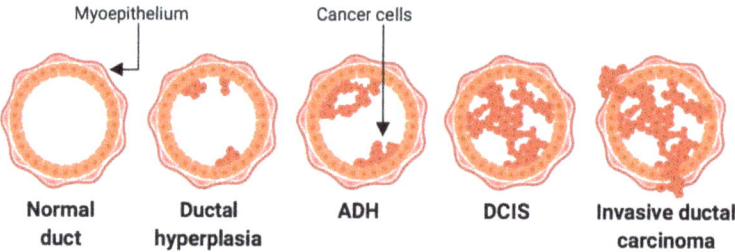

Figure 1. Stages of breast cancer development. Tumour cell initiation and expansion within the mammary ducts characterises atypical ductal hyperplasia (ADH). This progresses to ductal carcinoma in situ (DCIS), which is identified as a complete filling of the mammary duct with tumour cells. Once the myoepithelium is breached and tumour cells escape beyond the mammary duct confinement, the cancer is classified as an invasive ductal carcinoma [7].

DCIS lesions are characterized into low, intermediate, and high grade. The grades are distinguished by cellular features including the presence of calcifications and necrosis within the duct, the regularity and uniformity of the cells and their nuclei, and the extent of proliferation causing distortion of the duct [8]. Irregularity of the tumour cell nuclei, mitotic figures, and the extent of necrosis within the duct all dictate higher lesion grading [9]. DCIS lesions are typically surgically removed, but their diagnosis confers a risk of both DCIS recurrence and progression to invasive disease. This occurs for each DCIS grade, however the risk of recurrence or progression is highest in the high-grade lesions, and lowest in the low-grade lesions [10–13].

Tumours are characterized as invasive ductal carcinoma (IDC) once the cells are no longer confined to the affected duct, but have broken through the basement membrane and subsequently have invaded the surrounding stroma [2]. The presence of hormone or growth factor receptors can divide the invasive cancers into distinct subtypes. These include estrogen receptor-positive (ER+), human epidermal growth factor receptor 2 (HER2)-positive, and triple negative (TNBC) BCa [14]. TNBC expresses neither hormone nor growth factor receptors. BCa can also be classified by molecular characteristics into luminal (which can be ER+ or ER− and also ER+HER2+), or HER2+ (which expresses amplification of the human epidermal growth factor receptor 2 (HER2) gene, but are negative for ER). Finally, there are 2 subtypes that lacks all growth factors and are referred to as Basal and Claudin low [15].

3. The role of the Immune System in Cancer

Alongside the traditional hallmarks of cancer such as unregulated cell growth and apoptosis evasion, immune-manipulating mechanisms are also considered pivotal characteristics of cancer cells [16]. Tumours have the ability to influence their immune microenvironment either by exerting immunosuppressive signalling, evading immune recognition, or fuelling tumour-promoting inflammation as a means of driving cancer progression. Given the appropriate conditions, leukocyte activation initiated by mutated cells can advance neoplastic transformations into malignant tumour cells [16].

This gives rise to the cancer immunoediting hypothesis. Here, it is postulated that the immune system exerts both host-protective and tumour-stimulating actions [17]. Cancer immunoediting is multifaceted and composed of three fundamental phases: elimination, equilibrium and escape (Figure 2) [18]. Initially, tumour-specific antigens are recognised by the innate and adaptive arms of the immune system and elicit a pro-inflammatory response [18]. The cancer immunosurveillance network acts in cohesion to eliminate developing tumour cells, thereby preventing further tumourigenesis. Tumours only progress to the equilibrium phase if immunosurveillance is unsuccessful or impaired. Subsequently, cancerous cells persisting habitually in equilibrium with their microenvironment are more equipped to mutate and produce new populations of tumour variants [18]. Modifications to tumour cells can allow them to ultimately employ immunosuppressive mechanisms, thus evading and essentially escaping the immune system in the final phase [18]. These immunologically sculpted tumours grow with fewer selective pressures, actively induce an immunosuppressive microenvironment and become evident clinically.

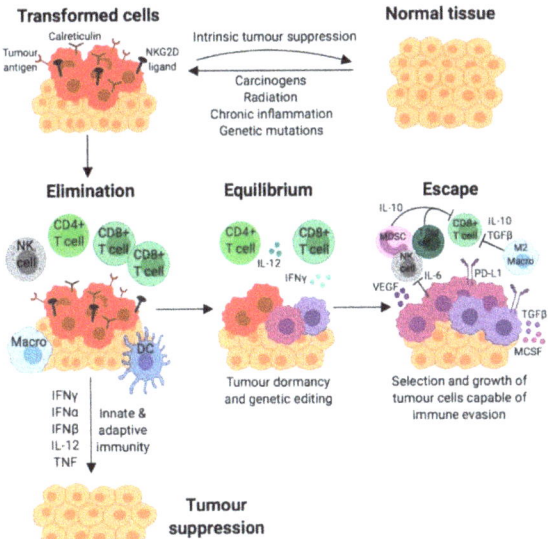

Figure 2. The three phases of cancer immunoediting. Normal cells transition to tumour cells expressing specific tumour antigens, calreticulin, and NKG2D ligands if subject to oncogenic mutational transformation. Elimination is the first phase of cancer immunoediting, where the cells of the innate and adaptive immune system are recruited to the site of the tumour antigens and attempt to destroy tumour cells via immune attack mechanisms (including secretion of cytokines IFNγ, IFNα, IFNβ, IL-12 and TNF). Any persisting tumour cells enter the second phase, equilibrium, where selection pressures instigate new tumour cell genetic variants. These genetic modifications allow tumour evasion of the immune system and promotion to the third phase, escape, where tumour cells progressively develop and become clinically detectable as a palpable mass. Immune evasion is influenced by factors including tumour cell PD-L1 upregulation, secretion of immuno-inhibitory cytokines (IL-6, IL-10, TGFβ and MCSF) and recruitment of inhibitory immune cells (M2 macrophages, Regulatory T (TReg) cells and Myeloid-derived suppressor cells (MDSCs)) that abrogate immune-mediated tumour cell killing via inhibition of Natural Killer (NK) cells and CD8+ T cells. Tumour cells also experience a downregulation of tumour antigen, calreticulin and NKG2D ligands, so are less susceptible to immune recognition [19].

4. The Innate and Adaptive Immune System

The immune system is an organism's natural defence mechanism that provides protection from a plethora of pathogens, infections and diseases. Immune regulation is tightly controlled, which enables appropriate recognition and response to foreign threats whilst avoiding unwanted inflammation towards healthy tissue and the body's natural microbial flora. The immune system is composed of a dynamic network of cells, tissues and organs that broadly function in two lines of defence: innate and adaptive immunity [20]. This division of the immune system is tailored directly towards the pathogenic threat encountered, and also confers immunological memory where long-lasting protection against the specific pathogen is established [20]. Both arms of the immune system are emerging to play key roles on BCa development and progression.

5. Tumour Infiltrating Lymphocytes (TILs) and BCa

Tumour infiltrating lymphocytes (TILs) are immune cells that have migrated to the tumour tissue and the local microenvironment. This population is indicative of an immune response generated by the patient against the malignancy. In TNBC and HER2+ disease in particular, the presence of TILs has been shown to correlate with a good prognosis and good response to chemotherapy. The relationship has not been as definitely proven for ER+ disease, indicating that the luminal subtypes may be less immunogenic than the others. This indicates that simple TIL counts are not as effective as a prognostic marker in these tumours [21–23]. TILs have also been found to be a prognostic indicator for higher rates of pathological complete responses (pCRs) to neoadjuvant chemotherapy [24–27].

Whilst TILs can be present within or around the tumour, TIL assessment is primarily concerned with stromal TILs counted in H&E-stained tumour sections as stated by The International TILs Working Group. While TILs in each compartment together constitute the population of lymphocytic infiltration and may contribute to prognostic significance, the majority of TILs are found in the stroma. Intratumoural TILs are difficult to quantify and low concordance between different scorers of the same sample have been reported [28]. To quantify the number of stromal TILs, the guidelines state that one should count the proportion of TILs in the stromal compartment in the visual field. Experts in the field have developed guidelines and tutorials for assessing TILs in invasive cancers and metastases, as well as DCIS lesions.

6. The Immune Regulation in Invasive BCa

TILs have been found to be elevated in primary invasive cancers compared to metastases. The TIL populations across BCa in general are predominantly made up of T lymphocytes, and in particular CD8+ cytotoxic T lymphocytes (CTLs). Due to this fact, CD8+ cells are a robust immune prognostic marker for the outcome of BCa patients, particularly the TN and HER2+ subtypes, because they represent an active, adaptive immune response to the neoantigens on the surface of the tumour cells and correlate positively with improved survival [29].

CTLs have the capacity to differentiate further into tissue-resident memory T (T_{RM}) cells that exist within the breast tissue without recirculating systemically. T_{RM} cells express high levels of immune checkpoint molecules that contribute to tumour elimination and have been shown to be actively involved in BCa immunosurveillance. T_{RM} status has been shown to be an even greater prognostic marker than CD8+ cells alone, and is significantly associated with improved TNBC patient survival [30]. The T helper cells present during acute inflammation are predominantly T helper cell type 1 (Th1) polarized and secrete cytokines such as IFNγ, TNFα and IL-2 which act to limit tumour growth, promote antigen processing and presentation, and activate macrophages. The T helper cells present during chronic inflammation and cancer are type 2 (Th2) polarized and express IL-4, IL-5, IL-6, IL-10 and IL-13 which inhibit T cell-mediated cytotoxicity [31]. T regulatory lymphocytes (Tregs) are characterised as T lymphocytes which are both CD4+ and FOXP3+ and have immunosuppressive functions. Tregs normally help to protect against autoimmunity [32]. In the context of breast carcinomas, these immune cells are largely agreed to contribute to the pro-tumour immune response and assist the tumour in subsequent immune escape, so are thus associated with a poor prognosis [21,33]. These lymphocytes allow the progression of the tumour by expressing inhibitory factors that inhibit the anti-tumour Th1 response [33].

In addition to T cells there are many other immune cell types that infiltrate breast cancers including macrophages, NK cells, and dendritic cells (DCs) (Figure 3) [19,34,35]. In brief, CD4+ T helper, CD8+ CTLs, NK cells, M1 macrophages, and DCs are protective against tumour growth [36]. Conversely, CD4+ FOXP3+ Th2 cells, M2 macrophages, and myeloid-derived suppressor cells (MDSCs) can drive tumour growth [36].

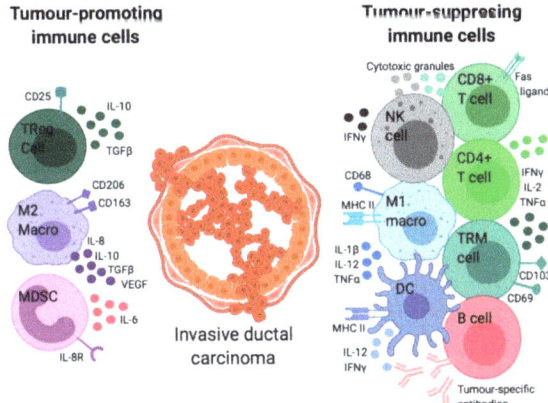

Figure 3. The immune microenvironment of invasive ductal carcinoma. Subsets of the immune system can elicit both tumour-promoting and tumour-suppressing effects. Immune inhibition of tumours is largely driven by the activity of CD8+ T cells, CD4+ T cells, Tissue-resident T (T_{RM}) cells, B cells, Natural Killer (NK) cells, M1 macrophages and dendritic cells (DC). The tumour-fighting immune landscape produces cytokines that inhibit tumour development (including IFNγ, TNFα, IL-1β, IL-2 and IL-12). CD8+ T cells and NK cells also secrete cytotoxic granules that trigger tumour cell apoptosis. Similarly, B cells secrete tumour-specific antibodies that target tumour cells for elimination. In contrast, the immune stimulation of tumours is promoted by Regulatory T (TReg) cells, M2 macrophages and Myeloid-derived suppressor cells (MDSCs), which act to suppress their anti-tumour immune counterparts and facilitate tumour growth. These cells release immuno-inhibitory pro-tumour cytokines (TGFβ, VEGF, IL-6, IL-8 and IL-10) [37–41].

Tissue-resident macrophages are typically found along the ductal system in the stroma of the normal breast, and are present prior to the development of any malignancy [42,43]. These are some of the first immune cells to encounter tumour cells when they begin to form a hyperplastic or neoplastic growth. The macrophages associated with tumours are referred to as tumour associated macrophages (TAM) and their infiltration accompanies a worse prognosis in many cancers [44,45]. TAMs in invasive BCa have been shown to express higher levels of the transcription factor hypoxia-inducible factor 2α (HIF-2α) in comparison to macrophages from the normal breast [46]. HIF-2α along with HIF-1α from the tumour cells [47] activate the expression of vascular endothelial growth factor (VEGF) which stimulates angiogenesis [48,49]. By vascularizing an early tumour, the TAMs ensure that the tumour receives the nourishment it requires for malignant growth and metastasis. In support of this positive feedback, microvessel density and VEGF expression have been found to be significantly correlated with TAM density in IDC [50].

Cytokines from the tumour microenvironment are also key players in this process, as they can induce phenotypic changes in macrophages. IL-10 and TGF-β switch the macrophages from an M1-like (proinflammatory or classically activated) state to an M2-like (anti-inflammatory or alternatively activated) state. M1 macrophages elicit anti-tumour immune signaling and are associated with tumour killing capacity. Conversely, M2 macrophages exert pro-tumour effects and are associated with fibrosis and the production of matrix proteins [51] as well as angiogenesis, metastasis, and the suppression of adaptive immunity [52,53]. Human BCa cell lines cultured in vitro are able to polarise macrophages towards the M2 phenotype [54]. In BCa patient samples, M2 macrophages in the stroma correlate with the presence of a lesion [54]. Retrospective studies of preserved human tumours have demonstrated that M2 macrophages are significantly associated with poor prognosis in both ER- and ER+ tumours [21].

MDSCs are a collection of progenitor and immature myeloid-lineage cell types which serve as a brake on immune system activation [55]. High levels of MDSCs have been identified as a poor prognostic marker for many cancers, and most likely participate in the pro-tumourigenic pathway through the suppression and inhibition of the host anti-tumour immune response [55,56]. BCa patients have higher circulating MDSC counts than their normal-matched counterparts [57]. Greater quantities of MDSCs isolated from the blood of these patients correlated with poor prognosis, and when cultured with T cells in vitro they were able to significantly inhibit proliferation of the lymphocytic population in comparison to MDSCs derived from normal subjects [57]. Looking at early-stage breast cancer, patients with greater neutrophil (a type of MDSC) counts had a higher neutrophil to lymphocyte ratio and were more likely to relapse [58].

DCs express MHC Class II and can present their antigenic peptides to CD4+ T cells. They prime tumour specific effector T cells to attack the tumour and are thought to play an important role in shaping the host response to the cancerous cells. DC maturation and survival are impaired in invasive tumours and the infiltration of plasmacytoid DCs (pDCs) in primary BCa is correlated with poor clinical outcome. This indicates that pDCs contribute to BCa progression [59].

Natural killer (NK) cells are unique in that they have both innate and adaptive immune properties [60]. NK cells participate in the anti-tumour immune response through the production of pro-inflammatory cytokines, which recruit and induce proliferation of other immune cells [61]. NK cells can also directly mediate anti-tumour immunity by killing the tumour cells themselves without prior sensitization, so therefore play an active role in cancer immunosurveillance [62,63]. However, the ability of NK cells to recognize and kill tumour cells is impaired in cancer patients, as tumour NK cells exhibit an inhibitory phenotype characterised by the expression of inhibitory markers [64–66]. In BCa patients, NK cell dysfunction correlates with tumour progression and invasiveness [65,67].

B lymphocytes are CD20+ adaptive immune cells which confer humoral immunity through the production and secretion of antibodies, which are made of the protein immunoglobulin and recognise specific tumour-antigens. Antibodies bind to these antigens and can inhibit the functionality of the receptor or ligand they are bound to. Additionally, antibodies can signal to other cancer-killing cells that they are bound to a tumour cell, thereby activating them to eliminate tumour cell populations [68]. B cells participate in immunity alongside the T cell response through their ability to present antigen and co-stimulatory molecules to these lymphocytes [69]. Furthermore, B cells can be found in the breast milk secreted by the lactating normal breast [42,43]. In IDC, B lymphocytes and immunoglobulin gene expression signatures have been associated with a favourable prognosis in retrospective studies [70,71]. Though this supports an anti-tumour role for B cells and antibodies, other studies have associated them with poor prognostic factors in BCa. Human BCa cells can induce a regulatory phenotype in B cells, instigating production of transforming growth factor beta (TGF-β), a cytokine that stimulates CD4+ T cells to become immunosuppressive T regulatory cells [72].

Although not strictly an immune cell, fibroblasts are present within the stromal microenvironment of the breast and serve to produce the extracelullar matrix (ECM) proteins (in particular collagen). They can also manufacture and respond to cytokines, allowing them to cooperate with the immune cells within the stromal microenvironment. However, fibroblasts can control epithelial cell polarity, proliferation, and to some extent, tumourigenic potential. Cancer associated fibroblasts (CAFs) have been shown to drive increased tumour growth compared to normal fibroblasts [73]. They contribute to cancer cell survival and progression by secreting high levels of nutrient-rich ECM proteins, or ECM-degrading proteases. These can promote persistent chronic inflammation within the tumour microenvironment and inducing the epithelial mesenchymal transition (EMT) of tumour cells [74–77].

CAFs have the capacity to produce pro-inflammatory cytokines. These CAF-secreted cytokines disrupt the normal cytokine balance to stimulate tumour growth by initiating angiogenesis and inhibiting CTLs. CAFs have been shown to secrete high levels of the pro-inflammatory cytokines IL-1β, IL-8, IL-10, tumour necrosis factor-alpha (TNFα), monocyte chemoattractant protein-1 (CCL2), stromal derived factor-1 (CXCL12) and interferon-beta (IFNβ) [78,79]. The importance of the CAFs in cancer growth has been highlighted by genetic analyses showing that their gene expression profiles are very different to normal breast fibroblasts. Moreover, the expression profiles of CAFs taken from tumours with poor (increased recurrence and shorter disease-free survival) versus good (reduced recurrence and longer disease-free survival) outcome are also very different [80]. The good-outcome fibroblasts were enriched for immune modulators such as those involved in the Th1 immune response. This includes expression of T cell receptor complexes (CD8a, CD247, CD3D), MHC class I protein binding and granzyme A/B activity. The poor-outcome stroma had increased levels of hypoxia and angiogenesis and decreased chemokines that stimulate NK migration and T cell survival [80].

7. Immune Regulation of DCIS

The pre-invasive DCIS stage of BCa also exhibits significant immune infiltration. Gorringe and colleagues showed that TILs are present in high grade DCIS lesions, with smaller numbers also observed in low and intermediate grade lesions [81]. A global study of 53 mastectomy samples demonstrated that T cell, B cell and macrophage levels were all elevated in DCIS compared with the normal breast and remained elevated across subsequent cancer progression [82]. Similarly, neutrophils have been found to be significantly higher in the breast of women with DCIS than in the normal breast [83]. Clinical research assessing specific subsets of immune cells in DCIS has indicated that CD68+ macrophages (in particular the M2 macrophages), CD4+ T cells and CD20+ B cells were elevated in the high-grade DCIS cases compared to low [84].

CAFs are also thought to play a role in the transition of DCIS to IDC via their secretion of factors which modify the surrounding stromal matrix. When fibroblasts sourced from the normal breast or IDC were injected alongside a DCIS cell line in xenografts, the IDC-derived fibroblasts (or CAFs) elicted a significant increase in tumour weight whilst normal fibroblasts had no effect on xenograft progression [85]. One mechanism through which CAFs may be accomplishing this in early BCa development is through the production of IL-10, which not only stimulates M2 polarisation of TAMs but additionally serves to modulate T cell and NK cell phenotypes [54,86]. Osula et al. have demonstrated that CAFs significantly upregulate expression of IL-6 in comparison to their normal counterparts. By culturing these fibroblasts with DCIS cell lines, Osula and colleagues revealed that DCIS cells grow faster, and that this growth is inhibited with treatment of an IL-6 neutralising antibody [87]. Paracrine IL-6 signalling between malignant cells and pro-tumour fibroblasts may thus be influential in the progression of DCIS to IDC.

Recurrent DCIS describes the reappearance of additional DCIS lesions after the primary diagnosis and treatment and/or progression to invasive disease [9]. The highest risk of DCIS recurrence correlates with patients displaying both low T cell numbers and elevated macrophages [84]. Of these recurrent cases, immunosuppressive CD206+ M2 macrophages were also prevalent, thus suggesting that their anti-inflammatory effects may abrogate tumour-fighting T cell functions in these early lesions [84]. Illustrating the pro-tumourigenic role of macrophages, mouse models transplanted with pre-invasive breast cancer cell lines have shown that metastatic progression is inhibited when the macrophages are depleted prior to transplantation [88]. When directly compared with invasive BCa, the inflammatory response to the malignant cells in DCIS is highly active. There are significantly more CTLs in DCIS expressing granzyme B and IFNγ, marking these cells as activated, effector cytotoxic T cells [83]. In the same study, the diversity of T cell receptor clonotypes were found to be significantly higher in DCIS than in IDC.

During a chronic infection, CD8+ T cells undergo a hierarchical loss of function and increase the expression of coinhibitory receptors in a process called exhaustion. Importantly, targeting coinhibitory receptors such as PD-1 and CTLA-4 using monoclonal antibodies, alone or in combination, has proven to be effective in restoring the function of exhausted T cells. When DCIS and IDC were compared, the T cell immunoglobulin and ITIM domain (TIGIT) co-inhibitory receptor was found to have higher expression in T cells from DCIS patients compared to HER2+ and TNBC IDC. However, PD-L1 was almost undetectable in DCIS and increased in IDC. CTLA-4 was also higher in T cells from IDCs compared with DCIS [83]. Together this indicates that the immune microenvironment becomes suppressive during invasive progression. but that each of the checkpoint molecules may play a distinct role.

8. Immune Regulation of Hyperplasia

The immune regulation of early hyperplastic breast tumourigenesis is understood to a considerably lesser degree than that of DCIS. Limited published data exists surrounding the immune infiltrate in ADH of the breast. Gorringe and colleagues have shown that in DCIS a higher Fraction of Genome Altered compared to normal (measured by copy number variation analysis) correlates with a higher infiltration of TILs in DCIS [81]. They have not yet assessed TIL numbers in ADH compared to the normal breast, but have shown that ADH lesions exhibit aneuploidy, loss of heterozygosity, gross chromosomal rearrangement (such as amplifications and large-scale deletion) and methylation changes. This indicates that the genomic changes present may activate the immune system early. In support of this, human studies in endometrial cancer have demonstrated that significant immune involvement enhanced the proliferative rate of hyperplastic tissue [89]. In particular, macrophage numbers and the inflammatory cytokines they produce were significantly associated with early malignancies and tumourigenesis.

Whilst the immune composition of ADH has not yet been explored, increased CD4+ T cells, CTLs and B cells have been observed in lobules with lobulitis [90]. Similarly, normal breast tissue from women with high breast density (which confers a 4-6-fold increased risk of BCa) exhibits increased macrophages, DCs, B cells and CD4+ T cells. High-density tissue also disaplayed increased IL-6 and IL-4 secretion, thereby suggesting pro-tumour Th2 polarization [91]. The lack of information in hyperplastic lesions may be due their small size (≤2 mm) [92–94] and close relationship to low grade DCIS. This means the ADH samples are only collected for diagnostic purposes and not research. It is also notable that there is a lack of concordance amongst pathologists in differentiating low-grade DCIS and ADH [94]. Further analysis of the immune landscape of pre-invasive lesions including ADH will hopefully reveal whether the microenvironment assists at this earliest stage of tumour escape from immune regulation.

Fibroblasts may also play a role in the earliest stages of tumour growth. This notion has been suggested by work demonstrating that stromal-specific inactivation of TGFβ-RII leads to pre-invasive prostate cancer lesions in mice [95], and that stromal phosphatase and tensin homolog (PTEN) loss can drive BCa growth [96]. In addition to stimulating the growth of early hyperplastic cells, CAFs may participate in the loss of epithelial characteristics of ductal lesions. Fibroblasts isolated from ADH-affected breast tissue exhibited an activated phenotype mirroring that of CAFs isolated from DCIS. When cultured with the BCa cell line MCF-7, these ADH-associated fibroblasts induced decreased expression of the epithelial protein e-cadherin and increased expression of the mesenchymal protein vimentin [97]. This indicates that even when precursor cells are merely hyperplastic, activation of fibroblasts under appropriate conditions may prime the lesion towards malignant transformation.

9. Immune-Based Therapies for BCa Growth and Progression

As mentioned above, it is well-established that in both IDC and DCIS, high numbers of stromal lymphocytes serve as a good prognostic factor in TNBC and HER2+ disease. This opens the door to potentially utilize immunotherapies to mobilize the immune system against BCa. The PD-1/PD-L1 inhibitory pathway is one of the most intensively investigated avenues in the development of immune-based therapeutics. PD-L1 is known to be expressed by primary and metastatic IDCs and has been identified as a poor prognostic indicator in these patients [98–100], likely serving to downregulate the T cell response to tumour cells. As TNBC has limited successful therapies, anti-PD-L1 therapy represents a promising new treatment option. In vivo models of TNBC demonstrate that treatment with antibodies targeting PD-L1 expressed on tumour cells reduces tumour volume whilst increasing tumour immunogenicity [101]. PD-L1 inhibition has additionally been investigated for use in DCIS. Expression of the immunosuppressive ligand is far less common in this earlier stage, though when expression is observed, it is most commonly in HER2+ lesions [81,102]. Several trials are currently underway investigating the use of anti-PD-L1 therapies both alone and in combination with HER2-specific treatments, as reviewed by Ubago et al. [103].

Combination immunotherapies have also been proven as potentially efficacious novel TNBC treatments. TNBC often upregulates activity of MEK, which contributes to an overactivation of the Ras/MAPK pathway and thus serves as a poor prognostic indicator for recurrence and survival in these patients. However, T cells also use MEK signaling for proliferation, activation, and differentiation, so simply inhibiting MEK activity reduces the potential utility of recruiting the immune system. When MEK inhibition was combined with agonist antibodies to activating receptors on T cells, or with anti-PD-1/PD-L1 therapies, survival and tumour size significantly improved in xenograft TNBC models [101,104].

Immunotherapies tend to particularly target T cells and the adaptive immune response. Innate immunity represents an alternative route through which to pursue immune-based therapies. One such novel therapy is anti-CSF1R, which inhibits the receptor found on TAMs responsible for their recruitment and M2 activation as pro-tumourigenic immune cells. Mixed data exists concerning the role of CSF1R inhibition and tumour growth in mice, with some studies demonstrating significant reductions in tumourigenesis and others showing limited effectiveness or stimulated cancer metastasis [105,106]. This avenue of innate immune modulation in cancer therapies therefore remains somewhat elusive, and requires further research to shed light on any possible therapeutic benefits.

10. Conclusions

The role of the immune microenvironment in BCa is becoming clearer. Infiltrating immune cells in invasive lesions are predominantly T lymphocytes, and in particular CTLs. The CD8+ CTLs are now viewed as a robust immune prognostic marker for the outcome of TN and HER2+ BCa patients. There are additional innate and adaptive cells that infiltrate BCa or remain in close proximity in the stromal microenvironment. CD4+ T helper, CD8+ CTLs, NK cells, M1 macrophages, and DCs are likely protecting against tumour growth whilst the CD4+ FOXP3+ Th2 cells, M2 macrophages, and myeloid-derived suppressor cells (MDSCs) simulate tumour growth. The cytokines present at the tumour site are also key players in this process, often controlling the infiltration as well as activation and polarization state of the immune cells. CAFs have altered gene expression profiles and function compared to normal breast fibroblasts and can drive increased tumour growth by aiding cancer cell survival and progression and by secreting high levels of nutrient-rich ECM proteins, or ECM-degrading proteases. Less is known about the pre-invasive stages of BCa development including DCIS and ADH. However, TILs are present in high-grade DCIS lesions, less so in low- and intermediate-grade lesions. Those pre-invasive lesions with the highest risk of recurrence correlates have been show to exhibit low T cell numbers and elevated macrophages. The TIL numbers at this time may be correlated with the level of genetic changes that are measured within the lesions. As ADH lesions already exhibit significant genetic changes (aneuploidy, loss of heterozygosity, gross chromosomal rearrangement and methylation changes) it is expected that the immune system will already be activated and in hyperplastic endometrial cancer this has been shown. As we increase our understanding of the earliest stages of BCa development and the interaction with the immune system, we will begin to define whether immune therapies can be delivered earlier for better disease control.

Author Contributions: H.T., M.R.; K.B. contributed to the Writing—Original Draft Preparation as well as Writing—Review & Editing.

Funding: H.T. was supported by a Peter MacCallum summer student scholarship and a Victorian Cancer Council summer studentship. MR was supported by a Peter MacCallum summer student scholarship and Frances Elizabeth Thompson Trust Scholarship. KB is supported by the Peter MacCallum Foundation.

Acknowledgments: All figures were created with BioRender.com.

Conflicts of Interest: The authors declare no conflict of interest.

References

1. Donaldson, A.R.; McCarthy, C.; Goraya, S.; Pederson, H.J.; Sturgis, C.D.; Grobmyer, S.R.; Calhoun, B.C. Breast cancer risk associated with atypical hyperplasia and lobular carcinoma in situ initially diagnosed on core-needle biopsy. *Cancer* **2018**, *124*, 459–465. [CrossRef]
2. Lerwill, M.F. Current practical applications of diagnostic immunohistochemistry in breast pathology. *Am. J. Surg. Pathol.* **2004**, *28*, 1076–1091. [CrossRef] [PubMed]
3. Kader, T.; Hill, P.; Rakha, E.A.; Campbell, I.G.; Gorringe, K.L. Atypical ductal hyperplasia: Update on diagnosis, management, and molecular landscape. *Breast Cancer Res.* **2018**, *20*, 39. [CrossRef] [PubMed]
4. Pinder, S.E.; Ellis, I.O. The diagnosis and management of pre-invasive breast disease: Ductal carcinoma in situ (DCIS) and atypical ductal hyperplasia (ADH)—Current definitions and classification. *Breast Cancer Res.* **2003**, *5*, 254–257. [CrossRef] [PubMed]
5. Hartmann, L.C.; Degnim, A.C.; Santen, R.J.; Dupont, W.D.; Ghosh, K. Atypical hyperplasia of the breast—Risk assessment and management options. *N. Engl. J. Med.* **2015**, *372*, 78–89. [CrossRef] [PubMed]
6. Coopey, S.B.; Hughes, K.S. *Breast Cancer Risk Prediction in Women with Atypical Breast Lesions*; Springer International Publishing: Berlin, Germany, 2018; pp. 103–113.
7. Malhotra, G.K.; Zhao, X.; Band, H.; Band, V. Histological, molecular and functional subtypes of breast cancers. *Cancer Biol. Ther.* **2010**, *10*, 955–960. [CrossRef] [PubMed]
8. Pinder, S.E.; Duggan, C.; Ellis, I.O.; Cuzick, J.; Forbes, J.F.; Bishop, H.; Fentiman, I.S.; George, W.D. A new pathological system for grading DCIS with improved prediction of local recurrence: Results from the UKCCCR/ANZ DCIS trial. *Br. J. Cancer* **2010**, *103*, 94–100. [CrossRef]
9. Gorringe, K.L.; Fox, S.B. Ductal Carcinoma In Situ Biology, Biomarkers, and Diagnosis. *Front. Oncol.* **2017**, *7*, 248. [CrossRef]
10. Lagios, M.D.; Margolin, F.R.; Westdahl, P.R.; Rose, M.R. Mammographically detected duct carcinoma in situ. Frequency of local recurrence following tylectomy and prognostic effect of nuclear grade on local recurrence. *Cancer* **1989**, *63*, 618–624. [CrossRef]
11. Maxwell, A.J.; Clements, K.; Hilton, B.; Dodwell, D.J.; Evans, A.; Kearins, O.; Pinder, S.E.; Thomas, J.; Wallis, M.G.; Thompson, A.M.; et al. Risk factors for the development of invasive cancer in unresected ductal carcinoma in situ. *Eur. J. Surg. Oncol.* **2018**, *44*, 429–435. [CrossRef]
12. Roka, S.; Rudas, M.; Taucher, S.; Dubsky, P.; Bachleitner-Hofmann, T.; Kandioler, D.; Gnant, M.; Jakesz, R. High nuclear grade and negative estrogen receptor are significant risk factors for recurrence in DCIS. *Eur. J. Surg. Oncol.* **2004**, *30*, 243–247. [CrossRef] [PubMed]
13. Sanders, M.E.; Schuyler, P.A.; Simpson, J.F.; Page, D.L.; Dupont, W.D. Continued observation of the natural history of low-grade ductal carcinoma in situ reaffirms proclivity for local recurrence even after more than 30 years of follow-up. *Mod. Pathol.* **2015**, *28*, 662–669. [CrossRef] [PubMed]
14. Prat, A.; Pineda, E.; Adamo, B.; Galvan, P.; Fernandez, A.; Gaba, L.; Diez, M.; Viladot, M.; Arance, A.; Munoz, M. Clinical implications of the intrinsic molecular subtypes of breast cancer. *Breast* **2015**, *24* (Suppl. 2), S26–S35. [CrossRef]
15. Dai, X.; Xiang, L.; Li, T.; Bai, Z. Cancer Hallmarks, Biomarkers and Breast Cancer Molecular Subtypes. *J. Cancer* **2016**, *7*, 1281–1294. [CrossRef] [PubMed]

16. Cavallo, F.; De Giovanni, C.; Nanni, P.; Forni, G.; Lollini, P.L. 2011: The immune hallmarks of cancer. *Cancer Immunol. ImmunoTher.* **2011**, *60*, 319–326. [CrossRef] [PubMed]
17. Dunn, G.P.; Old, L.J.; Schreiber, R.D. The immunobiology of cancer immunosurveillance and immunoediting. *Immunity* **2004**, *21*, 137–148. [CrossRef]
18. Dunn, G.P.; Old, L.J.; Schreiber, R.D. The three Es of cancer immunoediting. *Annu Rev. Immunol.* **2004**, *22*, 329–360. [CrossRef]
19. Mittal, D.; Gubin, M.M.; Schreiber, R.D.; Smyth, M.J. New insights into cancer immunoediting and its three component phases—Elimination, equilibrium and escape. *Curr. Opin. Immunol.* **2014**, *27*, 16–25. [CrossRef] [PubMed]
20. Sharpe, M.; Mount, N. Genetically modified T cells in cancer therapy: Opportunities and challenges. *Dis. Model Mech.* **2015**, *8*, 337–350. [CrossRef] [PubMed]
21. Ali, H.R.; Chlon, L.; Pharoah, P.D.; Markowetz, F.; Caldas, C. Patterns of Immune Infiltration in Breast Cancer and Their Clinical Implications: A Gene-Expression-Based Retrospective Study. *PLoS Med.* **2016**, *13*, e1002194. [CrossRef] [PubMed]
22. Dushyanthen, S.; Beavis, P.A.; Savas, P.; Teo, Z.L.; Zhou, C.; Mansour, M.; Darcy, P.K.; Loi, S. Relevance of tumor-infiltrating lymphocytes in breast cancer. *BMC Med.* **2015**, *13*, 202. [CrossRef] [PubMed]
23. Pruneri, G.; Gray, K.P.; Vingiani, A.; Viale, G.; Curigliano, G.; Criscitiello, C.; Lang, I.; Ruhstaller, T.; Gianni, L.; Goldhirsch, A.; et al. Tumor-infiltrating lymphocytes (TILs) are a powerful prognostic marker in patients with triple-negative breast cancer enrolled in the IBCSG phase III randomized clinical trial 22-00. *Breast Cancer Res. Treat.* **2016**, *158*, 323–331. [CrossRef] [PubMed]
24. Denkert, C.; Loibl, S.; Noske, A.; Roller, M.; Muller, B.M.; Komor, M.; Budczies, J.; Darb-Esfahani, S.; Kronenwett, R.; Hanusch, C.; et al. Tumor-associated lymphocytes as an independent predictor of response to neoadjuvant chemotherapy in breast cancer. *J. Clin. Oncol.* **2010**, *28*, 105–113. [CrossRef] [PubMed]
25. Ladoire, S.; Arnould, L.; Apetoh, L.; Coudert, B.; Martin, F.; Chauffert, B.; Fumoleau, P.; Ghiringhelli, F. Pathologic complete response to neoadjuvant chemotherapy of breast carcinoma is associated with the disappearance of tumor-infiltrating foxp3+ regulatory T cells. *Clin. Cancer Res.* **2008**, *14*, 2413–2420. [CrossRef]
26. Menard, S.; Tomasic, G.; Casalini, P.; Balsari, A.; Pilotti, S.; Cascinelli, N.; Salvadori, B.; Colnaghi, M.I.; Rilke, F. Lymphoid infiltration as a prognostic variable for early-onset breast carcinomas. *Clin. Cancer Res.* **1997**, *3*, 817–819. [PubMed]
27. Ono, M.; Tsuda, H.; Shimizu, C.; Yamamoto, S.; Shibata, T.; Yamamoto, H.; Hirata, T.; Yonemori, K.; Ando, M.; Tamura, K.; et al. Tumor-infiltrating lymphocytes are correlated with response to neoadjuvant chemotherapy in triple-negative breast cancer. *Breast Cancer Res. Treat.* **2012**, *132*, 793–805. [CrossRef] [PubMed]
28. Salgado, R.; Denkert, C.; Demaria, S.; Sirtaine, N.; Klauschen, F.; Pruneri, G.; Wienert, S.; Van den Eynden, G.; Baehner, F.L.; Penault-Llorca, F.; et al. The evaluation of tumor-infiltrating lymphocytes (TILs) in breast cancer: Recommendations by an International TILs Working Group 2014. *Ann. Oncol.* **2015**, *26*, 259–271. [CrossRef] [PubMed]
29. Pruneri, G.; Vingiani, A.; Denkert, C. Tumor infiltrating lymphocytes in early breast cancer. *Breast* **2018**, *37*, 207–214. [CrossRef]
30. Savas, P.; Virassamy, B.; Ye, C.; Salim, A.; Mintoff, C.P.; Caramia, F.; Salgado, R.; Byrne, D.J.; Teo, Z.L.; Dushyanthen, S.; et al. Single-cell profiling of breast cancer T cells reveals a tissue-resident memory subset associated with improved prognosis. *Nat. Med.* **2018**, *24*, 986–993. [CrossRef]
31. Kohrt, H.E.; Nouri, N.; Nowels, K.; Johnson, D.; Holmes, S.; Lee, P.P. Profile of immune cells in axillary lymph nodes predicts disease-free survival in breast cancer. *PLoS Med.* **2005**, *2*, e284. [CrossRef]
32. Wieckiewicz, J.; Goto, R.; Wood, K.J. T regulatory cells and the control of alloimmunity: From characterisation to clinical application. *Curr. Opin. Immunol.* **2010**, *22*, 662–668. [CrossRef] [PubMed]
33. Schreiber, R.D.; Old, L.J.; Smyth, M.J. Cancer immunoediting: Integrating immunity's roles in cancer suppression and promotion. *Science* **2011**, *331*, 1565–1570. [CrossRef] [PubMed]
34. O'Sullivan, T.; Saddawi-Konefka, R.; Vermi, W.; Koebel, C.M.; Arthur, C.; White, J.M.; Uppaluri, R.; Andrews, D.M.; Ngiow, S.F.; Teng, M.W.; et al. Cancer immunoediting by the innate immune system in the absence of adaptive immunity. *J. Exp. Med.* **2012**, *209*, 1869–1882. [CrossRef] [PubMed]
35. Quezada, S.A.; Peggs, K.S.; Simpson, T.R.; Allison, J.P. Shifting the equilibrium in cancer immunoediting: From tumor tolerance to eradication. *Immunol. Rev.* **2011**, *241*, 104–118. [CrossRef]

36. Emens, L.A. Breast cancer immunobiology driving immunotherapy: Vaccines and immune checkpoint blockade. *Expert. Rev. Anticancer Ther.* **2012**, *12*, 1597–1611. [CrossRef]
37. Mittrucker, H.W.; Visekruna, A.; Huber, M. Heterogeneity in the differentiation and function of CD8(+) T cells. *Arch. Immunol. Ther. Exp. (Warsz)* **2014**, *62*, 449–458. [CrossRef]
38. Lanier, L.L. Up on the tightrope: Natural killer cell activation and inhibition. *Nat. Immunol.* **2008**, *9*, 495–502. [CrossRef]
39. LA, O.R.; Tai, L.; Lee, L.; Kruse, E.A.; Grabow, S.; Fairlie, W.D.; Haynes, N.M.; Tarlinton, D.M.; Zhang, J.G.; Belz, G.T.; et al. Membrane-bound Fas ligand only is essential for Fas-induced apoptosis. *Nature* **2009**, *461*, 659–663. [CrossRef]
40. Eibel, H.; Kraus, H.; Sic, H.; Kienzler, A.K.; Rizzi, M. B cell biology: An overview. *Curr. Allergy. Asthma. Rep.* **2014**, *14*, 434. [CrossRef]
41. Abbas, A.K.; Murphy, K.M.; Sher, A. Functional diversity of helper T lymphocytes. *Nature* **1996**, *383*, 787–793. [CrossRef]
42. Coussens, L.M.; Pollard, J.W. Leukocytes in mammary development and cancer. *Cold Spring Harb. Perspect. Biol.* **2011**, *3*. [CrossRef] [PubMed]
43. Inman, J.L.; Robertson, C.; Mott, J.D.; Bissell, M.J. Mammary gland development: Cell fate specification, stem cells and the microenvironment. *Development* **2015**, *142*, 1028–1042. [CrossRef] [PubMed]
44. Knutson, K.L.; Disis, M.L. Tumor antigen-specific T helper cells in cancer immunity and immunotherapy. *Cancer Immunol. ImmunoTher.* **2005**, *54*, 721–728. [CrossRef] [PubMed]
45. Mukhtar, R.A.; Nseyo, O.; Campbell, M.J.; Esserman, L.J. Tumor-associated macrophages in breast cancer as potential biomarkers for new treatments and diagnostics. *Expert. Rev. Mol. Diagn.* **2011**, *11*, 91–100. [CrossRef] [PubMed]
46. Leek, R.D.; Talks, K.L.; Pezzella, F.; Turley, H.; Campo, L.; Brown, N.S.; Bicknell, R.; Taylor, M.; Gatter, K.C.; Harris, A.L. Relation of hypoxia-inducible factor-2 alpha (HIF-2 alpha) expression in tumor-infiltrative macrophages to tumor angiogenesis and the oxidative thymidine phosphorylase pathway in Human breast cancer. *Cancer Res.* **2002**, *62*, 1326–1329.
47. Talks, K.L.; Turley, H.; Gatter, K.C.; Maxwell, P.H.; Pugh, C.W.; Ratcliffe, P.J.; Harris, A.L. The expression and distribution of the hypoxia-inducible factors HIF-1alpha and HIF-2alpha in normal human tissues, cancers, and tumor-associated macrophages. *Am. J. Pathol.* **2000**, *157*, 411–421. [CrossRef]
48. Ziello, J.E.; Jovin, I.S.; Huang, Y. Hypoxia-Inducible Factor (HIF)-1 regulatory pathway and its potential for therapeutic intervention in malignancy and ischemia. *Yale J. Biol. Med.* **2007**, *80*, 51–60.
49. Loboda, A.; Jozkowicz, A.; Dulak, J. *HIF-1* versus *HIF-2*—Is one more important than the other? *Vascul. Pharmacol.* **2012**, *56*, 245–251. [CrossRef]
50. Valkovic, T.; Dobrila, F.; Melato, M.; Sasso, F.; Rizzardi, C.; Jonjic, N. Correlation between vascular endothelial growth factor, angiogenesis, and tumor-associated macrophages in invasive ductal breast carcinoma. *Virchows Arch.* **2002**, *440*, 583–588. [CrossRef]
51. Mills, C.D.; Ley, K. M1 and M2 macrophages: The chicken and the egg of immunity. *J. Innate Immun.* **2014**, *6*, 716–726. [CrossRef]
52. Schmieder, A.; Michel, J.; Schonhaar, K.; Goerdt, S.; Schledzewski, K. Differentiation and gene expression profile of tumor-associated macrophages. *Semin. Cancer Biol.* **2012**, *22*, 289–297. [CrossRef] [PubMed]
53. Siveen, K.S.; Kuttan, G. Role of macrophages in tumour progression. *Immunol. Lett.* **2009**, *123*, 97–102. [CrossRef] [PubMed]
54. Sousa, S.; Brion, R.; Lintunen, M.; Kronqvist, P.; Sandholm, J.; Monkkonen, J.; Kellokumpu-Lehtinen, P.L.; Lauttia, S.; Tynninen, O.; Joensuu, H.; et al. Human breast cancer cells educate macrophages toward the M2 activation status. *Breast Cancer Res.* **2015**, *17*, 101. [CrossRef] [PubMed]
55. Gabrilovich, D.I.; Nagaraj, S. Myeloid-derived suppressor cells as regulators of the immune system. *Nat. Rev. Immunol.* **2009**, *9*, 162–174. [CrossRef] [PubMed]
56. Ostrand-Rosenberg, S.; Sinha, P. Myeloid-derived suppressor cells: Linking inflammation and cancer. *J. Immunol.* **2009**, *182*, 4499–4506. [CrossRef] [PubMed]
57. Safarzadeh, E.; Hashemzadeh, S.; Duijf, P.H.G.; Mansoori, B.; Khaze, V.; Mohammadi, A.; Kazemi, T.; Yousefi, M.; Asadi, M.; Mohammadi, H.; et al. Circulating myeloid-derived suppressor cells: An independent prognostic factor in patients with breast cancer. *J. Cell Physiol.* **2019**, *234*, 3515–3525. [CrossRef] [PubMed]

58. Mando, P.; Rizzo, M.; Roberti, M.P.; Julia, E.P.; Pampena, M.B.; Perez de la Puente, C.; Loza, C.M.; Ponce, C.; Nadal, J.; Colo, F.A.; et al. High neutrophil to lymphocyte ratio and decreased CD69(+)NK cells represent a phenotype of high risk in early-stage breast cancer patients. *Oncol. Targets Ther.* **2018**, *11*, 2901–2910. [CrossRef]
59. Treilleux, I.; Blay, J.Y.; Bendriss-Vermare, N.; Ray-Coquard, I.; Bachelot, T.; Guastalla, J.P.; Bremond, A.; Goddard, S.; Pin, J.J.; Barthelemy-Dubois, C.; et al. Dendritic cell infiltration and prognosis of early stage breast cancer. *Clin. Cancer Res.* **2004**, *10*, 7466–7474. [CrossRef]
60. Vivier, E.; Raulet, D.H.; Moretta, A.; Caligiuri, M.A.; Zitvogel, L.; Lanier, L.L.; Yokoyama, W.M.; Ugolini, S. Innate or adaptive immunity? The example of natural killer cells. *Science* **2011**, *331*, 44–49. [CrossRef]
61. Caligiuri, M.A. Human natural killer cells. *Blood* **2008**, *112*, 461–469. [CrossRef]
62. Cheng, M.; Chen, Y.; Xiao, W.; Sun, R.; Tian, Z. NK cell-based immunotherapy for malignant diseases. *Cell Mol. Immunol.* **2013**, *10*, 230–252. [CrossRef] [PubMed]
63. Ames, E.; Murphy, W.J. Advantages and clinical applications of natural killer cells in cancer immunotherapy. *Cancer Immunol. ImmunoTher.* **2014**, *63*, 21–28. [CrossRef] [PubMed]
64. Pasero, C.; Gravis, G.; Granjeaud, S.; Guerin, M.; Thomassin-Piana, J.; Rocchi, P.; Salem, N.; Walz, J.; Moretta, A.; Olive, D. Highly effective NK cells are associated with good prognosis in patients with metastatic prostate cancer. *Oncotarget* **2015**, *6*, 14360–14373. [CrossRef] [PubMed]
65. Mamessier, E.; Sylvain, A.; Thibult, M.L.; Houvenaeghel, G.; Jacquemier, J.; Castellano, R.; Goncalves, A.; Andre, P.; Romagne, F.; Thibault, G.; et al. Human breast cancer cells enhance self tolerance by promoting evasion from NK cell antitumor immunity. *J. Clin. Invest.* **2011**, *121*, 3609–3622. [CrossRef] [PubMed]
66. Costello, R.T.; Sivori, S.; Marcenaro, E.; Lafage-Pochitaloff, M.; Mozziconacci, M.J.; Reviron, D.; Gastaut, J.A.; Pende, D.; Olive, D.; Moretta, A. Defective expression and function of natural killer cell-triggering receptors in patients with acute myeloid leukemia. *Blood* **2002**, *99*, 3661–3667. [CrossRef] [PubMed]
67. Ascierto, M.L.; Idowu, M.O.; Zhao, Y.; Khalak, H.; Payne, K.K.; Wang, X.Y.; Dumur, C.I.; Bedognetti, D.; Tomei, S.; Ascierto, P.A.; et al. Molecular signatuRes. mostly associated with NK cells are predictive of relapse free survival in breast cancer patients. *J. Transl. Med.* **2013**, *11*, 145. [CrossRef] [PubMed]
68. Metzger, H.; Kinet, J.P. How antibodies work: Focus on Fc receptors. *FASEB J.* **1988**, *2*, 3–11. [CrossRef]
69. Crawford, A.; Macleod, M.; Schumacher, T.; Corlett, L.; Gray, D. Primary T cell expansion and differentiation in vivo requiRes. antigen presentation by B cells. *J. Immunol.* **2006**, *176*, 3498–3506. [CrossRef]
70. Mahmoud, S.M.; Paish, E.C.; Powe, D.G.; Macmillan, R.D.; Grainge, M.J.; Lee, A.H.; Ellis, I.O.; Green, A.R. Tumor-infiltrating CD8+ lymphocytes predict clinical outcome in breast cancer. *J. Clin. Oncol.* **2011**, *29*, 1949–1955. [CrossRef]
71. Schmidt, M.; Bohm, D.; von Torne, C.; Steiner, E.; Puhl, A.; Pilch, H.; Lehr, H.A.; Hengstler, J.G.; Kolbl, H.; Gehrmann, M. The humoral immune system has a key prognostic impact in node-negative breast cancer. *Cancer Res.* **2008**, *68*, 5405–5413. [CrossRef]
72. Olkhanud, P.B.; Damdinsuren, B.; Bodogai, M.; Gress, R.E.; Sen, R.; Wejksza, K.; Malchinkhuu, E.; Wersto, R.P.; Biragyn, A. Tumor-evoked regulatory B cells promote breast cancer metastasis by converting resting CD4(+) T cells to T-regulatory cells. *Cancer Res.* **2011**, *71*, 3505–3515. [CrossRef]
73. Orimo, A.; Gupta, P.B.; Sgroi, D.C.; Arenzana-Seisdedos, F.; Delaunay, T.; Naeem, R.; Carey, V.J.; Richardson, A.L.; Weinberg, R.A. Stromal fibroblasts present in invasive human breast carcinomas promote tumor growth and angiogenesis through elevated SDF-1/CXCL12 secretion. *Cell* **2005**, *121*, 335–348. [CrossRef]
74. Boire, A.; Covic, L.; Agarwal, A.; Jacques, S.; Sherifi, S.; Kuliopulos, A. PAR1 is a matrix metalloprotease-1 receptor that promotes invasion and tumorigenesis of breast cancer cells. *Cell* **2005**, *120*, 303–313. [CrossRef]
75. Sternlicht, M.D.; Lochter, A.; Sympson, C.J.; Huey, B.; Rougier, J.P.; Gray, J.W.; Pinkel, D.; Bissell, M.J.; Werb, Z. The stromal proteinase MMP3/stromelysin-1 promotes mammary carcinogenesis. *Cell* **1999**, *98*, 137–146. [CrossRef]
76. Stetler-Stevenson, W.G.; Aznavoorian, S.; Liotta, L.A. Tumor cell interactions with the extracellular matrix during invasion and metastasis. *Annu. Rev. Cell Biol.* **1993**, *9*, 541–573. [CrossRef]
77. Yu, Y.; Xiao, C.H.; Tan, L.D.; Wang, Q.S.; Li, X.Q.; Feng, Y.M. Cancer-associated fibroblasts induce epithelial-mesenchymal transition of breast cancer cells through paracrine TGF-beta signalling. *Br. J. Cancer* **2014**, *110*, 724–732. [CrossRef]
78. Kalluri, R.; Zeisberg, M. Fibroblasts in cancer. *Nat. Rev. Cancer* **2006**, *6*, 392–401. [CrossRef]

79. Buckley, C.D.; Pilling, D.; Lord, J.M.; Akbar, A.N.; Scheel-Toellner, D.; Salmon, M. Fibroblasts regulate the switch from acute resolving to chronic persistent inflammation. *Trends Immunol.* **2001**, *22*, 199–204. [CrossRef]
80. Finak, G.; Bertos, N.; Pepin, F.; Sadekova, S.; Souleimanova, M.; Zhao, H.; Chen, H.; Omeroglu, G.; Meterissian, S.; Omeroglu, A.; et al. Stromal gene expression predicts clinical outcome in breast cancer. *Nat. Med.* **2008**, *14*, 518–527. [CrossRef]
81. Hendry, S.; Pang, J.B.; Byrne, D.J.; Lakhani, S.R.; Cummings, M.C.; Campbell, I.G.; Mann, G.B.; Gorringe, K.L.; Fox, S.B. Relationship of the Breast Ductal Carcinoma In Situ Immune Microenvironment with Clinicopathological and Genetic Features. *Clin. Cancer Res.* **2017**, *23*, 5210–5217. [CrossRef]
82. Hussein, M.R.; Hassan, H.I. Analysis of the mononuclear inflammatory cell infiltrate in the normal breast, benign proliferative breast disease, in situ and infiltrating ductal breast carcinomas: Preliminary observations. *J. Clin. Pathol.* **2006**, *59*, 972–977. [CrossRef]
83. Gil Del Alcazar, C.R.; Huh, S.J.; Ekram, M.B.; Trinh, A.; Liu, L.L.; Beca, F.; Zi, X.; Kwak, M.; Bergholtz, H.; Su, Y.; et al. Immune Escape in Breast Cancer During In Situ to Invasive Carcinoma Transition. *Cancer Discov.* **2017**, *7*, 1098–1115. [CrossRef]
84. Campbell, M.J.; Baehner, F.; O'Meara, T.; Ojukwu, E.; Han, B.; Mukhtar, R.; Tandon, V.; Endicott, M.; Zhu, Z.; Wong, J.; et al. Characterizing the immune microenvironment in high-risk ductal carcinoma in situ of the breast. *Breast Cancer Res. Treat.* **2017**, *161*, 17–28. [CrossRef]
85. Hu, M.; Yao, J.; Carroll, D.K.; Weremowicz, S.; Chen, H.; Carrasco, D.; Richardson, A.; Violette, S.; Nikolskaya, T.; Nikolsky, Y.; et al. Regulation of in situ to invasive breast carcinoma transition. *Cancer Cell* **2008**, *13*, 394–406. [CrossRef]
86. Kalluri, R. The biology and function of fibroblasts in cancer. *Nat. Rev. Cancer* **2016**, *16*, 582–598. [CrossRef]
87. Osuala, K.O.; Sameni, M.; Shah, S.; Aggarwal, N.; Simonait, M.L.; Franco, O.E.; Hong, Y.; Hayward, S.W.; Behbod, F.; Mattingly, R.R.; et al. Il-6 signaling between ductal carcinoma in situ cells and carcinoma-associated fibroblasts mediates tumor cell growth and migration. *BMC Cancer* **2015**, *15*, 584. [CrossRef]
88. Carron, E.C.; Homra, S.; Rosenberg, J.; Coffelt, S.B.; Kittrell, F.; Zhang, Y.; Creighton, C.J.; Fuqua, S.A.; Medina, D.; Machado, H.L. Macrophages promote the progression of premalignant mammary lesions to invasive cancer. *Oncotarget* **2017**, *8*, 50731–50746. [CrossRef]
89. Ning, C.; Xie, B.; Zhang, L.; Li, C.; Shan, W.; Yang, B.; Luo, X.; Gu, C.; He, Q.; Jin, H.; et al. Infiltrating Macrophages Induce ERalpha Expression through an IL17A-mediated Epigenetic Mechanism to Sensitize Endometrial Cancer Cells to Estrogen. *Cancer Res.* **2016**, *76*, 1354–1366. [CrossRef]
90. Degnim, A.C.; Brahmbhatt, R.D.; Radisky, D.C.; Hoskin, T.L.; Stallings-Mann, M.; Laudenschlager, M.; Mansfield, A.; Frost, M.H.; Murphy, L.; Knutson, K.; et al. Immune cell quantitation in normal breast tissue lobules with and without lobulitis. *Breast Cancer Res. Treat.* **2014**, *144*, 539–549. [CrossRef]
91. Huo, C.W.; Hill, P.; Chew, G.; Neeson, P.J.; Halse, H.; Williams, E.D.; Henderson, M.A.; Thompson, E.W.; Britt, K.L. High mammographic density in women is associated with protumor inflammation. *Breast Cancer Res.* **2018**, *20*, 92. [CrossRef]
92. Lopez-Garcia, M.A.; Geyer, F.C.; Lacroix-Triki, M.; Marchio, C.; Reis-Filho, J.S. Breast cancer precursors revisited: Molecular featuRes. and progression pathways. *Histopathology* **2010**, *57*, 171–192. [CrossRef]
93. Page, D.L.; Dupont, W.D.; Rogers, L.W.; Rados, M.S. Atypical hyperplastic lesions of the female breast. A long-term follow-up study. *Cancer* **1985**, *55*, 2698–2708. [CrossRef]
94. Walia, S.; Ma, Y.; Lu, J.; Lang, J.E.; Press, M.F. Pathology and current management of borderline breast epithelial lesions. *Am. J. Hematol./Oncol.* **2017**, *14*, 24–31.
95. Bhowmick, N.A.; Chytil, A.; Plieth, D.; Gorska, A.E.; Dumont, N.; Shappell, S.; Washington, M.K.; Neilson, E.G.; Moses, H.L. TGF-beta signaling in fibroblasts modulates the oncogenic potential of adjacent epithelia. *Science* **2004**, *303*, 848–851. [CrossRef]
96. Trimboli, A.J.; Cantemir-Stone, C.Z.; Li, F.; Wallace, J.A.; Merchant, A.; Creasap, N.; Thompson, J.C.; Caserta, E.; Wang, H.; Chong, J.L.; et al. Pten in stromal fibroblasts suppresses mammary epithelial tumours. *Nature* **2009**, *461*, 1084–1091. [CrossRef]
97. Sun, Y.; Yang, D.; Xi, L.; Chen, Y.; Fu, L.; Sun, K.; Yin, J.; Li, X.; Liu, S.; Qin, Y.; et al. Primed atypical ductal hyperplasia-associated fibroblasts promote cell growth and polarity changes of transformed epithelium-like breast cancer MCF-7 cells via miR-200b/c-IKKbeta signaling. *Cell Death Dis.* **2018**, *9*, 122. [CrossRef]

98. Cimino-Mathews, A.; Thompson, E.; Taube, J.M.; Ye, X.; Lu, Y.; Meeker, A.; Xu, H.; Sharma, R.; Lecksell, K.; Cornish, T.C.; et al. PD-L1 (B7-H1) expression and the immune tumor microenvironment in primary and metastatic breast carcinomas. *Hum. Pathol.* **2016**, *47*, 52–63. [CrossRef]
99. Muenst, S.; Schaerli, A.R.; Gao, F.; Daster, S.; Trella, E.; Droeser, R.A.; Muraro, M.G.; Zajac, P.; Zanetti, R.; Gillanders, W.E.; et al. Expression of programmed death ligand 1 (PD-L1) is associated with poor prognosis in human breast cancer. *Breast Cancer Res. Treat.* **2014**, *146*, 15–24. [CrossRef]
100. Muenst, S.; Soysal, S.D.; Gao, F.; Obermann, E.C.; Oertli, D.; Gillanders, W.E. The presence of programmed death 1 (PD-1)-positive tumor-infiltrating lymphocytes is associated with poor prognosis in human breast cancer. *Breast Cancer Res. Treat.* **2013**, *139*, 667–676. [CrossRef]
101. Loi, S.; Dushyanthen, S.; Beavis, P.A.; Salgado, R.; Denkert, C.; Savas, P.; Combs, S.; Rimm, D.L.; Giltnane, J.M.; Estrada, M.V.; et al. RAS/MAPK Activation Is Associated with Reduced Tumor-Infiltrating Lymphocytes in Triple-Negative Breast Cancer: Therapeutic Cooperation Between MEK and PD-1/PD-L1 Immune Checkpoint Inhibitors. *Clin. Cancer Res.* **2016**, *22*, 1499–1509. [CrossRef]
102. Ubago, J.M.; Blanco, L.Z.; Shen, T.; Siziopikou, K.P. The PD-1/PD-L1 Axis in HER2+ Ductal Carcinoma In Situ (DCIS) of the Breast. *Am. J. Clin. Pathol.* **2019**, *152*, 169–176. [CrossRef]
103. Ayoub, N.M.; Al-Shami, K.M.; Yaghan, R.J. Immunotherapy for HER2-positive breast cancer: Recent advances and combination therapeutic approaches. *Breast Cancer* **2019**, *11*, 53–69. [CrossRef]
104. Dushyanthen, S.; Teo, Z.L.; Caramia, F.; Savas, P.; Mintoff, C.P.; Virassamy, B.; Henderson, M.A.; Luen, S.J.; Mansour, M.; Kershaw, M.H.; et al. Agonist immunotherapy restoRes. T cell function following MEK inhibition improving efficacy in breast cancer. *Nat. Commun.* **2017**, *8*, 606. [CrossRef]
105. Leftin, A.; Ben-Chetrit, N.; Joyce, J.A.; Koutcher, J.A. Imaging endogenous macrophage iron deposits reveals a metabolic biomarker of polarized tumor macrophage infiltration and response to CSF1R breast cancer immunotherapy. *Sci. Rep.* **2019**, *9*, 857. [CrossRef]
106. Swierczak, A.; Cook, A.D.; Lenzo, J.C.; Restall, C.M.; Doherty, J.P.; Anderson, R.L.; Hamilton, J.A. The promotion of breast cancer metastasis caused by inhibition of CSF-1R/CSF-1 signaling is blocked by targeting the G-CSF receptor. *Cancer Immunol. Res.* **2014**, *2*, 765–776. [CrossRef]

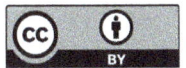

© 2019 by the authors. Licensee MDPI, Basel, Switzerland. This article is an open access article distributed under the terms and conditions of the Creative Commons Attribution (CC BY) license (http://creativecommons.org/licenses/by/4.0/).

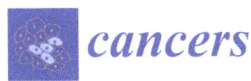

Review

Molecular Basis of Tumor Heterogeneity in Endometrial Carcinosarcoma

Susanna Leskela [1,2,*], Belen Pérez-Mies [2,3], Juan Manuel Rosa-Rosa [1,2], Eva Cristobal [1], Michele Biscuola [2,4,5], María L. Palacios-Berraquero [6], SuFey Ong [7], Xavier Matias-Guiu Guia [2,8,9,10] and José Palacios [1,2,11,*]

1. Department of Pathology, Institute Ramón y Cajal for Health Research, 28034 Madrid, Spain
2. CIBER-ONC, Instituto de Salud Carlos III, 28029 Madrid, Spain
3. Department of Pathology, Hospital Ramón y Cajal, 28034 Madrid, Spain
4. Department of Pathology, Instituto de Biomedicina de Sevilla (IBiS), 41013 Seville, Spain
5. Hospital Universitario Virgen del Rocío/CSIC/Universidad de Sevilla, 41013 Seville, Spain
6. Department of Hematology and Hemotherapy, Clínica Universidad de Navarra, 31008 Pamplona, Spain
7. NanoString Technologies, Inc, Seattle, WA 98109, USA
8. Department of Pathology, Hospital U Arnau de Vilanova, 25198 Lleida, Spain
9. Department of Pathology, Hospital U de Bellvitge, L'Hospitalet de Llobregat, 08907 Barcelona, Spain
10. IRBLLEIDA, IDIBELL, University of Lleida, 25003 Lleida, Spain
11. Faculty of Medicine, University of Alcalá de Henares, Alcalá de Henares, 28801 Madrid, Spain
* Correspondence: susanna.leskela@gmail.com (S.L.); jose.palacios@salud.madrid.org (J.P.); Tel.: +34-91-336-8140 (S.L.); +34-91-336-8337 (J.P.)

Received: 24 May 2019; Accepted: 2 July 2019; Published: 10 July 2019

Abstract: Endometrial carcinosarcoma (ECS) represents one of the most extreme examples of tumor heterogeneity among human cancers. ECS is a clinically aggressive, high-grade, metaplastic carcinoma. At the morphological level, intratumor heterogeneity in ECS is due to an admixture of epithelial (carcinoma) and mesenchymal (sarcoma) components that can include heterologous tissues, such as skeletal muscle, cartilage, or bone. Most ECSs belong to the copy-number high serous-like molecular subtype of endometrial carcinoma, characterized by the *TP53* mutation and the frequently accompanied by a large number of gene copy-number alterations, including the amplification of important oncogenes, such as *CCNE1* and *c-MYC*. However, a proportion of cases (20%) probably represent the progression of tumors initially belonging to the copy-number low endometrioid-like molecular subtype (characterized by mutations in genes such as *PTEN*, *PI3KCA*, or *ARID1A*), after the acquisition of the *TP53* mutations. Only a few ECS belong to the microsatellite-unstable hypermutated molecular type and the *POLE*-mutated, ultramutated molecular type. A common characteristic of all ECSs is the modulation of genes involved in the epithelial to mesenchymal process. Thus, the acquisition of a mesenchymal phenotype is associated with a switch from E- to N-cadherin, the up-regulation of transcriptional repressors of E-cadherin, such as Snail Family Transcriptional Repressor 1 and 2 (SNAI1 and SNAI2), Zinc Finger E-Box Binding Homeobox 1 and 2 (ZEB1 and ZEB2), and the down-regulation, among others, of members of the miR-200 family involved in the maintenance of an epithelial phenotype. Subsequent differentiation to different types of mesenchymal tissues increases tumor heterogeneity and probably modulates clinical behavior and therapy response.

Keywords: uterine carcinosarcoma; endometrial carcinoma; metaplastic carcinoma; epithelial-to-mesenchymal transition; clonality; mutation; *TP53*; PI3K/AKT pathway; gene expression; miRNA expression

1. Clinicopathological Characteristics

Endometrial carcinosarcoma (ECS), also known as malignant mixed Müllerian tumor (MMMT), is a high-grade tumor characterized by a biphasic growth of malignant epithelial (carcinomatous) and mesenchymal (sarcomatous) components (Figure 1) [1]. ECS is a rare aggressive neoplasm accounting for approximately 2% to 5% of gynecological carcinomas, but it causes around 16% of all deaths due to malignancies of the uterine corpus [2,3]. Although ECS shares similar risk factors with endometrial carcinoma, such as obesity, nulliparity, smoking, and exogenous estrogen use, they present at more advanced stages and have significantly worse survival than high-grade endometrial carcinomas [3–8].

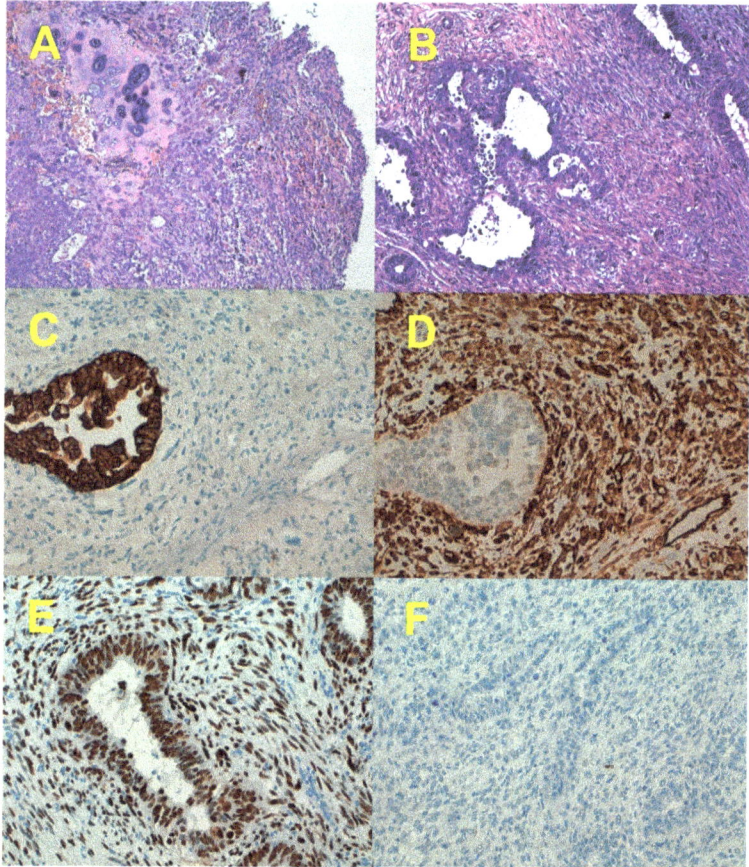

Figure 1. Morphological and immunohistochemical features of endometrial carcinosarcoma. (**A**) Hematoxylin-eosin staining of an endometrial carcinosarcoma showing the epithelial component surrounded by the heterologous mesenchymal component (chondrosarcoma). (**B**) Endometrial carcinosarcoma with homologous sarcoma (H&E). (**C**) Cytokeratin expression of the case depicted in b. (**D**) Vimentin expression in the case depicted in b. (**E**) p53 overexpression in both the carcinomatous and sarcomatous components. (**F**) p53 null pattern in both the carcinomatous and sarcomatous components. Only occasional normal stromal cells expressed p53. Original magnification 10× for (**A**,**B**), and 20× for (**C**–**F**).

Matsuo et al. [9] analyzed the incidence of ECS in the USA during 1973–2013 in 235,849 primary endometrial carcinomas (ECs) and observed that the proportion of ECS is now significantly higher than before and accounts for more than 5% of ECs. There was a significant rise in the proportion of ECS among primary ECs from 1.7% to 5.6% during this period. Moreover, among 76,118 type II ECs, the proportion of ECS also increased significantly from 6% to 17.5%; ECS was detected in 11,000 (4.7%) women. The percentage of black women with ECS was elevated from 11.9% to 20%, whereas the proportion of white women decreased from 86% to 60.5%. The possible factors associated with the increase of ECS include the increment in the number of older women and the obese population in the US, and the global increase in the incidence of breast cancer with a concordant increment in tamoxifen use [9].

Several studies have demonstrated that tamoxifen use may be associated with an increased incidence of ECS. In women with breast cancer, the incidence of ECS is 6.35-fold higher in those treated with tamoxifen [10]. Matsuo et al. [11] reported that ~6% of women with ECS have a history of tamoxifen use and that tamoxifen-related ECS was significantly associated with a higher proportion of stage IA disease (48.4% versus 29.9%) and a lower risk of stage IVB disease (7.8% versus 16%) compared to tamoxifen-unrelated ECS. Deep myometrial tumor invasion was less common in uterine carcinosarcoma related to tamoxifen use (28.3% versus 48.8%). However, in spite of these favorable tumor characteristics, tamoxifen-related ECS had comparable stage-specific survival outcomes compared to tamoxifen-unrelated ECS.

From a morphological point of view, the epithelial component of ECS could be endometrioid (most common in most series) or non-endometrioid (serous, clear cell, undifferentiated, or mixed) [3,4,12–15]. Matsuo et al. [16] reported that among 906 ECS evaluated for histological patterns in their series, high-grade carcinoma/homologous sarcoma (40.8%) was the most common type followed by high-grade carcinoma/heterologous sarcoma (30.9%), low-grade carcinoma/homologous sarcoma (18%), and low-grade-carcinoma/heterologous sarcoma (10.3%). In 75% to 95% of ECS, the epithelial component was of high grade [16,17]. The mesenchymal component could be minimal or extensive. Sarcoma dominance (SD) is defined by the presence of more than 50% of the tumor composed by the sarcomatous component. The mesenchymal component could be subdivided into homologous (fibrosarcoma, leiomyosarcoma, and endometrial stromal sarcoma) and heterologous, the latter including skeletal muscle, cartilage, fat, or osteoid, which is present in up to 60% of tumors [3,4,12–19]. Immunohistochemistry may be useful in confirming the presence of a heterologous mesenchymal component, which, as discussed later, is an adverse prognostic indicator in some series. For example, nuclear staining with myogenin and Myoblast determination protein 1 (myoD1) helps to confirm the presence of rhabdomyoblastic differentiation (Figure 2) [20].

Regarding other pathological features, 55% to 60% of ECS show less than 50% of myometrial invasion at diagnosis. Lymphovascular invasion (LVI) prevalence in ECS seems to be higher than in other types of endometrial cancer (60.4–62% vs. 26–52%) [21]. Matsuo et al. [21] reported that among LVI-positive cases, LVIs with a carcinomatous component alone was found in 76.8% and LVI containing a sarcomatous component with or without a carcinomatous component in the remaining 23.2%. Tumors in the LVI-sarcoma group were more likely to have SD (82.1% vs. 26.4%), heterologous sarcomatous component (51.3% vs. 37.9%), low-grade carcinoma (42.5% vs. 22.4%), and large tumor size (81% vs. 70.2%) in the primary tumor site compared with tumors in the LVI-carcinoma group.

Also, the pattern of metastasis differs between the epithelial and mesenchymal parts of the ECS. Thus, for example, Matsuo et al. [16] analyzed 1096 metastatic sites and showed that carcinoma components tended to spread lymphatically, while sarcoma components tended to spread locoregionally (cervix, vagina, etc.).

ECS follows an aggressive clinical course. Patients with International Federation of Gynecology and Obstetrics (FIGO) stage 1–2 disease have a five-year disease-specific survival of 59%, while those with stage 3 and 4 disease have a five-year disease-specific survival of 22% and 9%, respectively [2]. The most important prognostic factors in these tumors include FIGO stage and depth of myometrial invasion [5,7,8,13,15,22]. Other known clinicopathologic features associated with worse outcome are the grade and histology of the epithelial component and lymphovascular invasion [3,5,8,13]. Although the grade and the amount of the sarcomatous component and the presence of heterologous elements are not related to the overall outcome in some series [6,13,18,22], recent studies have shown the importance of the sarcomatous component in the prognosis and response to radiotherapy [17,23]. Thus, Matsuo et al. [24] reported that ECS with better prognosis were those composed of a low-grade carcinoma and homologous sarcoma without SD. In contrast, the worse prognosis corresponded to ECS composed of a high-grade carcinoma and heterologous sarcoma and SD. This latter type of tumor tended to occur in older, obese, and Caucasian patients, and they were more likely to have metastatic implants, large tumor sizes, LVI with sarcoma cells, and higher lymph node ratios. Also, SD seems to be a prognostic factor in some series [17,23], and it is associated with loco-regional tumor metastasis and recurrence with sarcoma. In addition, ECS with SD seems more sensitive to radiotherapy compared to ECS without sarcoma dominance [23]. Finally, different studies have reported a poor prognosis in ECS with rhabdomyoblastic differentiation [4,17,19].

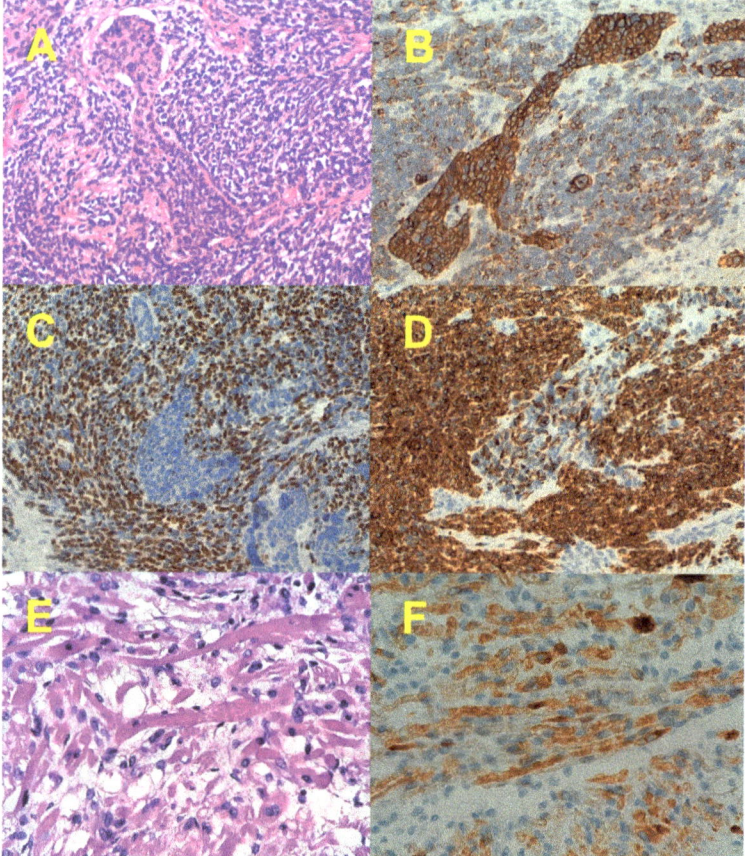

Figure 2. Endometrial carcinosarcoma with rhabdomyoblastic differentiation. Some cells showed an intermediate epithelial/mesenchymal differentiation as suggested by the expression pattern of cytokeratins, myogenin, and desmin. (**A**) Hematoxylin-eosin staining. (**B**) Cytokeratin (CK AE1/AE3) expression. (**C**) Myoblast determination protein 1 (MyoD1) expression. (**D**) Desmin expression. (**E**) Striated rhabdomyoblasts (H&E). (**F**) Desmin expression by striated rhabdomyoblasts. Original magnification 20× for A-D, and 40× for E and F.

Molecular studies have demonstrated similar genetic alterations in both the carcinomatous and sarcomatous components of ECS (Table 1). Thus, it is now accepted that most carcinosarcomas are in fact metaplastic carcinomas, in which the sarcomatous component is derived from the carcinomatous component as a result of transdifferentiation (epithelial-to-mesenchymal transition—EMT) during the evolution of the tumor as shown in several studies [25,26]. However, a small percentage of ECS probably represent real collision tumors, since they are molecularly biclonal and most likely develop from two independent cell populations [6,27].

Table 1. Comparison of gene mutation frequency among different histological types of endometrial cancer according to The Cancer Genome Atlas Program (TCGA).

GENE	Endometrioid Carcinoma	Serous Carcinoma	Carcinosarcoma
PTEN	82%	10%	19%
PIK3CA	54%	37%	35%
PIK3R1	36%	11%	11%
CTNNB1	34%	1%	2%
ARID1A	54%	8%	12%
KRAS	24%	3%	12%
CTCF	31%	2%	7%
TP53	21%	88%	91%
FBXW7	17%	24%	39%
PPP2R1A	11%	38%	28%
CHD4	9%	18%	17%
CCNE1 (ampl.)	16%	26%	41%
MYC (ampl.)	14%	24%	21%
MECOM (ampl.)	18%	33%	18%
PIK3CA (ampl.)	10%	22%	11%
ERBB2 (ampl.)	8%	19%	9%

2. Molecular Subtypes of ECS

Four molecular groups have been defined for ECs: the hypermutated (mismatch repair deficiency), the ultramutated (*POLE* mutated), the copy-number low, and the copy-number high groups. These groups not only have different molecular alterations but also different prognoses; patients from the ultramutated group show the best prognosis, whereas patients in the copy-number high group have the highest risk of recurrence [28].

Considering the mutational profile (Table 1; see below Section 2. Molecular Subtypes of ECS), most ECSs are similar to serous-like, copy-number high ECs. Thus, in the study by McConechy et al., most tumors had a molecular profile similar to endometrial serous carcinoma (characterized by the presence of *TP53*, *FBXW7*, and *PPP2R1A* mutations and the absence of *ARID1A*, *CTNNB1*, *KRAS*, or *PTEN* mutations), while part of the tumors displayed an endometrioid carcinoma-like mutation profile characterized by the presence of *ARID1A*, *CTNNB1*, *KRAS*, and *PTEN* mutations. Based on both combined genetic and immunohistochemical profiles in their cohort, 18 tumors presented serous-like and 11 tumors presented endometrioid-like molecular profiles. There was a good correlation between the histological subtyping (taking into account the morphology of the epithelial component) and the molecular subtyping in 27 of 29 uterine carcinosarcomas (93%) [29]. More recently Jones et al., applied this classification to their set of tumors, and were able to classify 55 out of 57 tumors, of which 22% were endometrioid and 78% serous-like ECS. One sample did not fit in the model due to an ultramutated phenotype caused by the *POLE* mutation, while another had no mutation in the genes used for classification. Interestingly, all 10 stage IV tumors were serous-like [30].

Most of the endometrioid-like ECSs also showed *TP53* mutations, implying that *TP53* could be involved in the progression of part of the copy-number low endometrioid-like carcinomas to ECSs, as we have previously reported in undifferentiated endometrial carcinoma [31]. Very few ECS belong to the microsatellite-unstable hypermutated molecular type and the *POLE*-mutated ultramutated molecular type used for the classification of endometrial carcinoma. The molecular heterogeneity present in ECS opens opportunities for targeted therapies.

3. Serous-Like Molecular Alterations in ECS

Previous studies combining aberrant expression of p53 and mutational analysis estimated a *TP53* mutation prevalence of 50–60% [3,12,22,27,32–35]. However, subsequent studies using Next Generation Sequencing (NGS) techniques have shown that the true frequency of *TP53* mutation in ECS is very high, between 64% and 91% [29,30,36–40]. In effect, *TP53* mutations are the most frequent molecular alterations in ECS (Table 1). The lack of nuclear p53 expression is most commonly detected with indel or nonsense mutations, while missense mutations usually lead to diffuse nuclear p53 immunostaining. Most of the mutations are located in the DNA binding domain, and very few are present in the translocation and tetramerization motifs. In the DNA binding domain, 32% of mutations are located on known hotspot residues, and the most frequent are the R248Q and R273C/H (12% and 7%, respectively) followed by H179R/D, H193R/Y, and S241Y (5% each), (http://cancergenome.nih.gov/) [41].

The carcinomatous and sarcomatous components show a concordance of 85% for the p53 protein overexpression and 96% for the *TP53* gene mutation, which points to a monoclonal origin of both components (Figure 1). p16 overexpression (in-block diffuse expression) occurs in about 60% of ECS simultaneously with TP53 mutations. The concordance of p16 expression between the carcinomatous and sarcomatous components was about 85% in different series [12,35,42–44]. In addition to *TP53*, ECSs show mutations in other genes that are also more frequently affected in endometrial serous carcinoma (ESC) than in endometrial endometrioid carcinoma (EEC). Accordingly, mutations of *FBXW7* and *PPP2R1A* have been reported in 19% to 39% and 1% to 38%, respectively, in different series [36–40].

Regarding the *BRCA1* and *BRCA2* genes, the frequency of ECS in patients carrying germinal *BRCA1/2* mutations has been analyzed in different studies. The estimated relative risk for mutation carriers is approximately 2% per year, most importantly among serous carcinoma [45–47]. A recent series has reported that *BRCA1/2* were found mutated in 18% and 27%, respectively of ECS [30], although in the TCGA (The Cancer Genome Atlas Program) series, only *BRCA2* mutations were detected and at a lower frequency (5%) [28]. Carcinosarcoma of the breast and ovary have been reported in some patients with *BRCA1/2* germline mutations [48–50].

Zhao et al. [51] found an excess of mutations in genes encoding *histone H2A* and *H2B*, as well as a significant amplification of the segment of chromosome 6p harboring the histone gene cluster containing these genes. Thus, mutations in histone *H2A/H2B* genes were significantly enriched in carcinosarcomas (CSs) compared with carcinomas (mutations in 21.2% of CSs and 5.2% of uterine and ovarian epithelial tumor). These findings implicate mutations in histone *H2A/H2B* genes in ECS.

Le Gallo et al. [40] have reported forkhead box A2 (*FOXA2*) mutations in 15.1% of ECS. *FOXA2* had not previously been implicated in ECSs and was predominated by frameshift and nonsense mutations. Sequencing of *FOXA2* in 160 primary endometrial carcinomas revealed somatic mutations in 5.7% of serous, 22.7% of clear cell, 9% of endometrioid, and 11.1% of mixed endometrial carcinomas, the majority of which were frameshift mutations. Collectively, the findings of the study of Le Gallo et al. [40] provide evidence that *FOXA2* is a pathogenic driver gene in the etiology of primary uterine cancers, including ECSs.

Similarly to ESC, ECS is characterized by aneuploidy and a high frequency of copy number variations (CNVs). Analysis of ploidy and whole-genome doubling has established a median ploidy of 3.3 and that 90% of ECS had undergone at least one whole-genome-doubling event. This percentage is significantly higher than in serous ovarian tumors, the tumor type with the next highest frequency of genomic doubling in the TCGA [38].

Recurring focal amplifications reported in the TCGA [38], some of which have also been observed in other series [51], include those containing known oncogenes such as *TERC* (3q26.2), *FGFR3* (4p16.3), *MYC* (8q24.21), *KAT6A* (10q22.2), *MDM2* (12q15), *ERBB2* (17q12), CCND1 (11q13), CCNE1 (19q12), *BCL2L1* (20q11.21), and *RIT1* (1q22) (Figure 3).

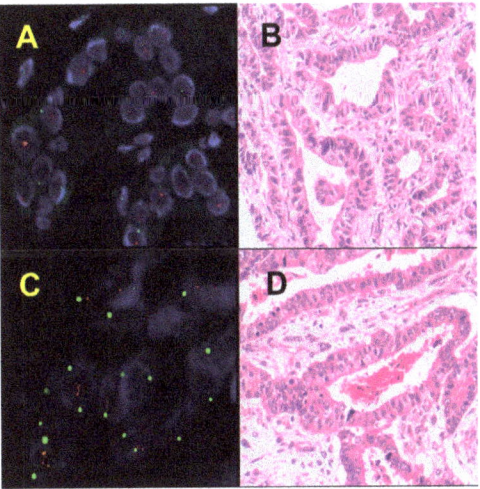

Figure 3. Amplification of oncogenes in endometrial carcinosarcomas analyzed by fluorescence in situ hybridization (FISH) (**A**) and (**B**), MYC proto-oncogene, bHLH transcription factor (*MYC*) amplification (**C**), and (**D**) Cyclin D1 (*CCND1*) amplification. Original magnification ×100 for A and C, and ×20 for B-D.

Cyclin D1 (*CCNE1*) is the most frequently amplified gene in ECS, 41% according to data derived from TCGA (Table 1). In other tumors, for example, ovarian high-grade serous carcinoma, amplification of *CCNE1* is associated with a worse prognosss and resistance to chemotherapy. According to Schipf et al., *c-MYC* amplification had a higher frequency in the carcinomatous compared to the sarcomatous tumor component. In their data on 30 carcinosarcomas of the ovary and uterus, *c-MYC* gene amplification was reported in 78% by fluorescence in situ hybridization (FISH) [52]. However, the TCGA data showed amplification of *c-MYC* in only 21% of ECSs [38].

The frequency of *ERBB2* amplification in ECS ranged from 3–20% [30,38,53–55]. Thus, ECS patients with *ERBB2* amplification could benefit from anti-HER2 (human epidermal growth factor receptor 2) therapies, such as Trastuzumab. For patients unresponsive to chemotherapy and Trastuzumab, T-DM1 (Trastuzumab emtansine) may offer an alternative treatment option, as recent studies show how ECS cell lines and derived xenografts with *ERBB2* amplification respond well to T-DM1 [56]. *PIK3CA* is amplified in 11% of ECS, further highlighting the importance of the phosphatidylinositol 3-kinase (PIK3) pathway (see Section 4. Endometrioid-Like Molecular Alterations).

Schipf et al. detected *ZNF217* amplification in 87% of gynecological CS [52]. Similarly to *c-MYC*, in the TCGA data set the frequency is much lower (9%) [28,38]. Two other frequently amplified oncogenes in ECS, *EGFR*, and *URI* (unconventional prefolding RPB5 interactor 1), have not been found in the TCGA data set. Biscuola et al. reported *EGFR* amplification by FISH in 19% of tumors [57], while in studies with smaller sample size, EGFR (epidermal growth factor receptor) protein overexpression has been reported in 45% to 82% of ECS, where a higher level of expression was seen in the sarcomatous component [53,58,59]. *URI1* amplification has been reported in 40% of ECS [60]. *URI1* amplification was also associated with poor survival and reduced response to adjuvant treatment. Likewise, in a cultured cell model, overexpression of *URI1* induced *ATM* (ATM Serine/Threonine Kinase) expression and resistance to cisplatin [60]. Recurring *GPC5* (Glypican 5) gain/amplification has been detected in a subset of ECS, mostly in the sarcoma component, and the authors linked the involvement of *GPC5* with sarcomatous transformation [61].

4. Endometrioid-Like Molecular Alterations

Mutations in genes encoding for the kinase or regulatory proteins of the PI3K/AKT (phosphatidylinositol 3-kinase/(Protein Kinase B) pathway have been detected in up to 67% of ECS [29]. Moreover, multiple PI3K/AKT pathway proteins have been found mutated in one tumor. *PIK3CA* mutations have been found in 11% to 40% [29,30,36,38,57,62,63] of the tumors. Unlike for *TP53*, with mutations concentrated on HotSpot regions, the mutations in *PIK3CA* are found scattered in the different functional domains. In addition to the traditional *PIK3CA* hotspots in exons 9 and 20, a smaller portion of ECS has mutations in exon 1, in the adaptor binding domain, helical domain, and C2 domain which increase kinase enzymatic activity [29,57].

The importance of mutations in this pathway comes from the fact that *PI3KCA* mutations have been detected in both the carcinoma and sarcoma components of the primary tumor and also in the metastatic tumor. This implies that they are important early events in the tumorigenesis of carcinosarcoma and thus could be targeted with PIK3CA/mTOR (Phosphatidylinositol-4,5-Bisphosphate 3-Kinase Catalytic Subunit Alpha /Mechanistic Target of Rapamycin Kinase) inhibitors [29,38]. PIK3CA inhibition has been applied successfully in advanced endometrial cancers [64].

Phosphatase And Tensin Homolog (*PTEN*) mutations are not as frequent as *PIK3CA*, but they are present in approximately 20% of ECS: 17% and 19% in the series reported by McConechy et al. [29] and the TCGA [38], respectively. However, Jones et al. reported that 47% of ECS carried *PTEN* mutation, but their series included only 17 cases [36]. *PTEN* and *PIK3CA* mutations frequently coexist in the same ECS [29].

Other genes with less frequency of mutations in the PI3K/AKT pathway in ECSs include Phosphatidylinositol 3-Kinase Regulatory Subunit 1 (*PIK3R1*) (10–17%), *PIK3R2, AKT1, AKT2,* and *AKT3* (less than 5% for each gene) [29,36,38,57].

AT-Rich Interaction Domain 1A (*ARID1A*) and Catenin Beta 1 (*CTNNB1*) are commonly mutated in EEC, and *ARID1A* mutations occur also in 10% to 15% of ECS, leading usually to loss of of protein expression, while mutations in *CTNNB1* are infrequent in ECS [36,38,63]. *KRAS* mutations were found in 12% and Cadherin 4 (*CDH4*) mutations in 18% [38].

Mismatch repair deficiency (MMR-def) and *POLE* mutations are more common in EEC than in ESC. MMR-def is due to germline or somatic even affecting mismatch repair genes, most frequently MutL Homolog 1 (*MLH1*), MutS Homolog 2 (*MSH2*), MutS Homolog 6 (*MSH6*), and Mismatch Repair Endonuclease PMS2 (*PMS2*). In sporadic EC, MMR-def is detected in 15–30% of cases [65], although a higher frequency has been detected among high-grade endometrioid carcinomas (45–63%) [31], most frequently due to *MLH1* promotor methylation. In addition, between 2–6% of endometrial carcinoma occurs in the context of Lynch syndrome due to germline mutations [66]. The frequency of MMR-def varies between 3% and 23% in ECS. The higher frequencies come from studies with a small sample size [36,67], while lower percentages have been observed in a bigger series [37,68]. *MLH1* promoter methylation is probably the major cause for MMR-def in most tumors [68], and accordingly, *MLH1* was epigenetically silenced in the two samples with MMR-def in the TCGA series [38].

Mutations in DNA Polymerase Epsilon, Catalytic Subunit (*POLE*) are present in some ECS, both of the most common HotSpot-mutations (P286R and V114L) have been identified in individual cases of ECS [38,69,70]. The most common mutations detected by NGS in recent studies are shown in Table 2.

Table 2. Comparison of gene mutation frequency among different series of Endometrial carcinosarcoma (ECS) analyzed by next-generation sequencing.

Gene	Cherniack (n = 57)	McConechy (n = 30)	Jones (n = 361)	Zhao (n = 64) *	Le Gallo (n = 53)
TP53	91%	80%	67%	~80%	76%
FBXW7	39%	20%		~22%	19%
PIK3CA	35%	40%	22%	~20%	34%
PPP2R1A	28%	13%		~25%	19%
PTEN	19%	27%		~7%	
CHD4	17%			~20%	17%
ARID1A	12%	10%		~4%	
KRAS	12%	10%		~4%	
PIK3R1	11%	17%		~4%	
AKT3		5%			
BRCA1			18%		
BRCA2			27%		
ZFHX3		7%			
CSMD3		23%			
HIST1H2BJ/G				21%	
FOXA2					15%

* approximated % in a combined series of endometrial and ovarian carcinosarcomas.

5. Gene Expression Profiles in ECS

Several studies have analyzed mRNA and microRNA (miRNA) expression profiles in ECS in comparison to other histological types of EC [71]. Regarding mRNA expression profiles, ECS differs from other EC histotypes in the expression, among others, of genes modulating epithelial-to-mesenchymal transition (EMT) and immune response (see Section 9. Immune Response in CS), and in the expression of cancer-testis antigens (CTA).

There are over 200 CTAs, which are classified into different families according to their sequence homology. In general, CTA genes are expressed only in normal testis and cancerous tissue. In many instances, CTA families are formed by clusters of nearly identical genes that are frequently located on the X-chromosome. A shared regulatory mechanism for related CTA clusters has been suggested as whole families of CTAs are often co-expressed together in tumors [72,73].

Overexpression of many members of the CTA family, such as melanoma antigen family A (*MAGEA*) members (*MAGEA6*, *MAGEA9*, *MAGEA12*), *XAGE2*, *CTCFL*, and *CTAG1A* (cancer/testis antigen 1A) has been reported in ECS [73]. *CTCF*, also known as the brother of the regulator of imprinted sites (*BORIS*), is an oncogene that deregulates the cancer epigenome, which is a common event in ECS [73,74]. Expression of CCCTC-Binding Factor Like (*CTCFL*) probably mediates the demethylation of another CTA gene, thus resulting in activation via repression [74]. Other genes of the CTA family associated with ECS, include, New York esophageal squamous cell carcinoma-1 (*NY-ESO-1*) and Preferentially Expressed Antigen In Melanoma (*PRAME*) [75,76]. Considering the tissue-restricted expression of CTA and its immunogenicity, immunotherapy based on CTA vaccines might be beneficial to ECS patients [73].

The miRNA signature of carcinosarcomas differs from endometrioid and serous carcinomas [77]. The function of miRNAs is to regulate gene expression by silencing. For this, they pair to the three prime untranslated region (3'UTR) of the target mRNA sequence and thereby direct their posttranscriptional repression. miRNAs are small noncoding RNAs, which in turn can be regulated by promotor methylation and transcription factors, or by miRNA processing and stability [78].

In addition to miRNAs related to EMT (see Section 7. Epithelial-to-Mesenchymal Transition), miR-20b, miR-301, and miR-487 are up-regulated in carcinosarcomas compared to both endometrioid and serous tumors, whereas miR-518b is down-regulated. Low expression of miR-20b seems to inhibit tumor cell growth but then again help the tumor cell to gain resistance to apoptosis in hypoxic conditions [79]. In another study, miR-888 overexpression was detected in ECS, and the progesterone receptor was its direct target [80]. Finally, lower cancer-specific survival has been associated with upregulation of miR-184 and downregulation of let-7b-5p and miR-124 [81].

6. Methylation Profiles in ECS

Similarly to other types of cancers, ECS displays abnormal DNA methylation patterns including genome-wide hypomethylation and site-specific hypermethylation, associated with increased expression of DNA methyltransferases (DNMT1, DNMT3a), when compared to the normal endometrium [38,82]. Regarding global hypomethylation, Li et al. [82] reported that in normal endometrium, the 80% of analyzed CpGs were methylated, whereas, in ECS samples, this ratio fell to 60% to 70%. In addition, all major classes of genomic transposable elements exhibited global DNA hypomethylation in ECS, with Long interspersed nuclear elements (LINEs) exhibiting the largest effect size. This effect was greater in ECS than in other histological types of endometrial carcinomas.

A number of tumor suppressor genes with recurrent hypermethylated promoters has also been reported in ECS, *KLF4*, *NDN*, *WT1*, *PROX1*, among others. Promoter hypermethylation of these genes is also common in other types of EC [38,82]. Interestingly, Cherniak et al. [38] reported that unsupervised cluster analysis of DNA methylation profiles of ECS grouped the tumors into three main classes according to their cancer-specific hypermethylation patterns. One group of tumors exhibited a hypermethylation pattern similar to that of EEC, whereas the others were much more similar to the ESC. Accordingly, the frequency of *PTEN* mutations was higher in the first group.

A constant characteristic of ECS is the aberrant DNA methylation of miR-200 genes (see discussion in Section 7. Epithelial-to-Mesenchymal Transition).

7. Epithelial-to-Mesenchymal Transition

EMT is a biological process that involves the acquisition of a mesenchymal/stem-cell-like phenotype by the (malignant) epithelial cells, endowing these cells with migratory and invasive properties, promoting cancer progression, preventing cell death and senescence, and inducing resistance to chemotherapy [83]. EMT has an important role in cancer, especially in tumor invasion and metastasis. During EMT, epithelial cells undergo a "cadherin switch" in which expression of N-cadherin is increased and E-cadherin expression reduced. E-cadherin can be repressed by either zinc-finger transcription factors (Snail1 (SNAI1), Slug/Snail2 (SNAI2), ZEB2 (SIP1) and ZEB1 (δ-EF1)) or basic helix–loop–helix transcription factors (E47 (TCF3), E2-2 (TCF4) or Twist). These EMT transcription factors (EMT-TF) can become activated through activation of different pathways such as Transforming Growth Factor Beta 1 (TGFβ), tyrosine kinase receptors and Wnt, among others [25].

We have previously suggested that EMT is activated in ECS [65,73,84,85]. Further studies have confirmed this suggestion [25,38,39,84,86]. For example, we used real-time PCR to measure the differences in the expression of, E-cadherin, cadherin-11, *SPARC*, *SNAIL*, *ZEB1*, *ZEB2*, *TWIST-1*, *TCF4*, *TGFβ1*, and *TGFβ2* between the epithelial and mesenchymal components of 23 ECSs. Also, we used immunohistochemistry to evaluate the expression of E-, P- and N-cadherin, cadherin-11, p120, vimentin, SPARC, fascin, and caveolin-1 in 76 ECS. In the mesenchymal component, a "cadherin switch" from E-cadherin to N-cadherin and cadherin 11 was observed. In addition, upregulation of all of E-cadherin repressors together with overexpression of all mesenchymal markers tested was demonstrated.

Also, High Mobility Group AT-Hook 2 (HMGA2) has a role in EMT as a regulator of SNAI1 expression and of other transcription factors downstream of SNAI1, such as Slug, ZEB1, and ZEB2. HMGA2 has been proposed to be regulated by the let-7/Lin28B pathway. Accordingly, we have previously demonstrated that an increase of Lin28B expression correlated with let-7b down-regulation and HMGA2 overexpression in ECS [73].

A role of the WNT pathway in the transition from an epithelial to a mesenchymal status is demonstrated by the fact that up to 23% of ECS showed nuclear β-catenin, not associated with *CTNNB1* mutation, in the sarcomatous but not in the carcinomatous component [57]. Nuclear β-catenin cooperates with Sox4 and p300 to transcriptionally up-regulate Slug to induce EMT [87].

Similarly to β-catenin, in another study, ALK tyrosine kinase receptor (ALK) was frequently over-expressed in the sarcomatous components of EC [87]. The authors suggest that ALK-related cascades could participate in divergent sarcomatous differentiation through the induction of EMT and inhibition of apoptosis [87]. In contrast, although the expression of L1CAM is a strong predictor of poor outcome in endometrial cancer and overexpression of L1CAM has been related to EMT in endometrial cancer cell lines [88], in clinical samples of ECS, only the epithelial component was positive in 65% of the cases, while no expression was seen in the mesenchymal part. Thus in ECS, L1CAM is not a marker for the mesenchymal phenotype [89].

MicroRNA signatures associated with EMT and their relationships with EMT markers in human carcinosarcomas have been studied by us and more recently by Cherniack et al. [25,38,84]. We used real-time PCR to measure the differences in the expression of 384 miRNAs, between the epithelial and mesenchymal components of ECS and found that miR-200 family members were down-regulated in the mesenchymal part of the ECS. The miR-200 family plays a major role in regulating epithelial plasticity, mainly through its involvement in double-negative feedback loops with the EMT-TFs ZEB1, ZEB2, SNAI1, and SNAI2, ultimately influencing E-cadherin expression levels [25,84,85]. Down-regulation of miR-200 family members in ECs is not only due to the transcriptional repression by EMT-TF, but also to promoter methylation [38,84]. In this sense, experimental studies have demonstrated a major role of ZEB1 in transcriptional repression and of SNAI1 and, to a lesser extent, SNAI2 in the epigenetic silencing through DNA hypermethylation of miR-200 genes [84]. Other down-regulated miRNAs in our studies included miR-23b and miR-29c, involved in the inhibition of mesenchymal markers, and miR-203 and miR-205 involved in the inhibition of cell stemness [25,84].

8. Beyond EMT: Stemness and Differentiation in ECS

It has been demonstrated that epithelial cells undergoing EMT to acquire mesenchymal features are more likely to possess stemness. In addition, some studies suggested that stemness can be associated with cells undergoing a partial EMT and showing a hybrid Epithelial/Mesenchymal phenotype. Jolly et al. postulated that the core EMT and stemness modules, miR-200/ZEB and Lin28/let7, govern EMT decision making [90]. According to this hypothesis, not only the miR-200/ZEB EMT module is active in ECS, as previously discussed, but also, we have previously demonstrated that the expression of the suppressor of miRNA biogenesis Lin28B was increased in ECS when compared with EEC samples (62.85-fold change). Moreover, we observed a significant inverse correlation between the expression of Lin28B and let-7b, supporting the hypothesis that they participate in the same regulatory pathway [73].

Cells with an Epithelial/Mesenchymal hybrid phenotype evolve to an epithelial or a mesenchymal phenotype depending on factors acting on the EMT and stemness modules [91]. Both routes would enable a secondary round of differentiation to specific epithelial or mesenchymal phenotypes [92]. ECS exemplified well this hypothesis since different types of mesenchymal tissues could develop. This is illustrated not only by the morphological evidence of striated muscle, cartilage, or bone tissue in ECS but also by molecular evidence. Thus, the presence of rhabdomyoblastic differentiation in ECS, the most common heterologous mesenchymal differentiation in ECS, is accompanied by the overexpression of genes that are characteristic of primary embryonic myocytes [93]. Romero-Perez et al. [73] demonstrated that in ECS there was an overexpression of the core network of transcription factors that control the myogenic program in primary myocytes, including Myf5, Myf6, MyoD, and MYOG (myogenin), in addition to other transcriptional factors involved in this process, such as SIX1 and EYE1/2. Moreover, overexpression of genes encoding specialized cytoskeletal proteins, such as slow (*Myh7*) and embryonic (*Myh3*) myosin heavy chains and skeletal α-actin (*Acta1*), was also observed. Similar to our previous results, Lu et al. [94] reported that 18 out of 57 ECS reported in the TCGA had a gene expression pattern enriched in genes involved in muscle development and morphogenesis, myoblast differentiation, and contraction regulation.

9. Immune Response in CS

The tumor microenvironment has an important role in cancer and immunomodulation of the microenvironment is a new focus in cancer medicine [95]. Accumulated evidence indicates that ECS is a rational target for immune therapy. In their study of gene expression, Romero-Peréz et al. found that over 10% of the genes differentially expressed between ECS and EEC were implicated in the immune response, suggesting differential immunomodulation between histotypes [73].

Ayers et al. have created a Tumor Inflammation Signature (TIS) using gene expression data from baseline tumor samples of pembrolizumab-treated patients. The signature includes 18 genes that reflect a suppressed adaptive immune response (antigen presentation, chemokine expression, cytotoxic activity, and adaptive immune resistance) and is enriched in tumors with sensitivity to Programmed cell death 1 ligand 1 (PD-L1) inhibitors [96]. In another study, Danaher et al. concluded that, although there was only a correlation between TIS and tumor mutational burden (TMB), the tumors could be classified equally well with either TIS or TMB [97]. Using data from TCGA, we compared the TIS between endometrioid and serous endometrial and ECS and observed that it is significantly lower in uterine carcinosarcoma ECS compared to both ECS and ESC (analysis of variance (ANOVA), $p < 0.001$, Figure 4). However, TIS varies more within than between tumor types, and although ECS has a relatively low score on average, more samples need to be studied to see if a group of patients might show association with prognosis or immunotherapy response prediction. For example in breast cancer, patients with the highest 10% of the TIS score had a markedly better prognosis [97].

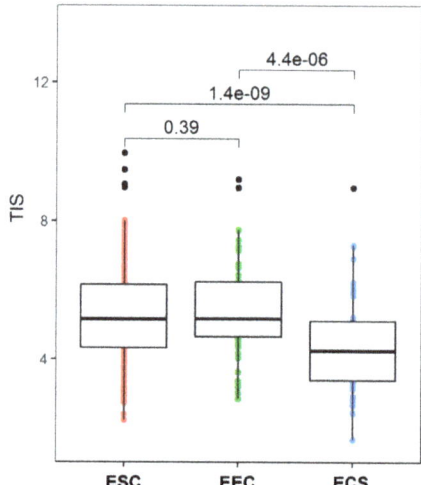

Figure 4. A boxplot histogram of Tumor Inflammation Signature (TIS) scores by endometrial cancer type in endometrial carcinosarcoma (ECS), endometrial serous carcinoma (ESC), and endometrial endometrioid carcinoma (EEC). *p* values from analysis of variance (ANOVA) test are shown for all comparisons.

Several studies have demonstrated that EMT contributes to evasion of immune surveillance [98–105]. PD-L1 has a major role in tumor immune escape and also in the development of a permissive immune microenvironment [105]. Different studies have observed an association between PD-L1 expression and mesenchymal characteristics in different tumor types, such as breast, lung, and pancreatic adenocarcinomas, among others. Also, it has been shown that miR-200 targets PD-L1. Moreover, the EMT-TF ZEB1 relieves miR-200 repression of PD-L1 on tumor cells, leading to CD8(+) T-cell immunosuppression and metastasis.

Regarding carcinosarcomas, PD-L1 expression was significantly higher in lung carcinosarcoma than in conventional non–small-cell lung carcinoma [106], providing a rationale for the potential use of immunotherapy. In this sense, a significant benefit of Nivolumab treatment in PD-L1 positive metastatic pulmonary carcinosarcoma has been reported in some patients [107]. In ovarian carcinosarcoma, PD-L1-positive expression was also observed in about 50% of the tumors, without differences between the epithelial and mesenchymal components [108]. To the best of our knowledge, there are only two studies on PD-L1 expression in ECS. Whereas in one study, PD-L1 was expressed in 25% of the tumors [30], in another, up to 86% of ECS expressed the biomarker [109]. This subset of tumors could benefit from drugs directed to the PD-1/PD-L1 pathway.

10. Conclusions and Perspectives

Carcinosarcoma is a heterogeneous aggressive endometrial carcinoma that probably represents the end-stage of the evolution of both endometrioid and serous carcinomas after triggering a stable EMT program (Figure 5). Molecular observations suggest that, although infrequent, endometrioid carcinomas associated with mutations in *PTEN* or *PIK3CA* are more prone to acquire *TP53* mutations than those associated with MMR-def, *POLE*, or *CTNNB1* mutations. Mutations in *TP53* seem to be essential, but not sufficient, to ECS development, since they are as frequent in ECS as in endometrial serous carcinoma. Although it is not clear what triggers EMT in tumors with *TP53* mutation, a common characteristic of all ECS is the switching of cadherins, the overexpression EMT-TF, and the down-regulation of miR-200 genes. Probably, the crosstalk of different EMT-TF and the differential regulation of miR-200 genes by transcriptional repression or by epigenetic silencing through DNA hypermethylation play a major role in fixing the mesenchymal phenotype. Subsequent activation of specific transcription programs could induce differentiation to diverse mesenchymal tissues.

At present, most patients with ECS are not stratified for treatment according to molecular alterations [110,111]. However, future clinical trials will most likely take into account this data. For example, a recent report has demonstrated the benefit provided when Traztuzumab is included in the treatment of ESC with HER2 amplification [112]. Considering the similarities between ESC and ECS, it is reasonable to think that anti-HER2 therapies would also benefit patients with HER2-positive ECS. Although the relatively low-frequency of ECS hinders efforts to design specific clinical trials, there are promising areas of research, such as the use of immunotherapy in tumors with *POLE* mutations, MMR-def, and high TMB, and also the use of Poly (ADP-ribose) polymerase (PARP) inhibitors in tumors with homologous recombination deficiency, especially due to germline or somatic *BRCA* mutations.

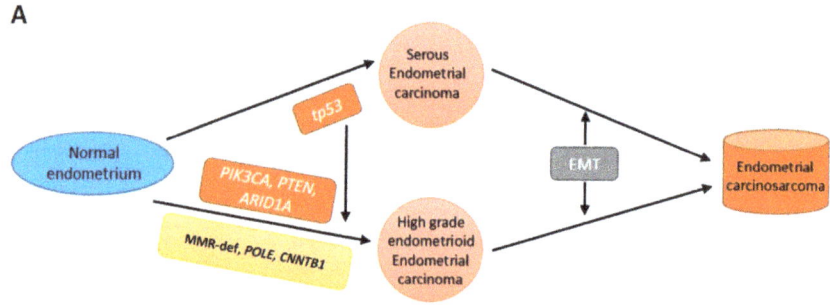

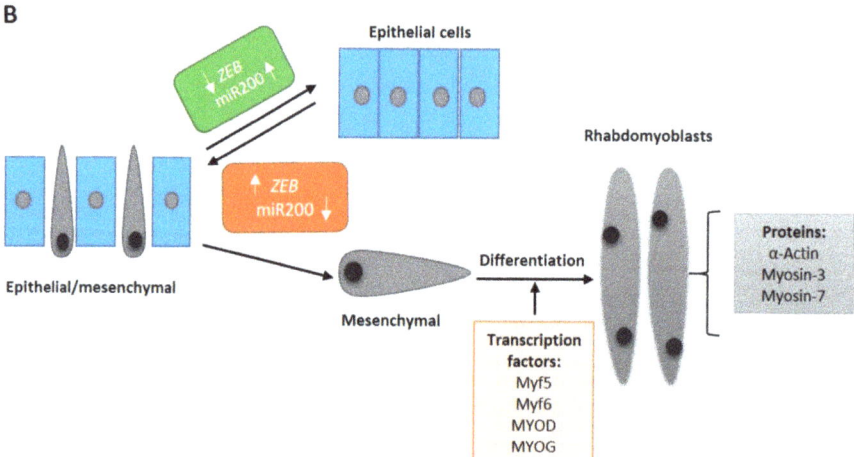

Figure 5. A proposed model of development of endometrial carcinosarcoma. (**A**) Evolution of both endometrioid and serous carcinomas to endometrial carcinosarcoma after eliciting a stable epithelial-to-mesenchymal transition (EMT) program. Transformation of normal endometrium to serous endometrial carcinoma is triggered by mutation in *TP53*. Endometrioid carcinomas with mutations in genes of the phosphatidylinositol 3-kinase (PIK3) pathway or *ARID1A* are more prone to acquire *TP53* mutations than those with mismatch repair deficiency or mutations in *POLE* and *CTNNB1*. (**B**) Endometrial carcinosarcomas are composed by a mixed population of cells representing diverse EMT states. The relative expression of some factors, such as miR-200 or ZEBs, dictate the specific cell state: epithelial, hybrid, or mesenchymal (adapted from Ref. 92).

Author Contributions: Conceptualization, S.L., and J.P.; Data curation, E.C. and J.M.R.-R.; Formal analysis, J.M.R.-R., S.F.O. and X.M.G.-G.; Funding acquisition, J.P.; Resources, J.P.; Supervision, B.P.-M., X.M.G.-G. and J.P.; Writing—original draft, S.L., B.P.-M., M.B., M.L.P.-B. and J.P.; Writing—review & editing, S.L., X.M.G.-G. and J.P.

Funding: This review was funded by grants from the Instituto de Salud Carlos III (ISCIII) (PIE15/00050 and PI16/00887) and CIBERONC (CB16/12/00316 and CB16/12/00231, CB16/12/00361), co-financed by the European Development Regional Fund. 'A way to achieve Europe' (FEDER), and by the Spanish Association Against Cancer Scientific Foundation (grants: AIO-aecc 2016 and Grupos Coordinados Traslacionales aecc 2018).

Conflicts of Interest: The authors declare no conflict of interest. The funders had no role in the design of the study; in the collection, analyses, or interpretation of data; in the writing of the manuscript, or in the decision to publish the results.

References

1. Tavassoli, F. *World Health Organization Classification of Tumours. Pathology and Genetics of Tumors of Breast and Female Genital Organs*; IARC Press: Lyon, France, 2003.
2. Gonzalez Bosquet, J.; Terstriep, S.A.; Cliby, W.A.; Brown-Jones, M.; Kaur, J.S.; Podratz, K.C.; Keeney, G.L. The impact of multi-modal therapy on survival for uterine carcinosarcomas. *Gynecol. Oncol.* **2010**, *116*, 419–423. [CrossRef] [PubMed]
3. De Jong, R.A.; Nijman, H.W.; Wijbrandi, T.F.; Reyners, A.K.; Boezen, H.M.; Hollema, H. Molecular markers and clinical behavior of uterine carcinosarcomas: Focus on the epithelial tumor component. *Mod. Pathol.* **2011**, *24*, 1368–1379. [CrossRef] [PubMed]
4. Ferguson, S.E.; Tornos, C.; Hummer, A.; Barakat, R.R.; Soslow, R.A. Prognostic features of surgical stage I uterine carcinosarcoma. *Am. J. Surg. Pathol.* **2007**, *31*, 1653–1661. [CrossRef] [PubMed]
5. Amant, F.; Cadron, I.; Fuso, L.; Berteloot, P.; de Jonge, E.; Jacomen, G.; Van Robaeys, J.; Neven, P.; Moerman, P.; Vergote, I. Endometrial carcinosarcomas have a different prognosis and pattern of spread compared to high-risk epithelial endometrial cancer. *Gynecol. Oncol.* **2005**, *98*, 274–280. [CrossRef] [PubMed]
6. George, E.; Lillemoe, T.J.; Twiggs, L.B.; Perrone, T. Malignant mixed mullerian tumor versus high-grade endometrial carcinoma and aggressive variants of endometrial carcinoma: A comparative analysis of survival. *Int. J. Gynecol. Pathol.* **1995**, *14*, 39–44. [CrossRef] [PubMed]
7. Callister, M.; Ramondetta, L.M.; Jhingran, A.; Burke, T.W.; Eifel, P.J. Malignant mixed mullerian tumors of the uterus: Analysis of patterns of failure, prognostic factors, and treatment outcome. *Int. J. Radiat. Oncol. Biol. Phys.* **2004**, *58*, 786–796. [CrossRef]
8. Bansal, N.; Herzog, T.J.; Seshan, V.E.; Schiff, P.B.; Burke, W.M.; Cohen, C.J.; Wright, J.D. Uterine carcinosarcomas and grade 3 endometrioid cancers: Evidence for distinct tumor behavior. *Obstet. Gynecol.* **2008**, *112*, 64–70. [CrossRef] [PubMed]
9. Matsuo, K.; Ross, M.S.; Machida, H.; Blake, E.A.; Roman, L.D. Trends of uterine carcinosarcoma in the United States. *J. Gynecol. Oncol.* **2018**, *29*, e22. [CrossRef] [PubMed]
10. Jeong, B.K.; Sung, C.O.; Kim, K.R. Uterine malignant mixed mullerian tumors following treatment with selective estrogen receptor modulators in patients with breast cancer: A report of 13 cases and their clinicopathologic characteristics. *J. Pathol. Transl. Med.* **2019**, *53*, 31–39. [CrossRef]
11. Matsuo, K.; Ross, M.S.; Bush, S.H.; Yunokawa, M.; Blake, E.A.; Takano, T.; Ueda, Y.; Baba, T.; Satoh, S.; Shida, M.; et al. Tumor characteristics and survival outcomes of women with tamoxifen-related uterine carcinosarcoma. *Gynecol. Oncol.* **2017**, *144*, 329–335. [CrossRef]
12. Buza, N.; Tavassoli, F.A. Comparative analysis of P16 and P53 expression in uterine malignant mixed mullerian tumors. *Int. J. Gynecol. Pathol.* **2009**, *28*, 514–521. [CrossRef] [PubMed]
13. Silverberg, S.G.; Major, F.J.; Blessing, J.A.; Fetter, B.; Askin, F.B.; Liao, S.Y.; Miller, A. Carcinosarcoma (malignant mixed mesodermal tumor) of the uterus. A gynecologic oncology group pathologic study of 203 cases. *Int. J. Gynecol. Pathol.* **1990**, *9*, 1–19. [CrossRef] [PubMed]
14. Sreenan, J.J.; Hart, W.R. Carcinosarcomas of the female genital tract. A pathologic study of 29 metastatic tumors: Further evidence for the dominant role of the epithelial component and the conversion theory of histogenesis. *Am. J. Surg. Pathol.* **1995**, *19*, 666–674. [CrossRef] [PubMed]
15. Costa, M.J.; Vogelsan, J.; Young, L.J. p53 gene mutation in female genital tract carcinosarcomas (malignant mixed mullerian tumors): A clinicopathologic study of 74 cases. *Mod. Pathol.* **1994**, *7*, 619–627. [PubMed]
16. Matsuo, K.; Takazawa, Y.; Ross, M.S.; Elishaev, E.; Podzielinski, I.; Yunokawa, M.; Sheridan, T.B.; Bush, S.H.; Klobocista, M.M.; Blake, E.A.; et al. Significance of histologic pattern of carcinoma and sarcoma components on survival outcomes of uterine carcinosarcoma. *Ann. Oncol.* **2016**, *27*, 1257–1266. [CrossRef] [PubMed]
17. Abdulfatah, E.; Lordello, L.; Khurram, M.; Van de Vijver, K.; Alosh, B.; Bandyopadhyay, S.; Oliva, E.; Ali-Fehmi, R. Predictive histologic factors in carcinosarcomas of the uterus: A multiinstitutional study. *Int. J. Gynecol. Pathol.* **2018**, *38*, 205–215. [CrossRef]
18. Costa, M.J.; Khan, R.; Judd, R. Carcinoma (malignant mixed mullerian [mesodermal] tumor) of the uterus and ovary. Correlation of clinical, pathologic, and immunohistochemical features in 29 cases. *Arch. Pathol. Lab. Med.* **1991**, *115*, 583–590. [PubMed]

19. Kurnit, K.C.; Previs, R.A.; Soliman, P.T.; Westin, S.N.; Klopp, A.H.; Fellman, B.M.; Lu, K.H.; Ramondetta, L.M.; Fleming, N.D. Prognostic factors impacting survival in early stage uterine carcinosarcoma. *Gynecol. Oncol.* **2019**, *152*, 31–37. [CrossRef]
20. McCluggage, W.G. A practical approach to the diagnosis of mixed epithelial and mesenchymal tumours of the uterus. *Mod. Pathol.* **2016**, *29* (Suppl. 1), S78–S91. [CrossRef]
21. Matsuo, K.; Takazawa, Y.; Ross, M.S.; Elishaev, E.; Yunokawa, M.; Sheridan, T.B.; Bush, S.H.; Klobocista, M.M.; Blake, E.A.; Takano, T.; et al. Significance of lymphovascular space invasion by the sarcomatous component in uterine carcinosarcoma. *Ann. Surg. Oncol.* **2018**, *25*, 2756–2766. [CrossRef]
22. Iwasa, Y.; Haga, H.; Konishi, I.; Kobashi, Y.; Higuchi, K.; Katsuyama, E.; Minamiguchi, S.; Yamabe, H. Prognostic factors in uterine carcinosarcoma: A clinicopathologic study of 25 patients. *Cancer* **1998**, *82*, 512–519. [CrossRef]
23. Matsuo, K.; Takazawa, Y.; Ross, M.S.; Elishaev, E.; Yunokawa, M.; Sheridan, T.B.; Bush, S.H.; Klobocista, M.M.; Blake, E.A.; Takano, T.; et al. Characterizing sarcoma dominance pattern in uterine carcinosarcoma: Homologous versus heterologous element. *Surg. Oncol.* **2018**, *27*, 433–440. [CrossRef] [PubMed]
24. Matsuo, K.; Takazawa, Y.; Ross, M.S.; Elishaev, E.; Yunokawa, M.; Sheridan, T.B.; Bush, S.H.; Klobocista, M.M.; Blake, E.A.; Takano, T.; et al. Proposal for a risk-based categorization of uterine carcinosarcoma. *Ann. Surg. Oncol.* **2018**, *25*, 3676–3684. [CrossRef] [PubMed]
25. Castilla, M.A.; Moreno-Bueno, G.; Romero-Perez, L.; Van De Vijver, K.; Biscuola, M.; López-García, M.Á.; Prat, J.; Matías-Guiu, X.; Cano, A.; Oliva, E.; et al. Micro-RNA signature of the epithelial-mesenchymal transition in endometrial carcinosarcoma. *J. Pathol.* **2011**, *223*, 72–80. [CrossRef] [PubMed]
26. Chiyoda, T.; Tsuda, H.; Tanaka, H.; Kataoka, F.; Nomura, H.; Nishimura, S.; Takano, M.; Susumu, N.; Saya, H.; Aoki, D. Expression profiles of carcinosarcoma of the uterine corpus-are these similar to carcinoma or sarcoma? *Genes Chromosomes Cancer* **2012**, *51*, 229–239. [CrossRef] [PubMed]
27. Wada, H.; Enomoto, T.; Fujita, M.; Yoshino, K.; Nakashima, R.; Kurachi, H.; Haba, T.; Wakasa, K.; Shroyer, K.R.; Tsujimoto, M.; et al. Molecular evidence that most but not all carcinosarcomas of the uterus are combination tumors. *Cancer Res.* **1997**, *57*, 5379–5385. [PubMed]
28. Talhouk, A.; McConechy, M.K.; Leung, S.; Li-Chang, H.H.; Kwon, J.S.; Melnyk, N.; Yang, W.; Senz, J.; Boyd, N.; Karnezis, A.N.; et al. A clinically applicable molecular-based classification for endometrial cancers. *Br. J. Cancer* **2015**, *113*, 299–310. [CrossRef] [PubMed]
29. McConechy, M.K.; Hoang, L.N.; Chui, M.H.; Senz, J.; Yang, W.; Rozenberg, N.; Mackenzie, R.; McAlpine, J.N.; Huntsman, D.G.; Clarke, B.A.; et al. In-depth molecular profiling of the biphasic components of uterine carcinosarcomas. *J. Pathol. Clin. Res.* **2015**, *1*, 173–185. [CrossRef] [PubMed]
30. Jones, N.L.; Xiu, J.; Chatterjee-Paer, S.; Buckley de Meritens, A.; Burke, W.M.; Tergas, A.I.; Wright, J.D.; Hou, J.Y. Distinct molecular landscapes between endometrioid and nonendometrioid uterine carcinomas. *Int. J. Cancer* **2017**, *140*, 1396–1404. [CrossRef] [PubMed]
31. Rosa-Rosa, J.M.; Leskela, S.; Cristobal-Lana, E.; Santón, A.; López-García, M.Á.; Muñoz, G.; Pérez-Mies, B.; Biscuola, M.; Prat, J.; Esther, O.E.; et al. Molecular genetic heterogeneity in undifferentiated endometrial carcinomas. *Mod. Pathol.* **2016**, *29*, 1390. [CrossRef] [PubMed]
32. Kounelis, S.; Jones, M.W.; Papadaki, H.; Bakker, A.; Swalsky, P.; Finkelstein, S.D. Carcinosarcomas (malignant mixed mullerian tumors) of the female genital tract: Comparative molecular analysis of epithelial and mesenchymal components. *Hum. Pathol.* **1998**, *29*, 82–87. [CrossRef]
33. Abeln, E.C.; Smit, V.T.; Wessels, J.W.; de Leeuw, W.J.; Cornelisse, C.J.; Fleuren, G.J. Molecular genetic evidence for the conversion hypothesis of the origin of malignant mixed mullerian tumours. *J. Pathol.* **1997**, *183*, 424–431. [CrossRef]
34. Liu, F.S.; Kohler, M.F.; Marks, J.R.; Bast, R.C., Jr.; Boyd, J.; Berchuck, A. Mutation and overexpression of the p53 tumor suppressor gene frequently occurs in uterine and ovarian sarcomas. *Obstet. Gynecol.* **1994**, *83*, 118–124. [PubMed]
35. Kanthan, R.; Senger, J.L.; Diudea, D. Malignant mixed Mullerian tumors of the uterus: Histopathological evaluation of cell cycle and apoptotic regulatory proteins. *World J. Surg. Oncol.* **2010**, *8*, 60. [CrossRef] [PubMed]
36. Jones, S.; Stransky, N.; McCord, C.L.; Cerami, E.; Lagowski, J.; Kelly, D.; Angiuoli, S.V.; Sausen, M.; Kann, L.; Shukla, M.; et al. Genomic analyses of gynaecologic carcinosarcomas reveal frequent mutations in chromatin remodelling genes. *Nat. Commun.* **2014**, *5*, 5006. [CrossRef] [PubMed]

37. McConechy, M.K.; Ding, J.; Cheang, M.C.; Wiegand, K.; Senz, J.; Tone, A.; Yang, W.; Prentice, L.; Tse, K.; Zeng, T.; et al. Use of mutation profiles to refine the classification of endometrial carcinomas. *J. Pathol.* **2012**, *228*, 20–30. [CrossRef] [PubMed]
38. Cherniack, A.D.; Shen, H.; Walter, V.; Stewart, C.; Murray, B.A.; Bowlby, R.; Hu, X.; Ling, S.; Soslow, R.A.; Broaddus, R.R.; et al. Integrated molecular characterization of uterine carcinosarcoma. *Cancer Cell* **2017**, *31*, 411–423. [CrossRef]
39. Liu, Y.; Weber, Z.; San Lucas, F.A.; Deshpande, A.; Jakubek, Y.A.; Sulaiman, R.; Fagerness, M.; Flier, N.; Sulaiman, J.; Davis, C.M.; et al. Assessing inter-component heterogeneity of biphasic uterine carcinosarcomas. *Gynecol. Oncol.* **2018**, *151*, 243–249. [CrossRef]
40. Le Gallo, M.; Rudd, M.L.; Urick, M.E.; Hansen, N.F.; National Institutes of Health Intramural Sequencing Center Comparative Sequencing Program; Merino, M.J.; Mutch, D.G.; Goodfellow, P.J.; Mullikin, J.C.; Bell, D.W. The FOXA2 transcription factor is frequently somatically mutated in uterine carcinosarcomas and carcinomas. *Cancer* **2018**, *124*, 65–73. [CrossRef]
41. D'Brot, A.; Kurtz, P.; Regan, E.; Jakubowski, B.; Abrams, J.M. A platform for interrogating cancer-associated p53 alleles. *Oncogene* **2017**, *36*, 286–291. [CrossRef]
42. Semczuk, A.; Skomra, D.; Chyzynska, M.; Szewczuk, W.; Olcha, P.; Korobowicz, E. Immunohistochemical analysis of carcinomatous and sarcomatous components in the uterine carcinosarcoma: A case report. *Pathol. Res. Pract.* **2008**, *204*, 203–207. [CrossRef] [PubMed]
43. Reid-Nicholson, M.; Iyengar, P.; Hummer, A.J.; Linkov, I.; Asher, M.; Soslow, R.A. Immunophenotypic diversity of endometrial adenocarcinomas: Implications for differential diagnosis. *Mod. Pathol.* **2006**, *19*, 1091–1100. [CrossRef] [PubMed]
44. Robinson-Bennett, B.; Belch, R.Z.; Han, A.C. Loss of p16 in recurrent malignant mixed mullerian tumors of the uterus. *Int. J. Gynecol. Cancer* **2006**, *16*, 1354–1357. [PubMed]
45. Saule, C.; Mouret-Fourme, E.; Briaux, A.; Becette, V.; Rouzier, R.; Houdayer, C.; Stoppa-Lyonnet, D. Risk of serous endometrial carcinoma in women with pathogenic BRCA1/2 variant after risk-reducing salpingo-oophorectomy. *J. Natl. Cancer Inst.* **2018**, *110*, 213–215. [CrossRef] [PubMed]
46. De Jonge, M.M.; Mooyaart, A.L.; Vreeswijk, M.P.; de Kroon, C.D.; van Wezel, T.; van Asperen, C.J.; Smit, V.T.; Dekkers, O.M.; Bosse, T. Linking uterine serous carcinoma to BRCA1/2-associated cancer syndrome: A meta-analysis and case report. *Eur. J. Cancer* **2017**, *72*, 215–225. [CrossRef]
47. Shu, C.A.; Pike, M.C.; Jotwani, A.R.; Friebel, T.M.; Soslow, R.A.; Levine, D.A.; Nathanson, K.L.; Konner, J.A.; Arnold, A.G.; Bogomolniy, F.; et al. Uterine cancer after risk-reducing salpingo-oophorectomy without hysterectomy in women with BRCA mutations. *JAMA Oncol.* **2016**, *2*, 1434–1440. [CrossRef] [PubMed]
48. Sonoda, Y.; Saigo, P.E.; Federici, M.G.; Boyd, J. Carcinosarcoma of the ovary in a patient with a germline BRCA2 mutation: Evidence for monoclonal origin. *Gynecol. Oncol.* **2000**, *76*, 226–229. [CrossRef]
49. Carnevali, I.W.; Cimetti, L.; Sahnane, N.; Libera, L.; Cavallero, A.; Formenti, G.; Riva, C.; Tibiletti, M.G. Two cases of carcinosarcomas of the ovary involved in hereditary cancer syndromes. *Int. J. Gynecol. Pathol.* **2017**, *36*, 64–70. [CrossRef]
50. Ghilli, M.; Mariniello, D.M.; Fanelli, G.; Cascione, F.; Fontana, A.; Cristaudo, A.; Cilotti, A.; Caligo, A.M.; Manca, G.; Colizzi, L.; et al. Carcinosarcoma of the breast: An aggressive subtype of metaplastic cancer. Report of a rare case in a young BRCA-1 mutated woman. *Clin. Breast Cancer* **2017**, *17*, e31–e35. [CrossRef]
51. Zhao, S.; Bellone, S.; Lopez, S.; Thakral, D.; Schwab, C.; English, D.P.; Black, J.; Cocco, E.; Choi, J.; Zammataro, L.; et al. Mutational landscape of uterine and ovarian carcinosarcomas implicates histone genes in epithelial-mesenchymal transition. *Proc. Natl. Acad. Sci USA* **2016**, *113*, 12238–12243. [CrossRef]
52. Schipf, A.; Mayr, D.; Kirchner, T.; Diebold, J. Molecular genetic aberrations of ovarian and uterine carcinosarcomas–a CGH and FISH study. *Virchows Arch.* **2008**, *452*, 259–268. [CrossRef] [PubMed]
53. Livasy, C.A.; Reading, F.C.; Moore, D.T.; Boggess, J.F.; Lininger, R.A. EGFR expression and HER2/neu overexpression/amplification in endometrial carcinosarcoma. *Gynecol. Oncol.* **2006**, *100*, 101–106. [CrossRef] [PubMed]
54. Raspollini, M.R.; Susini, T.; Amunni, G.; Paglierani, M.; Taddei, A.; Marchionni, M.; Scarselli, G.; Taddei, G.L. COX-2, c-KIT and HER-2/neu expression in uterine carcinosarcomas: Prognostic factors or potential markers for targeted therapies? *Gynecol. Oncol.* **2005**, *96*, 159–167. [CrossRef] [PubMed]

55. Sawada, M.; Tsuda, H.; Kimura, M.; Okamoto, S.; Kita, T.; Kasamatsu, T.; Yamada, T.; Kikuchi, Y.; Honjo, H.; Matsubara, O. Different expression patterns of KIT, EGFR, and HER-2 (c-erbB-2) oncoproteins between epithelial and mesenchymal components in uterine carcinosarcoma. *Cancer Sci.* **2003**, *94*, 986–991. [CrossRef]

56. Nicoletti, R.; Lopez, S.; Bellone, S.; Cocco, E.; Schwab, C.L.; Black, J.D.; Centritto, F.; Zhu, L.; Bonazzoli, E.; Buza, N.; et al. T-DM1, a novel antibody-drug conjugate, is highly effective against uterine and ovarian carcinosarcomas overexpressing HER2. *Clin. Exp. Metastasis* **2015**, *32*, 29–38. [CrossRef] [PubMed]

57. Biscuola, M.; Van de Vijver, K.; Castilla, M.A.; Romero-Pérez, L.; López-García, M.Á.; Díaz-Martín, J.; Matias-Guiu, X.; Oliva, E.; Palacios Calvo, J. Oncogene alterations in endometrial carcinosarcomas. *Hum. Pathol.* **2013**, *44*, 852–859. [CrossRef] [PubMed]

58. Cimbaluk, D.; Rotmensch, J.; Scudiere, J.; Gown, A.; Bitterman, P. Uterine carcinosarcoma: Immunohistochemical studies on tissue microarrays with focus on potential therapeutic targets. *Gynecol. Oncol.* **2007**, *105*, 138–144. [CrossRef] [PubMed]

59. Hayes, M.P.; Douglas, W.; Ellenson, L.H. Molecular alterations of EGFR and PIK3CA in uterine serous carcinoma. *Gynecol. Oncol.* **2009**, *113*, 370–373. [CrossRef] [PubMed]

60. Wang, Y.; Garabedian, M.J.; Logan, S.K. URI1 amplification in uterine carcinosarcoma associates with chemo-resistance and poor prognosis. *Am. J. Cancer Res.* **2015**, *5*, 2320–2329. [PubMed]

61. Chui, M.H.; Have, C.; Hoang, L.N.; Shaw, P.; Lee, C.H.; Clarke, B.A. Genomic profiling identifies GPC5 amplification in association with sarcomatous transformation in a subset of uterine carcinosarcomas. *J. Pathol. Clin. Res.* **2018**, *4*, 69–78. [CrossRef]

62. Murray, S.; Linardou, H.; Mountzios, G.; Manoloukos, M.; Markaki, S.; Eleutherakis-Papaiakovou, E.; Dimopoulos, M.A.; Papadimitriou, C.A. Low frequency of somatic mutations in uterine sarcomas: A molecular analysis and review of the literature. *Mutat. Res.* **2010**, *686*, 68–73. [CrossRef] [PubMed]

63. Growdon, W.B.; Roussel, B.N.; Scialabba, V.L.; Foster, R.; Dias-Santagata, D.; Iafrate, A.J.; Ellisen, L.W.; Tambouret, R.H.; Rueda, B.R.; Borger, D.R. Tissue-specific signatures of activating PIK3CA and RAS mutations in carcinosarcomas of gynecologic origin. *Gynecol. Oncol.* **2011**, *121*, 212–217. [CrossRef] [PubMed]

64. Makker, V.; Recio, F.O.; Ma, L.; Matulonis, U.A.; Lauchle, J.O.; Parmar, H.; Gilbert, H.N.; Ware, J.A.; Zhu, R.; Lu, S.; et al. A multicenter, single-arm, open-label, phase 2 study of apitolisib (GDC-0980) for the treatment of recurrent or persistent endometrial carcinoma (MAGGIE study). *Cancer* **2016**, *122*, 3519–3528. [CrossRef] [PubMed]

65. López-García, M.Á.; Begoña, V.; Castilla, M.A.; Romero-Pérez, L.; Díaz-Martín, J.; Biscuola, M.; Palacios, C.J. Genetics of endometrial carcinoma. *Cancer Genomics* **2013**, *11*, 51.

66. Mills, A.M.; Liou, S.; Ford, J.M.; Berek, J.S.; Pai, R.K.; Longacre, T.A. Lynch syndrome screening should be considered for all patients with newly diagnosed endometrial cancer. *Am. J. Surg. Pathol.* **2014**, *38*, 1501–1509. [CrossRef]

67. Taylor, N.P.; Zighelboim, I.; Huettner, P.C.; Powell, M.A.; Gibb, R.K.; Rader, J.S.; Mutch, D.G.; Edmonston, T.B.; Goodfellow, P.J. DNA mismatch repair and TP53 defects are early events in uterine carcinosarcoma tumorigenesis. *Mod. Pathol.* **2006**, *19*, 1333–1338. [CrossRef] [PubMed]

68. Hoang, L.N.; Ali, R.H.; Lau, S.; Gilks, C.B.; Lee, C.H. Immunohistochemical survey of mismatch repair protein expression in uterine sarcomas and carcinosarcomas. *Int. J. Gynecol. Pathol.* **2014**, *33*, 483–491. [CrossRef]

69. Hembree, T.N.; Teer, J.K.; Hakam, A.; Chiappori, A.A. Genetic investigation of uterine carcinosarcoma: Case report and cohort analysis. *Cancer Control* **2016**, *23*, 61–66. [CrossRef]

70. Bhangoo, M.S.; Boasberg, P.; Mehta, P.; Elvin, J.A.; Ali, S.M.; Wu, W.; Klempner, S.J. Tumor mutational burden guides therapy in a treatment refractory POLE-mutant uterine carcinosarcoma. *Oncologist* **2018**, *23*, 518–523. [CrossRef]

71. Maxwell, G.L.; Chandramouli, G.V.; Dainty, L.; Litzi, T.J.; Berchuck, A.; Barrett, J.C.; Risinger, J.I. Microarray analysis of endometrial carcinomas and mixed mullerian tumors reveals distinct gene expression profiles associated with different histologic types of uterine cancer. *Clin. Cancer Res.* **2005**, *11*, 4056–4066. [CrossRef]

72. Whitehurst, A.W. Cause and consequence of cancer/testis antigen activation in cancer. *Annu. Rev. Pharmacol. Toxicol.* **2014**, *54*, 251–272. [CrossRef] [PubMed]

73. Romero-Perez, L.; Castilla, M.A.; Lopez-Garcia, M.A.; Díaz-Martín, J.; Biscuola, M.; Ramiro-Fuentes, S.; Oliva, E.; Matias-Guiu, X.; Prat, J.; Cano, A.; et al. Molecular events in endometrial carcinosarcomas and the role of high mobility group AT-hook 2 in endometrial carcinogenesis. *Hum. Pathol.* **2013**, *44*, 244–254. [CrossRef] [PubMed]
74. Risinger, J.I.; Chandramouli, G.V.; Maxwell, G.L.; Custer, M.; Pack, S.; Loukinov, D.; Aprelikova, O.; Litzi, T.; Schrump, D.S.; Murphy, S.K.; et al. Global expression analysis of cancer/testis genes in uterine cancers reveals a high incidence of BORIS expression. *Clin. Cancer Res.* **2007**, *13*, 1713–1719. [CrossRef] [PubMed]
75. Resnick, M.B.; Sabo, E.; Kondratev, S.; Kerner, H.; Spagnoli, G.C.; Yakirevich, E. Cancer-testis antigen expression in uterine malignancies with an emphasis on carcinosarcomas and papillary serous carcinomas. *Int. J. Cancer* **2002**, *101*, 190–195. [CrossRef] [PubMed]
76. Roszik, J.; Wang, W.L.; Livingston, J.A.; Roland, C.L.; Ravi, V.; Yee, C.; Hwu, P.; Futreal, A.; Lazar, A.J.; Patel, S.R.; et al. Overexpressed PRAME is a potential immunotherapy target in sarcoma subtypes. *Clin. Sarcoma Res.* **2017**, *7*, 11. [CrossRef] [PubMed]
77. Ratner, E.S.; Tuck, D.; Richter, C.; Nallur, S.; Patel, R.M.; Schultz, V.; Hui, P.; Schwartz, P.E.; Rutherford, T.J.; Weidhaas, J.B. MicroRNA signatures differentiate uterine cancer tumor subtypes. *Gynecol. Oncol.* **2010**, *118*, 251–257. [CrossRef] [PubMed]
78. Gulyaeva, L.F.; Kushlinskiy, N.E. Regulatory mechanisms of microRNA expression. *J. Transl. Med.* **2016**, *14*, 143. [CrossRef] [PubMed]
79. Lei, Z.; Li, B.; Yang, Z.; Fang, H.; Zhang, G.M.; Feng, Z.H.; Huang, B. Regulation of HIF-1alpha and VEGF by miR-20b tunes tumor cells to adapt to the alteration of oxygen concentration. *PLoS ONE* **2009**, *4*, e7629. [CrossRef] [PubMed]
80. Hovey, A.M.; Devor, E.J.; Breheny, P.J.; Mott, S.L.; Dai, D.; Thiel, K.W.; Leslie, K.K. miR-888: A novel cancer-testis antigen that targets the progesterone receptor in endometrial cancer. *Transl. Oncol.* **2015**, *8*, 85–96. [CrossRef]
81. Gonzalez Dos Anjos, L.; de Almeida, B.C.; Gomes de Almeida, T.; Mourão Lavorato Rocha, A.; De Nardo Maffazioli, G.; Soares, F.A.; Werneck da Cunha, I.; Chada Baracat, E.; Candido Carvalho, K. Could miRNA signatures be useful for predicting uterine sarcoma and carcinosarcoma prognosis and treatment? *Cancers* **2018**, *10*, 315. [CrossRef]
82. Li, J.; Xing, X.; Li, D.; Zhang, B.; Mutch, D.G.; Hagemann, I.S.; Wang, T. Whole-genome DNA methylation profiling identifies epigenetic signatures of uterine carcinosarcoma. *Neoplasia* **2017**, *19*, 100–111. [CrossRef] [PubMed]
83. Thiery, J.P.; Acloque, H.; Huang, R.Y.; Nieto, M.A. Epithelial-mesenchymal transitions in development and disease. *Cell* **2009**, *139*, 871–890. [CrossRef] [PubMed]
84. Diaz-Martin, J.; Diaz-Lopez, A.; Moreno-Bueno, G.; Castilla, M.Á.; Rosa-Rosa, J.M.; Cano, A.; Palacios, J. A core microRNA signature associated with inducers of the epithelial-to-mesenchymal transition. *J. Pathol.* **2014**, *232*, 319–329. [CrossRef] [PubMed]
85. Diaz-Lopez, A.; Diaz-Martin, J.; Moreno-Bueno, G.; Cuevas, E.P.; Santos, V.; Olmeda, D.; Portillo, F.; Palacios, J.; Cano, A. Zeb1 and Snail1 engage miR-200f transcriptional and epigenetic regulation during EMT. *Int. J. Cancer* **2015**, *136*, E62–E73. [CrossRef] [PubMed]
86. Berger, A.C.; Korkut, A.; Kanchi, R.S.; Hegde, A.M.; Lenoir, W.; Liu, W.; Liu, Y.; Fan, H.; Shen, H.; Ravikumar, V.; et al. A comprehensive pan-cancer molecular study of gynecologic and breast cancers. *Cancer Cell* **2018**, *33*, 690–705. [CrossRef] [PubMed]
87. Inoue, H.; Hashimura, M.; Akiya, M.; Chiba, R.; Saegusa, M. Functional role of ALK-related signal cascades on modulation of epithelial-mesenchymal transition and apoptosis in uterine carcinosarcoma. *Mol. Cancer* **2017**, *16*, 37. [CrossRef] [PubMed]
88. Chen, J.; Gao, F.; Liu, N. L1CAM promotes epithelial to mesenchymal transition and formation of cancer initiating cells in human endometrial cancer. *Exp. Ther. Med.* **2018**, *15*, 2792–2797. [CrossRef]
89. Versluis, M.; Plat, A.; de Bruyn, M.; Matias-Guiu, X.; Trovic, J.; Krakstad, C.; Nijman, H.W.; Bosse, T.; de Bock, G.H.; Hollema, H. L1CAM expression in uterine carcinosarcoma is limited to the epithelial component and may be involved in epithelial-mesenchymal transition. *Virchows Arch.* **2018**, *473*, 591–598. [CrossRef]
90. Jolly, M.K.; Jia, D.; Boareto, M.; Mani, S.A.; Pienta, K.J.; Ben-Jacob, E.; Levine, H. Coupling the modules of EMT and stemness: A tunable 'stemness window' model. *Oncotarget* **2015**, *6*, 25161–25174. [CrossRef]

91. Pastushenko, I.; Blanpain, C. EMT transition states during tumor progression and metastasis. *Trends Cell Biol.* **2019**, *29*, 212–226. [CrossRef]
92. Wang, H.; Unternaehrer, J.J. Epithelial-mesenchymal transition and cancer stem cells: At the crossroads of differentiation and dedifferentiation. *Dev. Dyn.* **2019**, *248*, 10–20. [CrossRef] [PubMed]
93. Chal, J.; Pourquie, O. Making muscle: Skeletal myogenesis in vivo and in vitro. *Development* **2017**, *144*, 2104–2122. [CrossRef] [PubMed]
94. Lu, X.; Zhang, L.; Zhao, H.; Chen, C.; Wang, Y.; Liu, S.; Lin, X.; Wang, Y.; Zhang, Q.; Lu, T.; et al. Molecular classification and subtype-specific drug sensitivity research of uterine carcinosarcoma under multi-omics framework. *Cancer Biol. Ther.* **2019**, *20*, 227–235. [CrossRef] [PubMed]
95. Longoria, T.C.; Eskander, R.N. Immunotherapy in endometrial cancer–an evolving therapeutic paradigm. *Gynecol. Oncol. Res. Pract.* **2015**, *2*, 11. [CrossRef] [PubMed]
96. Ayers, M.; Lunceford, J.; Nebozhyn, M.; Murphy, E.; Loboda, A.; Kaufman, D.R.; Albright, A.; Cheng, J.D.; Kang, S.P.; Shankaran, V.; et al. IFN-gamma-related mRNA profile predicts clinical response to PD-1 blockade. *J. Clin. Invest.* **2017**, *127*, 2930–2940. [CrossRef] [PubMed]
97. Danaher, P.; Warren, S.; Lu, R.; Samayoa, J.; Sullivan, A.; Pekker, I.; Wallden, B.; Marincola, F.M.; Cesano, A. Pan-cancer adaptive immune resistance as defined by the Tumor Inflammation Signature (TIS): Results from The Cancer Genome Atlas (TCGA). *J. Immunother. Cancer* **2018**, *6*, 63. [CrossRef] [PubMed]
98. Dongre, A.; Rashidian, M.; Reinhardt, F.; Bagnato, A.; Keckesova, Z.; Ploegh, H.L.; Weinberg, R.A. Epithelial-to-mesenchymal transition contributes to immunosuppression in breast carcinomas. *Cancer Res.* **2017**, *77*, 3982–3989. [CrossRef]
99. Ueno, T.; Tsuchikawa, T.; Hatanaka, K.C.; Hatanaka, Y.; Mitsuhashi, T.; Nakanishi, Y.; Noji, T.; Nakamura, T.; Okamura, K.; Matsuno, Y.; et al. Prognostic impact of programmed cell death ligand 1 (PD-L1) expression and its association with epithelial-mesenchymal transition in extrahepatic cholangiocarcinoma. *Oncotarget* **2018**, *9*, 20034–20047. [CrossRef] [PubMed]
100. Noman, M.Z.; Janji, B.; Abdou, A.; Hasmim, M.; Terry, S.; Tan, T.Z.; Mami-Chouaib, F.; Thiery, J.P.; Chouaib, S. The immune checkpoint ligand PD-L1 is upregulated in EMT-activated human breast cancer cells by a mechanism involving ZEB-1 and miR-200. *Oncoimmunology* **2017**, *6*, e1263412. [CrossRef]
101. Kim, S.; Koh, J.; Kim, M.Y.; Kwon, D.; Go, H.; Kim, Y.A.; Jeon, Y.K.; Chung, D.H. PD-L1 expression is associated with epithelial-to-mesenchymal transition in adenocarcinoma of the lung. *Hum. Pathol.* **2016**, *58*, 7–14. [CrossRef]
102. Ock, C.Y.; Kim, S.; Keam, B.; Kim, M.; Kim, T.M.; Kim, J.H.; Jeon, Y.K.; Lee, J.S.; Kwon, S.K.; Hah, J.H.; et al. PD-L1 expression is associated with epithelial-mesenchymal transition in head and neck squamous cell carcinoma. *Oncotarget* **2016**, *7*, 15901–15914. [CrossRef] [PubMed]
103. Mak, M.P.; Tong, P.; Diao, L.; Cardnell, R.J.; Gibbons, D.L.; William, W.N.; Skoulidis, F.; Parra, E.R.; Rodriguez-Canales, J.; Wistuba, I.I.; et al. A patient-derived, pan-cancer EMT signature identifies global Molecular alterations and immune target enrichment following epithelial-to-mesenchymal transition. *Clin. Cancer Res.* **2016**, *22*, 609–620. [CrossRef] [PubMed]
104. Chen, L.; Gibbons, D.L.; Goswami, S.; Cortez, M.A.; Ahn, Y.H.; Byers, L.A.; Zhang, X.; Yi, X.; Dwyer, D.; Lin, W.; et al. Metastasis is regulated via microRNA-200/ZEB1 axis control of tumour cell PD-L1 expression and intratumoral immunosuppression. *Nat. Commun.* **2014**, *5*, 5241. [CrossRef] [PubMed]
105. Dong, P.; Xiong, Y.; Yue, J.; Hanley, S.J.B.; Watari, H. Tumor-intrinsic PD-L1 signaling in cancer initiation, development and treatment: Beyond immune evasion. *Front. Oncol.* **2018**, *8*, 386. [CrossRef] [PubMed]
106. Velcheti, V.; Rimm, D.L.; Schalper, K.A. Sarcomatoid lung carcinomas show high levels of programmed death ligand-1 (PD-L1). *J. Thorac. Oncol.* **2013**, *8*, 803–805. [CrossRef] [PubMed]
107. Zhang, Z.; Chen, Y.; Ma, M.; Hao, J.; Ding, R.; Han, L.; Zou, J.; Zhang, L.; Meng, Q.; Qu, X.; et al. Significant benefit of Nivolumab treating PD-L1 positive metastatic pulmonary carcinosarcoma: A case report and literature review. *Oncotarget* **2017**, *8*, 96453–96459. [CrossRef]
108. Zhu, J.; Wen, H.; Ju, X.; Bi, R.; Zuo, W.; Wu, X. Clinical significance of programmed death ligand1 and intra-tumoral CD8+ T lymphocytes in ovarian carcinosarcoma. *PLoS ONE* **2017**, *12*, e0170879.
109. Pinto, A.; Mackrides, N.; Nadji, M. PD-L1 expression in carcinosarcomas of the gynecologic tract: A potentially actionable biomarker. *Appl. Immunohistochem. Mol. Morphol.* **2018**, *26*, 393–397. [CrossRef]
110. Remmerie, M.; Janssens, V. Targeted therapies in type II endometrial cancers: Too little, but not too late. *Int. J. Mol. Sci.* **2018**, *19*, 2380. [CrossRef]

111. Clinical Trials. Available online: clinicaltrials.gov (accessed on 26 June 2019).
112. Fader, A.N.; Roque, D.M.; Siegel, E.; Buza, N.; Hui, P.; Abdelghany, O.; Chambers, S.K.; Secord, A.A.; Havrilesky, L.; O'Malley, D.M.; et al. Randomized phase II trial of carboplatin-paclitaxel versus carboplatin-paclitaxel-trastuzumab in uterine serous carcinomas that overexpress human epidermal growth factor receptor 2/neu. *J. Clin. Oncol.* **2018**, *36*, 2044–2051. [CrossRef]

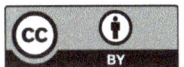

© 2019 by the authors. Licensee MDPI, Basel, Switzerland. This article is an open access article distributed under the terms and conditions of the Creative Commons Attribution (CC BY) license (http://creativecommons.org/licenses/by/4.0/).

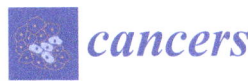

Review

Biological Significance of Tumor Heterogeneity in Esophageal Squamous Cell Carcinoma

Lehang Lin and De-Chen Lin *

Guangdong Provincial Key Laboratory of Malignant Tumor Epigenetics and Gene Regulation, Medical Research Center, Sun Yat-Sen University, Guangzhou 510120, China
* Correspondence: lindch5@mail.sysu.edu.cn; Tel.: +86-20-89205573; Fax: +86-20-81332601

Received: 15 July 2019; Accepted: 7 August 2019; Published: 12 August 2019

Abstract: Esophageal squamous cell carcinoma (ESCC) is a common and aggressive malignancy, with hitherto dismal clinical outcome. Genomic analyses of patient samples reveal a complex heterogeneous landscape for ESCC, which presents in both intertumor and intratumor forms, manifests at both genomic and epigenomic levels, and contributes significantly to tumor evolution, drug resistance, and metastasis. Here, we review the important molecular characteristics underlying ESCC heterogeneity, with an emphasis on genomic aberrations and their functional contribution to cancer evolutionary trajectories. We further discuss how novel experimental tools, including single-cell sequencing and three-dimensional organoids, may advance our understanding of tumor heterogeneity. Lastly, we suggest that deciphering the mechanisms governing tumor heterogeneity holds the potential to developing precision therapeutics for ESCC patients.

Keywords: esophageal squamous cell carcinoma; tumor heterogeneity; tumor evolution; precision medicine

1. Introduction

Esophageal carcinoma is the sixth most lethal cancer type worldwide, responsible for over 400,000 deaths annually [1,2]. Esophageal squamous cell carcinoma (ESCC) is the predominant histological subtype, accounting for 90% of cases [3,4]. Despite noteworthy advances in both cancer diagnosis and therapy, the clinical outlook for ESCC patients remains dismal, with a five-year survival rate below 30% [5,6]. A number of lines of evidence have demonstrated that this poor clinical outcome is at least partially attributed to the substantial intertumor and intratumor heterogeneity in ESCC [7,8].

The concept of tumor heterogeneity contains both intertumor and intratumor forms. Intertumor heterogeneity concerns the phenotypic and molecular differences among tumors from different patients, while intratumor heterogeneity refers to biological variations within the same tumor [9–13]. Heterogeneity is an important attribute of cancer and a major contributor to tumor progression. It manifests at two major levels: genomic (somatic mutations, copy number alterations, chromosomal rearrangements, etc.) and non-genomic (epigenomic changes, microenvironmental variabilities, etc.) [14,15]. The degree and complexity of tumor heterogeneity influence the strategy of tumor biopsy, cancer diagnosis, and treatment planning [7,9,14,16–18]. Increasingly, advances in sequencing technology and analysis algorithms have substantially promoted the understanding of both intertumor and intratumor heterogeneity in many cancer types, including ESCC [7,19,20]. However, translation of the accumulated knowledge on ESCC heterogeneity into clinical practice is still challenging. A systematic understanding of ESCC heterogeneity with respect to its composition, function, and implication is therefore urgently needed.

In this review, we summarized the evidence for both genomic and non-genomic sources of ESCC heterogeneity and discussed their biological and clinical significance in the context of tumor evolution.

We also described new technologies and methodologies that might further our understanding and management of ESCC heterogeneity and shared our perspectives on the future of this field.

2. Intertumor Heterogeneity

Taxonomy of cancer subtypes by specific molecular characteristics significantly improves the conventional histopathological classification and guides subtype-specific precision medicine. As exemplified in breast cancer (e.g., luminal, basal-like, Her2+), lung cancer (e.g., EGFR+, ALK fusion+), and gastric cancer (e.g., Epstein–Barr virus+, microsatellite unstable), intertumor heterogeneity has been widely studied and successfully translated into clinical knowledge in various cancer types [21–23]. However, the stratification of ESCC patients based on intertumoral molecular heterogeneity remains comparatively understudied.

In 2017, through an integrative multi-omics analysis, The Cancer Genome Atlas (TCGA) consortium classified 90 ESCC specimens into three subtypes, designated as ESCC1–3 [4]. ESCC1, mostly Asian samples, was enriched in genomic alterations in the *NRF2* pathway (*NFE2L2*, *KEAP1*, *CUL3*, and *ATG7*) and amplifications of *SOX2* and/or *TP63*; ESCC2, mainly Eastern European and South American samples, was characterized by higher rates of *NOTCH1* and *ZNF750* mutations, *CDK6* amplification, and inactivation of *KDM6A*, *KDM2D*, *PTEN*, and *PIK3R1*; only four cases were classified into ESCC3, which were all from North America and featured in *SMARCA4* mutation. Although these subtypes showed notable geographical trends, their associations with particular biological and/or clinical features were not extensively elucidated. In addition, because of the relatively small number of samples, these classifications need further validation in larger cohorts.

In addition to the effort from TCGA consortium, several individual laboratories have attempted to subgroup ESCC based on transcriptomic data. Upon analyzing tumor samples from African patients, Liu et al. [24] reported three ESCC subtypes based on their distinct expression patterns of cell cycle and neural transcripts. In another study, ESCC specimens from 360 East Asian individuals were divided into four molecular subtypes associated with distinct clinical metrics [25]. Most recently, a new research work has categorized Asian ESCCs into two subtypes, with subtype I overexpressing genes in immune response process and subtype II linked to ectoderm development, cell proliferation, and glycolysis process [26]. Additionally, Tanaka et al. [27] reported the presence of an immune-reactive subtype of ESCC patients with cytotoxic T-lymphocyte signatures activated by chemoradiotherapy.

Despite the fact that no consensus molecular subtypes of ESCC have been established, the above subtyping results are sufficient to confirm the existence of extensive intertumor heterogeneity among ESCC individuals, and further demonstrate heterogeneity amongst different ESCC ethnic groups. This is in line with the well-established dramatic geographic and demographic features of ESCC [28,29]. It should also be noted that the molecular factors and causes underlying intertumor heterogeneity are likely similar with those involved in intratumor diversity. In order to fully capture the tumor spectrum, and to further improve ESCC subclassification and treatment stratification, the molecular features of ESCC intratumor heterogeneity need to be comprehensively integrated.

3. Intratumor Heterogeneity

In the milestone paper published in 1976, Peter C. Nowell [30] proposed a model for cancer development: the Darwinian clonal evolution and selection of tumor cells. Since then, this model has been widely accepted and the phenomenon of intratumor heterogeneity has been highlighted as a cancer hallmark to reflect the non-uniformity and intricacy within tumor ecosystems [31–33]. To date, it is well established that intratumor heterogeneity is represented by the presence of distinct cell populations, which can occupy specific microenvironmental niches, behave as communities, and extensively interact with each other as well as with components of the tumor microenvironment [12]. Therefore, intratumor heterogeneity arises not only from genomic and epigenomic disorders of tumor cells themselves, but also from the influence of the tumor microenvironment [9]. Importantly, intratumor heterogeneity exists among different geographical regions of the same tumor (spatial heterogeneity), as well as between the primary tumor and subsequent local or distant recurrence in the same patient (temporal heterogeneity). As a cumulative result, tumor cells display remarkable variability in numerous phenotypic traits, including clinically important phenotypes such as the ability to seed metastases and to survive therapy (Figure 1) [34].

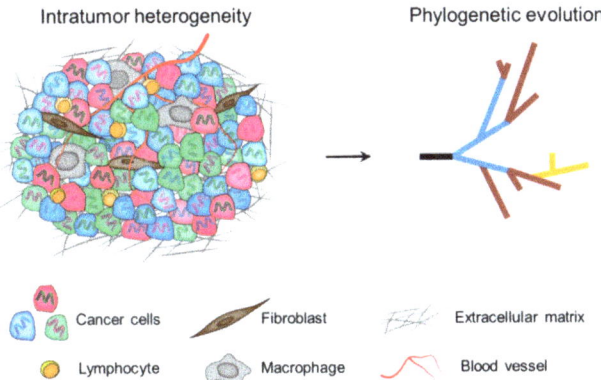

Figure 1. Multiple layers of intratumor heterogeneity. **Left**: Phenotypically distinct cancer cells with both genomic (DNA color) and epigenomic (cell color) heterogeneity are admixed with diversified microenvironmental components. **Right**: A phylogenetic framework helps to understand the nature and biological significance of tumor spatiotemporal heterogeneity.

3.1. Clonal Evolution of Tumors

According to the clonal evolution hypothesis, cancer arises from a single founder cell, and tumor progression is accompanied by the resultant succession of clonal expansions that follow the Darwinian logic [30]. This evolutionary perspective underlines genomic alterations as an essential substrate for fueling tumor transformation and evolution.

During each cell cycle, regardless of normal or cancer cells, DNA mutations may be acquired. Thus, the acquisition of mutations is a stochastic and random process. Consequently, innumerable rounds of cell divisions required for the formation of macroscopic tumors offer plenty of opportunities for Darwinian selection and emergence of clonal diversity in tumor cell populations. During clonal evolution, only a few "jackpot" mutations that activate oncogenic pathways and/or inactivate tumor suppressors are selectively advantageous, allowing the mutant clones to achieve selective sweeps. These functionally significant mutations are termed "drivers". In contrast, the vast majority of mutations are functionally neutral since they do not confer competitive fitness advantage. These mutations are so-called "passengers" and are mainly responsible for intratumor heterogeneity [35]. Importantly, clonal evolution often proceeds in a branching rather than in a linear manner, further contributing to variegated tumor subclones and the complexity of tumor evolution [14]. In fact, many neutral or mildly deleterious mutations during clonal expansion can be retained in the population, or even undergo expansions due to the genetic drift [32,35]. Moreover, given the fact that the Darwinian selection is context-specific, and the evolutionary dynamics of tumor microenvironment and epigenomic events could translate into heterogeneous selective pressures experienced by tumor cells, the selective effect of given mutations (either driver or passenger) can change substantially at different stages of tumor progression [14].

3.2. Spatial Intratumor Heterogeneity

Spatial intratumor heterogeneity has been elucidated at high resolution in many cancer types [15,36–40]. Recently, several groups have performed multi-regional deep-sequencing, and have presented a comprehensive heterogeneous landscape of ESCC [41–44]. Through analyzing

51 sub-tumor regions from 13 ESCC patients, Hao et al. [42] proposed that approximately 40% of driver mutations were spatially heterogeneous, including oncogenes such as *KIT*, and members of the *PI3K/MTOR* (*PIK3CA* and *MTOR*) and *NFE2L2* pathways (*NFE2L2* and *KEAP1*). In addition, significant spatial heterogeneity was observed in copy number alterations, including *EGFR* amplification and *CDKN2A/B* deletions [42]. Furthermore, taking into consideration the multi-step progression of ESCC, Zeng's team [43] sequenced different segments of ESCC tumors and their matched dysplasia samples in a cohort of 20 patients. Their analyses showed that esophagus dysplasia also carried high mutation load and, remarkably, more heterogeneous mutations were seen in dysplasia than in tumor samples from each patient. Moreover, through sequencing 682 micro-scale esophageal samples, Yokoyama et al. [45] reported very recently that pervasive expansions of multiple independent clones were more commonly present within physiologically normal esophagus in comparison to ESCCs. These seemingly surprising data indicate that diversified mutational backgrounds were already established in the precursor lesion or even normal esophageal epithelia, conferring on the esophageal cells the ability to evade selection pressure during ESCC development. Moreover, the degree and complexity of spatial heterogeneity was found to be highly correlated with ESCC aggressiveness [44]. Specifically, clinical stage of ESCC was negatively correlated with the proportion of ubiquitous mutations, and significantly more heterogeneous mutations were observed in ESCC patients with local metastasis, compared to those without.

Regionally segregated somatic mutations and copy number alterations have important clinical implications in ESCC. Firstly, they complicate pathological evaluation of tumor samples. Owing to potential sampling bias caused by spatial heterogeneity, the representability of tumor regions subject to pathological assessment is increasingly considered as a key factor. It is possible that diagnostic and therapeutic targets located in uninspected regions are missed by chance, and the heterogeneous spectrum of the tumor is inevitably underestimated. Additionally, spatial genomic heterogeneity is an important determinant for therapeutic responses. Although most cancers initially respond to treatment, they almost always relapse with the outgrowth of cancer cells that are no longer sensitive to the therapy. Many cases have demonstrated that resistance to targeted drugs may result from the preexisting heterogeneous cells. Examples include the impaired efficiency of EGFR inhibitor for lung cancer patients with heterogeneous driver status [46,47]. Lung cancers initially containing rare mutations of *EGFR*, e.g., T790M, or low frequency of *MET* amplification, are capable of rendering resistance to targeted therapy [18,31,48,49]. Another well-understood case is chronic myeloid leukemia, in which mutant forms of the BCR-ABL fusion protein have been implicated in the relapse of disease under imatinib treatment [50–52]. In ESCC, heterogeneous amplifications of *EGFR*, *FGFR1*, and *PD-L1* have been reported [42–44], accounting partially for the unsatisfactory efficacy of targeting such genomic lesions [53–55]. Spatial genomic heterogeneity, therefore, greatly challenges both accurate diagnosis and efficient cancer treatment.

In addition to genomic alterations, epigenomic dysregulation also contributes to spatial diversity within a tumor. Mechanistically, epigenomic heterogeneity may arise from changes in chromatin status (e.g., DNA methylation, histone modification), deregulation of microRNAs, and transcription regulators, etc. These alterations potentially provide fitness benefit, leading to intratumor heterogeneity either independently or in conjunction with genomic alterations [56–64]. For example, DNA methylation status within promoters of transcription factors SIM2 and SIX1 was strongly correlated with their heterogeneous expression pattern, which was further associated with ESCC differentiation, progression, and prognosis [65–67]. Dynamic changes of mutational status and promoter DNA methylation were also observed in the SWI/SNF chromatin remodeling complex and were shown to involve in ESCC carcinogenesis [68]. Moreover, epigenomic and genomic heterogeneity have been integratively analyzed in three ESCC patients [42]. Noticeably, the spatial heterogeneous pattern of DNA methylation closely recapitulated that of somatic mutations, indicating functional interplay between genomic and epigenomic alterations in ESCC.

The tumor microenvironment, consisting of fibroblasts, extracellular matrix, immune cells (e.g., macrophages, infiltrating lymphocytes), etc., imposes yet another layer of heterogeneity [44,69–75]. Tumor microenvironment can shape tumor cell phenotypes by augmenting both the intrinsic variability of cancer cells (e.g., by inducing stress responses and genomic instability) and the extrinsic diversity of microenvironmental contexts (e.g., different densities of blood and lymphatic vasculature, different numbers and types of infiltrating cells) [7]. In ESCC, the tumor microenvironment itself is indeed highly heterogeneous, as evidenced by recent reports of intratumor heterogeneity of tumor infiltrating T and B cells [44,70,75]. Additionally, Yan et al. [44] observed a tight association between genomic heterogeneity and variation of T cell repertoire in ESCC primary tumors. These results demonstrate that the intratumor genomic heterogeneity may have clinical relevance in ESCC through affecting tumor microenvironment. Meanwhile, ESCC cells could also benefit from the microenvironmental heterogeneity, which supports cellular diversity and influences evolutionary trajectories [14,62,76,77].

3.3. Temporal Intratumor Heterogeneity

Accumulating evidence suggests that intratumor heterogeneity contributes to tumor growth through a process called branched evolution. This model suggests that tumorigenesis is analogous to a growing tree, whose trunk gives rise to numerous branches [9,14,78]. Phylogenetic analysis is a useful approach to delineate such tree structure of cancer evolution [19,38,79–81]. Accordingly, in the phylogenetic tree, truncal (ubiquitous) events shared by the entire tumor population likely reflect processes involved before and during tumor initiation and early development, whereas branched (heterogeneous) events present in only some regions of the tumor reveal factors shaping the genome during tumor maintenance and progression. Characterization of the relative timing of key somatic events with possible biological relevance is therefore essential for deciphering the evolutionary processes of tumors, as well as further improving precision medicine strategies.

In ESCC, driver mutations were significantly more truncal/clonal than passenger mutations, in accordance with findings in other tumor types. Importantly, the majority of driver mutations in tumor suppressors (including *TP53*, *KMT2D*, *ZNF750*, etc.) had a tendency to locate in the trunks of phylogenetic trees, indicating that tumor suppressors are lost as relatively early events during ESCC development. In contrast, half of the driver mutations in the branches were in oncogenes, including potential actionable targets, *PIK3CA* and *MTOR*, suggesting that they are late events in ESCC [42]. This observation highlights the extra caution needed when considering inhibiting such oncogenic mutants in ESCC, given previous studies showing that suppressing subclonal drivers could otherwise lead to outgrowth of non-mutated subpopulations [82].

Esophageal squamous cell carcinoma evolution is a multi-step process that begins from low-grade dysplasia, high-grade dysplasia, carcinoma in situ to invasive tumor and metastasis [44]. To further explore the genomic dynamics during this process, recent studies applied multi-region sequencing on samples covering different stages of ESCC from the same patients and constructed phylogenetic trees that mapped mutations and copy number alterations chronologically [43,44,83]. Notably, only a small fraction of total genomic alterations was conserved from squamous dysplasia to ESCC tumors, implying the distinct evolutionary trajectories taken by precursor and neoplastic cells [43,83]. Phylogenetic analysis confirmed truncal mutations of *TP53* and *CDKN2A* and truncal copy number alterations of 11q13 (*CCND1*), 3q27 (*SOX2*), 2q31 (*NFE2L2*), and 9p21 (*CDKN2A*), validating that they are early changes during esophagus neoplastic transformation [83]. Independently, Chen et al. [43] also reported early emergence of copy number alterations in precursor lesions of ESCC and highlighted this phenomenon as a prominent genomic feature distinct from the development of esophageal adenocarcinoma, another pathological subtype of esophageal cancer. When considering alterations at pathway level, genes involved in cell cycle regulation (such as *TP53*, *CCND1*, *CDK6*, *RB1*, and *CDKN2A*) were frequently altered in the early stage of ESCC, whereas genes in *RTK/RAS/PI3K* tended to undergo alterations throughout the process of ESCC evolution [44].

Taking into consideration of the timing of metastatic outgrowth and the role of the intratumor heterogeneity, two distinct models for the derivation of ESCC metastasis have been proposed: the stepwise progression model and the parallel progression model (Figure 2) [43,44]. The stepwise progression model was characterized by tumor cells disseminated at the late stages of ESCC. Accordingly, metastases could be considered as direct descendants of the most malignant and aggressive clones that dominated primary tumors. This model was also described as the linear spread pattern by Yan et al. [44]. By comparison, in the parallel progression model, early spread of metastases during ESCC tumor progression was highlighted. Specifically, divergent evolutionary trajectories were found between primary tumors and metastatic lesions, as well as among metastatic lesions. This model was represented as both explosive spread and metastasis-to-metastasis patterns by Yan and colleagues [44].

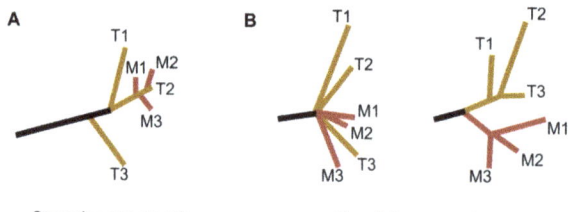

Figure 2. Phylogenic models for ESCC metastasis. (**A**) The stepwise progression model, in which metastases are seeded at the late stages of ESCC progression. This model was also described as the linear spread pattern by Yan et al. [44]. (**B**) The parallel progression model, in which tumor dissemination occurs at the early stages of ESCC progression. In this situation, dissemination of metastases could happen either (**Left**) explosively (explosive spread pattern) or via (**Right**) metastasis-to-metastasis pattern (T, Tumor; M, Metastasis).

More studies are required to elucidate the clonal relationship between ESCC primary and metastatic tumor cell populations, which will not only illuminate the evolutionary history of ESCC, but also create a more solid ground for therapeutic decision making. Ultimately, decoding the extent of differences between ESCC primary and metastases is crucial for the improved management of metastatic ESCC patients.

4. New Technologies for the Investigation of Intratumor Heterogeneity

It is with great excitement that we are witnessing novel technologies and methodologies being developed at a fast pace for the investigation of intratumor heterogeneity. These advances will uncover the molecular and biological features of intratumor heterogeneity with unprecedented resolution and they hold the potential to revolutionize our understanding of the complex intrinsic and extrinsic heterogeneity of ESCC.

4.1. Heterogeneity Studies at the Single-Cell Level

Technical advances in single-cell sequencing have been heralding a new era in resolving tumor heterogeneity and understanding the dynamics of subclonal architecture during tumor progression [31,36,84–88]. For instance, single-cell RNA sequencing of glioblastomas revealed that cell-to-cell inherent variability was evident in regulatory axes central to glioblastoma biology, prognosis, and therapy [88]. Single-cell DNA sequencing of a large number of breast cancer cells unraveled the punctuated evolution pattern of copy number alterations during tumor development [36,86,87]. In ESCC, single-cell RNA sequencing has been recently performed on three specimens, and substantial intratumor heterogeneity contributed by both tumor-intrinsic and microenvironmental alterations has been observed [89]. Nevertheless, more extensive single cell-based studies of ESCC are still lacking.

Compared to conventional bulk-tissue analysis, single-cell profiling is superior in its robust sensitivity in detecting subclonal/private genomic alterations at true single-cell resolution. Thus, single-cell sequencing is of pivotal importance in discovering subtle diversification and rare tumor clones. Looking to the future, we anticipate that the application of single-cell multi-omics technologies (e.g., transcriptome, methylome [90,91], and chromatin [92,93] assays) to both cancerous cells and infiltrating stromal cells will finally provide us with a panoramic view of ESCC heterogeneity.

4.2. Three-Dimensional Organoid Culture

Organoid cultures are three-dimensional multicellular constructs wherein cells can self-assemble to faithfully represent the physiological states of parent tissues or organs. Derived from patients, 3D organoids are crucial tools for disease modeling, especially cancers. Briefly, the generation of patient-derived organoids involves disintegration or digestion of the tumor tissue into single-cell suspensions or cell aggregates, followed by implantation of the cells in growth factor-optimized media and 3D basement membrane matrix (Matrigel) [94]. Currently, 3D organoids have been developed for several cancer types and been proven to successfully recapitulate tumor spatiotemporal heterogeneity [95–100]. Particularly, the generation of clonal organoids from different locations from the same tumors allows the study of tumor heterogeneity and evolution [100–103]. Specific driver and passenger mutations could be introduced by the CRISPR-Cas9 genome-editing system with the resultant organoids valuable for dissecting tumor progression mechanisms [104–107]. Importantly, organoid technology has also been leveraged to facilitate the development of personalized medicine, including drug screening and therapy response evaluation, which is in urgent need to overcome tumor heterogeneity [98,101,108–112].

In ESCC, Kijima and colleagues [113] have successfully generated and characterized 3D organoids from ESCC patients and provided proof-of-principle regarding their utility as a robust platform for analyzing cancer cell heterogeneity, evaluating drug sensitivity, and exploring mechanisms of drug resistance. However, given the importance of the tumor microenvironment, future work will require the investigation of ESCC-relevant niche factors and optimization of conditions for co-culturing with stromal and immune cells in the 3D organoids [114]. It also needs to be determined whether the 3D organoids could faithfully recapitulate the entire heterogeneity of ESCC, and to what extent could the heterogeneity be maintained after extended ex vivo culture. Additionally, future applications of 3D organoids in the clinical setting should include analysis of both ESCC precancerous and metastatic lesions. With such improvements in the organoid system, we believe that 3D organoid culture will become a powerful tool to model the biological function of intratumor heterogeneity. Through this tool, we can gain more insights into ESCC evolution in time and space and develop more effective precision medicine against this deadly disease.

5. Conclusions and Future Directions

It is now clear that heterogeneity is a hallmark of ESCC. However, a significant lag still exists between the knowledge advance of tumor heterogeneity and its clinical translation regarding to diagnostic, prognostic, and therapy. Firstly, it is worth investigating whether the heterogeneity degree by itself could serve as an important biomarker in predicting ESCC progression and guiding treatment decisions. Notably, the extent of clonal diversity predicts the probability of malignant progression in Barrett's esophagus [115]. The quantitative evaluation of cellular diversity has also been used as a biomarker in breast cancer [116]. These examples suggest that diagnostic value of heterogeneity may have universal applicability in cancers irrespective of tumor anatomy. Secondly, given that a heterogeneous tumor is the resulting accumulation of both genomic and non-genomic diversities, the heterogeneity of both cellular and non-cellular components (e.g., epigenome, tumor microenvironment) should be more extensively explored, together with their associations with ESCC biology and clinical outcomes. This entails chronological studies assessing heterogeneity along disease progression of the same patient, from squamous dysplasia to cancer metastases. Moreover, longitudinal studies evaluating intratumor heterogeneity changes during and following therapeutic interventions are required to support identifying early resistant disease and limiting iatrogenic impacts of therapy on ESCC evolution. Thirdly, although heterogeneity undoubtedly poses a formidable obstruction to therapeutic success, there exists a potential to reach drug-sensitive states by strategies of reducing or even exploiting tumor heterogeneity. Current promising therapeutics include targeting epigenetic modifications of cancer cells (e.g., histone deacetylase inhibitors), modulating the tumor microenvironment (e.g., anti-angiogenic therapy, immune therapy), as well as multiplex-targeted therapy and adaptive therapy. Importantly, there is also a significant progress in the development of anti-cancer stem cell (CSC) treatments, since CSCs constitute a new research focus in tumor heterogeneity [117–119]. Particularly, CSCs not only contribute to the phenotypic heterogeneity of primary tumor but can persist under treatment and provoke drug-resistant recurrence and distant metastasis. In conclusion, advanced theoretical understanding of the tumor heterogeneity along with the rapid development of associated technologies will help develop more innovative and effective precision medicine against ESCC.

Author Contributions: L.L. and D.-C.L. conceived and wrote the review.

Funding: This study was supported by grants from the National Natural Science Foundation of China (81672786, 81872306, 81802692), China Postdoctoral Science Foundation (2018M640867, 2019T120774), and Guangdong Science and Technology Department (2017B030314026).

Acknowledgments: We thank Dong Yin for his discussion regarding the manuscript.

Conflicts of Interest: The authors declare no conflict of interest.

References

1. Torre, L.A.; Bray, F.; Siegel, R.L.; Ferlay, J.; Lortet-Tieulent, J.; Jemal, A. Global cancer statistics, 2012. *CA Cancer J. Clin.* **2015**, *65*, 87–108. [CrossRef] [PubMed]
2. Lin, D.C.; Wang, M.R.; Koeffler, H.P. Genomic and Epigenomic Aberrations in Esophageal Squamous Cell Carcinoma and Implications for Patients. *Gastroenterology* **2018**, *154*, 374–389. [CrossRef] [PubMed]
3. Rustgi, A.K.; El-Serag, H.B. Esophageal carcinoma. *N. Engl. J. Med.* **2014**, *371*, 2499–2509. [CrossRef]
4. Cancer Genome Atlas Research Network. Integrated genomic characterization of oesophageal carcinoma. *Nature* **2017**, *541*, 169–175. [CrossRef] [PubMed]
5. Pennathur, A.; Gibson, M.K.; Jobe, B.A.; Luketich, J.D. Oesophageal carcinoma. *Lancet* **2013**, *381*, 400–412. [CrossRef]
6. Napier, K.J.; Scheerer, M.; Misra, S. Esophageal cancer: A Review of epidemiology, pathogenesis, staging workup and treatment modalities. *World J. Gastrointest. Oncol.* **2014**, *6*, 112–120. [CrossRef] [PubMed]
7. Yap, T.A.; Gerlinger, M.; Futreal, P.A.; Pusztai, L.; Swanton, C. Intratumor heterogeneity: Seeing the wood for the trees. *Sci. Transl. Med.* **2012**, *4*, 127ps10. [CrossRef] [PubMed]
8. Gerlinger, M.; Swanton, C. How Darwinian models inform therapeutic failure initiated by clonal heterogeneity in cancer medicine. *Br. J. Cancer* **2010**, *103*, 1139–1143. [CrossRef] [PubMed]
9. Gerashchenko, T.S.; Denisov, E.V.; Litviakov, N.V.; Zavyalova, M.V.; Vtorushin, S.V.; Tsyganov, M.M.; Perelmuter, V.M.; Cherdyntseva, N.V. Intratumor heterogeneity: Nature and biological significance. *Biochemistry* **2013**, *78*, 1201–1215. [CrossRef]
10. Visvader, J.E. Cells of origin in cancer. *Nature* **2011**, *469*, 314–322. [CrossRef]
11. Wolman, S.R.; Heppner, G.H. Genetic heterogeneity in breast cancer. *J. Natl. Cancer Inst.* **1992**, *84*, 469–470. [CrossRef] [PubMed]
12. Tabassum, D.P.; Polyak, K. Tumorigenesis: It takes a village. *Nat. Rev. Cancer* **2015**, *15*, 473–483. [CrossRef] [PubMed]
13. Axelrod, R.; Axelrod, D.E.; Pienta, K.J. Evolution of cooperation among tumor cells. *Proc. Natl. Acad. Sci. USA* **2006**, *103*, 13474–13479. [CrossRef] [PubMed]
14. Marusyk, A.; Almendro, V.; Polyak, K. Intra-tumour heterogeneity: A looking glass for cancer? *Nat. Rev. Cancer* **2012**, *12*, 323–334. [CrossRef] [PubMed]

15. Navin, N.; Krasnitz, A.; Rodgers, L.; Cook, K.; Meth, J.; Kendall, J.; Riggs, M.; Eberling, Y.; Troge, J.; Grubor, V.; et al. Inferring tumor progression from genomic heterogeneity. *Genome Res.* **2010**, *20*, 68–80. [CrossRef]
16. Swanton, C. Intratumor heterogeneity: Evolution through space and time. *Cancer Res.* **2012**, *72*, 4875–4882. [CrossRef]
17. Horswell, S.; Matthews, N.; Swanton, C. Cancer heterogeneity and "the struggle for existence": Diagnostic and analytical challenges. *Cancer Lett.* **2013**, *340*, 220–226. [CrossRef]
18. Fisher, R.; Pusztai, L.; Swanton, C. Cancer heterogeneity: Implications for targeted therapeutics. *Br. J. Cancer* **2013**, *108*, 479–485. [CrossRef]
19. Gerlinger, M.; Rowan, A.J.; Horswell, S.; Math, M.; Larkin, J.; Endesfelder, D.; Gronroos, E.; Martinez, P.; Matthews, N.; Stewart, A.; et al. Intratumor heterogeneity and branched evolution revealed by multiregion sequencing. *N. Engl. J. Med.* **2012**, *366*, 883–892. [CrossRef]
20. Van Nistelrooij, A.M.; van Marion, R.; Koppert, L.B.; Biermann, K.; Spaander, M.C.; Tilanus, H.W.; van Lanschot, J.J.; Wijnhoven, B.P.; Dinjens, W.N. Molecular clonality analysis of esophageal adenocarcinoma by multiregion sequencing of tumor samples. *BMC Res. Notes* **2017**, *10*, 144. [CrossRef]
21. Cancer Genome Atlas Research Network. Comprehensive molecular characterization of gastric adenocarcinoma. *Nature* **2014**, *513*, 202–209. [CrossRef] [PubMed]
22. Cancer Genome Atlas Research Network. Comprehensive molecular profiling of lung adenocarcinoma. *Nature* **2014**, *511*, 543–550. [CrossRef] [PubMed]
23. Heiser, L.M.; Sadanandam, A.; Kuo, W.L.; Benz, S.C.; Goldstein, T.C.; Ng, S.; Gibb, W.J.; Wang, N.J.; Ziyad, S.; Tong, F.; et al. Subtype and pathway specific responses to anticancer compounds in breast cancer. *Proc. Natl. Acad. Sci. USA* **2012**, *109*, 2724–2729. [CrossRef] [PubMed]
24. Liu, W.; Snell, J.M.; Jeck, W.R.; Hoadley, K.A.; Wilkerson, M.D.; Parker, J.S.; Patel, N.; Mlombe, Y.B.; Mulima, G.; Liomba, N.G.; et al. Subtyping sub-Saharan esophageal squamous cell carcinoma by comprehensive molecular analysis. *JCI Insight* **2016**, *1*, e88755. [CrossRef] [PubMed]
25. Xiong, T.; Wang, M.; Zhao, J.; Liu, Q.; Yang, C.; Luo, W.; Li, X.; Yang, H.; Kristiansen, K.; Roy, B.; et al. An esophageal squamous cell carcinoma classification system that reveals potential targets for therapy. *Oncotarget* **2017**, *8*, 49851–49860. [CrossRef] [PubMed]
26. Wang, F.; Yan, Z.; Lv, J.; Xin, J.; Dang, Y.; Sun, X.; An, Y.; Qi, Y.; Jiang, Q.; Zhu, W.; et al. Gene Expression Profiling Reveals Distinct Molecular Subtypes of Esophageal Squamous Cell Carcinoma in Asian Populations. *Neoplasia* **2019**, *21*, 571–581. [CrossRef] [PubMed]
27. Tanaka, Y.; Aoyagi, K.; Minashi, K.; Komatsuzaki, R.; Komatsu, M.; Chiwaki, F.; Tamaoki, M.; Nishimura, T.; Takahashi, N.; Oda, I.; et al. Discovery of a Good Responder Subtype of Esophageal Squamous Cell Carcinoma with Cytotoxic T-Lymphocyte Signatures Activated by Chemoradiotherapy. *PLoS ONE* **2015**, *10*, e0143804. [CrossRef]
28. Malhotra, G.K.; Yanala, U.; Ravipati, A.; Follet, M.; Vijayakumar, M.; Are, C. Global trends in esophageal cancer. *J. Surg. Oncol.* **2017**, *115*, 564–579. [CrossRef]
29. Wheeler, J.B.; Reed, C.E. Epidemiology of esophageal cancer. *Surg. Clin. N. Am.* **2012**, *92*, 1077–1087. [CrossRef]
30. Nowell, P.C. The clonal evolution of tumor cell populations. *Science* **1976**, *194*, 23–28. [CrossRef]
31. Zheng, X.; Zhang, G.; Li, P.; Zhang, M.; Yan, X.; Zhang, X.; Yang, J.; Li, H.; Liu, X.; Ma, Z.; et al. Mutation tracking of a patient with EGFR-mutant lung cancer harboring de novo MET amplification: Successful treatment with gefitinib and crizotinib. *Lung Cancer* **2019**, *129*, 72–74. [CrossRef] [PubMed]
32. Merlo, L.M.; Pepper, J.W.; Reid, B.J.; Maley, C.C. Cancer as an evolutionary and ecological process. *Nat. Rev. Cancer* **2006**, *6*, 924–935. [CrossRef] [PubMed]
33. Michor, F.; Iwasa, Y.; Nowak, M.A. Dynamics of cancer progression. *Nat. Rev. Cancer* **2004**, *4*, 197–205. [CrossRef]
34. Bedard, P.L.; Hansen, A.R.; Ratain, M.J.; Siu, L.L. Tumour heterogeneity in the clinic. *Nature* **2013**, *501*, 355–364. [CrossRef] [PubMed]
35. Marusyk, A.; Polyak, K. Tumor heterogeneity: Causes and consequences. *Biochim. Biophys. Acta* **2010**, *1805*, 105–117. [CrossRef] [PubMed]
36. Navin, N.; Kendall, J.; Troge, J.; Andrews, P.; Rodgers, L.; McIndoo, J.; Cook, K.; Stepansky, A.; Levy, D.; Esposito, D.; et al. Tumour evolution inferred by single-cell sequencing. *Nature* **2011**, *472*, 90–94. [CrossRef]

37. Sottoriva, A.; Spiteri, I.; Piccirillo, S.G.; Touloumis, A.; Collins, V.P.; Marioni, J.C.; Curtis, C.; Watts, C.; Tavare, S. Intratumor heterogeneity in human glioblastoma reflects cancer evolutionary dynamics. *Proc. Natl. Acad. Sci. USA* **2013**, *110*, 4009–4014. [CrossRef]
38. Zhang, J.; Fujimoto, J.; Zhang, J.; Wedge, D.C.; Song, X.; Zhang, J.; Seth, S.; Chow, C.W.; Cao, Y.; Gumbs, C.; et al. Intratumor heterogeneity in localized lung adenocarcinomas delineated by multiregion sequencing. *Science* **2014**, *346*, 256–259. [CrossRef]
39. Xue, R.; Li, R.; Guo, H.; Guo, L.; Su, Z.; Ni, X.; Qi, L.; Zhang, T.; Li, Q.; Zhang, Z.; et al. Variable Intra-Tumor Genomic Heterogeneity of Multiple Lesions in Patients With Hepatocellular Carcinoma. *Gastroenterology* **2016**, *150*, 998–1008. [CrossRef]
40. Gerlinger, M.; Horswell, S.; Larkin, J.; Rowan, A.J.; Salm, M.P.; Varela, I.; Fisher, R.; McGranahan, N.; Matthews, N.; Santos, C.R.; et al. Genomic architecture and evolution of clear cell renal cell carcinomas defined by multiregion sequencing. *Nat. Genet.* **2014**, *46*, 225–233. [CrossRef]
41. Cao, W.; Wu, W.; Yan, M.; Tian, F.; Ma, C.; Zhang, Q.; Li, X.; Han, P.; Liu, Z.; Gu, J.; et al. Multiple region whole-exome sequencing reveals dramatically evolving intratumor genomic heterogeneity in esophageal squamous cell carcinoma. *Oncogenesis* **2015**, *4*, e175. [CrossRef]
42. Hao, J.J.; Lin, D.C.; Dinh, H.Q.; Mayakonda, A.; Jiang, Y.Y.; Chang, C.; Jiang, Y.; Lu, C.C.; Shi, Z.Z.; Xu, X.; et al. Spatial intratumoral heterogeneity and temporal clonal evolution in esophageal squamous cell carcinoma. *Nat. Genet.* **2016**, *48*, 1500–1507. [CrossRef]
43. Chen, X.X.; Zhong, Q.; Liu, Y.; Yan, S.M.; Chen, Z.H.; Jin, S.Z.; Xia, T.L.; Li, R.Y.; Zhou, A.J.; Su, Z.; et al. Genomic comparison of esophageal squamous cell carcinoma and its precursor lesions by multi-region whole-exome sequencing. *Nat. Commun.* **2017**, *8*, 524. [CrossRef]
44. Yan, T.; Cui, H.; Zhou, Y.; Yang, B.; Kong, P.; Zhang, Y.; Liu, Y.; Wang, B.; Cheng, Y.; Li, J.; et al. Multi-region sequencing unveils novel actionable targets and spatial heterogeneity in esophageal squamous cell carcinoma. *Nat. Commun.* **2019**, *10*, 1670. [CrossRef]
45. Yokoyama, A.; Kakiuchi, N.; Yoshizato, T.; Nannya, Y.; Suzuki, H.; Takeuchi, Y.; Shiozawa, Y.; Sato, Y.; Aoki, K.; Kim, S.K.; et al. Age-related remodelling of oesophageal epithelia by mutated cancer drivers. *Nature* **2019**, *565*, 312–317. [CrossRef]
46. Chen, Z.Y.; Zhong, W.Z.; Zhang, X.C.; Su, J.; Yang, X.N.; Chen, Z.H.; Yang, J.J.; Zhou, Q.; Yan, H.H.; An, S.J.; et al. EGFR mutation heterogeneity and the mixed response to EGFR tyrosine kinase inhibitors of lung adenocarcinomas. *Oncologist* **2012**, *17*, 978–985. [CrossRef]
47. Mok, T.S.; Wu, Y.L.; Thongprasert, S.; Yang, C.H.; Chu, D.T.; Saijo, N.; Sunpaweravong, P.; Han, B.; Margono, B.; Ichinose, Y.; et al. Gefitinib or carboplatin-paclitaxel in pulmonary adenocarcinoma. *N. Engl. J. Med.* **2009**, *361*, 947–957. [CrossRef]
48. Engelman, J.A.; Zejnullahu, K.; Mitsudomi, T.; Song, Y.; Hyland, C.; Park, J.O.; Lindeman, N.; Gale, C.M.; Zhao, X.; Christensen, J.; et al. MET amplification leads to gefitinib resistance in lung cancer by activating ERBB3 signaling. *Science* **2007**, *316*, 1039–1043. [CrossRef]
49. Su, K.Y.; Chen, H.Y.; Li, K.C.; Kuo, M.L.; Yang, J.C.; Chan, W.K.; Ho, B.C.; Chang, G.C.; Shih, J.Y.; Yu, S.L.; et al. Pretreatment epidermal growth factor receptor (EGFR) T790M mutation predicts shorter EGFR tyrosine kinase inhibitor response duration in patients with non-small-cell lung cancer. *J. Clin. Oncol.* **2012**, *30*, 433–440. [CrossRef]
50. Hofmann, W.K.; Komor, M.; Wassmann, B.; Jones, L.C.; Gschaidmeier, H.; Hoelzer, D.; Koeffler, H.P.; Ottmann, O.G. Presence of the BCR-ABL mutation Glu255Lys prior to STI571 (imatinib) treatment in patients with Ph+ acute lymphoblastic leukemia. *Blood* **2003**, *102*, 659–661. [CrossRef]
51. Deininger, M. Resistance to imatinib: Mechanisms and management. *J. Natl. Compr. Cancer Netw.* **2005**, *3*, 757–768. [CrossRef]
52. Linev, A.J.; Ivanov, H.J.; Zhelyazkov, I.G.; Ivanova, H.; Goranova-Marinova, V.S.; Stoyanova, V.K. Mutations Associated with Imatinib Mesylate Resistance—Review. *Folia Med.* **2018**, *60*, 617–623. [CrossRef]
53. Pectasides, E. Immune checkpoint blockade in esophageal squamous cell carcinoma: Is it ready for prime time? *J. Thorac. Dis.* **2018**, *10*, 1276–1279. [CrossRef]
54. Kang, X.; Chen, K.; Li, Y.; Li, J.; D'Amico, T.A.; Chen, X. Personalized targeted therapy for esophageal squamous cell carcinoma. *World J. Gastroenterol.* **2015**, *21*, 7648–7658. [CrossRef]

55. Guagnano, V.; Kauffmann, A.; Wohrle, S.; Stamm, C.; Ito, M.; Barys, L.; Pornon, A.; Yao, Y.; Li, F.; Zhang, Y.; et al. FGFR genetic alterations predict for sensitivity to NVP-BGJ398, a selective pan-FGFR inhibitor. *Cancer Discov.* **2012**, *2*, 1118–1133. [CrossRef]
56. Ng, C.K.; Pemberton, H.N.; Reis-Filho, J.S. Breast cancer intratumor genetic heterogeneity: Causes and implications. *Expert Rev. Anticancer Ther.* **2012**, *12*, 1021–1032. [CrossRef]
57. Van Vlodrop, I.J.; Niessen, H.E.; Derks, S.; Baldewijns, M.M.; van Criekinge, W.; Herman, J.G.; van Engeland, M. Analysis of promoter CpG island hypermethylation in cancer: Location, location, location! *Clin. Cancer Res.* **2011**, *17*, 4225–4231. [CrossRef]
58. Fraga, M.F.; Ballestar, E.; Villar-Garea, A.; Boix-Chornet, M.; Espada, J.; Schotta, G.; Bonaldi, T.; Haydon, C.; Ropero, S.; Petrie, K.; et al. Loss of acetylation at Lys16 and trimethylation at Lys20 of histone H4 is a common hallmark of human cancer. *Nat. Genet.* **2005**, *37*, 391–400. [CrossRef]
59. Farazi, T.A.; Hoell, J.I.; Morozov, P.; Tuschl, T. MicroRNAs in human cancer. *Adv. Exp. Med. Biol.* **2013**, *774*, 1–20.
60. Meacham, C.E.; Morrison, S.J. Tumour heterogeneity and cancer cell plasticity. *Nature* **2013**, *501*, 328–337. [CrossRef]
61. Podlaha, O.; Riester, M.; De, S.; Michor, F. Evolution of the cancer genome. *Trends Genet.* **2012**, *28*, 155–163. [CrossRef]
62. Tian, T.; Olson, S.; Whitacre, J.M.; Harding, A. The origins of cancer robustness and evolvability. *Integr. Biol.* **2011**, *3*, 17–30. [CrossRef]
63. Feinberg, A.P.; Ohlsson, R.; Henikoff, S. The epigenetic progenitor origin of human cancer. *Nat. Rev. Genet.* **2006**, *7*, 21–33. [CrossRef]
64. Baylin, S.B.; Ohm, J.E. Epigenetic gene silencing in cancer—A mechanism for early oncogenic pathway addiction? *Nat. Rev. Cancer* **2006**, *6*, 107–116. [CrossRef]
65. Komatsu, M.; Sasaki, H. DNA methylation is a key factor in understanding differentiation phenotype in esophageal squamous cell carcinoma. *Epigenomics* **2014**, *6*, 567–569. [CrossRef]
66. Tamaoki, M.; Komatsuzaki, R.; Komatsu, M.; Minashi, K.; Aoyagi, K.; Nishimura, T.; Chiwaki, F.; Hiroki, T.; Daiko, H.; Morishita, K.; et al. Multiple roles of single-minded 2 in esophageal squamous cell carcinoma and its clinical implications. *Cancer Sci.* **2018**, *109*, 1121–1134. [CrossRef]
67. Nishimura, T.; Tamaoki, M.; Komatsuzaki, R.; Oue, N.; Taniguchi, H.; Komatsu, M.; Aoyagi, K.; Minashi, K.; Chiwaki, F.; Shinohara, H.; et al. SIX1 maintains tumor basal cells via transforming growth factor-beta pathway and associates with poor prognosis in esophageal cancer. *Cancer Sci.* **2017**, *108*, 216–225. [CrossRef]
68. Nakazato, H.; Takeshima, H.; Kishino, T.; Kubo, E.; Hattori, N.; Nakajima, T.; Yamashita, S.; Igaki, H.; Tachimori, Y.; Kuniyoshi, Y.; et al. Early-Stage Induction of SWI/SNF Mutations during Esophageal Squamous Cell Carcinogenesis. *PLoS ONE* **2016**, *11*, e0147372. [CrossRef]
69. Kashima, H.; Noma, K.; Ohara, T.; Kato, T.; Katsura, Y.; Komoto, S.; Sato, H.; Katsube, R.; Ninomiya, T.; Tazawa, H.; et al. Cancer-associated fibroblasts (CAFs) promote the lymph node metastasis of esophageal squamous cell carcinoma. *Int. J. Cancer* **2019**, *144*, 828–840. [CrossRef]
70. Zhang, C.; Huang, H.; Miao, Y.; Xiong, H.; Lu, Z. Clonal distribution and intratumour heterogeneity of the B-cell repertoire in oesophageal squamous cell carcinoma. *J. Pathol.* **2018**, *246*, 323–330. [CrossRef]
71. Xiao, J.; Yang, W.; Xu, B.; Zhu, H.; Zou, J.; Su, C.; Rong, J.; Wang, T.; Chen, Z. Expression of fibronectin in esophageal squamous cell carcinoma and its role in migration. *BMC Cancer* **2018**, *18*, 976. [CrossRef]
72. Zhang, H.; Yue, J.; Jiang, Z.; Zhou, R.; Xie, R.; Xu, Y.; Wu, S. CAF-secreted CXCL1 conferred radioresistance by regulating DNA damage response in a ROS-dependent manner in esophageal squamous cell carcinoma. *Cell Death Dis.* **2017**, *8*, e2790. [CrossRef]
73. Zhang, H.; Xie, C.; Yue, J.; Jiang, Z.; Zhou, R.; Xie, R.; Wang, Y.; Wu, S. Cancer-associated fibroblasts mediated chemoresistance by a FOXO1/TGFbeta1 signaling loop in esophageal squamous cell carcinoma. *Mol. Carcinog.* **2017**, *56*, 1150–1163. [CrossRef]
74. Xing, S.; Zheng, X.; Zeng, T.; Zeng, M.S.; Zhong, Q.; Cao, Y.S.; Pan, K.L.; Wei, C.; Hou, F.; Liu, W.L. Chitinase 3-like 1 secreted by peritumoral macrophages in esophageal squamous cell carcinoma is a favorable prognostic factor for survival. *World J. Gastroenterol.* **2017**, *23*, 7693–7704. [CrossRef]
75. Chen, Z.; Zhang, C.; Pan, Y.; Xu, R.; Xu, C.; Chen, Z.; Lu, Z.; Ke, Y. T cell receptor beta-chain repertoire analysis reveals intratumour heterogeneity of tumour-infiltrating lymphocytes in oesophageal squamous cell carcinoma. *J. Pathol.* **2016**, *239*, 450–458. [CrossRef]

76. Junttila, M.R.; de Sauvage, F.J. Influence of tumour micro-environment heterogeneity on therapeutic response. *Nature* **2013**, *501*, 346–354. [CrossRef]
77. Hanahan, D.; Coussens, L.M. Accessories to the crime: Functions of cells recruited to the tumor microenvironment. *Cancer Cell* **2012**, *21*, 309–322. [CrossRef]
78. Greaves, M.; Maley, C.C. Clonal evolution in cancer. *Nature* **2012**, *481*, 306–313. [CrossRef]
79. Wu, X.; Northcott, P.A.; Dubuc, A.; Dupuy, A.J.; Shih, D.J.; Witt, H.; Croul, S.; Bouffet, E.; Fults, D.W.; Eberhart, C.G.; et al. Clonal selection drives genetic divergence of metastatic medulloblastoma. *Nature* **2012**, *482*, 529–533. [CrossRef]
80. Anderson, K.; Lutz, C.; van Delft, F.W.; Bateman, C.M.; Guo, Y.; Colman, S.M.; Kempski, H.; Moorman, A.V.; Titley, I.; Swansbury, J.; et al. Genetic variegation of clonal architecture and propagating cells in leukaemia. *Nature* **2011**, *469*, 356–361. [CrossRef]
81. De Bruin, E.C.; McGranahan, N.; Mitter, R.; Salm, M.; Wedge, D.C.; Yates, L.; Jamal-Hanjani, M.; Shafi, S.; Murugaesu, N.; Rowan, A.J.; et al. Spatial and temporal diversity in genomic instability processes defines lung cancer evolution. *Science* **2014**, *346*, 251–256. [CrossRef]
82. Lohr, J.G.; Stojanov, P.; Carter, S.L.; Cruz-Gordillo, P.; Lawrence, M.S.; Auclair, D.; Sougnez, C.; Knoechel, B.; Gould, J.; Saksena, G.; et al. Widespread genetic heterogeneity in multiple myeloma: Implications for targeted therapy. *Cancer Cell* **2014**, *25*, 91–101. [CrossRef]
83. Liu, X.; Zhang, M.; Ying, S.; Zhang, C.; Lin, R.; Zheng, J.; Zhang, G.; Tian, D.; Guo, Y.; Du, C.; et al. Genetic Alterations in Esophageal Tissues From Squamous Dysplasia to Carcinoma. *Gastroenterology* **2017**, *153*, 166–177. [CrossRef]
84. Xu, X.; Hou, Y.; Yin, X.; Bao, L.; Tang, A.; Song, L.; Li, F.; Tsang, S.; Wu, K.; Wu, H.; et al. Single-cell exome sequencing reveals single-nucleotide mutation characteristics of a kidney tumor. *Cell* **2012**, *148*, 886–895. [CrossRef]
85. Hou, Y.; Song, L.; Zhu, P.; Zhang, B.; Tao, Y.; Xu, X.; Li, F.; Wu, K.; Liang, J.; Shao, D.; et al. Single-cell exome sequencing and monoclonal evolution of a JAK2-negative myeloproliferative neoplasm. *Cell* **2012**, *148*, 873–885. [CrossRef]
86. Gao, R.; Davis, A.; McDonald, T.O.; Sei, E.; Shi, X.; Wang, Y.; Tsai, P.C.; Casasent, A.; Waters, J.; Zhang, H.; et al. Punctuated copy number evolution and clonal stasis in triple-negative breast cancer. *Nat. Genet.* **2016**, *48*, 1119–1130. [CrossRef]
87. Wang, Y.; Waters, J.; Leung, M.L.; Unruh, A.; Roh, W.; Shi, X.; Chen, K.; Scheet, P.; Vattathil, S.; Liang, H.; et al. Clonal evolution in breast cancer revealed by single nucleus genome sequencing. *Nature* **2014**, *512*, 155–160. [CrossRef]
88. Patel, A.P.; Tirosh, I.; Trombetta, J.J.; Shalek, A.K.; Gillespie, S.M.; Wakimoto, H.; Cahill, D.P.; Nahed, B.V.; Curry, W.T.; Martuza, R.L.; et al. Single-cell RNA-seq highlights intratumoral heterogeneity in primary glioblastoma. *Science* **2014**, *344*, 1396–1401. [CrossRef]
89. Wu, H.; Yu, J.; Li, Y.; Hou, Q.; Zhou, R.; Zhang, N.; Jing, Z.; Jiang, M.; Li, Z.; Hua, Y.; et al. Single-cell RNA sequencing reveals diverse intratumoral heterogeneities and gene signatures of two types of esophageal cancers. *Cancer Lett.* **2018**, *438*, 133–143. [CrossRef]
90. Gravina, S.; Ganapathi, S.; Vijg, J. Single-cell, locus-specific bisulfite sequencing (SLBS) for direct detection of epimutations in DNA methylation patterns. *Nucleic Acids Res.* **2015**, *43*, e93. [CrossRef]
91. Smallwood, S.A.; Lee, H.J.; Angermueller, C.; Krueger, F.; Saadeh, H.; Peat, J.; Andrews, S.R.; Stegle, O.; Reik, W.; Kelsey, G. Single-cell genome-wide bisulfite sequencing for assessing epigenetic heterogeneity. *Nat. Methods* **2014**, *11*, 817–820. [CrossRef]
92. Cusanovich, D.A.; Daza, R.; Adey, A.; Pliner, H.A.; Christiansen, L.; Gunderson, K.L.; Steemers, F.J.; Trapnell, C.; Shendure, J. Multiplex single cell profiling of chromatin accessibility by combinatorial cellular indexing. *Science* **2015**, *348*, 910–914. [CrossRef]
93. Buenrostro, J.D.; Wu, B.; Litzenburger, U.M.; Ruff, D.; Gonzales, M.L.; Snyder, M.P.; Chang, H.Y.; Greenleaf, W.J. Single-cell chromatin accessibility reveals principles of regulatory variation. *Nature* **2015**, *523*, 486–490. [CrossRef]
94. Lancaster, M.A.; Knoblich, J.A. Organogenesis in a dish: Modeling development and disease using organoid technologies. *Science* **2014**, *345*, 1247125. [CrossRef]

95. Sachs, N.; de Ligt, J.; Kopper, O.; Gogola, E.; Bounova, G.; Weeber, F.; Balgobind, A.V.; Wind, K.; Gracanin, A.; Begthel, H.; et al. A Living Biobank of Breast Cancer Organoids Captures Disease Heterogeneity. *Cell* **2018**, *172*, 373–386. [CrossRef]
96. Li, X.; Francies, H.E.; Secrier, M.; Perner, J.; Miremadi, A.; Galeano-Dalmau, N.; Barendt, W.J.; Letchford, L.; Leyden, G.M.; Goffin, E.K.; et al. Organoid cultures recapitulate esophageal adenocarcinoma heterogeneity providing a model for clonality studies and precision therapeutics. *Nat. Commun.* **2018**, *9*, 2983. [CrossRef]
97. Lee, S.H.; Hu, W.; Matulay, J.T.; Silva, M.V.; Owczarek, T.B.; Kim, K.; Chua, C.W.; Barlow, L.J.; Kandoth, C.; Williams, A.B.; et al. Tumor Evolution and Drug Response in Patient-Derived Organoid Models of Bladder Cancer. *Cell* **2018**, *173*, 515–528. [CrossRef]
98. Huch, M.; Gehart, H.; van Boxtel, R.; Hamer, K.; Blokzijl, F.; Verstegen, M.M.; Ellis, E.; van Wenum, M.; Fuchs, S.A.; de Ligt, J.; et al. Long-term culture of genome stable bipotent stem cells from adult human liver. *Cell* **2015**, *160*, 299–312. [CrossRef]
99. Jung, P.; Sato, T.; Merlos-Suarez, A.; Barriga, F.M.; Iglesias, M.; Rossell, D.; Auer, H.; Gallardo, M.; Blasco, M.A.; Sancho, E.; et al. Isolation and in vitro expansion of human colonic stem cells. *Nat. Med.* **2011**, *17*, 1225–1227. [CrossRef]
100. Hubert, C.G.; Rivera, M.; Spangler, L.C.; Wu, Q.; Mack, S.C.; Prager, B.C.; Couce, M.; McLendon, R.E.; Sloan, A.E.; Rich, J.N. A Three-Dimensional Organoid Culture System Derived from Human Glioblastomas Recapitulates the Hypoxic Gradients and Cancer Stem Cell Heterogeneity of Tumors Found In Vivo. *Cancer Res.* **2016**, *76*, 2465–2477. [CrossRef]
101. Aboulkheyr Es, H.; Montazeri, L.; Aref, A.R.; Vosough, M.; Baharvand, H. Personalized Cancer Medicine: An Organoid Approach. *Trends Biotechnol.* **2018**, *36*, 358–371. [CrossRef]
102. Yachida, S.; Jones, S.; Bozic, I.; Antal, T.; Leary, R.; Fu, B.; Kamiyama, M.; Hruban, R.H.; Eshleman, J.R.; Nowak, M.A.; et al. Distant metastasis occurs late during the genetic evolution of pancreatic cancer. *Nature* **2010**, *467*, 1114–1117. [CrossRef]
103. Drost, J.; Clevers, H. Organoids in cancer research. *Nat. Rev. Cancer* **2018**, *18*, 407–418. [CrossRef]
104. Drost, J.; van Boxtel, R.; Blokzijl, F.; Mizutani, T.; Sasaki, N.; Sasselli, V.; de Ligt, J.; Behjati, S.; Grolleman, J.E.; van Wezel, T.; et al. Use of CRISPR-modified human stem cell organoids to study the origin of mutational signatures in cancer. *Science* **2017**, *358*, 234–238. [CrossRef]
105. Roper, J.; Tammela, T.; Cetinbas, N.M.; Akkad, A.; Roghanian, A.; Rickelt, S.; Almeqdadi, M.; Wu, K.; Oberli, M.A.; Sanchez-Rivera, F.J.; et al. In vivo genome editing and organoid transplantation models of colorectal cancer and metastasis. *Nat. Biotechnol.* **2017**, *35*, 569–576. [CrossRef]
106. Neal, J.T.; Kuo, C.J. Organoids as Models for Neoplastic Transformation. *Annu. Rev. Pathol.* **2016**, *11*, 199–220. [CrossRef]
107. Matano, M.; Date, S.; Shimokawa, M.; Takano, A.; Fujii, M.; Ohta, Y.; Watanabe, T.; Kanai, T.; Sato, T. Modeling colorectal cancer using CRISPR-Cas9-mediated engineering of human intestinal organoids. *Nat. Med.* **2015**, *21*, 256–262. [CrossRef]
108. Jabs, J.; Zickgraf, F.M.; Park, J.; Wagner, S.; Jiang, X.; Jechow, K.; Kleinheinz, K.; Toprak, U.H.; Schneider, M.A.; Meister, M.; et al. Screening drug effects in patient-derived cancer cells links organoid responses to genome alterations. *Mol. Syst. Biol.* **2017**, *13*, 955. [CrossRef]
109. Broutier, L.; Mastrogiovanni, G.; Verstegen, M.M.; Francies, H.E.; Gavarro, L.M.; Bradshaw, C.R.; Allen, G.E.; Arnes-Benito, R.; Sidorova, O.; Gaspersz, M.P.; et al. Human primary liver cancer-derived organoid cultures for disease modeling and drug screening. *Nat. Med.* **2017**, *23*, 1424–1435. [CrossRef]
110. Verissimo, C.S.; Overmeer, R.M.; Ponsioen, B.; Drost, J.; Mertens, S.; Verlaan-Klink, I.; Gerwen, B.V.; van der Ven, M.; Wetering, M.V.; Egan, D.A.; et al. Targeting mutant RAS in patient-derived colorectal cancer organoids by combinatorial drug screening. *Elife* **2016**, *5*, e18489. [CrossRef]
111. Van de Wetering, M.; Francies, H.E.; Francis, J.M.; Bounova, G.; Iorio, F.; Pronk, A.; van Houdt, W.; van Gorp, J.; Taylor-Weiner, A.; Kester, L.; et al. Prospective derivation of a living organoid biobank of colorectal cancer patients. *Cell* **2015**, *161*, 933–945. [CrossRef]
112. Roerink, S.F.; Sasaki, N.; Lee-Six, H.; Young, M.D.; Alexandrov, L.B.; Behjati, S.; Mitchell, T.J.; Grossmann, S.; Lightfoot, H.; Egan, D.A.; et al. Intra-tumour diversification in colorectal cancer at the single-cell level. *Nature* **2018**, *556*, 457–462. [CrossRef]

113. Kijima, T.; Nakagawa, H.; Shimonosono, M.; Chandramouleeswaran, P.M.; Hara, T.; Sahu, V.; Kasagi, Y.; Kikuchi, O.; Tanaka, K.; Giroux, V.; et al. Three-Dimensional Organoids Reveal Therapy Resistance of Esophageal and Oropharyngeal Squamous Cell Carcinoma Cells. *Cell. Mol. Gastroenterol. Hepatol.* **2019**, *7*, 73–91. [CrossRef]
114. Whelan, K.A.; Muir, A.B.; Nakagawa, H. Esophageal 3D Culture Systems as Modeling Tools in Esophageal Epithelial Pathobiology and Personalized Medicine. *Cell. Mol. Gastroenterol. Hepatol.* **2018**, *5*, 461–478. [CrossRef]
115. Maley, C.C.; Galipeau, P.C.; Finley, J.C.; Wongsurawat, V.J.; Li, X.; Sanchez, C.A.; Paulson, T.G.; Blount, P.L.; Risques, R.A.; Rabinovitch, P.S.; et al. Genetic clonal diversity predicts progression to esophageal adenocarcinoma. *Nat. Genet.* **2006**, *38*, 468–473. [CrossRef]
116. Park, S.Y.; Lee, H.E.; Li, H.; Shipitsin, M.; Gelman, R.; Polyak, K. Heterogeneity for stem cell-related markers according to tumor subtype and histologic stage in breast cancer. *Clin. Cancer Res.* **2010**, *16*, 876–887. [CrossRef]
117. Kreso, A.; Dick, J.E. Evolution of the cancer stem cell model. *Cell Stem Cell* **2014**, *14*, 275–291. [CrossRef]
118. Boesch, M.; Sopper, S.; Zeimet, A.G.; Reimer, D.; Gastl, G.; Ludewig, B.; Wolf, D. Heterogeneity of Cancer Stem Cells: Rationale for Targeting the Stem Cell Niche. *Biochim. Biophys. Acta* **2016**, *1866*, 276–289. [CrossRef]
119. Zhang, H.F.; Wu, C.; Alshareef, A.; Gupta, N.; Zhao, Q.; Xu, X.E.; Jiao, J.W.; Li, E.M.; Xu, L.Y.; Lai, R. The PI3K/AKT/c-MYC Axis Promotes the Acquisition of Cancer Stem-Like Features in Esophageal Squamous Cell Carcinoma. *Stem Cells* **2016**, *34*, 2040–2051. [CrossRef]

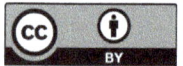

© 2019 by the authors. Licensee MDPI, Basel, Switzerland. This article is an open access article distributed under the terms and conditions of the Creative Commons Attribution (CC BY) license (http://creativecommons.org/licenses/by/4.0/).

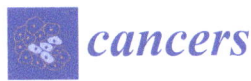

Review

The Impact of Tumor Eco-Evolution in Renal Cell Carcinoma Sampling

Estíbaliz López-Fernández [1,2] and José I. López [3,4,*]

1. FISABIO Foundation, 46020 Valencia, Spain; estibaliz.lopez@yahoo.es
2. Department of Health Sciences, European University of Valencia, Laureate Universities, 46023 Valencia, Spain
3. Department of Pathology, Cruces University Hospital, Biomarkers in Cancer Unit, Biocruces-Bizkaia Health Research Institute, Plaza de Cruces s/n, 48903 Barakaldo, Bizkaia, Spain
4. Department of Medical-Surgical Specialties, University of the Basque Country (UPV/EHU), 48940 Leioa, Spain
* Correspondence: jilpath@gmail.com; Tel.: +34-94-600-6084

Received: 5 November 2018; Accepted: 30 November 2018; Published: 4 December 2018

Abstract: Malignant tumors behave dynamically as cell communities governed by ecological principles. Massive sequencing tools are unveiling the true dimension of the heterogeneity of these communities along their evolution in most human neoplasms, clear cell renal cell carcinomas (CCRCC) included. Although initially thought to be purely stochastic processes, very recent genomic analyses have shown that temporal tumor evolution in CCRCC may follow some deterministic pathways that give rise to different clones and sub-clones randomly spatially distributed across the tumor. This fact makes each case unique, unrepeatable and unpredictable. Precise and complete molecular information is crucial for patients with cancer since it may help in establishing a personalized therapy. Intratumor heterogeneity (ITH) detection relies on the correctness of tumor sampling and this is part of the pathologist's daily work. International protocols for tumor sampling are insufficient today. They were conceived decades ago, when ITH was not an issue, and have remained unchanged until now. Noteworthy, an alternative and more efficient sampling method for detecting ITH has been developed recently. This new method, called multisite tumor sampling (MSTS), is specifically addressed to large tumors that are impossible to be totally sampled, and represent an opportunity to improve ITH detection without extra costs.

Keywords: clear cell renal cell carcinoma; tumor evolution; tumor ecology; intratumor heterogeneity; multisite tumor sampling; targeted therapy

1. Introduction

Clear cell renal cell carcinoma (CCRCC) is nowadays a health problem of major concern in developed societies. The tumor is an aggressive histologic subtype of renal cancer whose incidence is expected to be increased in the future due to the increasing rate of obesity and the ageing population occurring in Western countries [1]. CCRCC shows a well-known resistance to radio- and chemotherapy [2]. However, anti-angiogenic drugs and immune checkpoint blockade are showing promising therapeutic results. At present, three therapeutic options have demonstrated an overall survival improvement: cabozantinib and nivolumab in second or subsequent lines [3], and the combination of nivolumab and ipilimumab in first line therapy [4].

Pathologists are the medical specialists who handle surgical specimens and decide which parts of the tumor must be included for microscopic, immunohistochemical (IHC) and molecular analyses. Tumor representativeness is becoming a critical issue in modern pathology, either when selecting fragments from large resected tumors or when obtaining tissue cores from tumors prior to surgical resection for diagnostic and/or therapeutic purposes. Increasing evidences are showing in the last times that current sampling strategies may not be giving a complete information about the histological and/or molecular alterations that are present in many tumors of different topographies [5–9]. These inconsistencies rise serious concerns among oncologists [10]. Pathologists, however, seem not to be aware of this central problem since sampling protocols still remain unmodified in routine work.

Intratumor heterogeneity (ITH) is at the basis of the lack of tumor representativeness in many tumor samplings. Although well known for decades, the ITH molecular information is having a significant clinical impact in the last years. The arrival of targeted therapies has increased the need of very precise information about ITH since it is observed in many tumor types and represents a major hurdle for effective therapy, provoking therapeutic resistance and metastatic recurrence [11]. In this sense, Gerlinger et al. [12] unveiled in 2012 to what extent this phenomenon is present in clear cell renal cell carcinomas, describing the molecular heterogeneity of these tumors across different regions within the same tumor.

A new tumor sampling strategy has been developed very recently to improve ITH detection in routine practice [13]. This new method, termed multi-site tumor sampling (MSTS), has been successfully applied to CCRCC, although it can be applied to any tumor large enough as to make impossible a total sampling. Interestingly, MSTS outperforms routine sampling protocols in detecting ITH while keeping the cost fixed [14].

The present paper focuses on the importance of tumor representativeness in modern Oncology. A correct tumor sampling is mandatory for this purpose. CCRCC is a good example since it is a well-known paradigm of ITH. More specifically, this paper revisits some basic concepts and applied clinical issues of CCRCC evolution. Tumor ecology and spatial and temporal evolution constrains are then reviewed to contextualize the urgent need of an appropriate tumor analysis. Also, this overview details a more advantageous alternative for tumor sampling supported by a in silico modeling with clinical validation.

2. Tumors as Dynamic Cell Communities Guided by Ecological Principles

Neoplasia encompasses a number of complex and largely unknown processes with a metabolic background [15]. Although pathologists risk thinking of tumors under the microscope as static combinations of cells arranged in different backgrounds organized in varied architectural structures, malignant tumors are complex communities of cells evolving in time with individuals permanently interacting each other. The idea of comparing malignant tumors with other biological communities behaving in a swarm-like manner [16] following similar ecological rules [17,18] is not new. The adaptive mechanisms of tumor cells to their ever-changing habitat are a crucial issue to survive, grow and progress. Epithelial-mesenchymal transition (EMT), and its reversal process (mesenchymal-epithelial transition), are good examples of this dynamic adaptative capacity that can be eventually targeted [19]. A paradoxical effect of EMT is, for example, the development of low-grade metastases in high-grade CCRCC [20]. This tumor behavior, as defined in Ecology, can be synthesized in four models: predation, mutualism, commensalism and parasitism [21]. ITH is known to be induced genetically and epigenetically by interaction with the local tumor microenvironment. Interestingly, tumor microenvironment changes from tumor to tumor, from organ to organ, and even from region to region within the same tumor.

Swarming is defined as the collective behavior of a community of individuals without any centralized guidance or government. This behavior is based essentially on the sum of myriads of neighbor-to-neighbor communications, and is very common in Nature. Tumor cells reproduce this behavior when a specific subgroup within a community of malignant cells of a tumor decides to invade neighbor tissues or metastasize to other organs far away [16]. The collective acquisition of specific properties of tumor cells composing specific tumor compartments is a well-documented event in most tumors, CCRCC included [22]. This phenomenon applies also for tumor microenvironment.

For example, a selective loss of PD-L1 expression has been detected in tumor infiltrating lymphocytes (TIL) taking part of the vein/caval tumor thrombi compartment of CCRCC [23].

Predation refers to an inter-individual relationship in which one individual benefits the other killing it. The attack of some T-cells co-localized with tumor cells that is so evident under the microscope in some CCRCC is a good example of predation. This phenomenon has been investigated mainly in breast tumors. For example, a high co-localization of immune and tumor cells was associated to higher 10-year survival in Her2$^+$ breast carcinomas [24]. In the same sense, the pattern of the PD-1/PD-L1 axis expression in tumor cells and in TIL predicts tumor aggressiveness and survival also in Her2$^+$ breast cancer [25]. Although PD-1/PD-L1 axis blockade is being used with great promise for advanced CCRCC treatment, none study of co-localization of immune and cancer cells in these neoplasms has been published so far.

Cancer cells not always compete for scarce resources. Mutualism applied to cancer refers to the cooperation of two different cell clones for the same benefit thus favoring tumor growth and invasion. This process usually implicates extracellular matrix proteins, such as metalloproteinases and fibronectin, as happens in a zebrafish-melanoma xenograft model [26]. Interestingly, this cooperation has also been identified between tumor cells and stromal inflammatory cells [27].

Examples of commensalism have also been reported in neoplasia. Commensalism describes the relationship of two different cell clones for the benefit of one of them, although the other being not damaged. Also, this process refers to tumor cells and microenvironment cells interactions, for example, the cooperation between tumor cells and tumor-associated fibroblasts favoring tumor progression and metastases [28,29]. High levels of fibroblast activation protein (FAP) have been correlated with tumor size, high grade, high stage and shorter survival in CCRCC, both in primary tumors [30] and in its paired metastases [31]. In this regard, the IHC detection of FAP in the stromal tumor fibroblasts could be a potential biomarker of early lymph node metastatic status and therefore could account for the poor prognosis of FAP positive CCRCC [29]. Even more, recent evidences have shown that tumor microenvironment may vary in an organ-related way along the multiple disseminated metastases of the same tumor [32].

In these collective relationships, some situations lead to an individual to benefit from another damaging it, although not enough so as to destroy it (as happens in predation). In Ecology, this situation is termed parasitism and also occurs in tumor cell communities, for example, when considering the systemic damage generated by the local invasiveness and the metastatic spread of a tumor. This situation could be conceived as a reversal manifestation of the Warburg effect [33], and may explain the frequent association of tumor desmoplasia and biological aggressiveness that occur in many neoplasms.

3. Spatial and Temporal Evolution in Clear Cell Renal Cell Carcinomas

As mentioned in previous paragraphs, several researchers have shown how cancer can be regarded from an ecological perspective that governs tumor evolution [17,34,35]. Obvious ethical reasons do not allow the analysis of the temporal evolution of any tumor. However, bioinformatic tools can infer this process by reconstructing the past chronology. Data coming from the molecular analysis of the tumor tissue obtained from the patient can be phylogenetically analyzed. For example, a mathematical modeling has recently defined the timing in the evolution of CCRCC showing that the tumor originates as soon as in the childhood or adolescence of the patient, and remains silent for decades until appearing symptomatic [36]. More exactly, these early events in CCRCC consist in 3p loss with concurrent 5q gain as a result of chromothrypsis, a process that occurs only in a few hundreds of cells [36].

Four models of tumor evolution have been proposed: linear, branched, punctuated and neutral [37]. With respect to the evolutionary patterns, CCRCC may follow branched or punctuated models, as reported very recently [38].

In the linear evolution model, the new sequential driver mutations that appear across the time vanishes the previous ones due to a strong selective advantage. Such tumor evolution was proposed long time ago for some examples of colorectal adenocarcinomas [39]. Linear evolution is an example of Darwinian model.

Branched evolution model has been identified in many human tumors, CCRCC included [12], and basically consists in a truncal mutation shared by all tumor regions followed by clonal, sub-clonal and private mutations across the different tumor regions. The resulting evolutionary trees are shaped by the different accumulative clonal and sub-clonal divergences. Sub-clonal driver mutations and convergent evolution are two features observed in the branched evolution of CCRCC [12,40]. Interestingly, the coexistence of multiple sub-clones in branched tumors opens the door for the possibility of some type of sub-clonal cooperation following any of the ecological patterns described before. Branched evolution also follows a Darwinian model.

Also called the "Big Bang" model [41], the punctuated evolution model is characterized by a large number of genomic changes occurring at very early stages of tumor evolution. ITH is very high at the beginning but decreases progressively across the time as a result of the high selective predominance of very few clones. Typically, tumors developed in a punctuated model display low ITH and high amounts of single chromosomal rearrangements, a phenomenon termed chromothrypsis present in several human tumors, including a subset of CCRCC [36]. Punctuated evolution is also a Darwinian model of tumor evolution.

Neutral evolution is a paradigm of a non-Darwinian model with extremely high ITH in which natural selection driven by sub-clonal mutations and convergent evolution does no take place.

Most CCRCC follow either branched or punctuated evolution models. In this regard, a recent multicenter study analyzing 1206 regions from 101 patients has demonstrated that CCRCC display up to seven distinct evolutionary subtypes [38]. Three of these subtypes (multiple clonal drivers, *BAP1* driven and *VHL* wild type tumors) followed a punctuated model, were associated to aggressive clinical behavior and showed early 9p and 14q losses, high chromosomal complexity and low ITH. By contrast, three other subtypes (*PBRM1* → *SETD2*, *PBRM1* → *PI3K* and *PBRM1* → *SCNA* driven tumors) followed a branched model and were associated to a less aggressive behavior, with late 9p and 14q losses, low chromosomal complexity and high ITH. The sub-clonal acquisition of *BAP1* or other mutations linked to clinical aggressiveness marked the inflexion from indolence towards rapid evolution in this group of CCRCC. Finally, a seventh subtype (*VHL* mono-driver) was characterized by low chromosomal complexity and low ITH. Typically, this last subtype did not display 9p or 14q losses. These molecular subtypes were associated with classic gross (tumor diameter) and histological (Furhman's grade, TNM staging, presence of necrosis) parameters and have prognostic implications for patients [38].

With respect to the development of metastases, CCRCC have shown specific routes in a thorough analysis of 575 primary and 335 metastatic biopsies in 100 patients with metastatic CCRCC [42]. This multicenter study included three different cohorts of paired primary and metastatic samples of CCRCC with clinical follow up. The analysis also included samples obtained from the tumor thrombi in 24 cases. In summary, the aggressive evolutionary subtypes, that is, tumors with high chromosomal complexity and low ITH displayed a rapid progression to multiple metastases, whereas the opposite, that is, tumors with low chromosomal complexity but high ITH showed an attenuated temporal tumor progression, with tendency to develop late single metastasis. Finally, tumors within the seventh subtype never metastasized.

Although ITH is a main contributor to the development of therapeutic resistance, the mechanisms that underlie this causal inter-relation provide an example of natural selection through evolutionary adaptation [43]. Genetic and epigenetic changes contribute to modify and adapt tumor cell fitness to the new requirements, thus selecting specific clones not only to invade or metastasize, but also to resist to drugs. Targeted therapies, by definition, select tumor cell populations for resistance, this process being Darwinian in essence [44]. However, therapeutic resistance does not solely concern tumor cells;

the local tumor microenvironment also takes part in this process, for example, when the hypoxic status observed in some regions of many tumors applies additional pressure on tumors and contributes to the selection of cell clones adapted to survive under the new conditions [45]. Since drug resistances are a problem of major concern in Oncology and this issue is directly related to regional ITH, a more efficient sampling method to clarify this problem seems mandatory.

4. The Need for an Updated Tumor Sampling Adapted to Tumor Type

The only way to discover the complex spectrum of ecological relationships and the spatial and temporal evolution of tumors that have been revisited in previous paragraphs of this narrative is to improve significantly the tumor representativeness with an affordable sampling. In this sense, total tumor sampling would be the ideal solution, but it is not sustainable because many tumors are too large to be analyzed in their entirety. For these cases international accepted protocols were designed. At least theoretically, an effective sampling strategy must assure getting enough tissue so as to provide reliable information in a probable subsequent molecular analysis. The benefit of such strategy should necessarily be balanced with cost in a difficult sustainable equilibrium. At this point the key question is: How extensive must this sampling be to assure tumor representativeness while keeping the costs affordable? or, in other words, when to stop sampling? The answer is complex.

The strategy of getting one tissue fragment (roughly a piece of 1 cm^2 in dimension) per centimeter of tumor diameter is a rule applied to all tumors, comes from the early days of Pathology and is still followed by pathologists worldwide. When, how and why this strategy was chosen is difficult to know. Although our knowledge about neoplasms has dramatically improved since those days, astonishingly, nothing has changed in tumor sampling. Instead, pathologists focus their interest on the advances provided by -*omics* and other molecular advances brought by sophisticated devices and forget that the most expensive and advanced technique may miss the target if applied in an inappropriate or insufficient tissue sample. Once more, the simplest matters.

Internationally accepted protocols of tumor sampling state that one tumor tissue fragment per centimeter of tumor diameter must be got for histological analysis, plus a fragment of any *suspicious* area [46]. As many tumors appear homogeneous to the naked eye when sliced, tumor selection is usually performed by the pathologist in a blind way and hidden areas of heterogeneity that may be crucial for the patient are usually overlooked.

MSTS has been recently proposed for CCRCC (Figure 1) [13]. This approach follows the rationale *the more you sample the more you find* and applies the *divide and conquer* algorithm [47]. This algorithm has been already applied to resolve complex problems in physics [48], biology [49] and medicine [50], and is based on recursively breaking down a problem in smaller parts (divide) until these are simple enough to be solved directly (conquer). Then, partial solutions are combined to solve the original problem. MSTS has proved to outperform routine protocols in a in silico modeling [14] and in a clinical validation using classic histological parameters [51]. By using MSTS, it is possible to increase the number of samples while keeping the number of cassettes fixed. For such a purpose, the size of the samples must be trimmed from 1 cm^2 to 3 mm^2. This way each cassette can contain 8 small samples per cassette (80 in total in a tumor of 10 cm in diameter) obtained from very different, distant and representative regions of the tumor (Figure 2). A straightforward reasoning says that 80 small tissue fragments have a higher chance for detection of ITH as compared to 10 large samples.

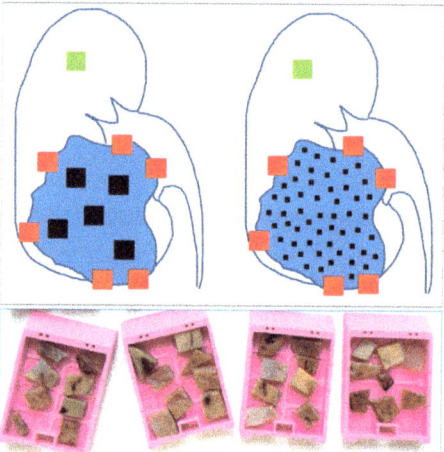

Figure 1. Schematic representation of routine and multisite tumor sampling (MSTS) concepts in renal tumors. The scheme shows the routine sampling (**left**) and the MSTS (**right**). Red cubes represent samples at the edges of the tumor (renal sinus, extrarenal extension and interface between non-tumor and tumor kidney) to detect tumor invasion at these levels. The green cube represents the preceptive sample of normal kidney. Black cubes represent the tumor sampling in both strategies making use of the same number of blocks (up to 8 small fragments can be introduced in one cassette in MSTS). Cassettes containing tumor tissue fragments from MSTS are shown at the bottom of the picture.

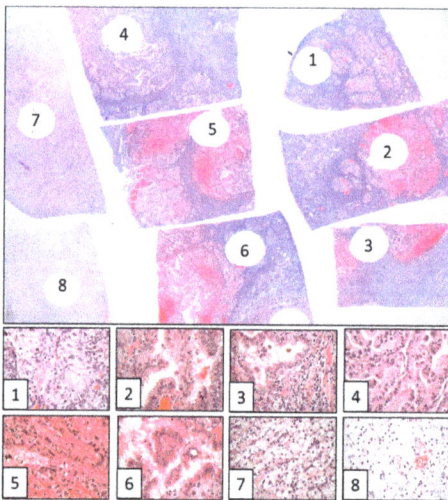

Figure 2. Multisite tumor sampling example in a clear cell renal cell carcinoma (CCRCC) showing the varied spectrum of histologies detected across the eight selected fragments in a single paraffin block, with clear cell high grade phenotype in sample 1, papillary eosinophilic in samples 2, 3, 4 and 6, solid eosinophilic in sample 5, and clear cell low grade in samples 7 and 8. (Hematoxylin & Eosin, original magnification, × 1.5 (large figure) and × 400 (figures 1 to 8)).

If it is accepted that the paraffin block can be the unit of cost in pathology laboratories, it can be assumed that MSTS is better than routine sampling protocol at the same cost [14]. Finally, this method allows the inclusion a small fragment of normal renal tissue in each cassette that can be useful as internal control for immunohistochemistry and/or molecular analyses. The storage of such amount of formalin-fixed and paraffin-embedded tumor tissue fragments in pathology laboratories may be very useful in the future when new technologies allow better analyses. However, pathologists may be reluctant to use MSTS because it takes a long time to collect 80 small samples in a tumor. The application of a cutting grid to the tumor slices in the grossing room will shorten significantly the process [52].

Also, an adaptation of MSTS to large tumors arising in hollow viscera has also been proposed, for example, for cancers arising along the digestive tract. In this particular setting, the anatomical barrier represented by the muscularis propria leads the tumors to grow with their long axes parallel to the wall of the viscera forming tumors with plate-like shapes, and not like spheroids as happens in the kidney, liver or other solid organs. Instead of tissue cubes, the sampling model here gets tissue bars including the whole thickness (from the lumen to the perivisceral adipose tissue) of the viscera [53]. MSTS has obtained here also better performances in detecting ITH compared with routine sampling [53].

As commented in previous paragraphs, temporal evolution in CCRCC follows several deterministic pathways that have been defined either as branched or punctuated models [37]. The discovering of branched CCRCC would benefit specially from MSTS. This possibility makes this strategy even more advantageous in these particular cases. Finally, the performance of MSTS to discover ITH has also proved to be superior at any time of tumor evolution and in all models compared with routine protocols [54].

Recent evidences, however, have demonstrated that tumor sampling must be adapted to the tumor type to be efficient because tumor evolution and the spectrum of ITH are in fact very different, as reflected by the range of evolutionary trees detected across different cancer types [55]. MSTS seems to be an advantageous approach in large tumors with high ITH because in these cases getting samples from many tumor regions will give more complete information of the whole mutational landscape. This happens specially in tumors following branched and neutral models. By contrast, tumors with low ITH levels, although sometimes more aggressive, apparently will not directly benefit from an exhaustive sampling across the tumor. This may happen in neoplasms following the linear and punctuated models.

5. Conclusions

This review is addressed to clinicians and pathologists that are involved in Oncology, and revisits the complexity of tumor evolution with a special mention to the reasons for which each tumor is truly unique. The definition of a more efficient method to discover this complexity is an urgent task. Pathologists, the medical specialists who handle surgical specimens, must reconsider if the currently accepted protocols for tumor sampling are appropriate enough to offer with reliability the expected answers that precision medicine needs today. In this regard, new sampling methods could provide substantial advantages for a more precise diagnosis in a subset of cases. MSTS could be a good option since it keeps the balance cost/benefit sustainable.

Author Contributions: E.L.-F. and J.I.L. conceived and wrote the review.

Funding: This work has been partially funded by the grant SAF2016-79847-R from Ministerio de Economía y Competitividad (MINECO), Spain (J.I.L.).

Conflicts of Interest: The authors declare no conflicts of interests.

References

1. Turajlic, S.; Swanton, C.; Boshoff, C. Kidney cancer: The next decade. *J. Exp. Med.* **2018**, *215*, 2477–2479. [CrossRef] [PubMed]
2. Hsieh, J.J.; Purdue, M.P.; Signoretti, S.; Swanton, C.; Albiges, L.; Schmidinger, M.; Heng, D.Y.; Larkin, J.; Ficarra, V. Renal cell carcinoma. *Nat. Rev. Dis. Primers* **2017**, *3*, 17009. [CrossRef] [PubMed]
3. Tannir, N.M.; Pal, S.K.; Atkins, M.B. Second-Line Treatment Landscape for Renal Cell Carcinoma: A Comprehensive Review. *Oncologist* **2018**, *23*, 540–555. [CrossRef] [PubMed]

4. Wu, B.; Zhang, Q.; Sun, J. Cost-effectiveness of nivolumab plus ipilimumab as first-line therapy in advanced renal-cell carcinoma. *J. Immunother. Cancer* **2018**, *6*, 124. [CrossRef]
5. Blumenfeld, A.J.; Guru, K.; Fuchs, G.J.; Kim, H.L. Percutaneous biopsy of renal cell carcinoma underestimates nuclear grade. *Urology* **2010**, *76*, 610–613. [CrossRef]
6. Tomaszewski, J.J.; Uzzo, R.G.; Smaldone, M.C. Heterogeneity and renal mass biopsy: A review of its role and reliability. *Cancer Biol. Med.* **2014**, *11*, 162–172. [CrossRef]
7. Beltrame, L.; di Martino, M.; Fruscio, R.; Calura, E.; Chapman, B.; Clivio, L.; Sina, F.; Mele, C.; Iatropoulos, P.; Grassi, T.; et al. Profiling cancer gene mutations in longitudinal epithelial ovarian cancer biopsies by targeted next-generation sequencing: A retrospective study. *Ann. Oncol.* **2015**, *26*, 1363–1371. [CrossRef]
8. Bettoni, F.; Masotti, C.; Habr-Gama, A.; Correa, B.R.; Gama-Rodrigues, J.; Vianna, M.R.; Vailati, B.B.; Sao Juliao, G.P.; Fernandez, L.M.; Galante, P.A.; et al. Intratumoral genetic heterogeneity in rectal cancer. Are single biopsies representative of the entirety of the tumor? *Ann. Surg.* **2017**, *265*, e4–e6. [CrossRef]
9. Ellsworth, R.E.; Blackburn, H.L.; Shriver, C.D.; Soon-Shiong, P.; Ellsworth, D.L. Molecular heterogeneity in breast cancer: State of the science and implications for patient care. *Semin. Cell Dev. Biol.* **2017**, *64*, 65–72. [CrossRef]
10. Soultati, A.; Stares, M.; Swanton, C.; Larkin, J.; Turajlic, S. How should clinicians address intratumor heterogeneity in clear cell renal cell carcinoma? *Curr. Opin. Urol.* **2015**, *25*, 358–366. [CrossRef]
11. Marusyk, A.; Almendro, V.; Polyak, K. Intra-tumour heterogeneity: A looking glass for cancer? *Nat. Rev. Cancer* **2012**, *12*, 323–334. [CrossRef] [PubMed]
12. Gerlinger, M.; Rowan, A.J.; Horswell, S.; Math, M.; Larkin, J.; Endesfelder, D.; Gronroos, E.; Martinez, P.; Matthews, N.; Stewart, A.; et al. Intratumor heterogeneity and branched evolution revealed by multiregion sequencing. *N. Eng. J. Med.* **2012**, *366*, 883–892. [CrossRef]
13. López, J.I.; Cortés, J.M. Multi-site tumor sampling (MSTS): A new tumor selection method to enhance intratumor heterogeneity detection. *Hum. Pathol.* **2017**, *64*, 1–6. [CrossRef] [PubMed]
14. López, J.I.; Cortés, J.M. A divide and conquer strategy in tumor sampling enhances detection of intratumor heterogeneity in pathology routine: A modeling approach in clear cell renal cell carcinoma. *F1000Research* **2016**, *5*, 385. [CrossRef]
15. De la Fuente, I.M. Elements of the cellular metabolic structure. *Front. Mol. Biosci.* **2015**, *2*, 16. [CrossRef] [PubMed]
16. Diesboeck, T.S.; Couzin, I.D. Collective behavior in cancer cell populations. *BioEssays* **2009**, *31*, 190–197. [CrossRef] [PubMed]
17. Merlo, L.M.F.; Pepper, J.M.; Reid, B.J.; Maley, C.C. Cancer as an evolutionary and ecological process. *Nat. Rev. Cancer* **2006**, *6*, 924–935. [CrossRef]
18. Horswell, S.; Matthews, N.; Swanton, C. Cancer heterogeneity and the "struggle for existence": Diagnostic and analytical challenges. *Cancer Lett.* **2013**, *340*, 220–226. [CrossRef]
19. Marcucci, F.; Stassi, G.; De Maria, R. Epithelial-mesenchymal transition: A new target in anticancer drug discovery. *Nat. Rev.* **2016**, *15*, 311–325. [CrossRef]
20. Lopez, J.I.; Mosteiro, L.; Guarch, R.; Larrinaga, G.; Pulido, R.; Angulo, J.C. Low-grade metastases in high-grade clear cell renal cell carcinomas. A clinicopathologic study of 4 cases with an insight into the role of mesenchymal-to-epithelial transition process. *Ann. Diagn. Pathol.* **2016**, *20*, 13–18. [CrossRef]
21. Nawaz, S.; Yuan, Y. Computational pathology: Exploring the spatial dimension of tumor ecology. *Cancer Lett.* **2016**, *380*, 296–303. [CrossRef] [PubMed]
22. Warsow, G.; Hübschmann, D.; Kleinheinz, K.; Nientiedt, C.; Heller, M.; Van Coile, L.; Tolstov, Y.; Trennheuser, L.; Wieczorek, K.; Pecqueux, C.; et al. Genomic features of renal cell carcinoma with venous tumor thrombus. *Sci. Rep.* **2018**, *8*, 7477. [CrossRef] [PubMed]
23. López, J.I.; Pulido, R.; Lawrie, C.H.; Angulo, J.C. Loss of PD-L1 (SP-142) expression characterizes renal vein tumor thrombus microenvironment in clear cell renal cell carcinoma. *Ann. Diagn. Pathol.* **2018**, *34*, 89–93. [CrossRef] [PubMed]
24. Maley, C.C.; Koelble, K.; Natrajan, R.; Aktipis, A.; Yuan, Y. An ecological measure of immune-cancer colocalization as a prognostic factor for breast cancer. *Breast Cancer Res.* **2015**, *17*, 131. [CrossRef] [PubMed]
25. Tsang, J.Y.S.; Au, W.L.; Lo, K.Y.; Ni, Y.B.; Hlaing, T.; Hu, J.; Chan, S.K.; Chan, K.F.; Cheung, S.Y.; Tse, G.M. PD-L1 expression and tumor infiltrating PD-1+ lymphocytes associated with outcome in HER2+ breast cancer patients. *Breast Cancer Res. Treat.* **2017**, *162*, 19–30. [CrossRef]

26. Chapman, A.; del Ama, L.F.; Ferguson, J.; Kamarashev, J.; Wellbrock, C.; Hurlstone, A. Heterogeneous tumor subpopulations cooperate to drive invasion. *Cell Rep.* **2014**, *8*, 688–695. [CrossRef] [PubMed]
27. Sica, A.; Mantovani, A. Macrophage plasticity and polarization: In vivo veritas. *J. Clin. Invest.* **2012**, *122*, 787–795. [CrossRef] [PubMed]
28. Hwang, R.F.; Moore, T.; Arumugam, T.; Ramachandran, V.; Amos, K.D.; Rivera, A.; Ji, B.; Evans, D.B.; Logsdon, C.D. Cancer-associated stromal fibroblasts promote pancreatic tumor progression. *Cancer Res.* **2008**, *68*, 918–926. [CrossRef] [PubMed]
29. Zhang, Y.; Tang, H.; Cai, J.; Zhang, T.; Guo, J.; Feng, D.; Wang, Z. Ovarian cancer-associated fibroblasts contribute to epithelial ovarian carcinoma metastasis by promoting angiogenesis, lymphangiogenesis and tumor cell invasion. *Cancer Lett.* **2011**, *303*, 47–55. [CrossRef]
30. Lopez, J.I.; Errarte, P.; Erramuzpe, A.; Guarch, R.; Cortes, J.M.; Angulo, J.C.; Pulido, R.; Irazusta, J.; Llarena, R.; Larrinaga, G. Fibroblast activation protein predicts prognosis in clear cell renal cell carcinoma. *Hum. Pathol.* **2016**, *54*, 100–105. [CrossRef]
31. Errarte, P.; Guarch, R.; Pulido, R.; Blanco, L.; Nunes-Xavier, C.E.; Beitia, M.; Gil, J.; Angulo, J.C.; Lopez, J.I.; Larrinaga, G. The expression of fibroblast activation protein in clear cell renal cell carcinomas is associated with synchronous lymph node metastases. *PLoS ONE* **2016**, *11*, e0169105. [CrossRef] [PubMed]
32. Jimenez-Sanchez, A.; Memon, D.; Pourpe, S.; Veeraraghavan, H.; Li, Y.; Vargas, H.A.; Gill, M.B.; Park, K.J.; Zivanovic, O.; Konner, J.; et al. Heterogeneous tumor-immune microenvironments among differentially growing metastases in an ovarian cancer patient. *Cell* **2017**, *170*, 927–938. [CrossRef] [PubMed]
33. Pavlides, S.; Whitaker-Menezes, D.; Castello-Cros, R.; Flomenberg, N.; Vitkiewicz, A.K.; Frank, P.G.; Casimiro, M.C.; Wang, C.; Fortina, P.; Addya, S.; et al. The reverse Warburg effect: Aerobic glycolysis in cancer associated fibroblasts and the tumor stroma. *Cell Cycle* **2009**, *8*, 3984–4001. [CrossRef] [PubMed]
34. Marusyk, A.; Polyak, K. Tumor heterogeneity: Causes and consequences. *Biochim. Biophys. Acta* **2010**, *1805*, 105–117. [CrossRef] [PubMed]
35. McGranahan, N.; Swanton, C. Biological and therapeutic impact of intratumor heterogeneity in cancer evolution. *Cancer Cell* **2015**, *27*, 15–26. [CrossRef] [PubMed]
36. Mitchell, T.J.; Turajlic, S.; Rowan, A.; Nicol, D.; Farmery, J.H.R.; O'Brien, T.; Martincorena, I.; Tarpey, P.; Angelopoulos, N.; Yates, L.; et al. Timing the landmark events in the evolution of clear cell renal cell cancer: TRACERx Renal. *Cell* **2018**, *173*, 611–623. [CrossRef]
37. Davis, A.; Gao, R.; Navin, N. Tumor evolution: Linear, branching, neutral or punctuated? *Biochim. Biophys. Acta* **2017**, *1867*, 151–161. [CrossRef]
38. Turajlic, S.; Xu, H.; Litchfield, K.; Rowan, A.; Horswell, S.; Chambers, T.; O'Brien, T.; Lopez, J.I.; Watkins, T.B.K.; Nicol, N.; et al. Deterministic evolutionary trajectories influence primary tumor growth: TRACERx Renal. *Cell* **2018**, *173*, 595–610. [CrossRef]
39. Fearon, E.R.; Vogelstein, B. A genetic model for colorectal tumorigenesis. *Cell* **1990**, *61*, 759–767. [CrossRef]
40. Gerlinger, M.; Horswell, S.; Larkin, A.J.; Rowan, A.J.; Salm, M.P.; Varela, I.; Fisher, R.; McGranahan, N.; Matthews, N.; Santos, C.R.; et al. Genomic architecture and evolution of clear cell renal cell carcinomas defined by multiregion sequencing. *Nat. Genet.* **2014**, *46*, 225–233. [CrossRef]
41. Sottoriva, A.; Kang, H.; Ma, Z.; Graham, T.A.; Salomon, M.P.; Zhao, J.; Marjoram, P.; Siegmund, K.; Press, M.F.; Shibata, D.; et al. A Big Bang model of human colorectal tumor growth. *Nat. Genet.* **2015**, *47*, 209–216. [CrossRef] [PubMed]
42. Turajlic, S.; Xu, H.; Litchfied, K.; Rowan, A.; Chambers, T.; Lopez, J.I.; Nicol, D.; O'Brien, T.; Larkin, J.; Horswell, S.; et al. Tracking cancer evolution reveals constrained routes to metastases: TRACERx Renal. *Cell* **2018**, *173*, 581–594. [CrossRef] [PubMed]
43. Arnal, A.; Ujvari, B.; Crespi, B.; Gatenby, R.A.; Tissot, T.; Vittecoq, M.; Ewald, P.W.; Casali, A.; Ducasse, H.; Jacqueline, C.; et al. Evolutionary perspective of cancer: Myth, metaphors, and reality. *Evol. Appl.* **2015**, *8*, 541–544. [CrossRef] [PubMed]
44. Pepper, J.W. *Darwinian Strategies to Avoid the Evolution of Drug Resistance during Cancer Treatment. Evolutionary Thinking in Medicine*; Alvergne, A., Ed.; Springer: Cham, Switzerland, 2016; pp. 167–176.
45. Lloyd, M.C.; Cunningham, J.J.; Bui, M.M.; Gillies, R.J.; Brown, J.S.; Gatenby, R.A. Darwinian dynamics of intratumoral heterogeneity: Not solely random mutations but also variable environmental selection forces. *Cancer Res.* **2016**, *76*, 3136–3144. [CrossRef] [PubMed]

46. Trpkov, K.; Grignon, D.J.; Bonsib, S.M.; Amin, M.B.; Billis, A.; Lopez-Beltran, A.; Samaratunga, H.; Tamboli, P.; Delahunt, B.; Egevad, L.; et al. Handling and staging of renal cell carcinoma: The International Society of Urological Pathology Consensus (ISUP) conference recommendations. *Am. J. Surg. Pathol.* **2013**, *37*, 1505–1517. [CrossRef] [PubMed]
47. Cormen, T.H.; Leiserson, C.E.; Rivest, R.L.; Stein, C. *Introduction to Algorithms*, 2nd ed.; MIT Press: Cambridge, MA, USA, 2001.
48. Ming, D.; Yang, W. A divide and conquer strategy to improve diffusion sampling in generalized ensemble simulators. *J. Chem. Phys.* **2008**, *128*, 094106. [CrossRef]
49. Eisenstein, M. Cell sorting: Divide and conquer. *Nature* **2006**, *441*, 1179–1185. [CrossRef]
50. Kristensen, V.N. Divide and conquer: The genetic basis of molecular subclassification of breast cancer. *EMBO Mol. Med.* **2011**, *3*, 183–185. [CrossRef]
51. Guarch, R.; Cortés, J.M.; Lawrie, C.H.; Lopez, J.I. Multi-site tumor sampling (MSTS) significantly improves the performance of histological detection of intratumor heterogeneity in clear cell renal cell carcinoma. *F1000Research* **2016**, *5*, 2020. [CrossRef]
52. López, J.I.; Cortés, J.M. A multi-site cutting device implements efficiently the divide-and-conquer strategy in tumor sampling. *F1000Research* **2016**, *5*, 1587. [CrossRef]
53. Cortés, J.M.; de Petris, G.; López, J.I. Detection of intratumor heterogeneity in modern pathology: A multisite tumor sampling perspective. *Front. Med.* **2017**, *4*, 25. [CrossRef] [PubMed]
54. Erramuzpe, A.; Cortés, J.M.; López, J.I. Multisite tumor sampling enhances the detection of intratumor heterogeneity at all different temporal stages of tumor evolution. *Virchows Arch.* **2018**, *472*, 187–194. [CrossRef] [PubMed]
55. McGranahan, N.; Swanton, C. Clonal heterogeneity and tumor evolution: Past, present, and the future. *Cell* **2017**, *168*, 613–628. [CrossRef] [PubMed]

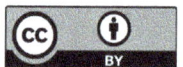

© 2018 by the authors. Licensee MDPI, Basel, Switzerland. This article is an open access article distributed under the terms and conditions of the Creative Commons Attribution (CC BY) license (http://creativecommons.org/licenses/by/4.0/).

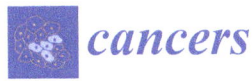

Review

Exploring Tumor Heterogeneity Using PET Imaging: The Big Picture

Clément Bailly [1,2], Caroline Bodet-Milin [1,2], Mickaël Bourgeois [1,2,3], Sébastien Gouard [1], Catherine Ansquer [2], Matthieu Barbaud [2], Jean-Charles Sébille [2], Michel Chérel [1,3,4], Françoise Kraeber-Bodéré [1,2,4] and Thomas Carlier [1,2,*]

1. CRCINA, INSERM, CNRS, Université d'Angers, Université de Nantes, 44093 Nantes, France
2. Nuclear Medicine Department, University Hospital, 44093 Nantes, France
3. Groupement d'Intérêt Public Arronax, 44800 Saint-Herblain, France
4. Nuclear Medicine Department, ICO-René Gauducheau Cancer Center, 44800 Saint-Herblain, France
* Correspondence: thomas.carlier@chu-nantes.fr; Tel.: +33-240-084-136; Fax: +33-240-084-218

Received: 25 June 2019; Accepted: 28 August 2019; Published: 31 August 2019

Abstract: Personalized medicine represents a major goal in oncology. It has its underpinning in the identification of biomarkers with diagnostic, prognostic, or predictive values. Nowadays, the concept of biomarker no longer necessarily corresponds to biological characteristics measured ex vivo but includes complex physiological characteristics acquired by different technologies. Positron-emission-tomography (PET) imaging is an integral part of this approach by enabling the fine characterization of tumor heterogeneity in vivo in a non-invasive way. It can effectively be assessed by exploring the heterogeneous distribution and uptake of a tracer such as 18F-fluoro-deoxyglucose (FDG) or by using multiple radiopharmaceuticals, each providing different information. These two approaches represent two avenues of development for the research of new biomarkers in oncology. In this article, we review the existing evidence that the measurement of tumor heterogeneity with PET imaging provide essential information in clinical practice for treatment decision-making strategy, to better select patients with poor prognosis for more intensive therapy or those eligible for targeted therapy.

Keywords: PET; heterogeneity; radiomics; radiopharmaceuticals; SUV; nuclear medicine

1. Introduction

Heterogeneity is a concept familiar to pathologists. Phenotypical and functional differences arise among cancer cells during the course of the disease because of genetic changes [1]. Similarly, the interactions of cancer cells with their microenvironment or the local variation in angiogenesis and hypoxia are not uniform in the tumor. Not to mention the perpetual clonal remodeling under the pressure of microenvironment and treatments. This large biological, cellular, and tissue heterogeneity exist at the intratumoral level (molecular differences within one tumor), intrapatient level (variation of tumor features between lesions within one patient), and interpatient level (variation of tumor features between patients). This heterogeneity conditions tumor aggressiveness and therapeutic resistance and represents a significant challenge in the design of effective treatment strategies [2]. The prerequisite for personalized medicine relies on the report of such heterogeneities. Yet, the realization of multi-region sampling from each tumor of a single patient raises ethical or technical questions. Positron-emission-tomography (PET) imaging appears as a perfect tool to overcome this obstacle, providing a whole-body non-invasive method of assessing tumor heterogeneity, through the use of multiple radiopharmaceuticals, each providing different information. In parallel, the information derived from the uptakes' analysis of a tracer such as 18F-fluoro-deoxyglucose (FDG) has enabled the emergence of a wide variety of PET quantitative metrics including simple semi-quantitative approaches such as standardized uptake value (SUV) and "high-order metrics" that involve a segmentation step and supplementary image processing. These parameters, besides their utility for therapeutic response, should play a key role in the prognostic characterization of tumors, along with the development of personalized medicine. Radiomics—the high throughput extraction of large amounts of imaging elements from radiographic images—tackles this challenge and is one of the most promising strategies [3,4]. The purpose of this short review is to present the latest developments in the exploration of tumor heterogeneity in PET imaging. Different examples of neoplasias are presented during the three developed axes. Nevertheless, to emphasize to the reader that these tools can be used in all diseases, lymphoma is used as a common thread throughout this review.

2. Inter- and Intra-patient Tumor Heterogeneity Exploration through Multiple Tracers PET Imaging

Nuclear medicine is one of the most dynamic medical fields, in constant evolution over the past decades. The main strength of this discipline lies in its incredible catalog of radiopharmaceuticals allowing exploration of virtually every major organ system in the body (Table 1). Personalized medicine has never been so relevant today and nuclear medicine is on its leading edge, probing deep inside each patient or tumor to reveal its inner workings. Predictive biomarkers are an essential tool of precision medicine and individualized treatment. Yet, as mentioned above, tumor heterogeneity contributes to sampling error, especially for metastatic diseases; target's expression at one site does not guarantee expression at all sites. Moreover, target accessibility of drugs is not assessed by biopsy, and target expression does not provide evidence of targeted-therapy impact on the target. In this context, PET imaging overcomes many of these limitations exploring target heterogeneity, assessing target expression and potential accessibility across the whole disease burden, to aid clinical decision making. A perfect example was recently published by Bensch et al. with the initial results from the first-in-human imaging with 89Zirconium-labeled atezolizumab [5]. The programmed cell death protein 1 (PD1)/programmed death-ligand 1 (PD-L1) axis is an important immune checkpoint for T-cell activation. PD-L1 overexpression is associated with a poor prognosis in a variety of cancers yet these patients typically have a stronger response to anti-PD-L1 therapy such as atezolizumab [6–9]. The PD-L1 expression is usually evaluated using immunohistochemistry or RNA sequencing. In Bensch et al. study, clinical responses were better correlated with PET uptake before treatment than these two evaluations.

Table 1. Main validated positron-emission-tomography (PET) tracers and their principal indications (based on [10,11]).

Tracer	Metabolic Process	Principal Oncological Indications
11C-Methionine	Amino acid transport and protein synthesis	Diagnosis and grading of brain tumors
18F-Choline (FCH)	Phosphatidylcholine metabolism and cellular membrane turnover	Biopsy guidance of prostate cancer recurrence/primary staging in high-risk prostate cancer before surgical procedures or planning external beam radiation
18F-Fluoro-Deoxyglucose (FDG)	Glucose metabolism	Diagnosis/restaging of lung cancer, colorectal cancer, breast cancer, lymphoma, sarcoma, melanoma, head and neck cancer
18F-DOPA	Dopamine uptake and metabolism	Diagnosis of neuroendocrine tumors (NET)/documented NET metastasis in unknown primary
68Ga-DOTA-Peptides	Somatostatin receptors	Identification of primary tumor in patients with documented NET metastasis/assessment of NET disease extent before treatment
18F-Fluoroestradiol (FES)	Estrogen receptor	Status of tumor lesions to determine need for endocrine therapy in breast cancer

Table 1. Cont.

Tracer	Metabolic Process	Principal Oncological Indications
18F-Fluorothymidine (FLT)	Cellular proliferation and	Differential diagnosis between benign and malignant lesions/lymphoma staging and therapeutic evaluation
18-Sodium Fluoride (NaF)	Bone metabolism	Detection of bone involvement in tumors with elevated risk of bone metastasis
68Ga-Prostate-Specific Membrane Antigen (PSMA)	PSMA expression	Localization of tumor tissue in recurrent prostate cancer

Breast cancer also represents a great model for this type of approach [12,13]. Indeed, in this pathology, 18F-fluoroestradiol (FES) PET has been validated as an accurate method for providing information on estrogen receptor (ER) status of tumor lesions to determine need for endocrine therapy [14–17]. Indeed, the uptake of FES has been proven to correlate with ER expression in biopsy sample [16]. Similarly, several works showed that radiolabeled monoclonal antibodies could non-invasively identify lesions with positive or over-expression of the human epidermal growth factor receptor 2 (HER2) and predict response to anti-HER2 antibody-based therapy [18–21]. In particular, Gebhart et al. recently reported the promising results of the ZEPHIR trial. This work successfully evaluated two PET imaging as tools to investigate heterogeneity of advanced HER2-positive breast cancer (PET imaging using trastuzumab radiolabeled with 89Zirconium) and to predict patient outcome under trastuzumab emtansine (PET imaging with FDG) [22,23]. This innovative study showed the clear benefit of combining both imaging methods in predicting whether adequate tumor targeting is followed by sufficient efficacy and cytotoxicity.

Beyond the "simple" search for the expression of a target before initiating a treatment directed against it, the use of several radiotracers in the same patient can allow to comprehensively assess disease activity, extent, and heterogeneity. Tumors derived from cells of the neural crest represent the perfect historical model for this approach [24]. This large group of neoplasms includes a large variety of tumors, such as gastroenteropancreatic neuroendocrine tumors (GEPs), neuroblastoma, paraganglioma, pheochromocytoma, medullary thyroid carcinoma, and small cell lung cancer. These tumors are characterized by similar appearances and expression of different peptides and amines. Prognostic criteria of this group are generally related to the metastatic extension of the disease but also to the functional activity, degree of differentiation of the tumor and proliferative indices. These parameters are essential in the management of these patients. Today, multiple molecular imaging methods are available to explore these various biologic and histologic characteristics with very high specificity and can be performed at the whole-body scale [25,26]. Tracers used can be grouped in three different categories. 123-metaiodobenzylguanidine (123MIBG), an analog of norepinephrine and 18F-fluorodihydroxyphenylalanine (FDOPA), an amine precursor, exploit catecholamine synthesis, storage, and secretion pathways. 111In-pentetreotide and 68Gallium-labeled somatostatin analog peptides (68Ga-DOTA-TOC, 68Ga-DOTA-NOC, 68Ga-DOTA-TATE) assess the somatostatin receptors expression. Finally, FDG uptake has been found to correlate with de-differentiation, increasing aggressiveness and proliferation rate, and poor prognosis. This phenomenon was first described in differentiated thyroid carcinomas. Indeed, de-differentiated thyroid carcinomas lose their capacity to capture radioiodine and can be detected by FDG-PET since glycolysis increase at the same time. Thus, imaging assessment of two or more tracers may yield more clinical information than each alone [27–32] (Figures 1 and 2).

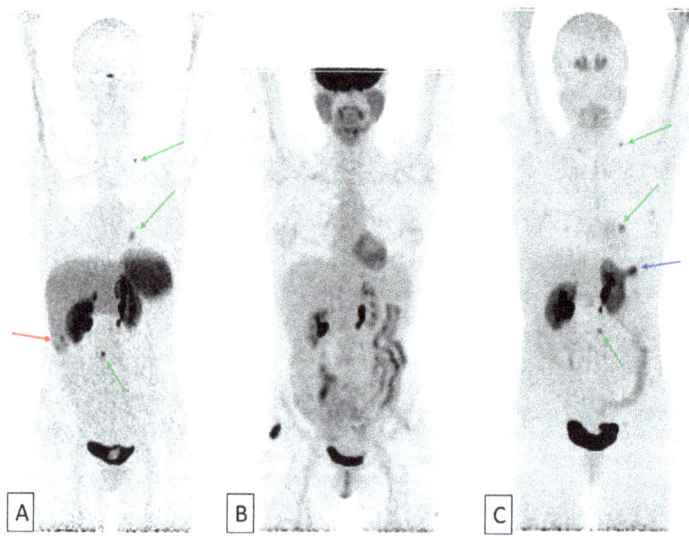

Figure 1. An example of a 46-year-old patient with pluri-metastatic intestinal neuroendocrine tumor (grade 2, ki67 at 4%). 68Ga DOTA-TOC (**A**), FDG-PET (18F-fluoro-deoxyglucose-positron-emission-tomography) (**B**) and FDOPA (18F-fluorodihydroxyphenylalanine) (**C**) imaging were realized. MIP (maximum intensity projections) images from the respective PET data sets are shown. The subject has positive on both FDOPA and somatostatine-receptor imaging, dominant disease which exhibits no FDG uptake (green arrows). One hepatic lesion was FDOPA-negative and 68Ga-DOTA-TOC-positive (red arrow) and one gastric lesion was FDOPA-positive and 68Ga-DOTA-TOC negative (blue arrow). Images courtesy of Pr C. Bodet-Milin.

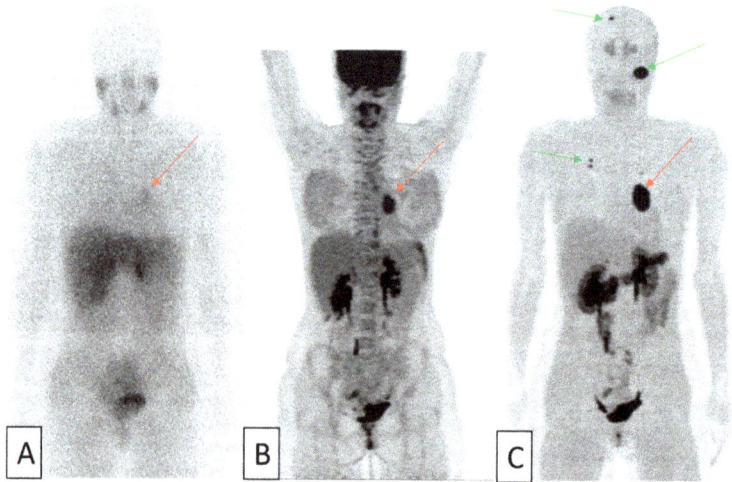

Figure 2. An example of 37-year-old patient with pluri-metastatic paraganglioma. MIP (maximum intensity projections) images of the realized 123MIBG-scintigraphy (**A**), FDG-PET (**B**) and FDOPA-PET (**C**) are shown. The subject has a mediastinal lesion, barely seen on 123MIBG-scintigraphy and clearly positive with the others tracers (red arrows). Pulmonary and skull lesions (green arrows) were only visible on FDOPA-PET. Images courtesy of Dr C. Ansquer © Catherine Ansquer

Lymphomas represent another cancer group where multiple tracers' exploration might allow a better potential characterization of tumor heterogeneity. Indeed, today, FDG-PET occupies a central position in accurate staging and therapeutic evaluation of lymphomas [33]. Nevertheless, a certain number of crucial questions remain regarding its optimal application. While risk-based strategies may appear to enhance patients' outcomes for those with Hodgkin's lymphoma, findings are not so impressive in non-Hodgkin's lymphoma [33]. Similarly, novel therapies that may generate an immune response may lead to false-positive FDG-PET results, requiring the incorporation of these flare-ups reactions in existing interpretation criteria [34]. Therefore, the development of other radiotracers with different uptake mechanisms from FDG could be of interest [35]. 18F-fluorothymidine (FLT) and 11C-methionine (MET), for instance, were both reported to correlate with cellular proliferation activity and lymphoma histological grade of malignancy, respectively, through the exploration of DNA and protein synthesis [36,37]. Moreover, FLT showed excellent results in treatment monitoring and particularly in the setting of early interim evaluation, with more specific and accurate analyses than FDG [38,39]. In the same way, 18F-fludarabine, an adenine nucleoside analog, owing to its specificity for lymphoid cells and its absence of uptake in inflammatory tissues, holds great promise for therapeutic evaluation [40]. Finally, the first in-human study of 68Ga-CXCR4, targeting chemokine receptor CXCR4, which is frequently overexpressed in various tumor types, showed high lesions' uptake [41,42]. Moreover, voxel-by-voxel analysis in one patient identified striking inter- and intralesional heterogeneity in the uptake of 68Ga CXCR4 and FDG, implying that the biological information given by the two probes may be complementary even in lesions that show avidity for both [42].

Systematic multiple tracers imaging could be used to reveal different profiles with highly different prognoses. This multiple-tracers imaging associated with an appropriate scoring system might also influence patients' management and help selecting between different therapy options [28,43,44]. Indeed, these tumors may be treated with molecular radiotherapy using the same pathways: 131-metaiodobenzylguanidine (131-MIBG) and 177Lutetium-DOTA-TATE. Impressive reports were reported with these targeted therapies in GEPs and neuroblastoma [45–49]. A theranostic approach, integrating imaging and therapy in the same system, providing individualized tailored treatment, despite intratumor and interlesional heterogeneities, is expected to play an increasingly pivotal role in this large tumor group [50,51].

The theranostic approach indeed represents a formidable field of expansion for nuclear medicine in an era where targeted therapies have become essential tools in oncology pharmacopoeia [52,53]. As described above in breast cancer and neuroendocrine tumors, it offers a non-invasive method for quantitatively evaluating target expression in vivo, selecting patients for costly and potentially toxic treatments, and monitoring responses [50,51,54–56]. In addition, this approach constitutes a valuable asset in the development of new drugs by pharmaceutical companies. Drug development being a fairly time-consuming and costly process, it represents an effective solution to rapidly monitor drug candidates' pharmacokinetics and biodistribution. This strategy can improve the strength and effectiveness of early trials by enhancing patient selection, optimizing dose, and rationalizing treatment reactions [54].

3. Intrapatient Tumor Heterogeneity Exploration through Quantitative Analysis of PET Imaging

FDG-PET has become an essential tool for cancer diagnosis, staging, and therapeutic evaluation. It has undoubtedly changed the landscape of lymphoma, lung, head and neck or breast cancers management [57–59]. This spread of the PET imaging technique was particularly enabled by its quantification ability which allows the use of a reproducible metric for cancer monitoring. The SUV and particularly SUVmax (defined as the SUV value of the maximum intensity voxel within a region of interest) is widely used in everyday clinical practice. It is popularly adopted as a surrogate of tissue accumulation of tracers and particularly as the overall net rate of FDG uptake. It is defined as the ratio between the radiopharmaceutical concentration (expressed in Bq/mL) and the decay-corrected injected activity normalized by a given factor (mass of the patient, body surface area or lean body mass) [60]. The precise description of underlying technical limitations of this metric is beyond the scope of this short review and is already largely discussed in the literature [60–62]. Only its use under clinical situation is highlighted here. Indeed, the computation of intrapatient tumor heterogeneity in FDG-PET imaging using SUV has been already applied in a wide variety of indications even if not intentionally or explicitly. FDG uptake heterogeneity may reflect different tumor profiles with different aggressiveness and consequently prognosis. This contribution offered by the calculation of SUV has been particularly investigated in lymphoma.

Some histological subtypes of lymphoma such as follicular and mantle cell lymphomas are heterogeneous diseases with a variety of clinical, genetic, biological features and related different outcomes. In these pathologies, the intensity of FDG uptake on PET imaging at baseline varies greatly between patients [33]. Some present barely detectable uptakes while others exhibit very intense fixations. Yet, this spectrum of SUV, from very low to very high uptakes, provides clinically relevant information. Indeed, several reports demonstrated that the level of FDG uptake on PET imaging is largely correlated to lymphoma histology [63,64]. More particularly, indolent disease with low proliferation rate is generally associated with low uptake, while a more aggressive disease presented higher FDG uptake. In the same way, very intense FDG uptake associated to a clear uptake gradient may pertain transformation from indolent to aggressive lymphoma. These findings were confirmed in a prospective study conducted to evaluate the value of FDG-PET as an accurate guide for biopsies in suspected transformed tissues [65]. In patients with newly diagnosed indolent lymphoma, low SUV numbers may reduce the suspicion of transformation in disease sites that were not biopsied. Conversely, in patients with histologically proven indolent lymphoma, an uncharacteristically higher than expected SUV may herald an aggressive subtype, warranting a targeted biopsy. Our team reported similar findings in mantle cell lymphomas. A broad inter-individual tumor cell heterogeneity regarding FDG avidity was observed in several works with a strong prognostic value on survival of quantitative parameters such as SUVmax of the lesions with the highest uptake determined at diagnosis [66–69]. This close relationship between high SUVmax values and a more aggressive mantle cell lymphoma behavior was also supported by the concordance between SUVmax, aggressive variants, and high percentage (> 30%) of Ki67 positive cells.

This hypothesis that the prognosis of the disease is linked to the most aggressive contingent corresponding to the lesion with the highest FDG uptake is also reinforced by some studies exploring the predictive prognostic value of FDG-PET during treatment. Since the development of normalized criteria for assessment of tumor burden changes, the required number of lesions to consider for response determination remained a fundamental question [70–72]. The RECIST criteria used for radiological evaluation recommended the measurement of five target-lesions, selected "randomly," only on their suitability for accurate repeated measures [70]. On the contrary, several works using PET imaging showed that only the most metabolically active lesions, representing the most aggressive portions of tumors, are critical to consider [73–77]. This approach implies taking the single hottest area as the reference point on the pre-treatment and post-treatment studies, even if not necessarily the same area, considering only the worst biologic behaviors of the malignancy. This controversial concept was explored in many cancers and was applied both in solid tumors with the PERCIST criteria and in lymphomas. For example, Lin et al. were the first to measure the reduction of SUVmax in the "hottest" lesion before and during the treatment, in diffuse large B-cell lymphoma (Figure 3). In their study, they also investigated the FDG uptake changes on interim FDG-PET within the initial hottest tumor site on baseline FDG-PET (18% of 92 patients) which resulted in more false-negative exams in predicting PFS [76].

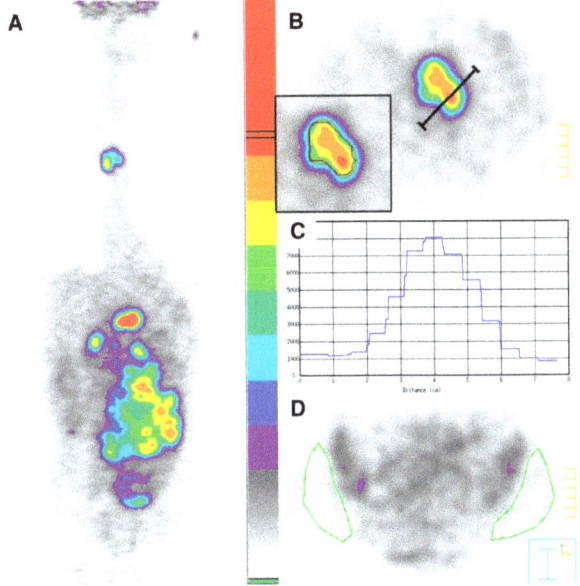

Figure 3. Selection of regions of interest in 57-y-old patient before chemotherapy. (**A**) Graded color-scaled parametric analysis applied in reconstructed coronal PET image shows most active tumor in upper abdomen. (**B**) Transverse PET image with a higher scale reveals celiac tumor (T) with activity profile crossing the hottest point (red spot). (**C**) Corresponding activity profile in counts-per-pixel. Isocontours are drawn with lower autocontour threshold of 4500 counts-per-pixel (red isocontour at inset in B). (**D**) Normal background tissue (N): two large ROIs are manually selected on gluteal muscles, avoiding iliac bone marrow activity. This research was originally published in JNM [76]. © SNMMI.

This approach was also recently reported in multiple myeloma patients [78]. In this pathology, multi-clonal heterogeneity remains one of the main challenges in developing effective strategies. Multiple myeloma is indeed characterized by spatial differences in the clonal architecture, with potential non-homogeneous distribution of high-risk disease for which multi-region investigations appear critical [79–81]. Yet, in a study by our team, the percentage difference of SUVmax between baseline and interim FDG-PET was a powerful tool to predict long-term outcomes in patients with FDG-avid multiple myeloma [78]. There again, similar to previous work in lymphomas or in solid tumors, the hottest lesion in any region was used for comparison even if its location differed from the initial hottest lesion on PET at diagnosis, to assess the most aggressive portion of the disease on each PET examination, to free oneself from intrapatient heterogeneity.

4. Intratumor Heterogeneity Exploration through Quantitative Analysis of PET Imaging

In addition to conventional measurements of SUV, a new class of metrics has recently emerged in PET imaging and is currently being clinically investigated [61]. A simple visual analysis of the FDG uptake in PET images indeed suggests that the spatial distribution of voxels of different intensities in a selected region and thus the spatial distribution of the radiotracer can be extremely heterogeneous. And one can assume that this localized heterogeneity in medical images "partly" reflects heterogeneity on a lower scale and underlying variations in metabolism, cellular proliferation or necrosis [82]. Advanced image analysis of a tumor could then capture additional information and some researchers suggested that genomic, proteomics, and other -omics patterns could be expressed in terms of macroscopic image-based features [83]. This concept requiring the extraction of a large number of quantitative data from medical multimodal images has become popular under the term "radiomics" [3,84,85]. In recent years, considerable efforts have been made by the medical imaging community to obtain correlations between these image characteristics and tumor heterogeneity. Those metrics are often referred to as "textural features" and belong to "high order parameters" (Table 2) along with shape-descriptors or other descriptors based on fractal analysis or wavelet decomposition [61,86]. They measure the relationships between groups of two or more voxels in the image (Figure 4). Numerous textural features can be extracted from medical images, yet only a handful are sufficiently reliable, robust, and reproducible. Texture analysis remains limited and biased by many methodological and technical factors inherent to PET images' acquisition, reconstruction algorithms, or segmentation technique that can affect the quantification of image heterogeneity [86]. A number of recommendations are available to help and guide researchers in making the right choices in the calculation and selection of parameters [86–89].

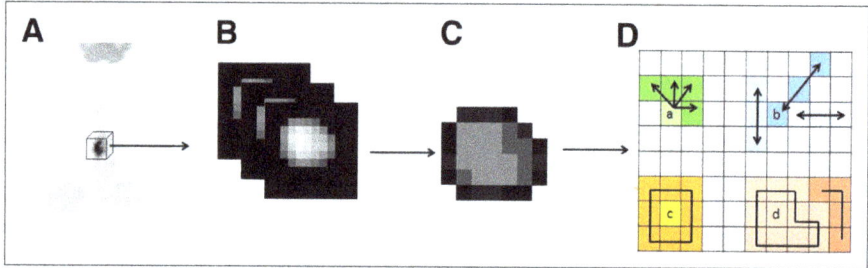

Figure 4. Whole-body 18F-FDG PET scan (**A**) tumor segmentation (**B**) and voxel-intensity resampling (**C**) allowing extraction of different features (**D**) by analysis of consecutive voxels in a direction (for cooccurrence matrices) (a), alignment of voxels with same intensity (b), difference between voxels and their neighbors (c), and zones of voxels with same intensity (d). This research was originally published in JNM [90]. © SNMMI.

Table 2. Common imaging heterogeneity parameters. (Based on [61,91]).

Order	Matrix	Name of the Parameter	Description of the Parameter
First Order		SUVmax	SUV value of the maximum intensity voxel within a region of interest (ROI)
		SUVpeak	Average SUV within a small ROI (usually, a 1-cm^3 spherical volume)
		SUVmean	Average measure of SUV within a defined ROI
		Metabolic tumor volume (MTV)	Volume of a defined ROI
		Total lesion glycolysis (TLG)	Product of SUVmean × MTV
Second Order	Grey-Level Co-Occurrence Matrix (GLCM)	Contrast	Local variations in the GLCM
		Correlation	Joint probability occurrence of the specified pixel pairs
		Entropy	Texture randomness or irregularity
		Energy	Sum of squared elements in the GLCM
		Homogeneity	Closeness of the distribution of elements to the diagonal
High Order	Gray-Level Run-Length Matrix (GLRLM)	Short run emphasis (SRE)	Distribution of short runs
		Long run emphasis (LRE)	Distribution of long runs
		High gray level run emphasis (HGRE)	Distribution of high grey level values runs
		Grey-level non-uniformity (GLNU)	Similarity of grey level values throughout the image
		Run percentage (RP)	Homogeneity and distribution of runs of an image in a specific direction

Table 2. Cont.

Order	Matrix	Name of the Parameter	Description of the Parameter
	Gray-Level Zone Size Encoding Method (GLZSM)	High gray-level zone emphasis (HGZE)	Distribution of high grey level values zones
		Zone length non uniformity (ZLNU)	Similarity of zone length throughout the image
		Zone percentage (ZP)	Homogeneity and distribution of zones of an image in a specific direction
		Short zone emphasis (SZE)	Distribution of small zones
	Neighborhood Grey Tone Difference Matrix (NGTDM)	Coarseness	Granularity within an image.

To date, numerous studies explored the potential value of textural features in PET imaging with encouraging results in a number of cancers [86,92]. However, only a limited number adopted rigorous methodological choices with particularly large cohorts of patients and robust statistical analysis [93,94]. Keeping in mind these limitations, the evidence supporting the additional value of advanced image features from FDG-PET continues to expand year after year. Several of the most recent studies have used techniques such as external cohort validation [95–97], or even machine-learning technique [98,99] and concluded in the usefulness of textural analysis regarding patient management. Several method were also proposed to minimize the effect of inter-center variability related to textural features computation [95,100,101] with encouraging results both on a methodological and prognostic level. One should keep in mind that several hundred, if not thousands of handcrafted features can be extracted, when the number of patients used to construct the predictive model is often several order of magnitude lower than the number of features analyzed. The use of machine learning approaches in this context is thus very useful but opens other issues related to the choice of suitable algorithm for selecting features and subsequent classifier which were shown to be not unique [102] The use of more complex approaches relying on deep learning (especially convolutional neural networks) may alleviate most of the difficulties raised by handcrafted features even if other challenges arise like the number of data used for training and tuning hyper-parameters of the model. A very good overview of the available technique that may be potentially clinically efficient in a near future can be found in [103].

Finally, a few studies have investigated the potential combination of image-derived features from multimodal imaging or associated to clinical data [95,104–106]. One example of a nomogram construction, published by Desseroit et al. [104], combining tumor and heterogeneity features extracted from both PET and CT components of routinely acquired FDG-PET scans in non-small cell lung cancers is shown in Figure 5. Reports in patients with mantle cell lymphoma also successfully applied this approach [107–109]. In this pathology, as demonstrated in a prospective study [107,108] and confirmed in a recent work by Mayerhoefer et al. [109], the combination of radiomic features with bio-clinical scores may possibly improve risk stratification. All these approaches form the basis for future works investigating the value of textural features in PET imaging and combining these methods will only reinforce the validity of the studies. In this regard, a recent study focused on this topic and successfully applied some of these approaches. In this work [95], Lucia et al. validated in two independent external cohorts of patients previously developed textural features-based models [110] relying on FDG PET and MRI for prediction of disease-free survival and locoregional control in locally advanced cervical cancer. Moreover, to adjust for the multicenter effects, they used the ComBat method, derived from genomic data analysis. They were able to identify two radiomics features indeed associated with worse outcome, confirming that more heterogeneous tumors have a poorer prognosis [95].

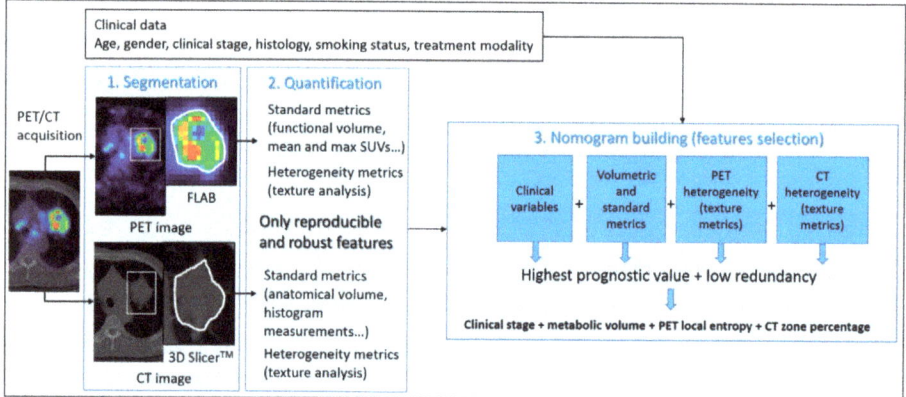

Figure 5. Workflow of a nomogram construction combining tumor and heterogeneity features extracted from both PET and CT components of routinely acquired FDG-PET scans in non-small cell lung cancers, allowing for better stratification among patients with stage II–III, compared to stage I. This research was originally published in EJNMMI [104]. © Springer.

Radiomic is a promising field. Unlike histological biomarkers derived from invasive biopsy which sample only a small limited tumor region, as described above, radiomics non-invasively interrogate the whole tumor. Visualization of tumor heterogeneity is essential in the assessment of tumor aggressiveness and prognosis. Radiomic has an exceptional potential and may prove critical toward personalized medicine [83].

5. Conclusions

Nuclear medicine is one of the most dynamic medical fields. Advances in cancer biology knowledge together with the rise of new imaging techniques (new detection system and progress in imaging analysis) make this discipline a domain of tremendous and growing evolution. This dynamism is a real asset as personalized medicine has never been so relevant today. Indeed, PET imaging appears as an essential tool for non-invasive exploration of intratumoral and interlesional heterogeneity through the exploration of the distribution and uptake of a tracer or by using multiple radiopharmaceuticals, each providing different information. There is convincing evidence that the integration of PET imaging "profiling," combining these approaches, associated to clinical, biological, or genomic data could improve tumor characterization and prognosis prediction to allow adequate patients stratification to therapeutic regimens. By combining at least one metabolic tracer with a phenotypic one, and by quoting Mankoff et Dehdashti [31], "it may then be possible to show that when it comes to molecular imaging, 1 plus 1 is greater than 2."

Author Contributions: All authors have directly participated in the review process and in the writing of this paper, and have read and approved the final version submitted.

Funding: This research was funded in part by grants from the French National Agency for Research, called "Investissements d'Avenir" IRON LabEx n° ANR-11-LABX-0018-01, IGO LabEx n° ANR-11-LABX-0016-01, Siric ILIAD, ArronaxPlus Equipex n° ANR-11-EQPX-0004 and NExT n° ANR-16-IDEX-0007.

Acknowledgments: Figure 2 was reproduced with permission from Catherine Ansquer © Catherine Ansquer. Figure 3 was originally published in JNM by Chieh Lin et al. Figure 4 was originally published in JNM by Florent Tixier et al. Figure 5 was originally published in EJNMMI by Desseroit et al.

Conflicts of Interest: The authors declare no conflict of interest.

References

1. Tabassum, D.P.; Polyak, K. Tumorigenesis: It takes a village. *Nat. Rev. Cancer* **2015**, *15*, 473–483. [CrossRef] [PubMed]
2. Dagogo-Jack, I.; Shaw, A.T. Tumour heterogeneity and resistance to cancer therapies. *Nat. Rev. Clin. Oncol.* **2018**, *15*, 81–94. [CrossRef] [PubMed]
3. Lambin, P.; Rios-Velazquez, E.; Leijenaar, R.; Carvalho, S.; Van Stiphout, R.G.; Granton, P.; Zegers, C.M.; Gillies, R.; Boellard, R.; Dekker, A.; et al. Radiomics: Extracting more information from medical images using advanced feature analysis. *Eur. J. Cancer* **2012**, *48*, 441–446. [CrossRef] [PubMed]
4. Aerts, H.J.W.L.; Velazquez, E.R.; Leijenaar, R.T.H.; Parmar, C.; Grossmann, P.; Cavalho, S.; Bussink, J.; Monshouwer, R.; Haibe-Kains, B.; Rietveld, D.; et al. Decoding tumour phenotype by noninvasive imaging using a quantitative radiomics approach. *Nat. Commun.* **2014**, *5*, 4006. [CrossRef] [PubMed]
5. Bensch, F.; Van Der Veen, E.L.; Hooge, M.N.L.-D.; Jorritsma-Smit, A.; Boellaard, R.; Kok, I.C.; Oosting, S.F.; Schröder, C.P.; Hiltermann, T.J.N.; Van Der Wekken, A.J.; et al. 89Zr-atezolizumab imaging as a non-invasive approach to assess clinical response to PD-L1 blockade in cancer. *Nat. Med.* **2018**, *24*, 1852–1858. [CrossRef] [PubMed]
6. Mu, C.-Y.; Huang, J.-A.; Chen, Y.; Chen, C.; Zhang, X.-G. High expression of PD-L1 in lung cancer may contribute to poor prognosis and tumor cells immune escape through suppressing tumor infiltrating dendritic cells maturation. *Med. Oncol.* **2011**, *28*, 682–688. [CrossRef] [PubMed]
7. Chen, L.; Han, X. Anti–PD-1/PD-L1 therapy of human cancer: Past, present, and future. *J. Clin. Investig.* **2015**, *125*, 3384–3391. [CrossRef]
8. Krishnamurthy, A.; Jimeno, A. Atezolizumab: A novel PD-L1 inhibitor in cancer therapy with a focus in bladder and non-small cell lung cancers. *Drugs Today* **2017**, *53*, 217–237. [CrossRef]
9. Fehrenbacher, L.; Spira, A.; Ballinger, M.; Kowanetz, M.; Vansteenkiste, J.; Mazieres, J.; Park, K.; Smith, D.; Artal-Cortes, A.; Lewanski, C.; et al. Atezolizumab versus docetaxel for patients with previously treated non-small-cell lung cancer (POPLAR): A multicentre, open-label, phase 2 randomised controlled trial. *Lancet* **2016**, *387*, 1837–1846. [CrossRef]
10. Jadvar, H.; Delgado-Bolton, R.; Nadel, H.; Rohren, E.; Zukotynski, K.; Kauffman, J.; Ahuja, S.; Colletti, P.M.; Esposito, G.; Krause, B.J.; et al. Appropriate Use Criteria for 18 F-FDG PET/CT in Restaging and Treatment Response Assessment of Malignant Disease. *J. Nucl. Med.* **2017**, *58*, 2026–2037. [CrossRef]
11. Lopci, E.; Nanni, C.; Castellucci, P.; Montini, G.C.; Allegri, V.; Rubello, D.; Chierichetti, F.; Ambrosini, V.; Fanti, S. Imaging with non-FDG PET tracers: Outlook for current clinical applications. *Insights Imaging* **2010**, *1*, 373–385. [CrossRef] [PubMed]
12. Chudgar, A.V.; Mankoff, D.A. Molecular Imaging and Precision Medicine in Breast Cancer. *PET Clin.* **2017**, *12*, 39–51. [CrossRef] [PubMed]
13. Koleva-Kolarova, R.G.; Greuter, M.J.; Feenstra, T.L.; Vermeulen, K.M.; De Vries, E.F.; Parkin, D.; Buskens, E.; De Bock, G.H. Molecular imaging with positron emission tomography and computed tomography (PET/CT) for selecting first-line targeted treatment in metastatic breast cancer: A cost-effectiveness study. *Oncotarget* **2018**, *9*, 19836–19846. [CrossRef] [PubMed]
14. Kurland, B.F.; Peterson, L.M.; Lee, J.H.; Schubert, E.K.; Currin, E.R.; Link, J.M.; Krohn, K.A.; Mankoff, D.A.; Linden, H.M. Estrogen receptor binding (FES PET) and glycolytic activity (FDG PET) predict progression-free survival on endocrine therapy in patients with ER+ breast cancer. *Clin. Cancer Res.* **2017**, *23*, 407–415. [CrossRef] [PubMed]
15. Mortimer, J.E.; Dehdashti, F.; Siegel, B.A.; Katzenellenbogen, J.A.; Fracasso, P.; Welch, M.J. Positron emission tomography with 2-[18F]Fluoro-2-deoxy-D-glucose and 16alpha-[18F]fluoro-17beta-estradiol in breast cancer: Correlation with estrogen receptor status and response to systemic therapy. *Clin. Cancer Res.* **1996**, *2*, 933–939.
16. Liao, G.J.; Clark, A.S.; Schubert, E.K.; Mankoff, D.A. 18F-Fluoroestradiol PET: Current Status and Potential Future Clinical Applications. *J. Nucl. Med.* **2016**, *57*, 1269–1275. [CrossRef] [PubMed]
17. Van Kruchten, M.; Glaudemans, A.W.J.M.; De Vries, E.F.J.; Beets-Tan, R.G.H.; Schröder, C.P.; Dierckx, R.A.; De Vries, E.G.E.; Hospers, G.A.P. PET Imaging of Estrogen Receptors as a Diagnostic Tool for Breast Cancer Patients Presenting with a Clinical Dilemma. *J. Nucl. Med.* **2012**, *53*, 182–190. [CrossRef]

18. Dijkers, E.C.; Kosterink, J.G.; Rademaker, A.P.; Perk, L.R.; Van Dongen, G.A.; Bart, J.; De Jong, J.R.; De Vries, E.G.; Hooge, M.N.L.-D. Development and Characterization of Clinical-Grade 89Zr-Trastuzumab for HER2/neu ImmunoPET Imaging. *J. Nucl. Med.* **2009**, *50*, 974–981. [CrossRef]
19. Baum, R.P.; Prasad, V.; Schuchardt, C.; Orlova, A.; Wennborg, A.; Tolmachev, V.; Feldwisch, J.; Müller, D. Molecular Imaging of HER2-Expressing Malignant Tumors in Breast Cancer Patients Using Synthetic 111In- or 68Ga-Labeled Affibody Molecules. *J. Nucl. Med.* **2010**, *51*, 892–897. [CrossRef]
20. Tamura, K.; Kurihara, H.; Yonemori, K.; Tsuda, H.; Suzuki, J.; Kono, Y.; Honda, N.; Kodaira, M.; Yamamoto, H.; Yunokawa, M.; et al. 64Cu-DOTA-Trastuzumab PET Imaging in Patients with HER2-Positive Breast Cancer. *J. Nucl. Med.* **2013**, *54*, 1869–1875. [CrossRef]
21. Jauw, Y.W.S.; Oordt, C.W.M.-V.D.H.V.; Hoekstra, O.S.; Hendrikse, N.H.; Vugts, D.J.; Zijlstra, J.M.; Huisman, M.C.; Van Dongen, G.A.M.S. Immuno-Positron Emission Tomography with Zirconium-89-Labeled Monoclonal Antibodies in Oncology: What Can We Learn from Initial Clinical Trials? *Front. Pharmacol.* **2016**, *7*, 35. [CrossRef] [PubMed]
22. Gebhart, G.; Lamberts, L.E.; Wimana, Z.; Garcia, C.; Emonts, P.; Ameye, L.; Stroobants, S.; Huizing, M.; Aftimos, P.; Tol, J.; et al. Molecular imaging as a tool to investigate heterogeneity of advanced HER2-positive breast cancer and to predict patient outcome under trastuzumab emtansine (T-DM1): The ZEPHIR trial. *Ann. Oncol.* **2016**, *27*, 619–624. [CrossRef] [PubMed]
23. Clark, A.S.; DeMichele, A.; Mankoff, D. HER2 imaging in the ZEPHIR study. *Ann. Oncol.* **2016**, *27*, 555–557. [CrossRef] [PubMed]
24. Maguire, L.H.; Thomas, A.R.; Goldstein, A.M. Tumors of the neural crest: Common themes in development and cancer: Tumors of the Neural Crest. *Dev. Dyn.* **2015**, *244*, 311–322. [CrossRef] [PubMed]
25. Bar-Sever, Z.; Biassoni, L.; Shulkin, B.; Kong, G.; Hofman, M.S.; Lopci, E.; Manea, I.; Koziorowski, J.; Castellani, R.; Boubaker, A.; et al. Guidelines on nuclear medicine imaging in neuroblastoma. *Eur. J. Nucl. Med. Mol. Imaging* **2018**, *45*, 2009–2024. [CrossRef] [PubMed]
26. Kennedy, A.S.; Dezarn, W.A.; McNeillie, P.; Coldwell, D.; Nutting, C.; Carter, D.; Murthy, R.; Rose, S.; Warner, R.R.P.; Liu, D.; et al. Radioembolization for Unresectable Neuroendocrine Hepatic Metastases Using Resin 90Y-Microspheres: Early Results in 148 Patients. *Am. J. Clin. Oncol.* **2008**, *31*, 271–279. [CrossRef] [PubMed]
27. Liu, Y.-L.; Lu, M.-Y.; Chang, H.-H.; Lu, C.-C.; Lin, D.-T.; Jou, S.-T.; Yang, Y.-L.; Lee, Y.-L.; Huang, S.-F.; Jeng, Y.-M.; et al. Diagnostic FDG and FDOPA positron emission tomography scans distinguish the genomic type and treatment outcome of neuroblastoma. *Oncotarget* **2016**, *7*, 18774–18786. [CrossRef] [PubMed]
28. Chan, D.L.; Pavlakis, N.; Schembri, G.P.; Bernard, E.J.; Hsiao, E.; Hayes, A.; Barnes, T.; Diakos, C.; Khasraw, M.; Samra, J.; et al. Dual Somatostatin Receptor/FDG PET/CT Imaging in Metastatic Neuroendocrine Tumours: Proposal for a Novel Grading Scheme with Prognostic Significance. *Theranostics* **2017**, *7*, 1149–1158. [CrossRef] [PubMed]
29. Zhang, P.; Yu, J.; Li, J.; Shen, L.; Li, N.; Zhu, H.; Zhai, S.; Zhang, Y.; Yang, Z.; Lu, M. Clinical and Prognostic Value of PET/CT Imaging with Combination of 68Ga-DOTATATE and 18F-FDG in Gastroenteropancreatic Neuroendocrine Neoplasms. *Contrast Media Mol. Imaging* **2018**, *2018*, 2340389. [CrossRef]
30. Cistaro, A.; Quartuccio, N.; Caobelli, F.; Piccardo, A.; Paratore, R.; Coppolino, P.; Sperandeo, A.; Arnone, G.; Ficola, U. 124I-MIBG: A new promising positron-emitting radiopharmaceutical for the evaluation of neuroblastoma. *Nucl. Med. Rev.* **2015**, *18*, 102–106. [CrossRef]
31. Mankoff, D.A.; Dehdashti, F. Imaging Tumor Phenotype: 1 Plus 1 Is More than 2. *J. Nucl. Med.* **2009**, *50*, 1567–1569. [CrossRef] [PubMed]
32. Waseem, N.; Aparici, C.M.; Kunz, P.L.; Waseem, N.L. Evaluating the Role of Theranostics in Grade 3 Neuroendocrine Neoplasms. *J. Nucl. Med.* **2019**, *60*, 882–891. [CrossRef] [PubMed]
33. Barrington, S.F.; Mikhaeel, N.G.; Kostakoglu, L.; Meignan, M.; Hutchings, M.; Müeller, S.P.; Schwartz, L.H.; Zucca, E.; Fisher, R.I.; Trotman, J.; et al. Role of imaging in the staging and response assessment of lymphoma: Consensus of the International Conference on Malignant Lymphomas Imaging Working Group. *J. Clin. Oncol.* **2014**, *32*, 3048–3058. [CrossRef] [PubMed]
34. Cheson, B.D.; Ansell, S.; Schwartz, L.; Gordon, L.I.; Advani, R.; Jacene, H.A.; Hoos, A.; Barrington, S.F.; Armand, P. Refinement of the Lugano Classification lymphoma response criteria in the era of immunomodulatory therapy. *Blood* **2016**, *128*, 2489–2496. [CrossRef] [PubMed]

35. Kong, F.-L.; Ford, R.J.; Yang, D.J. Managing Lymphoma with Non-FDG Radiotracers: Current Clinical and Preclinical Applications. Available online: https://www.hindawi.com/journals/bmri/2013/626910/ (accessed on 20 August 2019).
36. Buck, A.K.; Bommer, M.; Stilgenbauer, S.; Juweid, M.; Glatting, G.; Schirrmeister, H.; Mattfeldt, T.; Tepsic, D.; Bunjes, D.; Mottaghy, F.M.; et al. Molecular Imaging of Proliferation in Malignant Lymphoma. *Cancer Res.* **2006**, *66*, 11055–11061. [CrossRef] [PubMed]
37. Nuutinen, J.; Leskinen, S.; Lindholm, P.; Söderström, K.-O.; Någren, K.; Huhtala, S.; Minn, H. Use of carbon-11 methionine positron emission tomography to assess malignancy grade and predict survival in patients with lymphomas. *Eur. J. Nucl. Med.* **1998**, *25*, 729–735. [CrossRef] [PubMed]
38. Minamimoto, R.; Fayad, L.; Advani, R.; Vose, J.; Macapinlac, H.; Meza, J.; Hankins, J.; Mottaghy, F.; Juweid, M.; Quon, A. Diffuse Large B-Cell Lymphoma: Prospective Multicenter Comparison of Early Interim FLT PET/CT versus FDG PET/CT with IHP, EORTC, Deauville, and PERCIST Criteria for Early Therapeutic Monitoring. *Radiology* **2016**, *280*, 220–229. [CrossRef]
39. Herrmann, K.; Buck, A.K.; Schuster, T.; Abbrederis, K.; Blümel, C.; Santi, I.; Rudelius, M.; Wester, H.-J.; Peschel, C.; Schwaiger, M.; et al. Week one FLT-PET response predicts complete remission to R-CHOP and survival in DLBCL. *Oncotarget* **2014**, *5*, 4050–4059. [CrossRef]
40. Chantepie, S.; Hovhannisyan, N.; Guillouet, S.; Pelage, J.-P.; Ibazizene, M.; Bodet-Milin, C.; Carlier, T.; Gac, A.-C.; Reboursière, E.; Vilque, J.-P.; et al. 18F-Fludarabine PET for Lymphoma Imaging: First-in-Humans Study on DLBCL and CLL Patients. *J. Nucl. Med.* **2018**, *59*, 1380–1385. [CrossRef]
41. Gourni, E.; Demmer, O.; Schottelius, M.; D'Alessandria, C.; Schulz, S.; Dijkgraaf, I.; Schumacher, U.; Schwaiger, M.; Kessler, H.; Wester, H.-J. PET of CXCR4 Expression by a 68Ga-Labeled Highly Specific Targeted Contrast Agent. *J. Nucl. Med.* **2011**, *52*, 1803–1810. [CrossRef]
42. Herrmann, K.; Schottelius, M.; Lapa, C.; Osl, T.; Poschenrieder, A.; Hänscheid, H.; Lückerath, K.; Schreder, M.; Bluemel, C.; Knott, M.; et al. First-in-Human Experience of CXCR4-Directed Endoradiotherapy with 177Lu- and 90Y-Labeled Pentixather in Advanced-Stage Multiple Myeloma with Extensive Intra- and Extramedullary Disease. *J. Nucl. Med.* **2016**, *57*, 248–251. [CrossRef] [PubMed]
43. Hindié, E. The NETPET Score: Combining FDG and Somatostatin Receptor Imaging for Optimal Management of Patients with Metastatic Well-Differentiated Neuroendocrine Tumors. *Theranostics* **2017**, *7*, 1159–1163. [CrossRef] [PubMed]
44. Gains, J.E.; Sebire, N.J.; Moroz, V.; Wheatley, K.; Gaze, M.N. Immunohistochemical evaluation of molecular radiotherapy target expression in neuroblastoma tissue. *Eur. J. Nucl. Med. Mol. Imaging* **2018**, *45*, 402–411. [CrossRef] [PubMed]
45. Gains, J.E.; Bomanji, J.B.; Fersht, N.L.; Sullivan, T.; D'Souza, D.; Sullivan, K.P.; Aldridge, M.; Waddington, W.; Gaze, M.N. 177Lu-DOTATATE Molecular Radiotherapy for Childhood Neuroblastoma. *J. Nucl. Med.* **2011**, *52*, 1041–1047. [CrossRef] [PubMed]
46. Kayano, D.; Kinuya, S. Iodine-131 Metaiodobenzylguanidine Therapy for Neuroblastoma: Reports So Far and Future Perspective. *Sci. World J.* **2015**, *2015*, 1–9. [CrossRef]
47. Deubzer, H.; Hundsdoerfer, P.; Fuchs, J.; Prasad, V.; Timmermann, B.; Astrahantseff, K.; Berthold, F.; Simon, T.; Hero, B.; Schulte, J.H.; et al. 2017 GPOH Guidelines for Diagnosis and Treatment of Patients with Neuroblastic Tumors. *Klin. Pädiatr.* **2017**, *229*, 147–167.
48. Kong, G.; Hofman, M.S.; Murray, W.K.; Wilson, S.; Wood, P.; Downie, P.; Super, L.; Hogg, A.; Eu, P.; Hicks, R.J. Initial Experience with Gallium-68 DOTA-Octreotate PET/CT and Peptide Receptor Radionuclide Therapy for Pediatric Patients with Refractory Metastatic Neuroblastoma. *J. Pediatr. Hematol.* **2016**, *38*, 1–96. [CrossRef]
49. Strosberg, J.; El-Haddad, G.; Wolin, E.; Hendifar, A.; Yao, J.; Chasen, B.; Mittra, E.; Kunz, P.L.; Kulke, M.H.; Jacene, H.; et al. Phase 3 Trial of 177Lu-Dotatate for Midgut Neuroendocrine Tumors. *N. Engl. J. Med.* **2017**, *376*, 125–135. [CrossRef]
50. Navalkissoor, S.; Flux, G.; Bomanji, J. Molecular radiotheranostics for neuroendocrine tumours. *Clin. Med.* **2017**, *17*, 462–468. [CrossRef]
51. Lee, S.T.; Kulkarni, H.R.; Singh, A.; Baum, R.P. Theranostics of Neuroendocrine Tumors. *Visc. Med.* **2017**, *33*, 358–366. [CrossRef]
52. Bailly, C.; Cléry, P.-F.; Faivre-Chauvet, A.; Bourgeois, M.; Guérard, F.; Haddad, F.; Barbet, J.; Chérel, M.; Kraeber-Bodéré, F.; Carlier, T.; et al. Immuno-PET for Clinical Theranostic Approaches. *Int. J. Mol. Sci.* **2016**, *18*, 57. [CrossRef] [PubMed]

53. Giesen, D.; Jalving, M.; Moek, K.L.; Kok, I.C.; De Groot, D.J.A.; Fehrmann, R.S.; Hooge, M.N.L.-D.; Brouwers, A.H.; De Vries, E.G. Theranostics Using Antibodies and Antibody-Related Therapeutics. *J. Nucl. Med.* **2017**, *58*, 83–90.
54. Lamberts, L.E.; Williams, S.P.; Van Scheltinga, A.G.T.; Hooge, M.N.L.-D.; Schroder, C.P.; Gietema, J.A.; Brouwers, A.H.; De Vries, E.G. Antibody Positron Emission Tomography Imaging in Anticancer Drug Development. *J. Clin. Oncol.* **2015**, *33*, 1491–1504. [CrossRef] [PubMed]
55. Kraeber-Bodere, F.; Bailly, C.; Chérel, M.; Chatal, J.-F. ImmunoPET to help stratify patients for targeted therapies and to improve drug development. *Eur. J. Nucl. Med. Mol. Imaging* **2016**, *43*, 2166–2168. [CrossRef] [PubMed]
56. Sörensen, J.; Velikyan, I.; Sandberg, D.; Wennborg, A.; Feldwisch, J.; Tolmachev, V.; Orlova, A.; Sandström, M.; Lubberink, M.; Olofsson, H.; et al. Measuring HER2-Receptor Expression In Metastatic Breast Cancer Using [68Ga]ABY-025 Affibody PET/CT. *Theranostics* **2016**, *6*, 262–271. [CrossRef] [PubMed]
57. Fletcher, J.W.; Djulbegovic, B.; Soares, H.P.; Siegel, B.A.; Lowe, V.J.; Lyman, G.H.; Coleman, R.E.; Wahl, R.; Paschold, J.C.; Avril, N.; et al. Recommendations on the Use of 18F-FDG PET in Oncology. *J. Nucl. Med.* **2008**, *49*, 480–508. [CrossRef]
58. Czernin, J.; Allen-Auerbach, M.; Nathanson, D.; Herrmann, K. PET/CT in Oncology: Current Status and Perspectives. *Curr. Radiol. Rep.* **2013**, *1*, 177–190. [CrossRef]
59. Petersen, H.; Holdgaard, P.C.; Madsen, P.H.; Knudsen, L.M.; Gad, D.; Gravergaard, A.E.; Rohde, M.; Godballe, C.; Engelmann, B.E.; Bech, K.; et al. FDG PET/CT in cancer: Comparison of actual use with literature-based recommendations. *Eur. J. Nucl. Med. Mol. Imaging* **2016**, *43*, 695–706. [CrossRef]
60. Thie, J.A. Understanding the standardized uptake value, its methods, and implications for usage. *J. Nucl. Med.* **2004**, *45*, 1431–1434.
61. Carlier, T.; Bailly, C. State-Of-The-Art and Recent Advances in Quantification for Therapeutic Follow-Up in Oncology Using PET. *Front. Med.* **2015**, *2*, 18. [CrossRef]
62. Keyes, J.W. SUV: Standard uptake or silly useless value? *J. Nucl. Med.* **1995**, *36*, 1836–1839. [PubMed]
63. Okada, J.; Oonishi, H.; Yoshikawa, K.; Itami, J.; Uno, K.; Imaseki, K.; Arimizu, N. FDG-PET for predicting the prognosis of malignant lymphoma. *Ann. Nucl. Med.* **1994**, *8*, 187–191. [CrossRef] [PubMed]
64. Schöder, H.; Noy, A.; Gönen, M.; Weng, L.; Green, D.; Erdi, Y.E.; Larson, S.M.; Yeung, H.W.D. Intensity of 18fluorodeoxyglucose uptake in positron emission tomography distinguishes between indolent and aggressive non-Hodgkin's lymphoma. *J. Clin. Oncol.* **2005**, *23*, 4643–4651. [CrossRef] [PubMed]
65. Bodet-Milin, C.; Kraeber-Bodéré, F.; Moreau, P.; Campion, L.; Dupas, B.; Le Gouill, S.; Drouet, M.; Delaunay, C.; Grenier, N.; Garrigou, P.; et al. Investigation of FDG-PET/CT imaging to guide biopsies in the detection of histological transformation of indolent lymphoma. *Haematologica* **2008**, *93*, 471–472. [CrossRef] [PubMed]
66. Bodet-Milin, C.; Bailly, C.; Meignan, M.; Beriollo-Riedinger, A.; Casasnovas, R.-O.; Devillers, A.; Lamy, T.; Santiago-Ribeiro, M.; Gyan, E.; Gallazzini-Crépin, C.; et al. Predictive Power of FDG-PET Parameters at Diagnosis and after Induction in Patients with Mantle Cell Lymphoma, Interim Results from the LyMa-PET Project, Conducted on Behalf of the Lysa Group. *Blood* **2015**, *126*, 335.
67. Bodet-Milin, C.; Touzeau, C.; Leux, C.; Sahin, M.; Moreau, A.; Maisonneuve, H.; Morineau, N.; Jardel, H.; Gallazini-Crépin, C.; Gries, P.; et al. Prognostic impact of 18F-fluoro-deoxyglucose positron emission tomography in untreated mantle cell lymphoma: A retrospective study from the GOELAMS group. *Eur. J. Nucl. Med. Mol. Imaging* **2010**, *37*, 1633–1642. [CrossRef] [PubMed]
68. Bailly, C.; Carlier, T.; Touzeau, C.; Arlicot, N.; Kraeber-Bodéré, F.; Le Gouill, S.; Bodet-Milin, C. Interest of FDG-PET in the Management of Mantle Cell Lymphoma. *Front. Med.* **2019**, *6*, 70. [CrossRef]
69. Bailly, C.; Carlier, T.; Berriolo-Riedinger, A.; Casasnovas, O.; Gyan, E.; Meignan, M.; Moreau, A.; Burroni, B.; Djaileb, L.; Gressin, R.; et al. Prognostic value of FDG-PET in patients with mantle cell lymphoma: Results from the LyMa-PET Project. *Haematologica* **2019**. [CrossRef]
70. Eisenhauer, E.; Therasse, P.; Bogaerts, J.; Schwartz, L.; Sargent, D.; Ford, R.; Dancey, J.; Arbuck, S.; Gwyther, S.; Mooney, M.; et al. New response evaluation criteria in solid tumours: Revised RECIST guideline (Version 1.1). *Eur. J. Cancer* **2009**, *45*, 228–247. [CrossRef]
71. Therasse, P.; Arbuck, S.G.; Eisenhauer, E.A.; Wanders, J.; Kaplan, R.S.; Rubinstein, L.; Verweij, J.; Van Glabbeke, M.; Van Oosterom, A.T.; Christian, M.C.; et al. New Guidelines to Evaluate the Response to Treatment in Solid Tumors. *J. Natl. Cancer Inst.* **2000**, *92*, 205–216. [CrossRef]

72. Schwartz, L.H.; Litiere, S.; De Vries, E.; Ford, R.; Gwyther, S.; Mandrekar, S.; Shankar, L.; Bogaerts, J.; Chen, A.; Dancey, J.; et al. RECIST 1.1—Update and Clarification: From the RECIST Committee. *Eur. J. Cancer* **2016**, *62*, 132–137. [CrossRef] [PubMed]
73. Wahl, R.L.; Jacene, H.; Kasamon, Y.; Lodge, M.A. From RECIST to PERCIST: Evolving Considerations for PET Response Criteria in Solid Tumors. *J. Nucl. Med.* **2009**, *50*, 122S–150S. [CrossRef] [PubMed]
74. Al-Hajj, M.; Becker, M.W.; Wicha, M.; Weissman, I.; Clarke, M.F. Therapeutic implications of cancer stem cells. *Curr. Opin. Genet. Dev.* **2004**, *14*, 43–47. [CrossRef] [PubMed]
75. Huff, C.A.; Matsui, W.; Smith, B.D.; Jones, R.J. The paradox of response and survival in cancer therapeutics. *Blood* **2006**, *107*, 431–434. [CrossRef] [PubMed]
76. Lin, C.; Itti, E.; Haioun, C.; Petegnief, Y.; Luciani, A.; Dupuis, J.; Paone, G.; Talbot, J.-N.; Rahmouni, A.; Meignan, M. Early 18F-FDG PET for Prediction of Prognosis in Patients with Diffuse Large B-Cell Lymphoma: SUV-Based Assessment versus Visual Analysis. *J. Nucl. Med.* **2007**, *48*, 1626–1632. [CrossRef] [PubMed]
77. Wahl, R.L.; Zasadny, K.; Helvie, M.; Hutchins, G.D.; Weber, B.; Cody, R. Metabolic monitoring of breast cancer chemohormonotherapy using positron emission tomography: Initial evaluation. *J. Clin. Oncol.* **1993**, *11*, 2101–2111. [CrossRef] [PubMed]
78. Bailly, C.; Carlier, T.; Jamet, B.; Eugene, T.; Touzeau, C.; Attal, M.; Hulin, C.; Facon, T.; Leleu, X.; Perrot, A.; et al. Interim PET Analysis in First-Line Therapy of Multiple Myeloma: Prognostic Value of ΔSUVmax in the FDG-Avid Patients of the IMAJEM Study. *Clin. Cancer Res.* **2018**, *24*, 5219–5224. [CrossRef] [PubMed]
79. Matsui, W.; Huff, C.A.; Wang, Q.; Malehorn, M.T.; Barber, J.; Tanhehco, Y.; Smith, B.D.; Civin, C.I.; Jones, R.J. Characterization of clonogenic multiple myeloma cells. *Blood* **2004**, *103*, 2332–2336. [CrossRef] [PubMed]
80. Rasche, L.; Chavan, S.S.; Stephens, O.W.; Patel, P.H.; Tytarenko, R.; Ashby, C.; Bauer, M.; Stein, C.; Deshpande, S.; Wardell, C.; et al. Spatial genomic heterogeneity in multiple myeloma revealed by multi-region sequencing. *Nat. Commun.* **2017**, *8*, 268. [CrossRef]
81. Rasche, L.; Kortüm, K.M.; Raab, M.S.; Weinhold, N. The Impact of Tumor Heterogeneity on Diagnostics and Novel Therapeutic Strategies in Multiple Myeloma. *Int. J. Mol. Sci.* **2019**, *20*, 1248. [CrossRef]
82. Pugachev, A.; Ruan, S.; Carlin, S.; Larson, S.M.; Campa, J.; Ling, C.C.; Humm, J.L. Dependence of FDG uptake on tumor microenvironment. *Int. J. Radiat. Oncol.* **2005**, *62*, 545–553. [CrossRef] [PubMed]
83. Gillies, R.J.; Kinahan, P.E.; Hricak, H. Radiomics: Images Are More than Pictures, They Are Data. *Radiology* **2016**, *278*, 563–577. [CrossRef] [PubMed]
84. Lambin, P.; Leijenaar, R.T.; Deist, T.M.; Peerlings, J.; De Jong, E.E.; Van Timmeren, J.; Sanduleanu, S.; LaRue, R.T.; Even, A.J.; Jochems, A.; et al. Radiomics: The bridge between medical imaging and personalized medicine. *Nat. Rev. Clin. Oncol.* **2017**, *14*, 749–762. [CrossRef] [PubMed]
85. Hatt, M.; Tixier, F.; Visvikis, D.; Cheze Le Rest, C. Radiomics in PET/CT: More Than Meets the Eye? *J. Nucl. Med.* **2017**, *58*, 365–366. [CrossRef] [PubMed]
86. Hatt, M.; Tixier, F.; Pierce, L.; Kinahan, P.E.; Rest, C.C.L.; Visvikis, D. Characterization of PET/CT images using texture analysis: The past, the present ... any future? *Eur. J. Nucl. Med. Mol. Imaging* **2016**, 1–15. [CrossRef] [PubMed]
87. Vallières, M.; Zwanenburg, A.; Badic, B.; Cheze Le Rest, C.; Visvikis, D.; Hatt, M. Responsible Radiomics Research for Faster Clinical Translation. *J. Nucl. Med.* **2018**, *59*, 189–193. [CrossRef] [PubMed]
88. Berthon, B.; Spezi, E.; Galavis, P.; Shepherd, T.; Apte, A.; Hatt, M.; Fayad, H.; De Bernardi, E.; Soffientini, C.D.; Schmidtlein, C.R.; et al. Toward a standard for the evaluation of PET-Auto-Segmentation methods following the recommendations of AAPM task group No. 211: Requirements and implementation. *Med Phys.* **2017**, *44*, 4098–4111. [CrossRef] [PubMed]
89. Zwanenburg, A.; Leger, S.; Vallières, M.; Löck, S. Image biomarker standardisation initiative. *arXiv* **2016**, arXiv:1612.07003.
90. Tixier, F.; Le Rest, C.C.; Hatt, M.; Albarghach, N.M.; Pradier, O.; Metges, J.-P.; Corcos, L.; Visvikis, D. Intratumor heterogeneity characterized by textural features on baseline 18F-FDG PET images predicts response to concomitant radiochemotherapy in esophageal cancer. *J. Nucl. Med.* **2011**, *52*, 369–378. [CrossRef] [PubMed]
91. Cook, G.J.R.; Siddique, M.; Taylor, B.P.; Yip, C.; Chicklore, S.; Goh, V. Radiomics in PET: Principles and applications. *Clin. Transl. Imaging* **2014**, *2*, 269–276. [CrossRef]
92. Lee, J.W.; Lee, S.M. Radiomics in Oncological PET/CT: Clinical Applications. *Nucl. Med. Mol. Imaging* **2018**, *52*, 170–189. [CrossRef] [PubMed]

93. Chalkidou, A.; O'Doherty, M.J.; Marsden, P.K. False Discovery Rates in PET and CT Studies with Texture Features: A Systematic Review. *PLoS ONE* **2015**, *10*, e0124165. [CrossRef] [PubMed]
94. Welch, M.L.; McIntosh, C.; Haibe-Kains, B.; Milosevic, M.F.; Wee, L.; Dekker, A.; Huang, S.H.; Purdie, T.G.; O'Sullivan, B.; Aerts, H.J.; et al. Vulnerabilities of radiomic signature development: The need for safeguards. *Radiother. Oncol.* **2019**, *130*, 2–9. [CrossRef] [PubMed]
95. Lucia, F.; Visvikis, D.; Vallières, M.; Desseroit, M.-C.; Miranda, O.; Robin, P.; Bonaffini, P.A.; Alfieri, J.; Masson, I.; Mervoyer, A.; et al. External validation of a combined PET and MRI radiomics model for prediction of recurrence in cervical cancer patients treated with chemoradiotherapy. *Eur. J. Nucl. Med. Mol. Imaging* **2019**, *46*, 864–877. [CrossRef] [PubMed]
96. Wu, J.; Aguilera, T.; Shultz, D.; Gudur, M.; Rubin, D.L.; Loo, B.W.; Diehn, M.; Li, R. Early-Stage Non–Small Cell Lung Cancer: Quantitative Imaging Characteristics of 18F Fluorodeoxyglucose PET/CT Allow Prediction of Distant Metastasis. *Radiology* **2016**, *281*, 270–278. [CrossRef] [PubMed]
97. Carvalho, S.; Leijenaar, R.T.H.; Troost, E.G.C.; van Timmeren, J.E.; Oberije, C.; van Elmpt, W.; de Geus-Oei, L.-F.; Bussink, J.; Lambin, P. 18F-fluorodeoxyglucose positron-emission tomography (FDG-PET)-Radiomics of metastatic lymph nodes and primary tumor in non-small cell lung cancer (NSCLC)—A prospective externally validated study. *PLoS ONE* **2018**, *13*, e0192859. [CrossRef] [PubMed]
98. Ypsilantis, P.-P.; Siddique, M.; Sohn, H.-M.; Davies, A.; Cook, G.; Goh, V.; Montana, G. Predicting Response to Neoadjuvant Chemotherapy with PET Imaging Using Convolutional Neural Networks. *PLoS ONE* **2015**, *10*, e0137036. [CrossRef] [PubMed]
99. Arimura, H.; Soufi, M.; Kamezawa, H.; Ninomiya, K.; Yamada, M. Radiomics with artificial intelligence for precision medicine in radiation therapy. *J. Radiat. Res.* **2019**, *60*, 150–157. [CrossRef] [PubMed]
100. Orlhac, F.; Boughdad, S.; Philippe, C.; Stalla-Bourdillon, H.; Nioche, C.; Champion, L.; Soussan, M.; Frouin, F.; Frouin, V.; Buvat, I. A Postreconstruction Harmonization Method for Multicenter Radiomic Studies in PET. *J. Nucl. Med.* **2018**, *59*, 1321–1328. [CrossRef] [PubMed]
101. Chatterjee, A.; Vallieres, M.; Dohan, A.; Levesque, I.R.; Ueno, Y.; Saif, S.; Reinhold, C.; Seuntjens, J. Creating Robust Predictive Radiomic Models for Data from Independent Institutions Using Normalization. *IEEE Trans. Radiat. Plasma Med Sci.* **2019**, *3*, 210–215. [CrossRef]
102. Upadhaya, T.; Vallieres, M.; Chatterjee, A.; Lucia, F.; Bonaffini, P.A.; Masson, I.; Mervoyer, A.; Reinhold, C.; Schick, U.; Seuntjens, J.; et al. Comparison of Radiomics Models Built Through Machine Learning in a Multicentric Context with Independent Testing: Identical Data, Similar Algorithms, Different Methodologies. *IEEE Trans. Radiat. Plasma Med Sci.* **2019**, *3*, 192–200. [CrossRef]
103. Liu, L.; Chen, J.; Fieguth, P.; Zhao, G.; Chellappa, R.; Pietikäinen, M. From BoW to CNN: Two Decades of Texture Representation for Texture Classification. *Int. J. Comput. Vis.* **2019**, *127*, 74–109. [CrossRef]
104. Desseroit, M.-C.; Visvikis, D.; Tixier, F.; Majdoub, M.; Guillevin, R.; Perdrisot, R.; Le Rest, C.C.; Hatt, M. Development of a nomogram combining clinical staging with (18)F-FDG PET/CT image features in non-small-cell lung cancer stage I-III. *Eur. J. Nucl. Med. Mol. Imaging* **2016**, *43*, 1477–1485. [CrossRef] [PubMed]
105. Chan, S.-C.; Cheng, N.-M.; Hsieh, C.-H.; Ng, S.-H.; Lin, C.-Y.; Yen, T.-C.; Hsu, C.-L.; Wan, H.-M.; Liao, C.-T.; Chang, K.-P.; et al. Multiparametric imaging using 18F-FDG PET/CT heterogeneity parameters and functional MRI techniques: Prognostic significance in patients with primary advanced oropharyngeal or hypopharyngeal squamous cell carcinoma treated with chemoradiotherapy. *Oncotarget* **2017**, *8*, 62606–62621. [CrossRef] [PubMed]
106. Vallières, M.; Freeman, C.R.; Skamene, S.R.; El Naqa, I. A radiomics model from joint FDG-PET and MRI texture features for the prediction of lung metastases in soft-tissue sarcomas of the extremities. *Phys. Med. Boil.* **2015**, *60*, 5471–5496. [CrossRef] [PubMed]
107. Bodet-Milin, C.; Bailly, C.; Meignan, M.; Berriolo-riedinger, A.; Devillers, A.; Hermine, O.; Carlier, T.; Hatt, M.; Kraeber-Bodéré, F.; Gouill, S.L. Prognosis value of quantitative indices derived from initial FDG PET/CT in untreated mantle cell lymphoma patients enrolled in the Lyma trial, a LYSA study. Preliminary results. *J. Nucl. Med.* **2015**, *56*, 659.
108. Carlier, T.; Bailly, C.; Hatt, M.; Kraeber-Bodéré, F.; Visvikis, D.; Gouill, S.L.; Bodet-Milin, C. Quantification of intratumor heterogeneity derived from baseline FDG PET/CT in untreated mantle cell lymphoma patients enrolled in a prospective phase III trial of the LYSA group: Preliminary results. *J. Nucl. Med.* **2015**, *56*, 429.

109. Mayerhoefer, M.E.; Riedl, C.C.; Kumar, A.; Gibbs, P.; Weber, M.; Tal, I.; Schilksy, J.; Schöder, H. Radiomic features of glucose metabolism enable prediction of outcome in mantle cell lymphoma. *Eur. J. Nucl. Med. Mol. Imaging* **2019**, 1–10. [CrossRef]
110. Lucia, F.; Visvikis, D.; Desseroit, M.-C.; Miranda, O.; Malhaire, J.-P.; Robin, P.; Pradier, O.; Hatt, M.; Schick, U. Prediction of outcome using pretreatment 18F-FDG PET/CT and MRI radiomics in locally advanced cervical cancer treated with chemoradiotherapy. *Eur. J. Nucl. Med. Mol. Imaging* **2018**, *45*, 768–786. [CrossRef]

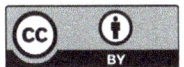

© 2019 by the authors. Licensee MDPI, Basel, Switzerland. This article is an open access article distributed under the terms and conditions of the Creative Commons Attribution (CC BY) license (http://creativecommons.org/licenses/by/4.0/).

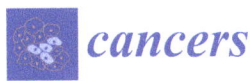

Review

Microsatellite Instability: Diagnosis, Heterogeneity, Discordance, and Clinical Impact in Colorectal Cancer

Camille Evrard [1], Gaëlle Tachon [2,3,4], Violaine Randrian [3,5], Lucie Karayan-Tapon [2,3,4] and David Tougeron [1,3,5,*]

1. Department of Medical Oncology, Poitiers University Hospital, 86021 Poitiers, France; camille.evrard@chu-poitiers.fr
2. Department of Cancer Biology, Poitiers University Hospital, 86021 Poitiers, France; gaelle.tachon@chu-poitiers.fr (G.T.); lucie.karayan-tapon@chu-poitiers.fr (L.K.-T.)
3. Faculty of Medicine, University of Poitiers, 86000 Poitiers, France; violaine.randrian@orange.fr
4. Laboratory of Experimental and Clinical Neuroscience, Institut national de la santé et de la recherche médicale (INSERM) 1084, F-86073 Poitiers, France
5. Department of Gastroenterology, Poitiers University Hospital, 86021 Poitiers, France
* Correspondence: david.tougeron@chu-poitiers.fr; Tel.: +33-5-4944-3751; Fax: +33-5-4944-3835

Received: 31 August 2019; Accepted: 13 October 2019; Published: 15 October 2019

Abstract: Tumor DNA mismatch repair (MMR) deficiency testing is important to the identification of Lynch syndrome and decision making regarding adjuvant chemotherapy in stage II colorectal cancer (CRC) and has become an indispensable test in metastatic tumors due to the high efficacy of immune checkpoint inhibitor (ICI) in deficient MMR (dMMR) tumors. CRCs greatly benefit from this testing as approximately 15% of them are dMMR but only 3% to 5% are at a metastatic stage. MMR status can be determined by two different methods, microsatellite instability (MSI) testing on tumor DNA, and immunohistochemistry of the MMR proteins on tumor tissue. Recent studies have reported a rate of 3% to 10% of discordance between these two tests. Moreover, some reports suggest possible intra- and inter-tumoral heterogeneity of MMR and MSI status. These issues are important to know and to clarify in order to define therapeutic strategy in CRC. This review aims to detail the standard techniques used for the determination of MMR and MSI status, along with their advantages and limits. We review the discordances that may arise between these two tests, tumor heterogeneity of MMR and MSI status, and possible explanations. We also discuss the strategies designed to distinguish sporadic versus germline dMMR/MSI CRC. Finally, we present new and accurate methods aimed at determining MMR/MSI status.

Keywords: microsatellite instability; colorectal cancer; immune checkpoints; deficient mismatch repair

1. Introduction

There are three major mechanisms in colorectal (CRC) carcinogenesis. The most common is chromosomal instability (CIN) in 75% of CRCs, the second is an epigenetic modification of DNA methylation, also called CpG island methylator phenotype (CIMP), in 20% of CRCs, and the third is microsatellite instability (MSI) or deficiency of DNA mismatch repair system (MMR) which occurs in approximately 15% of CRCs (Figure 1) [1]. It is worth noting that there is frequent overlap between CIMP and dMMR/MSI phenotype. CRC carcinogenesis is somewhat more complex, and while rare overlaps between CIN and CIMP or CIN and MSI phenotypes exist, they will not be developed here [2].

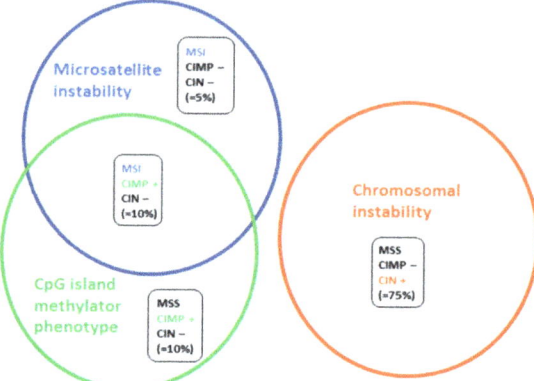

Figure 1. Simplified molecular subgroups of colorectal cancers. There are three major mechanisms of colorectal carcinogenesis, 75% of chromosomal instability, 20% of DNA methylation, and 15% of microsatellite instability or deficient DNA mismatch repair [1]. MSS: microsatellite stability, MSI: microsatellite instability, CIMP: CpG island methylator phenotype, CIN: chromosomal instability.

Microsatellites (also called "short tandem repeats") correspond to DNA sequences distributed throughout the genome (coding or non-coding sequences) with a repetitive structure, i.e., repetition, a variable number of times, of a single nucleotide or di-, tri-, or tetra-nucleotides. These repetitive structures are particularly prone to replication errors in the case of deficiency of the MMR system (dMMR status). An accumulation of errors in the sequence of these microsatellites, called microsatellite instability, highlights malfunction of the MMR system. Cancers with such phenotypes are said to be MSI or by extension, MMR-deficient (dMMR), which is the opposite of microsatellite stability (MSS), also known as MMR-proficient (pMMR).

The MMR system consists of four major proteins called MLH1, MSH2, MSH6, and PMS2. These proteins identify and correct DNA mismatches caused by DNA polymerase during replication, which occurs especially in microsatellites. These proteins work two by two, MLH1 with PMS2 and MSH2 with MSH6, and form the MutLα and MutSα complex, respectively. MutSα recognizes single base pair mismatch, creates a sliding clamp around DNA, and then binds the second complex, MutLα [3]. This combination interacts with many enzymes, including the DNA polymerase, to perform excision of the single mismatch and resynthesize the DNA strand (Figure 2). MutSα can also recognize other error patterns such as insertion and deletion loops and then preferably bind with MutL homologs, such as MutLβ (MLH1-PMS1) and MutLγ (MLH1-MLH3), thereby achieving error excision [4,5]. Loss of function of one of the four proteins (MLH1, PMS2, MSH2, or MSH6) leads to inactivation of the MMR system, resulting in a loss of fidelity of the replication and an accumulation of mutations. This ultra-mutated profile causes dMMR/MSI cancers, including dMMR/MSI CRC.

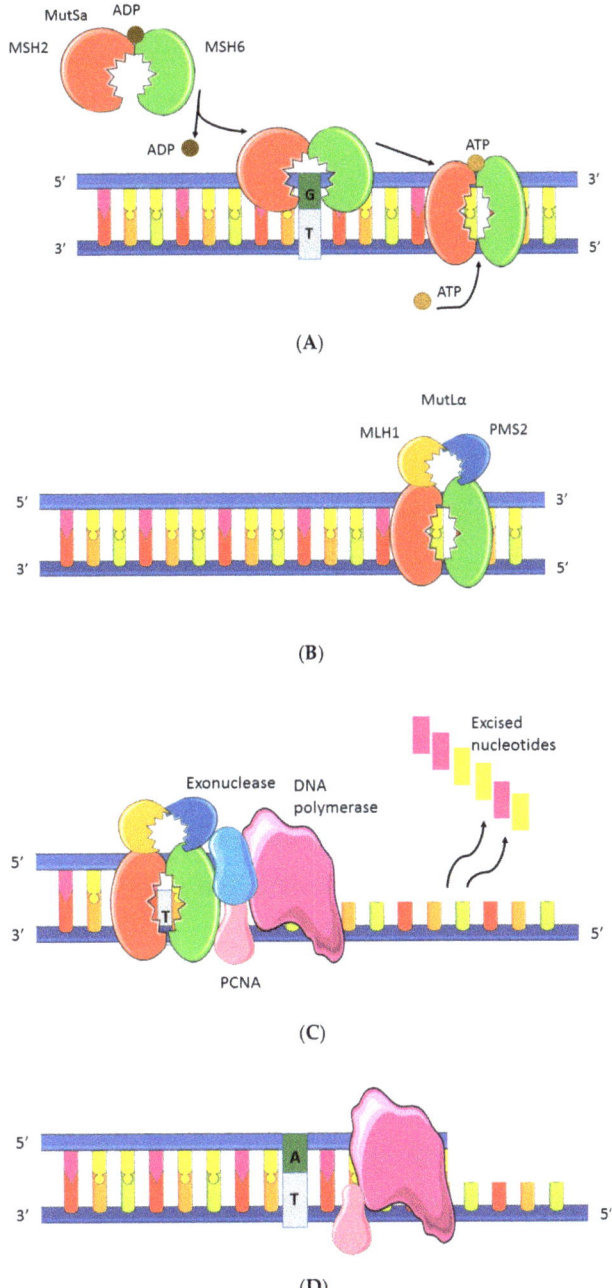

Figure 2. Mismatch repair mechanism. (**A**) Single mismatch, (**B**) DNA MMR protein sliding clamp, (**C**) exonuclease complex, and (**D**) resynthesis. The complex MutSα recognizes single base pair mismatch and surrounds the DNA like a clamp and then the MutL complex comes and links to MutSα. Different enzymes (PCNA and DNA polymerase) then intervene to excise the errors and to resynthesize the DNA. PCNA: proliferating cell nuclear antigen, ADP: adenosine diphosphate, ATP: adenosine triphosphate, and MMR: mismatch repair. Proteins from the DNA repair system: MSH2, MSH6, PMS2, and MLH1.

The dMMR/MSI phenotype can be acquired in sporadic CRC (75%) or constitutively in Lynch syndrome, due to germline mutation of one of the MMR genes (25%) [6]. Sporadic cases are due in most cases to a loss of expression of MLH1 caused by hypermethylation of the *MLH1* gene promoter. Indeed, dMMR/MSI detection is of major help to identify Lynch syndrome according to the revised Bethesda criteria (Table 1). Other clinical impacts of dMMR/MSI determination enter into decision making regarding adjuvant chemotherapy in stage II CRC and the use of immune checkpoint inhibitor (ICI) in chemoresistant metastatic dMMR/MSI tumors. About 20% of stage II and III CRCs present a dMMR/MSI phenotype and are associated with better prognosis than pMMR/MSS tumors [5]. Moreover, stage II dMMR/MSI CRCs do not benefit from adjuvant fluoropyrimidine chemotherapy [7,8]. Consequently, in view of a good prognosis for stage II dMMR/MSI CRCs and chemoresistance to fluoropyrimidine, adjuvant chemotherapy is not recommended. Nevertheless, for high-risk stage II dMMR/MSI CRCs with very poor prognosis criteria, such as T4 stage and vascular emboli, oxaliplatin-based adjuvant chemotherapy should be discussed case by case. In metastatic CRCs (mCRC), dMMR/MSI represents only around 3% to 5% of mCRCs and has been associated with poor prognosis and chemoresistance to standard treatment [9,10]. Nevertheless, recent series have reported prolonged overall survival in dMMR/MSI mCRC and a trend toward better outcomes of anti-vascular endothelial growth factor (anti-VEGF) as compared with anti-epidermal growth factor receptor (anti-EGFR), but no difference according to chemotherapy regimen, i.e., irinotecan-based chemotherapy as compared with oxaliplatin-based chemotherapy has been reported [11]. Finally, recent nonrandomized trials suggest high efficacy of immune checkpoint inhibitor (ICI) in chemoresistant dMMR/MSI metastatic tumors due to the high tumor mutational burden in these tumors, while the other predictor of response to ICI is the IHC labeling of the PD-L1 protein (programmed death-ligand 1) [12,13].

Table 1. Revised Bethesda criteria [14].

1. Colorectal cancer diagnosed in a patient less than 50 years of age
2. Presence of synchronous, metachronous colorectal, or other HNPCC-associated tumors *, regardless of age
3. Colorectal cancer with the MSI histology † diagnosed in a patient less than 60 years of age §
4. Colorectal cancer diagnosed in one or more first-degree relatives with an HNPCC-related tumor, with one of the cancers being diagnosed under age 50 years
5. Colorectal cancer diagnosed in two or more first- or second-degree relatives with HNPCC-related tumors, regardless of age

*: Hereditary nonpolyposis colorectal cancer (HNPCC)-related tumors include colorectal, endometrial, stomach, ovarian, pancreas, ureter and renal pelvis, biliary tract, and brain (usually glioblastoma as seen in Turcot syndrome) tumors, sebaceous gland adenomas and keratoacanthomas in Muir–Torre syndrome, and carcinoma of the small bowel. †: Presence of tumor-infiltrating lymphocytes, Crohn's-like lymphocytic reaction, mucinous/signet-ring differentiation, or medullary growth pattern. §: There was no consensus among the workshop participants on whether to include the age criteria in guideline three above; participants voted to keep less than 60 years of age in the guidelines.

To conclude, dMMR/MSI testing in CRC is indicated primarily in the following three circumstances: in stage II CRCs to define indications and modalities of adjuvant chemotherapy, in stage IV to treat with ICI, and for screening of Lynch syndrome based on the revised Bethesda criteria. However, in some centers, dMMR/MSI testing is performed in all CRCs given its interest in multiple circumstances.

2. Mismatch Repair System and Microsatellite Instability Testing

The status of dMMR and MSI can be determined by two different methods, molecular MSI testing based on DNA extracted from tumor tissue and immunohistochemistry (IHC) of the MMR proteins based on sections of formalin-fixed paraffin-embedded (FFPE) tumor block. Commonly, a tumor is called dMMR if it presents nuclear loss of expression of at least one of the MMR proteins (MLH1, PMS2, MSH2, or MSH6), in contrast to pMMR tumor. A tumor is called MSI (or MSI-high, MSI-H) if it presents instability (variation in the microsatellite length) of at least 40% of a panel of microsatellites tested on tumor DNA, in contrast to MSS tumor.

2.1. Microsatellite Instability Testing

Microsatellite instability testing is carried out on tumor DNA extracted from frozen or FFPE tumor tissue. A specific area with high tumor cellularity (>20%) has to be selected by an experienced pathologist to avoid false negative results [15]. Microsatellite instability is assessed by analyzing microsatellite loci, either mononucleotide repeats or a combination of dinucleotide and mononucleotide repeats as recommended [16].

The first reference panel, referred to as the Bethesda panel, consists of two mononucleotide loci (big adenine tract *BAT-25* and *BAT-26*) and three dinucleotide loci (*D2S123*, *D5S346*, and *D17S250*) [12]. *BAT-25* is found in intron 16 of the *c-KIT* gene and *BAT-26* in the intron 5 of the *MSH2* gene. *D2S123* (2p16) is telomeric to mismatch repair genes *MSH-2* and *MSH-6*, *D5S346* (5q21–22) is close to the locus for the *adenomatosis polyposis coli* (*APC*) tumor suppressor gene, and *D17S250* (17q11.2–12) is close to the locus for the tumor suppressor gene *BRCA-1* [17]. As dinucleotide repeats are less sensitive than mononucleotide repeats for MSI detection, a comparison with non-tumor matching DNA is always required (DNA extracted from non-tumor tissue from a surgical specimen). When using the Bethesda panel, tumors with instability of two or more of these loci are considered as MSI (i.e., MSI-high), and cancers with no instability at any of the five loci are considered MSS. Cancers with only one out of five unstable loci are interpreted as MSI-low, although it is unclear whether MSI-low represents a biologically distinct category or whether it simply reflects the inherent limitations of faithfully replicating these repetitive sequences. For the time being, these tumors are considered as MSS.

The second panel is the pentaplex panel, which consists of the following five consensus mononucleotide repeats: *BAT-25*, *BAT-26*, *NR-21* located in the untranslated 5′ region of the *SLC7AB* gene, *NR-24* located in the untranslated 5′ region of the *ZNF-2* gene, and *NR-27* (*MONO-27*) located in the untranslated 5′ region of the *IAP-1* gene. The quasi-monomorphic nature of these microsatellites facilitates their analysis; they have several repetitions and their size is highly homogeneous in the Caucasian population [18]. Using the pentaplex panel, a tumor will be called MSI if at least three markers out of five are unstable (Figure 3B). A tumor with no instability, or one unstable marker, is classified MSS (Figure 3A). In very rare cases, where two markers are unstable, a healthy tissue analysis is carried out to confirm or deny instability by comparing healthy and tumor tissue. This panel has become the new standard, in most international recommendations for MSI testing; contrary to the Bethesda panel, it does not require comparison with non-tumor tissue for MSI determination in CRC [19].

Both MSI techniques are based on the simultaneous amplification of five markers in a multiplex PCR. Amplification products then migrate on capillary electrophoresis, which enables marker distribution depending on their sizes. Taq polymerase is not faithful enough to reproduce the exact number of nucleotide repetitions, and therefore, at the expected size of a marker, the electrophoresis profile shows a multiple peak pattern. The reference size of the marker per sample is given by the main, higher peak and needs to be compared to its expected size in the general population [16]. If the size of the marker significantly differs from its expected size, it signifies instability. For non-colorectal tumor tissue, systematic double testing of tumor tissue and non-tumor tissue is performed for MSI testing. When compared with non-tumor tissue, the threshold to define MSI is lowered to two unstable markers out of five [20].

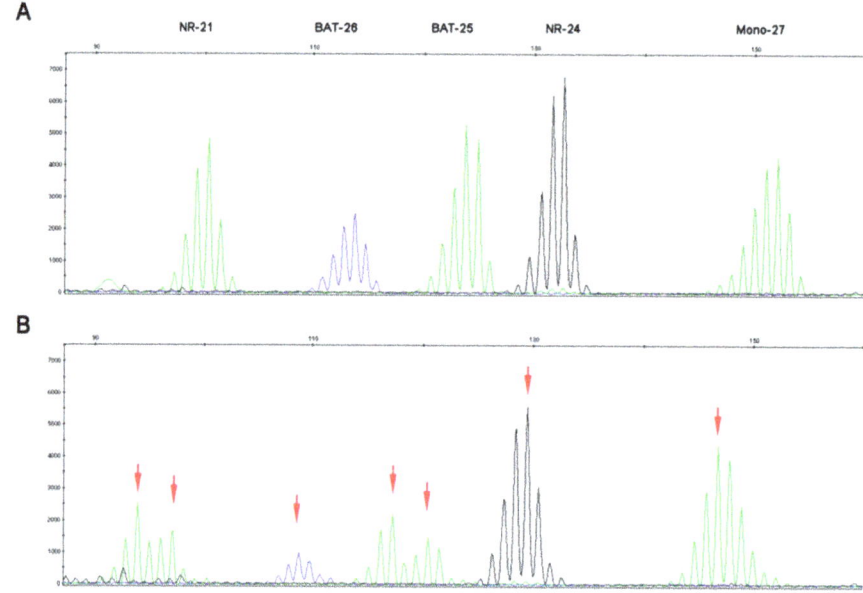

Figure 3. MSS and MSI profiles using the pentaplex panel. (**A**) MSS profile of the five consensus mononucleotide repeats and (**B**) MSI profile with 5 unstable mononucleotide repeats. Red arrows indicate microsatellite instability.

2.2. MMR Protein Testing

IHC is a technique detecting protein expression directly from tissue samples. As MMR proteins (MLH1, MSH2, MSH6, and PMS2) are in the nucleus, only nuclear staining is taken into account in MMR protein detection. MMR protein loss is defined by the absence of IHC staining in the nucleus of tumor cells, whereas normal cells remain stained, ensuring the technical validity of the experiment. Indeed, nuclear staining of non-cancerous stromal cells is considered a good internal positive control, even in Lynch syndrome, insofar as only one allele is mutated outside the tumor area (germline mutation of one allele of one MMR gene). A cell develops a DNA repair defect only when its second copy of the gene also becomes non-functional (Knudson's two-hit hypothesis) as a result of a random mutation (somatic mutation of the second allele of the same MMR gene). A loss of MMR protein expression means genomic alteration (loss of heterozygosity, mutations or epigenetic modifications) of the corresponding gene. A tumor is considered dMMR if one of the four MMR proteins is lost (absence of nuclear staining) (Figure 4).

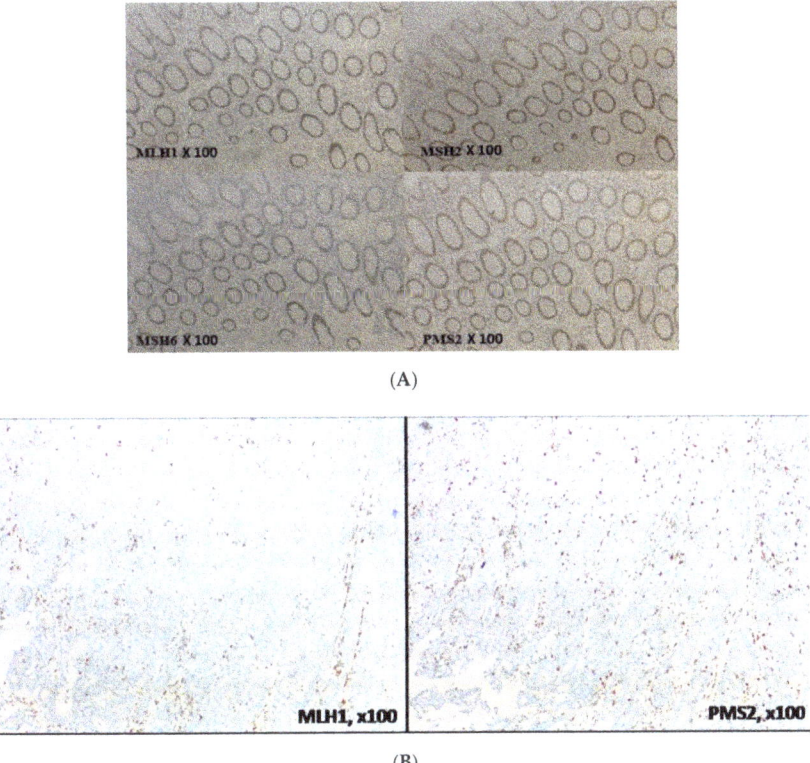

Figure 4. Immunochemistry of MMR proteins. (**A**) MMR-proficient (pMMR) tumor, normal colonic mucosa, no loss of expression of MMR proteins and (**B**) deficient MMR (dMMR) tumor with loss of MLH1 and PMS2 expression.

In the MMR system, protein functions are achieved by heterodimers, MLH1 being the PMS2 partner and MSH2 being the MSH6 partner. In their monomeric form, MMR proteins are degraded. Consequently, the loss of one MMR protein is usually accompanied by the loss of its partner. For instance, loss of MLH1 or MSH2 proteins will leave PMS2 and MSH6, respectively, in their monomeric forms, and they will be rapidly degraded. Consequently, loss of MLH1 expression is associated with PMS2 loss and loss of MSH2 expression is associated with MSH6 loss. However, the contrary is not true insofar as MLH1 and MSH2 proteins, in their monomeric forms, can interact with other proteins of the MMR system, i.e., MSH3, and thereby avoid degradation [21]. Indeed, isolated loss of PMS2 expression (≈5% to 10% of dMMR CRC [22]) or isolated loss of MSH6 expression (≈5% to 15% of dMMR CRC [23]) is not rare. In view of both economy and time saving, some pathologists have analyzed MMR expression of two proteins (MLH1 and MSH2) instead of four but have not been able to detect isolated loss of PMS2 or MSH6 expression. Indeed, most guidelines recommend performing IHC of all four MMR proteins to avoid misinterpretation [24].

2.3. Comparison of Molecular MSI Testing and MMR Proteins Immunohistochemistry

The molecular approach (MSI) presents the advantage of studying MMR system dysfunction and is not limited to protein expression. Indeed, some point mutations allow MMR protein expression (normal MMR proteins IHC), but without retaining the MMR function (MSI). However, MSI testing takes somewhat longer and costs a little more than the IHC technique and does not provide information as to which MMR gene is deficient.

While both MSI panels, the Bethesda and the pentaplex, use the two microsatellite markers *BAT-25* and *BAT-26*, polymorphisms have been reported for both, especially in African ethnicities [25]. To detect these polymorphisms and to avoid counting them as unstable markers, it is commonly admitted that an isolated unstable marker must be validated in comparison with the microsatellite profile of its matched non-tumor tissue, even for CRC using the pentaplex panel. In this case, MSI exploration will take longer. Finally, MSI interpretation requires trained molecular biologists, particularly to avoid misinterpretation of *BAT-25* or *BAT-26* microsatellites [25,26].

MMR protein IHC is easier and less expensive. Moreover, an isolated loss of MSH6 is not always responsible for MMR system deficiency, and hence not always detected by MSI technique [27,28]. Indeed, there exists functional redundancy of MMR proteins (PMS2 and PMS1, MSH6 and MSH3) with MMR protein expression loss at IHC loss, while MSS status is retained due to partial activity of the MMR system [22]. Moreover, MMR protein IHC can be difficult or misleading as it depends on staining processes, which are not standardized from one laboratory to another (antigen demasking, optimal antibody dilution, incubation time, etc.). Indeed, MMR protein IHC requires experienced pathologists [29]. The technique can give false positive results as a non-functional MMR protein can remain expressed in tumor tissue and detected by IHC even though the tumor is MSI. Indeed, although one third of *MLH1* mutations are missense mutations coding for non-functional proteins, MLH1 expression remains detected by IHC [28]. Heterogeneous loss of MMR protein expression has also been observed for MSH6 due to *MSH6* somatic mutations [30].

With regard to sensitivity and specificity of IHC, they vary from 81% to 100% and from 80% to 92%, respectively [31]. MSI analysis sensitivity ranges from 67% to 100% and specificity from 61% to 92% using the Bethesda panel. When using the pentaplex panel, sensitivity is better (89% to 100%) (no control with non-tumoral tissue) as is specificity (79% to 100%) [32,33].

3. Challenges for Determination of the dMMR/MSI Mechanism

3.1. How to Classify Sporadic versus Germline dMMR/MSI Colorectal Cancer?

MMR deficiency can be acquired in sporadic dMMR/MSI tumors or constitutively in Lynch syndrome-related dMMR/MSI tumors. About 75% of dMMR/MSI CRCs are sporadic cases. In most cases, observed loss of MLH1 expression is caused by hypermethylation of its promoter, acquired during tumorigenesis. This epigenetic modification is developed in the context of senescence with global hypermethylation of DNA, mainly at CpG islands [34]. CpG islands are regions of DNA that contain numerous Guanine Cytosine dinucleotides bound together by a phosphodiester and frequently found in gene promoters. Usually, when the cytosine is methylated in the promoter region, it causes inhibition of transcription of the gene. CRC with global DNA hypermethylation is called "hypermethylator" or CpG island methylator phenotype (CIMP). CIMP tumors are frequently associated with *BRAF* p.V600 mutation (from 77% to 95%) but their interconnections remain unclear [35,36]. Therefore, dMMR/MSI CRCs with MLH1 loss and *BRAF* mutation are considered as sporadic dMMR/MSI CRCs. In the case of dMMR/MSI CRC with MLH1 loss and *BRAF* wild type status, *MLH1* promoter methylation is determined and a *MLH1* promoter hypermethylation signs the sporadic trait of the tumor.

The second group of dMMR/MSI CRCs is primarily related to Lynch syndrome (LS), i.e., with detectable monoallelic germline mutation in one of the four MMR genes. The LS diagnosis is a confirmed mutation of one of the MMR genes. The percentage of mutations identified in the case of suspicion of LS is very variable according to the criteria selected, i.e., more than 90% in the case of loss of MSH2 or MSH6, about 70% if the Amsterdam II criteria are met, about 40% in case of loss of MLH1, and about 30% if the revised Bethesda criteria are met [37–39]. Most of the germline mutations in LS occur in *MLH1* or *MSH2* genes (90%) (Table 2). *MSH6* and *PMS2* genes are less frequently affected (about 10% of cases). In addition, the pathogenicity of *PMS2* mutations is more difficult to establish because of pseudogene interferences [40]. Pseudogenes are usually characterized by a combination of homology to a known gene and loss of some functionality. Indeed, a *PMS2* non-expressed pseudogene exists and is highly homologous in both intronic and exonic sequences to the *PMS2* gene, hence polymorphisms in this pseudogene can be mistaken for mutations in the *PMS2* gene.

Table 2. The mutation frequencies of mismatch repair gene in Lynch syndrome [37–39].

Mismatch Repair Gene	Mutation Frequency
MSH2	50%
MLH1	30–40%
MSH6	7–10%
PMS2	<5%
EPCAM	1–3%
Constitutional *MLH1* epimutation	1–3%

According to the model described by Knudson et al. for tumor suppressor genes such as MMR genes, one allele of the MMR gene has a germline mutation (first hit) and the second allele of the same MMR gene is inactivated at the somatic level (second hit) by various alterations (somatic mutation, genomic rearrangement, promoter hypermethylation, and loss of heterozygosity), which induce deficiency of the MMR system [41]. International guidelines have defined algorithms to efficiently identify LS patients among patients with sporadic dMMR/MSI tumors (Figure 5) [42].

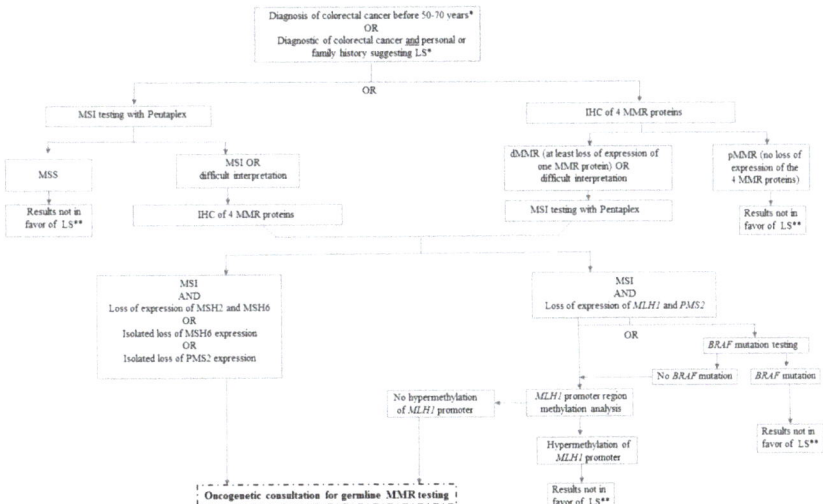

Figure 5. dMMR/MSI screening of colorectal cancer (CRC) for suspicion of Lynch syndrome. * According to the country and the guidelines, universal testing of CRC is recommended only if revised Bethesda criteria are met. ** A result that is not in favor of diagnosis of Lynch syndrome must be interpreted according to the patient's family history and if Lynch syndrome or another genetic predisposition is suspected, the patients must be referred to oncogenetic consultation. dMMR: deficient mismatch repair, IHC: immunohistochemistry, LS: Lynch syndrome, MSS: microsatellite stability, MSI: microsatellite instability, and pMMR: proficient mismatch repair.

3.2. MLH1 Promoter Hypermethylation

In dMMR/MSI CRC with loss of expression of MLH1, identification of the *MLH1* promoter hypermethylation and *BRAF* p.V600 mutation certifies the sporadic origin [24]. Conversely, if these alterations are not found, the patient should be referred to oncogenetics for MMR germline testing. Most teams initially limit their exploration to *BRAF* status due to cost and the time required for difficult

MLH1 promoter hypermethylation testing. In the event of dMMR/MSI CRC with loss of expression of MLH1 and *BRAF* wild-type status *MLH1* promoter hypermethylation testing is performed secondarily. Nevertheless, about 1% to 2% of LS cases (dMMR/MSI CRC with germline mutation) carry *BRAF* mutation [43]. These cases are rare but, at the individual level, the mis-screening of LS can have major consequences for the patient and his relatives. Indeed, dMMR/MSI *BRAF*-mutated CRC should be tested for *MLH1* promoter hypermethylation in the case of a high suspicion of LS to confirm, before germline MMR testing, that it is not a sporadic case.

Determination of somatic versus germline mechanism of dMMR/MSI CRC using methylation of the promoter of *MLH1* gene can sometimes be incorrect. While hypermethylation is mostly a somatic event, several cases of CRC with constitutional epimutations of the *MLH1* gene have been reported [44–46]. Constitutional *MLH1* epimutations cause severe LS phenotype, including young age of cancer onset and multiple primary tumors [45]. Usually, constitutional *MLH1* epimutation arises de novo with no or non-Mendelian inheritance and the second hit has a genetic, not an epigenetic basis (somatic mutation or loss of heterozygosity) [46]. Patients with dMMR/MSI CRC with *MLH1* promoter hypermethylation should be screened for constitutional *MLH1* epimutations in the case of early onset CRC (before 50 years) or with multiple tumors before 60 years [47].

3.3. Challenge in Determination of Lynch Syndrome

In approximately 60% to 70% of dMMR/MSI CRCs with suspected LS according to the revised Bethesda criteria, no mutation is identified (or variants of unknown significance) [48,49]. These tumors are called Lynch-like syndrome (LLS) and are a challenge for predisposition management of the patient and his family [48]. Indeed, the risk of colorectal cancer is higher in these families than in the general population but lower than in LS families [50]. LLS can be due to biallelic somatic inactivation of one MMR gene (or an allelic somatic mutation associated with loss of heterozygosity of the other allele), which means that the progeny of the patient has a risk of CRC equal to the general population. Indeed, upon excluding dMMR/MSI CRC patients with *MLH1* promoter hypermethylation and germline mutations, biallelic somatic inactivation is responsible for approximately 50% of the remaining dMMR/MSI CRCs [51]. Despite the evident interest of somatic exploration to avoid expensive and stressful screening protocol for a family with LLS, these tests are not routinely performed. Moreover, some of them remain unexplained and may be due to genetic alterations that have yet to be identified.

Another issue is the 3′ deletion of the *EPCAM* gene (epithelial cell adhesion molecule), also called *TACSTD1* (tumor-associated calcium signal transducer 1), which leads to a hypermethylator profile of its neighbor gene, *MSH2* [37]. The latter will not be expressed and a loss of MSH2/MSH6 protein will be detected by IHC. As no mutation in MMR genes will be detected by germline testing, the tumor can wrongly be classified as LLS with low cancer risk, whereas it is known that carriers of an *EPCAM* deletion have a cumulative risk of CRC similar to carriers of *MSH2* mutation [37]. Nevertheless, in most laboratories, germline *EPCAM* deletions are now analyzed primarily or secondarily in the absence of MMR mutation. The incidence of *EPCAM* deletions has appeared to vary between populations and may explain at least 1% to 3% of LS [52].

All in all, dMMR/MSI CRCs without evident sporadic mechanisms (i.e., *MLH1* promoter hypermethylation) and without germline mutation of *MLH1, PMS2, MSH2, MSH6*, deletion of *EPCAM* or germline *MLH1* promoter hypermethylation are considered unclassified as regards the molecular mechanism underlying the MMR deficiency, LS versus sporadic cases. This situation accounts for at least 30% of dMMR/MSI CRC patients with suspected LS [50,53]. These tumors are mostly 1-loss of MSH6 protein expression without *MSH6* germline mutation, 2-loss of MSH2 without *MSH2* germline mutation or *EPCAM* deletion, 3-loss of PMS2 with no loss of MLH1 and no *PMS2* germline mutation, and 4-loss of MLH1 protein expression with no *BRAF* mutation and no *MLH1* promoter hypermethylation and no *MLH1* germline mutation. These patients and their first-degree relatives must be considered as LS and monitored as such.

4. Discordance Between MMR Immunohistochemistry and DNA Microsatellites Testing

On the basis of the literature, discordances between IHC of MMR proteins and MSI molecular testing results range from 1% to 10% (Table 3).

Table 3. Rate of discordance between MMR immunohistochemistry and MSI testing in CRC.

Series *	Number of Patients	Population	MMR IHC	Molecular MSI Testing	Discordance Rates
Lindor NM et al., 2002 [54]	1144	From multiple centers from the Cooperative Family Registry for Colon Cancer Studies: USA, Australia, and Canada	2 proteins (MLH1 and MSH2)	10 markers: BAT25, BAT26, BAT40, BAT34C4, D5S346, D17S250, ACTC, D18S55, D10S197, and MYCL. or 6 markers: D5S346, TP53, D18S34, D18S49, D18S61, ACTC and BAT 26	2.4%
Hatch et al., 2005 [55]	262	CRC with complete resection	4 proteins (MLH1, MSH2, MSH6 and PMS2)	NCI panel (D5S346, BAT25, BAT26, D2S123, and D17S250)	5.4%
Pinol et al., 2005 [56]	1222	CRC in Spain	2 proteins (MSH2 and MLH1)	BAT26 ± BAT-25, D5S346, D2S123, and D17S250	2.8%
Watson et al., 2007 [57]	Cohort 1: 68 Cohort 2: 208	CRC patients younger than 60 years (BRAF mutated CRC are excluded in cohort 1)	4 proteins (MLH1, MSH2, MSH6 and PMS2)	Single microsatellite: BAT26	Cohort 1: 1.4% Cohort 2: 1%
Yuan L et al., 2015 [58]	296	CRC patients fulfilled revised Bethesda criteria	4 proteins (MLH1, MSH2, MSH6 and PMS2)	Bethesda panel	1%
Chen et al., 2018 [59]	569	Chinese monocentric study with only CRC	4 proteins (MLH1, MSH2, MSH6 and PMS2)	Bethesda panel	8.1%
Cohen et al., abstract ESMO 2018 [60]	92	CRC only	4 proteins (MLH1, MSH2, MSH6 and PMS2)	Pentaplex panel	9.1%
Jaffrelot M et al., abstract JFHOD 2019 [61]	2528	Patients with dMMR tumors (CRC, endometrium, non-colorectal digestive cancers and others)	4 proteins (MLH1, MSH2, MSH6 and PMS2)	Pentaplex panel	1.1%

CRC: colorectal cancer, IHC: immunohistochemistry, MMR: mismatch repair, MSI: microsatellite instability, and NCI: national institute cancer. * Only studies with more than 50 patients were included in the Table.

Studies evaluating discordances between molecular MSI and IHC tests in CRC are limited. Moreover, it is difficult to compare these studies with each other because the molecular panels used for MSI testing and the antibodies used for IHC are not the same. It is worth noting that the most frequently observed discordance was loss of MSH6 expression with MSS status [23]. Indeed, dMMR/MSS CRC with an isolated loss of MSH6 could be due to the partial redundancy of MSH6 and MSH3 protein function. When the MSH6 protein is impaired, the MSH2/MSH3 heterodimer continues to operate and DNA mismatch errors are partially corrected [26].

Unpublished data from our retrospective series of 1085 CRC patients showed 2.3% of discordances using IHC of the four MMR proteins and the pentaplex panel. Among the 25 discordant cases (2.3%), reviewing by expert biologists and pathologists enabled reclassification of seven cases, mostly because of misinterpretation of IHC due to poor quality of the staining or few tumor cells in the biopsy. The remaining 18 discordant cases (1.7%) were mainly dMMR/MSS tumors ($n = 15/18$) with isolated loss of MSH6 ($n = 6$). Indeed, pathologist and biologist expertise is crucial for accurate determination of dMMR and MSI status, as also described by Jaffrelot et al. [61]. They studied 2528 patients with different types of cancers with a discordance rate of 1.1%, using pentaplex panel for molecular biology and four proteins for IHC. Cohen et al. studied fewer patients ($n = 92$) but reported a higher discordance rate (9.8%) with the same two methods (pentaplex and four proteins) [60].

To avoid these discordances due to technical issues, it is necessary to follow some rules when performing the tests, mainly to use tumor samples with good quality, more than 20% of tumor cells and before any treatment, if possible (Table 4). Moreover, in cases of discordance, both tests must be repeated so as to detect errors or tumor heterogeneity.

Table 4. Main causes of discordances and quality criteria to prevent them.

Causes of Discordance	Quality Criteria to Prevent Discordance	
	MMR IHC	Molecular DNA testing
Low tumor cells [62]	Selection of a specific area with the highest rate of tumor cells	Macrodissection or selection of tumor sections enriched in tumor cells ($\geq 20\%$)
Pre-analytical difficulties [28]	Use formol 4% (not Bouin's fixative), protocol standardization efforts, participation in national and international quality assessment	Protocol standardization efforts, participation in national and international quality assessment
Non-expert physician [29]	Participation in training sessions and request for rereading by expert if necessary	
Neoadjuvant treatment [63]	Testing on pretherapeutic samples	
Polymorphisms in non-Caucasian ethnic groups	-	Testing of paired tumor and non-tumor tissues
Discordance of tumor biopsy	Testing of the complete surgical resection	
Heterogeneous IHC pattern (Tumor heterogeneity suspected) [64]	Multiple sampling	-

MMR: mismatch repair and IHC: immunohistochemistry.

Finally, 1% to 2% of discordances between MMR protein IHC and MSI molecular testing by pentaplex remain unexplained. In these cases, germline mutation testing of the MMR genes must be performed if LS is suspected. A diagnostic of LS implies a lifelong cancer screening protocol for the patient and their relatives. Moreover, a recent report suggests that half of the diagnoses of patients with mCRC and primary resistance to ICI are due to misinterpretation of the MMR IHC or MSI tests. Indeed, to avoid false positive of dMMR or MSI tests, both tests are recommended before ICI treatment, especially in clinical trials (Figure 6). Indeed, most trials with ICI now consider these discordances during patient inclusion. Whereas in previous studies, either dMMR or MSI status was required for patient inclusion [65,66], at present, both tests have to be performed with no discordance (dMMR and MSI) [67,68]. Patients with discordant tests are not eligible for these ongoing trials (pMMR/MSI or dMMR/MSS).

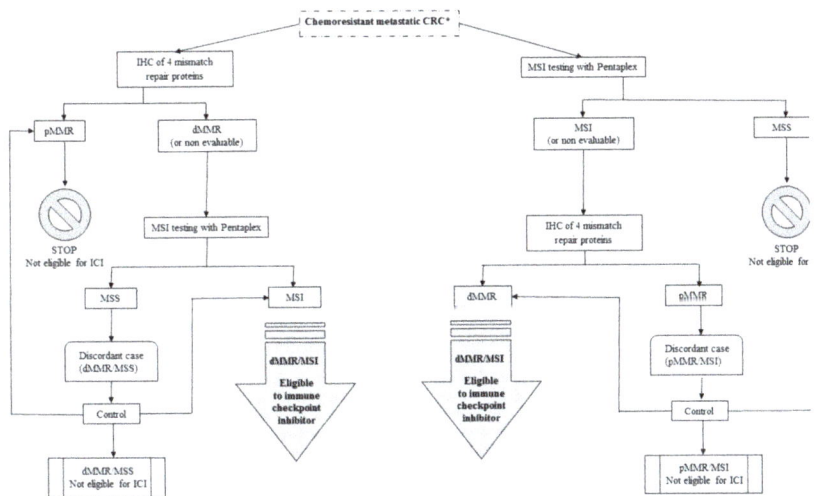

Figure 6. dMMR/MSI screening of metastatic CRC for eligibility to immune checkpoint inhibitors. * If no suspicion of Lynch syndrome. CRC: colorectal cancer, dMMR: deficient mismatch repair, IHC: immunohistochemistry, LS: Lynch syndrome, MSS: microsatellite stability, MSI: microsatellite instability, and pMMR: proficient mismatch repair.

Research is ongoing to improve detection of dMMR/MSI cases and to avoid discordant cases, with particular interest in the use of other microsatellite markers such as HSP110 [69] or an increased number of microsatellites analyzed using next-generation sequencing (NGS) [70] (see paragraph "perspective of MSI/MMR testing").

5. Focus on Tumor Heterogeneity

Although microsatellite instability is considered as an early event in CRC carcinogenesis, several recent studies have reported that microsatellite instability is not always a homogeneous event throughout the tumor in sporadic CRC [64,71]. Intra-tumoral heterogeneity is defined as the emergence of tumor subclones with different genotypes in the same tumor mass and inter-tumoral heterogeneity consists of the presence of at least two different tumor subclones on different tumor sites. Most studies in mCRC have reported good concordance in mutational profiles of major signaling pathways, such as *KRAS, TP53, APC, PIK3CA, BRAF,* and *NRAS,* between the primary tumor and its metastases, superior to 95% [72,73]. However, some recent studies using highly sensitive techniques or microdissection have identified tumor heterogeneity in CRC. Intra-tumoral and inter-tumoral heterogeneity of *KRAS* mutations is now well-known in mCRC and correlates with resistance or reduced efficacy of anti-EGFR therapies [74]. For instance, the Jeantet et al. study identified a high rate of *RAS* mutation heterogeneity in mCRCs with 33% of intra-tumoral heterogeneity and 36% of inter-tumoral heterogeneity [75]. Most articles about tumor heterogeneity have focused on common mutations such as *KRAS, TP53,* and *PIK3CA* while few data are available regarding MSI or MMR IHC tests and intra- and inter-tumoral heterogeneity, and its possible variations during the tumor growth process.

In Lynch syndrome, microsatellite instability is the primum movens of tumor carcinogenesis and all tumor cells should be dMMR/MSI with no heterogeneity. By contrast, in sporadic dMMR/MSI CRC and even if microsatellite instability is considered as an early event, MMR deficiency may emerge late in tumor progression with intra-tumoral or inter-tumoral heterogeneity. Indeed, according to Chapusot et al., among 100 sporadic proximal CRCs, eight present an uncommon MMR IHC pattern with loss of MMR expression (MLH1 and MSH6) restricted to small tumor areas and are MSI. Further analyses on other tumor areas finally established the presence of intra-tumoral heterogeneity [76].

Joost et al. collected 14 CRCs with heterogeneous IHC staining patterns that affected at least one of the MMR proteins, that is, MLH1/PMS2 in three tumors, PMS2 in two tumors, MSH2/MSH6 in 10 tumors (of which two also expressed heterogeneity for MLH1/PMS2), and MSH6 in one tumor. Analysis of these 14 sectioned tumor blocks by molecular biology using the pentaplex panel demonstrated intra-tumoral heterogeneity in three out of 14 tumors [71]. On the one hand, Tachon et al. reported a case of CRC with heterogeneous MLH1/PMS2 staining pattern in primary tumor confirmed by MSI testing, MSS in pMMR areas, and MSI in dMMR areas (intra-tumoral heterogeneity) [64]. By contrast, metastatic lymph nodes were pMMR/MSS. On the other hand, in a cohort of 271 CRC Asian patients, all MSI samples ($n = 39$) were dissected into three regions by tumors and analyzed using Bethesda panel and no intra-tumoral heterogeneity was detected [77].

Although they are rare, due to the prognostic and therapeutic impacts of dMMR and MSI status, detection of these atypical cases should be undertaken cautiously. Since most of these cases present atypical staining at MMR IHC, MSI will help to determine the major tumor subclones. In the case of discordance (dMMR/MSS), it may be useful to test at least two tumor areas of primary tumor or metastases with both techniques in order to identify tumor heterogeneity. Finally, large prospective studies are necessary to determine the rate of intra-tumoral and inter-tumoral heterogeneity of microsatellite instability and their impact on prognosis and treatment efficacy. As of now, there are no data concerning the efficacy of ICI in mCRC with intra- and inter-tumoral heterogeneity of dMMR and MSI status. Moreover, to our knowledge, there are no data concerning the dynamic evolution of MMR and MSI status during tumor progression, especially under treatment selection pressure.

6. Other Markers of Microsatellite Instability and Response to Immune Checkpoint Inhibitors

Finally, while MSI/dMMR reflects tumor genomic instability, it is not the only marker of response to ICI. Tumor mutational burden (TMB) has been described as predictive of response to ICI, in the subpopulation of MSI/dMMR mCRC [78], but not exclusively [79]. In dMMR CRC, due to frameshift mutations leading to abnormal truncated protein products, several immunogenic neoantigens are generated and explain the high number of tumor-infiltrating lymphocytes in these tumors [80]. For example, cytotoxic T lymphocytes specific to a neoantigen derived from *TGFbetaRII* frameshift mutation have been identified in dMMR CRC harboring this mutation [81]. Two triggering signals are required to initiate adaptive immune response by T cells: MHC-antigen (major histocompatibility complex) peptide recognition by the T-cell receptor and costimulation via a collection of receptors interacting with related ligands on antigen-presenting cells (APCs), thereby avoiding T-cell anergy [82]. CD28 is an example of costimulatory (positive) molecules and is constitutively expressed on the T-cell surface. It binds to B7.1 (CD80) or B7.2 (CD86), which are expressed on APCs and provides the positive costimulatory signal required for T-cell activation and survival [83]. In contrast, B7 molecules also interact with cytotoxic T-lymphocyte-associated antigen 4 (CTLA-4), which is expressed on T cells, to which it transmits an inhibitory costimulatory signal. In many cancers, especially dMMR/MSI mCRC, ligands of co-inhibitory immune checkpoint receptors are upregulated in a cancer cell or tumor microenvironment, leading to T-cell functional exhaustion and unresponsiveness (a state of anergy), and therefore to loss of tumor growth control (tumor escape). Other well-known immune checkpoints include PD-L1/PD-1, MHC class II and lymphocyte activation gene 3 (LAG-3), and galectin-9 and mucin domain-containing protein-3 (TIM-3). These interactions allow negative feedbacks and, using this rationale, several immune checkpoint inhibitors have been developed for cancer treatment (mAbs blocking co-inhibitory immune checkpoint receptors or their ligands). Indeed, hypermutated dMMR/MSI mCRCs, i.e., with high neoantigens load, have high sensitivity to immune checkpoint inhibitors, which reactivate cytotoxic T cells to kill dMMR/MSI tumors cells.

Alteration in *POLE* gene (DNA polymerase epsilon), observed in ≈0.5% of CRCs [84] can be detected somatically or constitutionally and is also responsible for tumor genomic instability, with an ultramutator phenotype and high TMB [85]. POLE encodes the major catalytic and proofreading subunits of the Polε DNA polymerase enzyme complex. The proofreading (exonuclease) function locates and replaces erroneous bases in the daughter strand through failed complementary pairing with the parental strand. High-fidelity incorporation of bases by POLE, coupled with its exonuclease proofreading function, ensures a low mutation rate. Clinically, patients in the POLE ultra-mutated group have been reported to have high sensitivity to ICI [85]. Recent reports suggest an overlap between dMMR and MSI status and POLE mutation.

A study has evaluated the relationship between MSI/dMMR, TMB, and PD-L1 expression in approximately 2000 tumor samples (1395 CRCs) [86]. About one-third of the MSI cases, all types of cancers combined, had TMB-low and only 26% of the MSI cases had positive PD-L1 status. All in all, only 0.6% of cancers combined the three positive markers (MSI, TMB high, and PD-L1 positive), although overlaps varied according to tumor type. Only 1.3% of CRCs combined the three positive markers (MSI, TMB high, and PD-L1 positive) but 5.7% were MSI, 6.7% TMB high, and 7.2% PD-L1 positive. In this CRC population, 5.4% of overlap MSI and TMB high and 1.6% of overlap MSI and PDL1 positive were observed [86]. For the moment, PD-L1 expression is not a proven biomarker to select mCRC patients for treatment with ICI [87] and TMB determination is too time-consuming and expensive for routine clinical practice. In spite of not being perfect, dMMR/MSI remains an established marker of response to ICI in mCRC and its determination is crucial [12]. Nevertheless, in mCRCs with discordances between IHC of MMR proteins and MSI, molecular testing determination of TMB could help to select mCRC patients for treatment with ICI. New biomarkers to select mCRC patients eligible for ICI are under investigation, especially immunoscore, which is being prospectively evaluated by our group in the Pochi trial (xelox, bevacizumab plus pembrolizumab in pMMR/MSS mCRC with high immunoscore).

Finally, molecular alterations associated with dMMR/MSI tumors, other than impairment of the four core MMR proteins, have recently been described. These alterations mostly impact histone methyltransferase or demethylase, with examples such as depletion of chromatin regulator SETD2 (set domain containing 2, methyltransferase) or deletion of FANCJ (Fanconi anemia, helicase) or overexpression of KDM4 (H3K36me2/me3 demethylase), which reduces the abundance of MSH6 [88–90]. In the Awwad et al. study, KMD4 overexpression led to disruption of MSH6 foci formation during S phase by demethylating its binding site, and resulted in a DNA mismatch repair system [90]. Genes involved in histone modification, such as SETD2, were significantly more mutated in older patients (≥65 years) and this enzyme modifies histone proteins associated with DNA that control the regulation of gene expression and DNA replication and prevent the association of MMR proteins with damaged DNA, thereby preventing DNA mismatch repair [91].

7. Perspectives of MMR Immunohistochemistry and DNA Microsatellites Testing

Aside from multiple tumor area testing and systematic double screening by MMR IHC and MSI tests, there are other ways to avoid false positives or false negatives, such as exploration of other microsatellite markers.

7.1. The Role of HSP110 Protein in the Diagnosis of Microsatellite Status

HSP110, a chaperon protein with a T_{17} mononucleotide repeat located within intron 8, described in CRC in 2011, shows a remarkably monomorphic profile in non-tumor tissue and is an interesting candidate for microsatellite instability assessment with IHC and in molecular biology (Figures 7 and 8) [69,92]. Buhard et al. have suggested that *HSP110 T_{17}* deletion is present in all true dMMR/MSI cases and should be used as a complementary test in discordant cases [69]. Indeed, from 70 patients with CRC considered to be at high risk of LS, 46 displayed unambiguous MSS status with the pentaplex panel and no aberrant HSP110 was detected in 45 of these 46 tumors (98%). For one patient with aberrant HSP110, MSI status was confirmed by IHC showing loss of MSH2 expression in the tumor. By contrast, in the Kim et al. study, 12% (n = 20/168) of MSI CRCs were not associated with instability of *HSP110 T_{17}* [93], however, based on our experience, establishment of HSP110 status by IHC or molecular technique (*HSP110 T_{17}* deletion) does not show 100% correlation and molecular determination of

$HSP110\ T_{17}$ deletion can be difficult. Finally, while more data are needed before using $HSP110\ T_{17}$ in routine clinical practice for MSI status determination, $HSP110\ T_{17}$ could be of help in difficult cases.

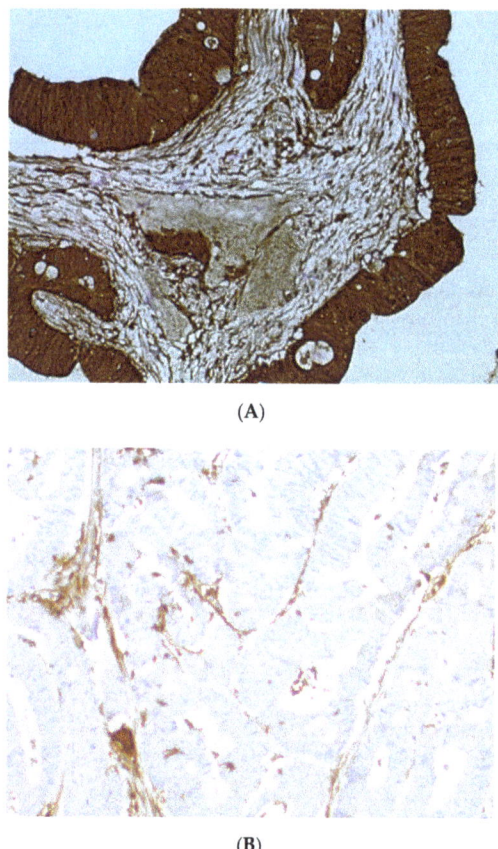

Figure 7. Immunohistochemistry of HSP110. (**A**) HSP110 expressed, ×20 and (**B**) loss of expression of HSP110, ×20.

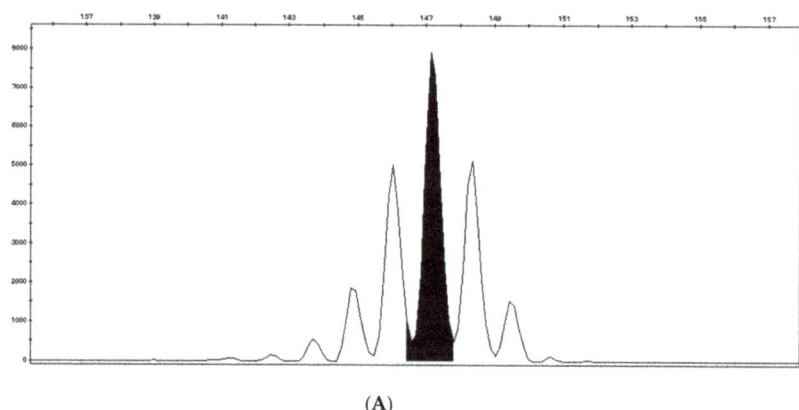

Figure 8. *Cont.*

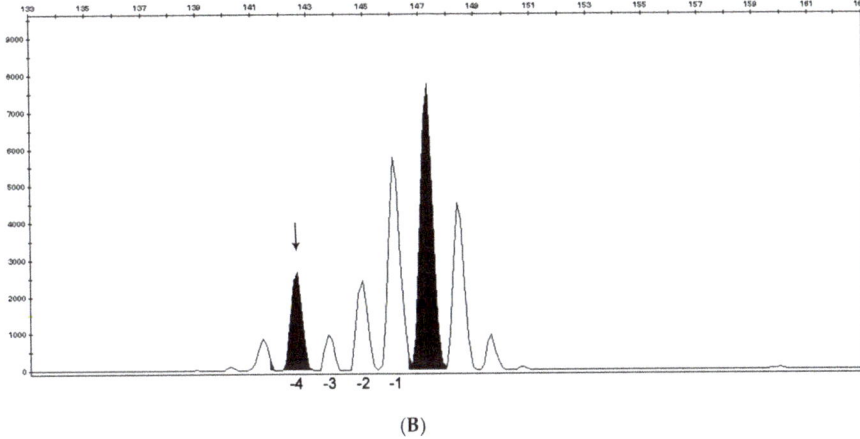

Figure 8. Microsatellite instability testing of *HSP110 T17*. (**A**) MSS tumor with T16/T16 phenotype (major peak at 147 bp) and (**B**) MSI tumor with large deletion of *HSP110 T17*, patient with a T16/T17 phenotype (peaks at 147 and 148 bps in the polymorphic zone). The major peak selected to determine size of the deletion is the peak at 147 bps and the black arrow corresponds to a deletion of 4 bps.

7.2. A Larger Panel of Microsatellites for Better Detection of Instability

To improve MSI detection, another way is to analyze a large panel of microsatellites instead of only five (i.e., pentaplex or Bethesda panels). Next-generation DNA sequencing (NGS), now routinely used for determination of molecular alterations in most cancers, can allow comprehensive investigation of multiple microsatellite loci simultaneously, while using appropriate computational tools. Several tools have been developed and compared to standard procedures [70,94,95]. The mSing method incorporating from 15 to 2957 microsatellite markers, has demonstrated 96.4% to 100% sensitivity and 97.2% to 100% specificity as compared to the pentaplex panel [94]. MSIsensor and MANTIS (microsatellite analysis for normal tumor instability), other computational tools for MSI detection with NGS, have also demonstrated their feasibility, although requiring non-tumor DNA [95,96]. MSIsensors scan a reference genome to locate homopolymers and microsatellites and then record homopolymers of at least 5 bp length and microsatellites of maximum repeat unit length five from the reference genome and each site is saved in a loci file for subsequent analysis. MANTIS uses a set of mono- to penta-nucleotide repeat microsatellites to detect MSI, by individually computing and aggregating the differences between the allele length distribution of each locus of matched tumor and normal samples to achieve an average distance score (zero, fully stable and two, fully unstable); a score threshold of 0.4 is recommended to diagnose MSI in tumors. MANTIS has displayed superior performance compared to the other tools (MANTIS, MSISensor, and mSINGS), having the highest overall sensitivity and specificity, even with loci panels of varying size. Nevertheless, interest in classifying cases with discordant MMR IHC and MSI results has never been explored. Moreover, NGS experiments are time-consuming and more expensive than standard MMR IHC/MSI techniques, notably due to the complex bioinformatic analysis required. The benefit and the place of this technique in this indication, therefore, remain to be precisely determined [97].

7.3. Tumor Circulating DNA to Overcome Tumor Heterogeneity

As previously highlighted, correct identification of dMMR and MSI status can be impaired by tumor heterogeneity, samples with few tumor cells or discordance between the two tests. Analysis of circulating tumor DNA (ctDNA) could be another method likely to easily determine MSI status. Tumor DNA is released into the bloodstream by exosome, secretion or necrosis and apoptosis. ctDNA allows direct analysis at a given time of all the molecular alterations present in the tumor and the metastases, in a minimally invasive way (blood test). To our knowledge, only two studies have reported the detection of MSI status using ctDNA [98,99]. In the Deng et al. study, 13 MSI CRCs based on standard MSI analysis (six mononucleotides: *NR-27, NR-21, BAT-26, BAT-25, NR-24,* and *MONO-27*), were correctly classified "MSI" using the NGS technique on tumoral tissue (analyses of the same microsatellite loci). On ctDNA of the same 13 patients, the standard MSI technique (by PCR) failed to detect MSI status while the NGS technique on ctDNA (the same as the one used for the tissue) correctly identified all MSI cases [98]. In the second study with pan-cancer, ctDNA testing using the Guardant360 (Guardant Health Clinical Laboratory, Redwood City, CA, US) NGS kit incorporating 99 putative microsatellite loci, accurately detected 87% (71/82) of tissue MSI-H and 99.5% of tissue microsatellite stability (863/867) with an overall accuracy of 98.4% (934/949) [99].

ctDNA testing allows non-invasive MSI testing at diagnosis and also provides an opportunity to follow the kinetics of MSI status. Monitoring MSI status at several time-points of tumor progression, especially at treatment start and at relapse or progression, may be of major interest for monitoring response to ICI (i.e., selection of pMMR/MSS subclones?) [100]. ctDNA testing could also help with regard to the tumor heterogeneity issue as it reflects all the tumor subclones at a specific time [101]. Multiple samplings would not be necessary as a single blood sample could detect all major clones located in the primary tumor and metastases as well. Nevertheless, as of now, we do not know whether dynamic change of MSI during carcinogenesis exists. Finally, as MMR IHC and MSI discordances are sometimes caused by insufficient sample quality or tumor cell quantity, ctDNA testing could also be an interesting substitute [102]. Nevertheless, more data are needed to validate MSI detection by ctDNA before application in routine clinical practice, which is ongoing in trials using ICI in dMMR/MSI tumors [98].

New techniques for MSI assessment will probably help to more accurately diagnose dMMR/MSI CRC and classify discordant cases such as MSI or MMS. However, while increasing the number of markers to define the MSI status, prognosis of the technique may not significantly improve. On the contrary, false positives may arise. Detection of cases with a low level of instability may be useful but can also be without a relevant impact on routine clinical practice. Indeed, one of the urgent questions to be addressed would be whether discordant cases or those with a low level of microsatellite instability could benefit from immune checkpoint inhibitor.

8. Conclusions

MMR/MSI screening is crucial not only for LS screening but also in therapeutic management, especially since the ICI revolution [89]. Indeed, patients with dMMR/MSI tumor have drawn a major benefit from immunotherapy, whatever the tumor type, with a rate of disease control reaching 80% and overall survival superior to three years in chemoresistant mCRC cases [10,12,103]. Consequently, all mCRCs should be tested for MMR and MSI status.

Since ICI is ineffective in pMMR/MSS CRC, as well as expensive and liable to induce severe side effects, it is essential to avoid false positive dMMR/MSI and false negative pMMR/MSS, and also to classify discordant cases (pMMR/MSI and dMMR/MSS) [104]. As recommended in recent trials with ICI, screening for ICI treatment in mCRC can be done by means of one test, MSI or MMR IHC, but in the case of a positive test or difficulties interpreting the results, the second test should be performed before treatment with ICI to confirm concordant dMMR/MSI results [67,68].

All the pitfalls of the different techniques must be known and any discordances should be investigated, in order to achieve the following: 1-control MMR IHC and MSI results, 2-check sample quality, 3-perform new tests on multiple tumor areas or sites, 4-test other microsatellites or ctDNA if techniques are available (or else, send sample to an expert team), and 5-perform MMR germline testing in the case of suspicion of LS. Indeed, rates of "true" discordant cases remain low. New techniques for MSI assessment (NGS, ctDNA, etc.) will probably help to more accurately diagnose dMMR/MSI CRC, which is a major challenge for these patients to have access to immunotherapy.

Author Contributions: Conceptualization, C.E. and D.T.; validation, C.E., G.T., V.R., L.K.-T., D.T.; investigation, C.E. and G.T.; resources, D.T.; data curation, C.E., G.T., V.R., L.K.-T., D.T.; writing—original draft preparation, C.E. and G.T.; writing—review and editing, C.E, G.T, V.R., L.K.-T., D.T.

Funding: This research received no external funding.

Acknowledgments: The authors wish to thank Vanessa Le Berre for her assistance in preparing the submission of the article and Jeffrey Arsham, an American medical translator, for reviewing our original English-language manuscript.

Conflicts of Interest: The authors have no relevant affiliations or financial involvement with any organization or entity with a financial interest in or financial conflict with the subject matter or materials discussed in the manuscript. This includes employment, consultancies, honoraria, stock ownership or options, expert testimony, grants or patents received or pending, or royalties. Peer reviewers on this manuscript have no relevant financial or other relationships to disclose.

Abbreviations

ADP	adenosine diphosphate
APC	*adenomatosis polyposis coli*
APCs	antigen-presenting cells
ATP	adenosine triphosphate
CRC	colorectal caner
ctDNA	circulating tumor DNA
dMMR	deficient mismatch repair
ICI	immune checkpoint inhibitor
IHC	immunohistochemistry
LS	Lynch syndrome
mCRC	metastatic colorectal cancer
MHC	major histocompatibility complex
MMR	mismatch repair
MSI	microsatellite instability
MSS	microsatellite stability
NGS	next-generation sequencing
NCI	national cancer institute
PCNA	proliferating cell nuclear antigen
PCR	polymerase chain reaction
PD-L1	programmed death ligand
pMMR	proficient mismatch repair
TMB	tumor mutational burden
LAG-3	lymphocyte activation gene 3
TIM-3	mucin domain-containing protein-3

References

1. Tariq, K.; Ghias, K. Colorectal cancer carcinogenesis: A review of mechanisms. *Cancer Biol. Med.* **2016**, *13*, 120. [CrossRef] [PubMed]
2. Snover, D.C. Update on the serrated pathway to colorectal carcinoma. *Hum. Pathol.* **2011**, *42*, 1–10. [CrossRef] [PubMed]
3. Fishel, R. Mismatch Repair. *J. Biol. Chem.* **2015**, *290*, 26395. [CrossRef] [PubMed]
4. Kawasoe, Y.; Tsurimoto, T.; Nakagawa, T.; Masukata, H.; Takahashi, T.S. MutSα maintains the mismatch repair capability by inhibiting PCNA unloading. *Elife* **2016**, *5*, e15155. [CrossRef] [PubMed]
5. Sinicrope, F.A.; Sargent, D.J. Molecular Pathways: Microsatellite Instability in Colorectal Cancer: Prognostic, Predictive, and Therapeutic Implications. *Clin. Cancer Res.* **2012**, *18*, 1506–1512. [CrossRef] [PubMed]
6. Hampel, H.; Frankel, W.L.; Martin, E.; Arnold, M.; Khanduja, K.; Kuebler, P.; Clendenning, M.; Sotamaa, K.; Prior, T.; Westman, J.A.; et al. Feasibility of Screening for Lynch Syndrome Among Patients with Colorectal Cancer. *J. Clin. Oncol.* **2008**, *26*, 5783. [CrossRef] [PubMed]

7. Ribic, C.M.; Sargent, D.J.; Moore, M.J.; Thibodeau, S.N.; French, A.J.; Goldberg, R.M.; Hamilton, S.R.; Laurent-Puig, P.; Gryfe, R.; Shepherd, L.E.; et al. Tumor Microsatellite-Instability Status as a Predictor of Benefit from Fluorouracil-Based Adjuvant Chemotherapy for Colon Cancer. *N. Engl. J. Med.* **2003**, *349*, 247. [CrossRef] [PubMed]
8. Tougeron, D.; Mouillet, G.; Trouilloud, I.; Lecomte, T.; Coriat, R.; Aparicio, T.; Des Guetz, G.; Lécaille, C.; Artru, P.; Sickersen, G.; et al. Efficacy of Adjuvant Chemotherapy in Colon Cancer with Microsatellite Instability: A Large Multicenter AGEO Study. *J. Natl. Cancer Inst.* **2016**, *108*, djv438. [CrossRef]
9. Venderbosch, S.; Nagtegaal, I.D.; Maughan, T.S.; Smith, C.G.; Cheadle, J.P.; Fisher, D.; Kaplan, R.; Quirke, P.; Seymour, M.T.; Richman, S.D.; et al. Mismatch repair status and BRAF mutation status in metastatic colorectal cancer patients: A pooled analysis of the CAIRO, CAIRO2, COIN and FOCUS studies. *Clin. Cancer Res.* **2014**, *20*, 5322–5330. [CrossRef]
10. Le, D.T.; Uram, J.N.; Wang, H.; Bartlett, B.R.; Kemberling, H.; Eyring, A.D.; Skora, A.D.; Luber, B.S.; Azad, N.S.; Laheru, D.; et al. PD-1 Blockade in Tumors with Mismatch-Repair Deficiency. *N. Engl. J. Med.* **2015**, *372*, 2509–2520. [CrossRef]
11. Tougeron, D.; Sueur, B.; Sefrioui, D.; Gentilhomme, L.; Lecomte, T.; Aparicio, T.; DES Guetz, G.; Artru, P.; De La Fouchardiere, C.; Moulin, V.; et al. A large multicenter study evaluating prognosis and chemosensitivity of metastatic colorectal cancers with microsatellite instability. *J. Clin. Oncol.* **2017**, *35*, 3536. [CrossRef]
12. Le, D.T.; Durham, J.N.; Smith, K.N.; Wang, H.; Bartlett, B.R.; Aulakh, L.K.; Lu, S.; Kemberling, H.; Wilt, C.; Luber, B.S.; et al. Mismatch repair deficiency predicts response of solid tumors to PD-1 blockade. *Science* **2017**, *357*, 409–413. [CrossRef] [PubMed]
13. Overman, M.J.; Lonardi, S.; Wong, K.Y.M.; Lenz, H.J.; Gelsomino, F.; Aglietta, M.; Morse, M.A.; Van Cutsem, E.; McDermott, R.; Hill, A.; et al. Durable Clinical Benefit with Nivolumab Plus Ipilimumab in DNA Mismatch Repair-Deficient/Microsatellite Instability-High Metastatic Colorectal Cancer. *J. Clin. Oncol.* **2018**, *36*, 773–779. [CrossRef] [PubMed]
14. Umar, A.; Boland, C.R.; Terdiman, J.P.; Syngal, S.; de la Chapelle, A.; Rüschoff, J.; Fishel, R.; Lindor, N.M.; Burgart, L.J.; Hamelin, R.; et al. Revised Bethesda Guidelines for Hereditary Nonpolyposis Colorectal Cancer (Lynch Syndrome) and Microsatellite Instability. *J. Natl. Cancer Inst.* **2004**, *96*, 261–268. [CrossRef] [PubMed]
15. Vasen, H.F.A.; Möslein, G.; Alonso, A.; Aretz, S.; Bernstein, I.; Bertario, L.; Blanco, I.; Bulow, S.; Burn, J.; Capella, G.; et al. Recommendations to improve identification of hereditary and familial colorectal cancer in Europe. *Fam. Cancer* **2010**, *9*, 109–115. [CrossRef] [PubMed]
16. Boland, C.R.; Thibodeau, S.N.; Hamilton, S.R.; Sidransky, D.; Eshleman, J.R.; Burt, R.W.; Meltzer, S.J.; Rodriguez-Bigas, M.A.; Fodde, R.; Ranzani, G.N.; et al. A National Cancer Institute Workshop on Microsatellite Instability for Cancer Detection and Familial Predisposition: Development of International Criteria for the Determination of Microsatellite Instability in Colorectal Cancer. *Cancer Res.* **1998**, *58*, 5248–5257.
17. Scarisbrick, J.J.; Mitchell, T.J.; Calonje, E.; Orchard, G.; Russell-Jones, R.; Whittaker, S.J. Microsatellite Instability Is Associated with Hypermethylation of the hMLH1 Gene and Reduced Gene Expression in Mycosis Fungoides. *J. Investig. Dermatol.* **2003**, *121*, 894–901. [CrossRef]
18. Murphy, K.M.; Zhang, S.; Geiger, T.; Hafez, M.J.; Bacher, J.; Berg, K.D.; Eshleman, J.R. Comparison of the Microsatellite Instability Analysis System and the Bethesda Panel for the Determination of Microsatellite Instability in Colorectal Cancers. *J. Mol. Diagn.* **2006**, *8*, 305–311. [CrossRef]
19. Suraweera, N.; Duval, A.; Reperant, M.; Vaury, C.; Furlan, D.; Leroy, K.; Seruca, R.; Iacopetta, B.; Hamelin, R. Evaluation of tumor microsatellite instability using five quasimonomorphic mononucleotide repeats and pentaplex PCR. *Gastroenterology* **2002**, *123*, 1804–1811. [CrossRef]
20. Wong, Y.F.; Cheung, T.H.; Lo, K.W.K.; Yim, S.F.; Chan, L.K.Y.; Buhard, O.; Duval, A.; Chung, T.K.H.; Hamelin, R. Detection of microsatellite instability in endometrial cancer: Advantages of a panel of five mononucleotide repeats over the National Cancer Institute panel of markers. *Carcinogenesis* **2006**, *27*, 951–955. [CrossRef]
21. Acharya, S.; Wilson, T.; Gradia, S.; Kane, M.F.; Guerrette, S.; Marsischky, G.T.; Kolodner, R.; Fishel, R. hMSH2 forms specific mispair-binding complexes with hMSH3 and hMSH6. *Proc. Natl. Acad. Sci. USA* **1996**, *93*, 13629–13634. [CrossRef] [PubMed]

22. Liu, W.; Zhang, D.; Tan, S.A.; Liu, X.; Lai, J. Sigmoid Colon Adenocarcinoma with Isolated Loss of PMS2 Presenting in a Patient with Synchronous Prostate Cancer with Intact MMR: Diagnosis and Analysis of the Family Pedigree. *Anticancer Res.* **2018**, *38*, 4847–4852. [CrossRef] [PubMed]
23. Verma, L.; Kane, M.F.; Brassett, C.; Schmeits, J.; Evans, D.G.R.; Kolodner, R.D.; Maher, E.R. Mononucleotide microsatellite instability and germline MSH6 mutation analysis in early onset colorectal cancer. *J. Med. Genet.* **1999**, *36*, 678–682. [PubMed]
24. INCA. *Tests Somatiques Recherchant une Déficience du Système MMR au Sein des Tumeurs du Spectre du Syndrome de Lynch*; Institut National du Cancer: Boulogne-Billancourt, France, 2016.
25. Pyatt, R.; Chadwick, R.B.; Johnson, C.K.; Adebamowo, C.; de la Chapelle, A.; Prior, T.W. Polymorphic Variation at the BAT-25 and BAT-26 Loci in Individuals of African Origin: Implications for Microsatellite Instability Testing. *Am. J. Pathol.* **1999**, *155*, 349–353. [CrossRef]
26. Zhang, L. Immunohistochemistry versus microsatellite instability testing for screening colorectal cancer patients at risk for hereditary nonpolyposis colorectal cancer syndrome. Part II. The utility of microsatellite instability testing. *J. Mol. Diagn.* **2008**, *10*, 301–307. [CrossRef] [PubMed]
27. Bao, F.; Panarelli, N.C.; Rennert, H.; Sherr, D.L.; Yantiss, R.K. Neoadjuvant therapy induces loss of MSH6 expression in colorectal carcinoma. *Am. J. Surg. Pathol.* **2010**, *34*, 1798–1804. [CrossRef] [PubMed]
28. Shia, J. Immunohistochemistry versus microsatellite instability testing for screening colorectal cancer patients at risk for hereditary nonpolyposis colorectal cancer syndrome. Part I. The utility of immunohistochemistry. *J. Mol. Diagn.* **2008**, *10*, 293–300. [CrossRef] [PubMed]
29. Overbeek, L.I.H.; Ligtenberg, M.J.L.; Willems, R.W.; Hermens, R.P.M.G.; Blokx, W.A.M.; Dubois, S.V.; van der Linden, H.; Meijer, J.W.R.; Mlynek-Kersjes, M.L.; Hoogerbrugge, N.; et al. Interpretation of Immunohistochemistry for Mismatch Repair Proteins is Only Reliable in a Specialized Setting. *Am. J. Surg. Pathol.* **2008**, *32*, 1246. [CrossRef]
30. McCarthy, A.J.; Capo-Chichi, J.M.; Spence, T.; Grenier, S.; Stockley, T.; Kamel-Reid, S.; Serra, S.; Sabatini, P.; Chetty, R. Heterogenous loss of mismatch repair (MMR) protein expression: A challenge for immunohistochemical interpretation and microsatellite instability (MSI) evaluation. *J. Pathol. Clin. Res.* **2019**, *5*, 115–129. [CrossRef]
31. Snowsill, T.; Coelho, H.; Huxley, N.; Jones-Hughes, T.; Briscoe, S.; Frayling, I.M.; Hyde, C. Molecular testing for Lynch syndrome in people with colorectal cancer: Systematic reviews and economic evaluation. *Health Technol. Assess. Winch. Engl.* **2017**, *21*, 1–238. [CrossRef]
32. Goel, A.; Nagasaka, T.; Hamelin, R.; Boland, C.R. An Optimized Pentaplex PCR for Detecting DNA Mismatch Repair-Deficient Colorectal Cancers. *PLoS ONE* **2010**, *5*, e9393. [CrossRef]
33. Xicola, R.M.; Llor, X.; Pons, E.; Castells, A.; Alenda, C.; Piñol, V.; Andreu, M.; Castellví-Bel, S.; Payá, A.; Jover, R.; et al. Performance of Different Microsatellite Marker Panels for Detection of Mismatch Repair–Deficient Colorectal Tumors. *J. Natl. Cancer Inst.* **2007**, *99*, 244–252. [CrossRef] [PubMed]
34. Robertson, K.D. DNA methylation and human disease. *Nat. Rev. Genet.* **2005**, *6*, 597–610. [CrossRef] [PubMed]
35. Weisenberger, D.J.; Siegmund, K.D.; Campan, M.; Young, J.; Long, T.I.; Faasse, M.A.; Kang, G.H.; Widschwendter, M.; Weener, D.; Buchanan, D.; et al. CpG island methylator phenotype underlies sporadic microsatellite instability and is tightly associated with *BRAF* mutation in colorectal cancer. *Nat. Genet.* **2006**, *38*, 787–793. [CrossRef] [PubMed]
36. Kambara, T.; Simms, L.A.; Whitehall, V.L.J.; Spring, K.J.; Wynter, C.V.A.; Walsh, M.D.; Barker, M.A.; Arnold, S.; McGivern, A.; Matsubara, N.; et al. BRAF mutation is associated with DNA methylation in serrated polyps and cancers of the colorectum. *Gut* **2004**, *53*, 1137–1144. [CrossRef] [PubMed]
37. Tutlewska, K.; Lubinski, J.; Kurzawski, G. Germline deletions in the EPCAM gene as a cause of Lynch syndrome—Literature review. *Hered. Cancer Clin. Pract.* **2013**, *11*, 9. [CrossRef]
38. Ward, R.L.; Dobbins, T.; Lindor, N.M.; Rapkins, R.W.; Hitchins, M.P. Identification of constitutional *MLH1* epimutations and promoter variants in colorectal cancer patients from the Colon Cancer Family Registry. *Genet. Med.* **2013**, *15*, 25–35. [CrossRef]
39. Crépin, M.; Dieu, M.C.; Lejeune, S.; Escande, F.; Boidin, D.; Porchet, N.; Morin, G.; Manouvrier, S.; Mathieu, M.; Buisine, M.P. Evidence of constitutional MLH1 epimutation associated to transgenerational inheritance of cancer susceptibility. *Hum. Mutat.* **2012**, *33*, 180–188. [CrossRef]

40. Chadwick, R.B.; Meek, J.E.; Prior, T.W.; Peltomaki, P.; de la Chapelle, A. Polymorphisms in a pseudogene highly homologous to PMS2. *Hum. Mutat.* **2000**, *16*, 530. [CrossRef]
41. Knudson, A.G. Two genetic hits (more or less) to cancer. *Nat. Rev. Cancer* **2001**, *1*, 157–162. [CrossRef]
42. Sinicrope, F.A. Lynch Syndrome–Associated Colorectal Cancer. *N. Engl. J. Med.* **2018**, *379*, 764–773. [CrossRef] [PubMed]
43. Parsons, M.T.; Buchanan, D.D.; Thompson, B.; Young, J.P.; Spurdle, A.B. Correlation of tumour BRAF mutations and MLH1 methylation with germline mismatch repair (MMR) gene mutation status: A literature review assessing utility of tumour features for MMR variant classification. *J. Med. Genet.* **2012**, *49*, 151–157. [CrossRef] [PubMed]
44. Dámaso, E.; Castillejo, A.; Arias, M.D.M.; Canet-Hermida, J.; Navarro, M.; Del Valle, J.; Campos, O.; Fernández, A.; Marín, F.; Turchetti, D.; et al. Primary constitutional MLH1 epimutations: A focal epigenetic event. *Br. J. Cancer* **2018**, *119*, 978–987. [CrossRef] [PubMed]
45. Goel, A.; Nguyen, T.P.; Leung, H.C.E.; Nagasaka, T.; Rhees, J.; Hotchkiss, E.; Arnold, M.; Banerji, P.; Koi, M.; Kwok, C.T.; et al. De novo constitutional MLH1 epimutations confer early-onset colorectal cancer in two new sporadic Lynch syndrome cases, with derivation of the epimutation on the paternal allele in one. *Int. J. Cancer* **2011**, *128*, 869–878. [CrossRef]
46. Hitchins, M.P.; Ward, R.L. Constitutional (germline) MLH1 epimutation as an aetiological mechanism for hereditary non-polyposis colorectal cancer. *J. Med. Genet.* **2009**, *46*, 793–802. [CrossRef]
47. Pineda, M.; Mur, P.; Iniesta, M.D.; Borràs, E.; Campos, O.; Vargas, G.; Iglesias, S.; Fernández, A.; Gruber, S.B.; Lázaro, C.; et al. MLH1 methylation screening is effective in identifying epimutation carriers. *Eur. J. Hum. Genet.* **2012**, *20*, 1256–1264. [CrossRef]
48. Carethers, J.M. Differentiating Lynch-like from Lynch Syndrome. *Gastroenterology* **2014**, *146*, 602–604. [CrossRef]
49. Antelo, M.; Golubicki, M.; Roca, E.; Mendez, G.; Carballido, M.; Iseas, S.; Cuatrecasas, M.; Moreira, L.; Sanchez, A.; Carballal, S.; et al. Lynch-like syndrome is as frequent as Lynch syndrome in early-onset nonfamilial nonpolyposis colorectal cancer. *Int. J. Cancer* **2019**, *145*, 705–713. [CrossRef]
50. Rodríguez-Soler, M.; Pérez-Carbonell, L.; Guarinos, C.; Zapater, P.; Castillejo, A.; Barberá, V.M.; Juárez, M.; Bessa, X.; Xicola, R.M.; Clofent, J.; et al. Risk of Cancer in Cases of Suspected Lynch Syndrome without Germline Mutation. *Gastroenterology* **2013**, *144*, 926–932. [CrossRef]
51. Geurts-Giele, W.R.R.; Leenen, C.H.M.; Dubbink, H.J.; Meijssen, I.C.; Post, E.; Sleddens, H.F.B.M.; Kuipers, E.J.; Goverde, A.; van den Ouweland, A.M.W.; van Lier, M.G.F.; et al. Somatic aberrations of mismatch repair genes as a cause of microsatellite-unstable cancers. *J. Pathol.* **2014**, *234*, 548–559. [CrossRef]
52. Kuiper, R.P.; Vissers, L.E.L.M.; Venkatachalam, R.; Bodmer, D.; Hoenselaar, E.; Goossens, M.; Haufe, A.; Kamping, E.; Niessen, R.C.; Hogervorst, F.B.L.; et al. Recurrence and variability of germline EPCAM deletions in Lynch syndrome. *Hum. Mutat.* **2011**, *32*, 407–414. [CrossRef] [PubMed]
53. Pearlman, R.; Haraldsdottir, S.; de la Chapelle, A.; Jonasson, J.G.; Liyanarachchi, S.; Frankel, W.L.; Rafnar, T.; Stefansson, K.; Pritchard, C.C.; Hampel, H. Clinical Characteristics of Colorectal Cancer Patients with Double Somatic Mismatch Repair Mutations Compared to Lynch Syndrome. *J. Med. Genet.* **2019**, *56*, 462. [CrossRef] [PubMed]
54. Lindor, N.M.; Burgart, L.J.; Leontovich, O.; Goldberg, R.M.; Cunningham, J.M.; Sargent, D.J.; Walsh-Vockley, C.; Petersen, G.M.; Walsh, M.D.; Leggett, B.A.; et al. Immunohistochemistry versus microsatellite instability testing in phenotyping colorectal tumors. *J. Clin. Oncol.* **2002**, *20*, 1043–1048. [CrossRef] [PubMed]
55. Hatch, S.B. Microsatellite Instability Testing in Colorectal Carcinoma: Choice of Markers Affects Sensitivity of Detection of Mismatch Repair-Deficient Tumors. *Clin. Cancer Res.* **2005**, *11*, 2180–2187. [CrossRef]
56. Piñol, V.; Castells, A.; Andreu, M.; Castellví-Bel, S.; Alenda, C.; Llor, X.; Xicola, R.M.; Rodríguez-Moranta, F.; Payá, A.; Jover, R.; et al. Accuracy of Revised Bethesda Guidelines, Microsatellite Instability, and Immunohistochemistry for the Identification of Patients with Hereditary Nonpolyposis Colorectal Cancer. *JAMA* **2005**, *293*, 1986–1994. [CrossRef]
57. Watson, N.; Grieu, F.; Morris, M.; Harvey, J.; Stewart, C.; Schofield, L.; Goldblatt, J.; Iacopetta, B. Heterogeneous Staining for Mismatch Repair Proteins during Population-Based Prescreening for Hereditary Nonpolyposis Colorectal Cancer. *J. Mol. Diagn.* **2007**, *9*, 472–478. [CrossRef]

58. Yuan, L.; Chi, Y.; Chen, W.; Chen, X.; Wei, P.; Sheng, W.; Zhou, X.; Shi, D. Immunohistochemistry and microsatellite instability analysis in molecular subtyping of colorectal carcinoma based on mismatch repair competency. *Int. J. Clin. Exp. Med.* **2015**, *8*, 20988.
59. Chen, M.; Chen, J.; Hu, J.; Chen, Q.; Yu, L.; Liu, B.; Qian, X.; Yang, M. Comparison of microsatellite status detection methods in colorectal carcinoma. *Int. J. Clin. Exp. Pathol.* **2018**, *11*, 1431–1438.
60. Cohen, R.; Hain, E.; Buhard, O.; Guilloux, A.; Bardier, A.; Kaci, R.; Bertheau, P.; Renaud, F.; Bibeau, F.; Fléjou, J.F. 537P Assessment of local clinical practice for testing of mismatch repair deficiency in metastatic colorectal cancer: The need for new diagnostic guidelines prior to immunotherapy. *Ann. Oncol.* **2018**, *29*, mdy281-083. [CrossRef]
61. Jaffrelot, M.; Laurenty, A.P.; Fares, N.; Staub, A.; Bonnet, D.; Danjoux, M.; Vande Perre, P.; Meilleroux, J.; Chipoulet, F.; Toulas, C.; et al. Fiabilité de l'étude du phénotype MMR tumoral: Étude a partir d'une cohorte de 4 948 cas de tests MSI et analyse des phénotypes atypiques. In Proceedings of the JFHOD, Paris, France, 21–24 March 2019.
62. Wang, Y. Differences in Microsatellite Instability Profiles between Endometrioid and Colorectal Cancers. *J. Mol. Diagn.* **2017**, *19*, 57–64. Available online: https://www-ncbi-nlm-nih-gov.gate2.inist.fr/pmc/articles/PMC5225298/ (accessed on 30 June 2019). [CrossRef]
63. Goldstein, J.B.; Wu, W.; Borras, E.; Masand, G.; Cuddy, A.; Mork, M.E.; Bannon, S.A.; Lynch, P.M.; Rodriguez-Bigas, M.; Taggart, M.W.; et al. Can Microsatellite Status of Colorectal Cancer Be Reliably Assessed after Neoadjuvant Therapy? *Clin. Cancer Res.* **2017**, *23*, 5246–5254. [CrossRef] [PubMed]
64. Tachon, G.; Frouin, E.; Karayan-Tapon, L.; Auriault, M.L.; Godet, J.; Moulin, V.; Wang, Q.; Tougeron, D. Heterogeneity of mismatch repair defect in colorectal cancer and its implications in clinical practice. *Eur. J. Cancer* **2018**, *95*, 112–116. [CrossRef] [PubMed]
65. Andre, T.; Lonardi, S.; Wong, K.Y.M.; Morse, M.; McDermott, R.S.; Hill, A.G.; Hendlisz, A.; Lenz, H.J.; Leach, J.W.; Moss, R.A.; et al. Combination of nivolumab (nivo) + ipilimumab (ipi) in the treatment of patients (pts) with deficient DNA mismatch repair (dMMR)/high microsatellite instability (MSI-H) metastatic colorectal cancer (mCRC): CheckMate 142 study. *J. Clin. Oncol.* **2017**, *35*, 3531. [CrossRef]
66. Diaz, L.A.; Le, D.T.; Yoshino, T.; Andre, T.; Bendell, J.C.; Koshiji, M.; Zhang, Y.; Kang, S.P.; Lam, B.; Jäger, D. KEYNOTE-177: Randomized phase III study of pembrolizumab versus investigator-choice chemotherapy for mismatch repair-deficient or microsatellite instability-high metastatic colorectal carcinoma. *J. Clin. Oncol.* **2017**, *35*, TPS815. [CrossRef]
67. Standard Chemotherapy vs. Immunotherapie in 2nd Line Treatment of MSI Colorectal Mestastatic Cancer. Full Text View. Available online: https://clinicaltrials.gov/ct2/show/NCT03186326 (accessed on 18 August 2019).
68. Interest of iRECIST Evaluation for DCR for Evaluation of Patients with Deficient MMR and /or MSI Metastatic Colorectal Cancer Treated with Nivolumab and Ipilimumab. Full Text View. Available online: https://clinicaltrials.gov/ct2/show/NCT03350126 (accessed on 18 August 2019).
69. Buhard, O.; Lagrange, A.; Guilloux, A.; Colas, C.; Chouchène, M.; Wanherdrick, K.; Coulet, F.; Guillerm, E.; Dorard, C.; Marisa, L.; et al. HSP110 T17 simplifies and improves the microsatellite instability testing in patients with colorectal cancer. *J. Med. Genet.* **2016**, *53*, 377–384. [CrossRef] [PubMed]
70. Zhu, L.; Huang, Y.; Fang, X.; Liu, C.; Deng, W.; Zhong, C.; Xu, J.; Xu, D.; Yuan, Y. A Novel and Reliable Method to Detect Microsatellite Instability in Colorectal Cancer by Next-Generation Sequencing. *J. Mol. Diagn.* **2018**, *20*, 225–231. [CrossRef] [PubMed]
71. Joost, P.; Veurink, N.; Holck, S.; Klarskov, L.; Bojesen, A.; Harbo, M.; Baldetorp, B.; Rambech, E.; Nilbert, M. Heterogenous mismatch-repair status in colorectal cancer. *Diagn. Pathol.* **2014**, *9*, 126. [CrossRef]
72. Kim, K.; Kim, J.E.; Hong, Y.S.; Ahn, S.M.; Chun, S.M.; Hong, S.M.; Jang, S.J.; Yu, C.S.; Kim, J.C.; Kim, T.W. Paired Primary and Metastatic Tumor Analysis of Somatic Mutations in Synchronous and Metachronous Colorectal Cancer. *Cancer Res. Treat. Off. J. Korean Cancer Assoc.* **2017**, *49*, 161–167. [CrossRef]
73. Jesinghaus, M.; Wolf, T.; Pfarr, N.; Muckenhuber, A.; Ahadova, A.; Warth, A.; Goeppert, B.; Sers, C.; Kloor, M.; Endris, V.; et al. Distinctive Spatiotemporal Stability of Somatic Mutations in Metastasized Microsatellite-stable Colorectal Cancer. *Am. J. Surg. Pathol.* **2015**, *39*, 1140–1147. [CrossRef]
74. Testa, U.; Pelosi, E.; Castelli, G. Colorectal cancer: Genetic abnormalities, tumor progression, tumor heterogeneity, clonal evolution and tumor-initiating cells. *Med. Sci.* **2018**, *6*, 31. [CrossRef]

75. Jeantet, M.; Tougeron, D.; Tachon, G.; Cortes, U.; Archambaut, C.; Fromont, G.; Karayan-Tapon, L. High Intra- and Inter-Tumoral Heterogeneity of RAS Mutations in Colorectal Cancer. *Int. J. Mol. Sci.* **2016**, *17*, 2015. [CrossRef] [PubMed]
76. Chapusot, C.; Martin, L.; Bouvier, A.M.; Bonithon-Kopp, C.; Ecarnot-Laubriet, A.; Rageot, D.; Ponnelle, T.; Laurent Puig, P.; Faivre, J.; Piard, F. Microsatellite instability and intratumoural heterogeneity in 100 right-sided sporadic colon carcinomas. *Br. J. Cancer* **2002**, *87*, 400–404. [CrossRef] [PubMed]
77. Bai, W.; Ma, J.; Liu, Y.; Liang, J.; Wu, Y.; Yang, X.; Xu, E.; Li, Y.; Xi, Y. Screening of MSI detection loci and their heterogeneity in East Asian colorectal cancer patients. *Cancer Med.* **2019**, *8*, 2157–2166. [CrossRef] [PubMed]
78. Schrock, A.B.; Ouyang, C.; Sandhu, J.; Sokol, E.; Jin, D.; Ross, J.S.; Miller, V.A.; Lim, D.; Amanam, I.; Chao, J.; et al. Tumor mutational burden is predictive of response to immune checkpoint inhibitors in MSI-high metastatic colorectal cancer. *Ann. Oncol.* **2019**, *30*, 1096–1103. [CrossRef] [PubMed]
79. Fabrizio, D.A.; George, T.J.; Dunne, R.F.; Frampton, G.; Sun, J.; Gowen, K.; Kennedy, M.; Greenbowe, J.; Schrock, A.B.; Hezel, A.F.; et al. Beyond microsatellite testing: Assessment of tumor mutational burden identifies subsets of colorectal cancer who may respond to immune checkpoint inhibition. *J. Gastrointest. Oncol.* **2018**, *9*, 610–617. [CrossRef] [PubMed]
80. Tougeron, D.; Fauquembergue, E.; Rouquette, A.; Le Pessot, F.; Sesboüé, R.; Laurent, M.; Berthet, P.; Mauillon, J.; Di Fiore, F.; Sabourin, J.C.; et al. Tumor-infiltrating lymphocytes in colorectal cancers with microsatellite instability are correlated with the number and spectrum of frameshift mutations. *Mod. Pathol.* **2009**, *22*, 1186–1195. [CrossRef]
81. Sæterdal, I.; Gjertsen, M.K.; Straten, P.; Eriksen, J.A.; Gaudernack, G. A TGFβRII frameshift-mutation-derived CTL epitope recognised by HLA-A2-restricted CD8+ T cells. *Cancer Immunol. Immunother.* **2001**, *50*, 469–476.
82. Colle, R.; Cohen, R.; Cochereau, D.; Duval, A.; Lascols, O.; Lopez-Trabada, D.; Afchain, P.; Trouilloud, I.; Parc, Y.; Lefevre, J.H.; et al. Immunotherapy and patients treated for cancer with microsatellite instability. *Bull. Cancer (Paris)* **2017**, *104*, 42–51. [CrossRef]
83. De Guillebon, E.; Roussille, P.; Frouin, E.; Tougeron, D. Anti program death-1/anti program death-ligand 1 in digestive cancers. *World J. Gastrointest. Oncol.* **2015**, *7*, 95–101. [CrossRef]
84. Müller, M.F.; Ibrahim, A.E.K.; Arends, M.J. Molecular pathological classification of colorectal cancer. *Virchows Arch.* **2016**, *469*, 125–134. [CrossRef]
85. Silberman, R.; Steiner, D.F.; Lo, A.A.; Gomez, A.; Zehnder, J.L.; Chu, G.; Suarez, C.J. Complete and Prolonged Response to Immune Checkpoint Blockade in POLE-Mutated Colorectal Cancer. *JCO Precis. Oncol.* **2019**, *3*, 1–5. [CrossRef]
86. Vanderwalde, A.; Spetzler, D.; Xiao, N.; Gatalica, Z.; Marshall, J. Microsatellite instability status determined by next-generation sequencing and compared with PD-L1 and tumor mutational burden in 11,348 patients. *Cancer Med.* **2018**, *7*, 746–756. [CrossRef] [PubMed]
87. Marginean, E.C.; Melosky, B. Is There a Role for Programmed Death Ligand-1 Testing and Immunotherapy in Colorectal Cancer with Microsatellite Instability? Part II-The Challenge of Programmed Death Ligand-1 Testing and Its Role in Microsatellite Instability-High Colorectal Cancer. *Arch. Pathol. Lab. Med.* **2018**, *142*, 26–34. [CrossRef] [PubMed]
88. Matsuzaki, K.; Borel, V.; Adelman, C.A.; Schindler, D.; Boulton, S.J. FANCJ suppresses microsatellite instability and lymphomagenesis independent of the Fanconi anemia pathway. *Genes Dev.* **2015**, *29*, 2532–2546. [CrossRef] [PubMed]
89. Li, F.; Mao, G.; Tong, D.; Huang, J.; Gu, L.; Yang, W.; Li, G.M. The Histone Mark H3K36me3 Regulates Human DNA Mismatch Repair through Its Interaction with MutSα. *Cell* **2013**, *153*, 590–600. [CrossRef] [PubMed]
90. Awwad, S.W.; Ayoub, N. Overexpression of KDM4 lysine demethylases disrupts the integrity of the DNA mismatch repair pathway. *Biol. Open* **2015**, *4*, 498. [CrossRef] [PubMed]
91. Puccini, A.; Lenz, H.J.; Marshall, J.L.; Arguello, D.; Raghavan, D.; Korn, W.M.; Weinberg, B.A.; Poorman, K.; Heeke, A.L.; Philip, P.A.; et al. Impact of Patient Age on Molecular Alterations of Left-Sided Colorectal Tumors. *Oncologist* **2019**, *24*, 319–326. [CrossRef]
92. Dorard, C.; de Thonel, A.; Collura, A.; Marisa, L.; Svrcek, M.; Lagrange, A.; Jego, G.; Wanherdrick, K.; Joly, A.L.; Buhard, O.; et al. Expression of a mutant HSP110 sensitizes colorectal cancer cells to chemotherapy and improves disease prognosis. *Nat. Med.* **2011**, *17*, 1283–1289. [CrossRef]

93. Kim, J.H.; Kim, K.J.; Rhee, Y.Y.; Oh, S.; Cho, N.Y.; Lee, H.S.; Kang, G.H. Expression status of wild-type HSP110 correlates with HSP110 T17 deletion size and patient prognosis in microsatellite-unstable colorectal cancer. *Mod. Pathol.* **2014**, *27*, 443–453. [CrossRef]
94. Salipante, S.J.; Scroggins, S.M.; Hampel, H.L.; Turner, E.H.; Pritchard, C.C. Microsatellite Instability Detection by Next Generation Sequencing. *Clin. Chem.* **2014**, *60*, 1192–1199. [CrossRef]
95. Niu, B.; Ye, K.; Zhang, Q.; Lu, C.; Xie, M.; McLellan, M.D.; Wendl, M.C.; Ding, L. MSIsensor: Microsatellite instability detection using paired tumor-normal sequence data. *Bioinformatics* **2014**, *30*, 1015. [CrossRef] [PubMed]
96. Kautto, E.A.; Bonneville, R.; Miya, J.; Yu, L.; Krook, M.A.; Reeser, J.W.; Roychowdhury, S. Performance evaluation for rapid detection of pan-cancer microsatellite instability with MANTIS. *Oncotarget* **2017**, *8*, 7452. [CrossRef] [PubMed]
97. Baudrin, L.G.; Deleuze, J.F.; How-Kit, A. Molecular and Computational Methods for the Detection of Microsatellite Instability in Cancer. *Front Oncol.* **2018**, *8*, 621. [CrossRef] [PubMed]
98. Deng, A.; Yang, J.; Lang, J.; Jiang, Z.; Wang, W.; Yuan, D.; Wang, X.; Tian, G. Monitoring microsatellite instability (MSI) in circulating tumor DNA by next-generation DNA-seq. *J. Clin. Oncol.* **2018**, *36*, 12025. [CrossRef]
99. Willis, J.; Lefterova, M.I.; Artyomenko, A.; Kasi, P.M.; Nakamura, Y.; Mody, K.; Catenacci, D.V.T.; Fakih, M.; Barbacioru, C.; Zhao, J.; et al. Validation of Microsatellite Instability Detection Using a Comprehensive Plasma-Based Genotyping Panel. *Clin. Cancer Res.* **2019**. [CrossRef]
100. Cabel, L.; Proudhon, C.; Romano, E.; Girard, N.; Lantz, O.; Stern, M.H.; Pierga, J.Y.; Bidard, F.C. Clinical potential of circulating tumour DNA in patients receiving anticancer immunotherapy. *Nat. Rev. Clin. Oncol.* **2018**, *15*, 639–650. [CrossRef]
101. Mattos-Arruda, L.D.; Weigelt, B.; Cortes, J.; Won, H.H.; Ng, C.K.Y.; Nuciforo, P.; Bidard, F.C.; Aura, C.; Saura, C.; Peg, V.; et al. Capturing intra-tumor genetic heterogeneity by de novo mutation profiling of circulating cell-free tumor DNA: A proof-of-principle. *Ann. Oncol.* **2014**, *25*, 1729. [CrossRef]
102. Day, D.; Frentzas, S.; Naidu, C.A.; Segelov, E.; Green, M. Current Utility and Future Applications of ctDNA in Colorectal Cancer. In *Advances in the Molecular Understanding of Colorectal Cancer*; Segelov, E., Ed.; IntechOpen: London, UK, 2019; Chapter 4; ISBN 978-1-78985-060-4.
103. Fader, A.N.; Diaz, L.A.; Armstrong, D.K.; Tanner, E.J.; Uram, J.; Eyring, A.; Wang, H.; Fisher, G.; Greten, T.; Le, D. Preliminary results of a phase II study: PD-1 blockade in mismatch repair–deficient, recurrent or persistent endometrial cancer. *Gynecol. Oncol.* **2016**, *141*, 206–207. [CrossRef]
104. Cohen, R.; Hain, E.; Buhard, O.; Guilloux, A.; Bardier, A.; Kaci, R.; Bertheau, P.; Renaud, F.; Bibeau, F.; Fléjou, J.F.; et al. Association of Primary Resistance to Immune Checkpoint Inhibitors in Metastatic Colorectal Cancer with Misdiagnosis of Microsatellite Instability or Mismatch Repair Deficiency Status. *JAMA Oncol.* **2019**, *5*, 551–555. [CrossRef]

© 2019 by the authors. Licensee MDPI, Basel, Switzerland. This article is an open access article distributed under the terms and conditions of the Creative Commons Attribution (CC BY) license (http://creativecommons.org/licenses/by/4.0/).

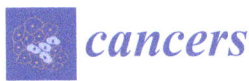

Review

Spatiotemporal pH Heterogeneity as a Promoter of Cancer Progression and Therapeutic Resistance

David E. Korenchan [1] and Robert R. Flavell [1,2,*]

[1] Department of Radiology and Biomedical Imaging, University of California, San Francisco, CA 94143, USA
[2] Department of Pharmaceutical Chemistry, University of California, San Francisco, CA 94143, USA
* Correspondence: Robert.Flavell@ucsf.edu; Tel.: +1-415-353-3638

Received: 21 June 2019; Accepted: 18 July 2019; Published: 20 July 2019

Abstract: Dysregulation of pH in solid tumors is a hallmark of cancer. In recent years, the role of altered pH heterogeneity in space, between benign and aggressive tissues, between individual cancer cells, and between subcellular compartments, has been steadily elucidated. Changes in temporal pH-related processes on both fast and slow time scales, including altered kinetics of bicarbonate-CO_2 exchange and its effects on pH buffering and gradual, progressive changes driven by changes in metabolism, are further implicated in phenotypic changes observed in cancers. These discoveries have been driven by advances in imaging technologies. This review provides an overview of intra- and extracellular pH alterations in time and space reflected in cancer cells, as well as the available technology to study pH spatiotemporal heterogeneity.

Keywords: tumor microenvironment; interstitial pH; acidosis; tumor heterogeneity; magnetic resonance imaging; hyperpolarized ^{13}C MRI; carbonic anhydrase; lactic acid; positron emission tomography

1. Introduction

In their seminal paper on the hallmarks of cancer [1], Hanahan and Weinberg proposed several common features of neoplasia, largely caused by genomic changes, that promote tumor development. Although genetic mutation is a necessary component of tumorigenesis, this must necessarily be accompanied by disruptions in cellular homeostasis, reflected in changes in metabolism and transport, which can be adapted according to cellular needs. These modifications both craft what has been referred to as the 'tumor microenvironment", an extracellular milieu that further promotes tumor development and inhibits antitumor immune activity, as well as cell–cell heterogeneity within tumors, which a growing body of research is supporting as a crucial factor in understanding overall tumor function [2].

Alterations in pH in cancer represent one of the principal known disruptions in cellular and tissue homeostasis. While initial interest was sparked by the observation that tumor tissues are significantly more acidic than their normal counterparts, recent research has delved into how intracellular and extracellular pH changes play a role in promoting tumor initiation, growth, survival, and metastasis. The body of research on pH suggests that global measurements of pH do not capture the full story; rather, the ability of cells to tune pH locally between organelles or between cells, as well as to respond to kinetic changes affecting pH, plays a crucial role in the development and maintenance of the cancer phenotype.

In this review article, we will summarize known findings on pH alterations in cancer and suggest how spatiotemporal heterogeneity in pH works to promote tumor survival and progression. We will also discuss the available methodologies for measuring pH on spatial and temporal scales, as well as potential opportunities for further technical development in elucidating how pH influences tumor behavior.

2. pH Heterogeneity in Space

Interstitial acidification in cancer has been known for several decades, based upon electrode pH measurements [3]. More recently, it has been suggested that interstitial acidification may be accompanied by cytosolic alkalinization. There is also growing interest in the altered pH of subcellular compartments, including endosomes and lysosomes. Several excellent reviews have summarized properties and associated phenotypic changes of both intra- and extracellular pH in the context of cancer [4–6]. Some salient details will be mentioned here. Normal tissue may demonstrate an intracellular pH (pH_i) and an extracellular pH (pH_e) of about 7.2 and 7.4, respectively. In cancer, pH_e decreases to 7.0 or lower, leading to a reversal in the pH_i–pH_e gradient across the cell membrane. Somewhat more controversial is the claim that pH_i significantly increases in the context of cancer, although in silico models based upon enzymatic pH-dependent activity profiles suggest that an alkaline pH_i confers maximal cell proliferation, upregulated glycolysis, and survival under hypoxia [7]. Changes in pH are closely linked with alterations in membrane transporter expression and function, which change transport kinetics of protons and small ions including sodium, chloride, bicarbonate, and lactate [8]. As will be discussed, $pH_{i,e}$ changes can lead to altered protein behavior and are associated with many phenotypic changes in cancer progression, including invasion, proliferation, stemness, aggressiveness, immune suppression, vascularization, and metastasis. Figure 1 summarizes pH-related changes in transporter expression, protein function, and cellular phenotype that are associated with cancer.

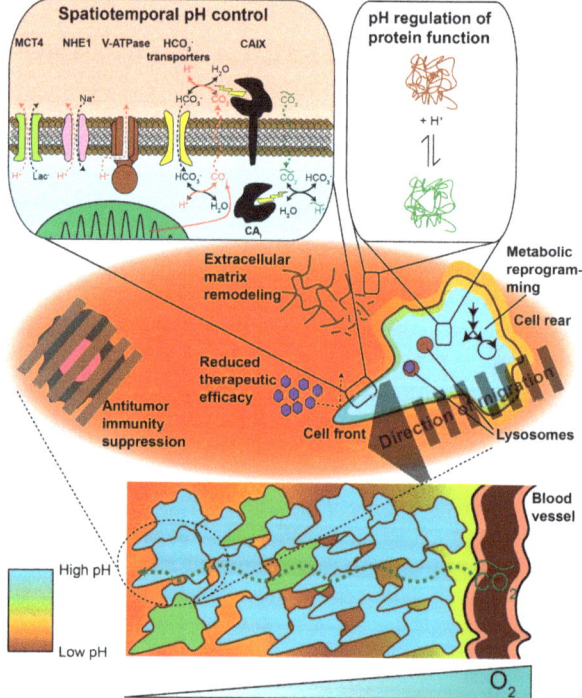

Figure 1. Spatiotemporal pH heterogeneity in cancer. Upper right inset: Proton extrusion mechanisms (red arrows and labels) employed by tumor cells include transport proteins such as monocarboxylate transporter 4 (MCT4), sodium-proton exchanger 1 (NHE1), or vacuolar-type ATPase. Alternatively, protons can be titrated with imported bicarbonate (HCO_3^-), which then diffuses out of the cell as CO_2.

Carbonic anhydrase 9 (CAIX) and potentially other extracellular isoforms catalyze bicarbonate-CO_2 exchange in order to reduce CO_2 back-diffusion into cells and induce interstitial proton release. High proton extrusion flux leads to an acidic pH_e. Cells may also experience systemic fluctuations in CO_2 (green arrows and labels), which induces pH_i fluctuations in cells expressing intracellular carbonic anhydrase isoforms. Upper left inset: Variations in pH lead to alterations in protonation states of proteins with pH-sensitive amino acid residues, thereby causing structural changes that affect protein function. Middle inset: Cancer cells may alter pH on a subcellular basis. Intracellular and extracellular pH spatial heterogeneity can promote focal adhesion formation and/or degradation for cellular migration. Additionally, altered lysosomal pH can facilitate drug resistance. An acidic pH_e is associated with immune cell anergy, drug localization to the extracellular space, and extracellular matrix remodeling. Lower section: pH heterogeneity may also exist on the level of tissues. Certain tumor cells may lower their pH_i in order to reduce proliferation and maintain capacity for differentiation. pH_e gradients can be sculpted in a tumor depending on metabolic differences between cells (e.g., glycolytic vs. oxidative metabolism) in combination with the proton extrusion mechanisms employed. Finally, systemic CO_2 fluctuations can alter pH depending on CA expression and localization.

2.1. Protonation as a Post-Translational Modification

Modulation of protein function based on pH represents a regulatory mechanism that can be rapid as well as locally constrained. Small changes in local pH can significantly affect the ratio of protonated versus deprotonated amino acid residues on a protein, depending on the acid dissociation constant (pK_a) of the side chain. Thus, single amino acid mutations in which the side chain pK_a moves in or out of the physiological pH range (e.g., arginine to histidine, or vice versa) can result in either a gain or loss of protein pH sensitivity. These pH-related changes in function are well-described for particular proteins in a recent review [9]. A few examples are detailed below. Proteins that contain pH-sensitive residues or domains affecting activity include calcineurin [10], sodium-proton exchanger 1 (NHE1) [11], cofilin [12], talin [13], and cancer signaling proteins including endothelial growth factor receptor (EGFR), and transcription factor p53 [14]. Proteins found in the extracellular space, notably proteases such as matrix metalloproteinase 3; urokinase-type plasminogen activator; and cathepsins B, D, and L, also exhibit pH-dependent activity and may in fact only be activated at low pH_e values [15]. Interestingly, arginine-to-histidine mutations feature prominently in a subset of cancers, including acute myeloid leukemia, colorectal, esophageal, low grade glioma, kidney chromophobe, medulloblastoma, pancreatic, prostate, stomach, and uterine malignancies, suggesting that these cancers may have accompanying changes in pH_i to regulate protein activity [16]. Thus, by tuning pH locally and temporally tumors can alter intracellular and extracellular protein functionality.

2.2. Intracellular pH

Generally speaking, interest in pH_i changes (including subcellular compartments other than the cytosol) has surrounded alterations in protein expression and function as a result of protonation state. We will discuss cellular changes that result from intracellular pH alterations.

2.2.1. Spatial Regulation of Protein Activity via Subcellular pH Heterogeneity

Localized control of pH_i within subcellular compartments can be accomplished based upon expression and localization of proton and other ion transporters. Spatial heterogeneity in pH_i can therefore contribute to phenotypic hallmarks of cancer. During cell migration, a high pH_i at the cell front induces formation of focal adhesion complexes, mitigated in particular by pH-dependent talin-actin binding [13], whereas a low pH_i at the cell rear promotes focal adhesion destabilization as well as myosin contraction [15]. Localization of NHE1 or MCT4 at the leading edge of migration can generate the higher pH_i required for cellular adhesion. Endosomes and lysosomes have a markedly reduced pH compared to the cytosol (6.2 and 4.5–5.0, respectively) [17], and the degree of acidity plays a crucial role in regulating lysosomal protein function. Lysosomal pH within tumor cells may therefore provide information regarding chemotherapeutic resistance, as increased vacuolar-type ATPase (V-ATPase) expression is linked with drug localization in lysosomes [18].

2.2.2. Intercellular pH_i Heterogeneity within Tumors

An intriguing area of investigation involves the influence of pH_i in cellular heterogeneity within a tumor. This is because an individual cell's fate and function can be strongly affected by pH_i. Studies of pH_i in the context of eye development in Drosophila melanogaster has revealed that increased proton efflux and a resultant rise in pH_i are sufficient to induce dysplasia, and that proton efflux inhibition in cancer cell lines induces lethality [19]. Additionally, extracellular ATP was shown to cause intracellular acidification in prostate cancer cells, leading to growth arrest via disruption of Ca^{2+} homeostasis [20]. pH_i is tightly regulated, and pharmacologic inhibition of proton export significantly reduces tumor growth [21]. These studies suggest a link between a high pH_i and oncogenic events and proliferation in mammalian cells. However, pH_i plays a role in both normal development and oncogenesis. Increases in pH_i were shown to be necessary for the efficient differentiation of both Drosophila follicle cells and mouse embryonic stem cells. Presumably, cancer stem cells might tend to promote a lower pH_i than surrounding cancer cells in order to prevent differentiation until necessary. Thus, measuring pH_i heterogeneity between cells in a tumor mass could potentially distinguish functional regions of the tumor for the purpose of designing therapeutic strategies to disrupt intercellular symbiosis.

2.3. Extracellular pH

Far from being merely a side-effect of increased metabolic fluxes, the lower pH_e observed in tumors can also vary spatially, forming gradients within the interstitial space as well as cooperating with the alkaline pH_i to generate a tumor environment favorable for therapeutic resistance and metastasis. We will briefly discuss the current mechanisms underlying interstitial acidification, then summarize the effects of pH_e spatial heterogeneity on tumors.

2.3.1. Metabolic and Physiological Contributors to Spatial Gradients and Acidic pH_e

Interstitial acidification, independent of its tumor-promoting properties, is generally viewed as a byproduct of altered metabolism coupled with changes in perfusion within tumors. Free protons diffuse with a diffusion constant of ~1×10^{-4} cm^2/s, which is fast enough compared to proton export rates to diminish the formation of spatial gradients outside the cell. However, proton diffusion through gels simulating the extracellular matrix has been measured as ~6×10^{-6} cm^2/s [22], almost two orders of magnitude slower than free proton diffusion and on the same order as water diffusion through biological tissue (~2×10^{-6} cm^2/s) [23]. This suggests that protons largely diffuse as mobile buffer species such as phosphate or carbon dioxide. As a cancer grows and outdistances its local blood supply, tumor regions become hypoxic, although they remain with diffusive distance of glucose [24]. This has traditionally been understood to lead to HIF-1α stabilization, which in turn induces overexpression of glycolytic enzymatic subunits (e.g., LDHA), proton-exporting transporters such as monocarboxylate transporter 4 (MCT4), and carbonic anhydrase 9 (CAIX). Increased lactate metabolic flux coupled with proton-lactate co-export via MCT4 is generally accepted to be a major mechanism of interstitial acidification, with a variety of other mechanisms also contributing (Figure 1). For example, V-ATPase and MCT4 are both major acidification mechanisms in human breast cancer cell lines [25]. Acidification has also been shown to occur in glycolysis-deficient Chinese hamster cells [26,27], suggesting that proton export pathways independent of lactate play a major role in this particular model. Therefore, depending upon the genetic and metabolic state of the tumor, a variety of mechanisms contribute to interstitial acidification.

Recent studies have suggested that pH_e gradients may be present throughout a tumor mass, and that these gradients, as well as the pH_i–pH_e gradient across the cell membrane, promote tumor growth and survival. Experimental evidence suggests that free proton diffusion through tumor interstitium is very small and that the majority of proton diffusion takes place by way of mobile buffers [22]. It has been hypothesized that various interstitial acidification mechanisms may be present throughout a tumor mass depending on oxygen/metabolite availability, transporter expression, and carbonic anhydrase (CA) activity, contributing to a pH gradient throughout the tumor [6]. Additionally, stromal cells near a lesion may shape pH_e gradients by forming a syncytium that can take up acidic byproducts and transport them away from the site of metabolism, as has been demonstrated in co-cultures of myofibroblasts and colorectal cancer cells [28]. An intriguing area of research is the contribution of CAIX to gradient sculpting of both pH_i and pH_e within cell spheroids and in vivo xenografts. HCT116 human colon carcinoma spheroids transfected to constitutively express CAIX diminish pH_i gradients between the spheroid core and periphery [29] while simultaneously increasing pH_e gradients [30]. When these cells were implanted in a mouse and imaged with a ^1H MRSI pH agent, the resulting tumors only demonstrated voxel pH_e values below 6.93, suggesting that CAIX acts as a "pH-stat" and keeps pH_e below a certain level [31]. Another interesting finding is that acid-extruding bicarbonate transporters such as solute carrier family 4, members 4 and 9 (SLC4A4 and SLC4A9) are hypoxia-inducible and are therefore likely expressed along with CAIX in hypoxic tumor regions [32]. Mathematical modeling of bicarbonate-CO_2 exchange, diffusion, and cellular metabolism predicts that the effect of CAIX catalysis on pH_i and pH_e heterogeneity is strongly dependent upon metabolic pathways and proton transport mechanisms. Whereas cells that mainly produce CO_2 or import HCO_3^- to titrate intracellular protons benefit greatly from higher CAIX activity, cells which export protons directly are minimally or even negatively affected by expressing CAIX [33]. Thus, interactions between cellular metabolism, proton export, CO_2 diffusion, and bicarbonate-CO_2 interconversion all give rise to the pH_e observed in tumors.

2.3.2. Acidic pH_e Can Alter Tumor Metabolism

Interstitial acidification that may be caused by altered metabolism can in turn affect metabolic pathways. Ippolito et al. discovered in a prostate neuroendocrine carcinoma (PNEC) cell line that glutamate decarboxylase (GAD) activity in cell lysates increased when the cells were incubated in acidic media (pH 6.5) and decreased in alkaline media (pH 8.5) [34]. Interestingly, glutamate-ammonia ligase (GLUL) demonstrated higher activity in both acidic and alkaline media relative to physiologic pH (pH 7.4). The measured activities correlated with changes in protein expression as well. In a following study, the group discovered that altering the culture media pH significantly altered metabolic pathways in the same cell line, with acidic pH favoring oxidative phosphorylation and alkaline pH stimulating nutrient consumption [35]. In keeping with this finding, they demonstrated that PNEC and human prostate cancer cell lines were more susceptible to niclosamide inhibition of mitochondrial function at acid pH and more susceptible to nutrient deprivation at alkaline pH. These findings are intriguing in that they suggest that pH_e measurements can aid in identifying metabolic heterogeneity within a tumor in order to devise therapeutic strategies against tumor subregions.

2.3.3. Spatial pH_e Gradients Promote Healthy Cell Death, Tumor Aggressiveness, and Therapeutic Resistance

Spatial regulation of tumor pH_e has a profound impact upon tumor aggressiveness, survival, and treatment resistance. The lower tumor pH_e forms a gradient with the less acidic interstitium of normal tissue, promoting a net proton flow that may in turn induce normal cell toxicity [36]. Normal cells may be unable to cope with the acid load because they are less able to remove intracellular protons as effectively as tumor cells. The resulting interstitial acidification could activate caspase activity, leading to apoptosis [37]. Interestingly, loss of p53 in cancer cells seems to protect against acidic pH_e-dependent induction of apoptosis as well [38]. Spatial fluctuations in pH_e can affect cellular migration and invasion. Prior in vivo studies of breast and colon cancer cells implanted in mice have established that tumors grow preferentially along gradients of decreasing pH_e, and that overexpression of glucose transporter 1 (GLUT1) and NHE1 transporters at the leading edge drives invasion [39]. The high transmembrane pH_i–pH_e gradient can also act as a defense mechanism against weakly basic chemotherapeutic agents, since these will preferentially protonate in the interstitium, pick up a net positive charge, and be prevented from cell internalization. This likely explains why extracellular alkalinization via bicarbonate buffer therapy was shown to enhance doxorubicin ($pK_a = 7.6$) uptake in MCF-7 xenografts in vivo [40]. Several effects of acidic pH_e on antitumor immune cell activity have been documented. Acid pH_e-dependent lactate import can induce anergy in human cytotoxic T-cells in vitro [41], and pH neutralization in vitro reverses anergy for human and murine infiltrating T-lymphocytes [42]. Acidosis leads to greater antigen uptake and presentation in dendritic cells (DCs) [43]; however, tumor-derived lactate could also play a role in inducing a tumor-favorable phenotype in DCs [44]. Bicarbonate therapy leads to more effective tumor cell killing by natural killer (NK) cells, suggesting a role for pH_e in modulating NK cell activity [45]. Finally, low pH_e also affects cellular differentiation status. Acid pH_e promotes the expression of glial stem cell markers [46] and promotes epithelial-to-mesenchymal transition in Lewis lung carcinoma cells [47].

Because transmembrane proton exporters and CA isoforms play a prominent role in cancer, several inhibitors have been designed against these targets. A good review on CA inhibitors has been written by Singh et al. [48]. Other inhibitors include amiloride derivatives against NHE1, proton pump inhibitors (PPIs) against V-ATPase, and MCT inhibitors such as 4,4'-di-isothiocyanostilbene-2,2'-disulfonate (DIDS) [49]. Additionally, a large body of literature exists on designing pH-sensitive drug delivery systems [50] or prodrugs [51] that release the drug or form the active therapeutic agent when they encounter the acidic tumor microenvironment.

3. pH Heterogeneity in Time

Studying alterations in pH distributions around, between, and within cells does not fully capture the underlying biological changes in cancer. Alterations in tumor pH happen on various timescales, ranging from transient, rapid fluctuations to slow, progressive changes. The fast-switching ability of pH-sensing protons potentially lends itself to respond to rapid changes in pH. Furthermore, tumor cells are known to undergo hypoxic-normoxic cycles as they outdistance their blood supply [24]. These cycles likely imply associated changes in pH, which can modulate cell behavior. Additionally, changes in regulation of carbonic anhydrase isoforms can affect the timescale of transient pH changes and thus increase or decrease tumor cell sensitivity to pH transients. The study of pH modulation kinetics represents an intriguing area of tumor biology that is only beginning to be elucidated. Finally, $pH_{i,e}$ in solid tumors can change over the course of disease progression in order to suit the changing needs and objectives of tumor cells. The following section highlights salient findings regarding temporal pH changes.

3.1. Carbonic Anhydrase Kinetics

The changes in protein expression for various isoforms of carbonic anhydrase, notably CAIX, are well-known for many cancers [52]. As alluded to in Section 2.2.1, CAIX activity can enable higher metabolic fluxes for rapidly-dividing cancer cells by accelerating HCO_3^-/CO_2-mediated "acid venting", which clears away acidic byproducts that might otherwise back up actively-utilized metabolic pathways. Biological studies and mathematical modeling of lactic acid-producing muscle tissue demonstrate the role of extracellular carbonic anhydrase in sustaining high metabolic flux and clearance to blood [53,54]. One of the important features of CAIX in particular is that because its expression is regulated via HIF1α, it is expressed along with other metabolism-related proteins such as LDHA, MCT4, and SLC4A4/9. Additionally, although CAIX and other hypoxia-induced proteins can be expressed through non-canonical HIF pathways, the catalytic activity of CAIX may be enhanced under hypoxic conditions [55]. As mentioned in Section 2.2.1, CAIX catalysis enhances metabolic fluxes depending upon the metabolic pathways utilized by cancer cells. Therefore, measuring bicarbonate-CO_2 exchange kinetics in vivo could serve as an indicator of metabolic capacity. Gallagher et al. measured differences in CAIX activity of HCT116 cells with and without constitutive CAIX expression implanted subcutaneously in mice. Although the CAIX-expressing cells demonstrated a faster rate of conversion in vitro, a slower interconversion was observed for these same cells in vivo, which they attributed to the lower in vivo tumor pH_e reducing overall CAIX enzymatic activity [56]. This highlights the complex phenomena that may contribute to pH regulation in vivo.

3.2. Effects of pH_i Transients on Tumor Cells

A very intriguing study was recently performed by Hulikova et al. regarding CA isoforms and coupling with CO_2 fluctuations [57]. The authors discovered that although expression of intracellular CA isoforms in various cell lines did not enhance proton diffusion throughout the cytosol, they did sensitize cytosolic pH_i to CO_2 fluctuations, enabling it to oscillate in response to oscillating pCO_2. Mathematical modeling of pCO_2-pH_i coupling revealed that the downregulation of intracellular CA_i acted as a sort of low-pass filter, reducing the amplitude of more rapid pH_i fluctuations. Intriguingly, the mammalian target of rapamycin complex 1 (mTORC1) pathway activation as measured by lower ribosomal protein S6 kinase (S6K) phosphorylation was achievable by exposing HCT116 cells to sharp pCO_2 fluctuations, whereas phosphorylation state did not significantly correlate with the average pH_i. CA inhibition with acetazolamide or knockdown of intracellular carbonic anhydrase 2 (CAII) significantly altered S6K phosphorylation state. The authors concluded that this coupling between pCO_2 and pH_i represents a potent signaling mechanism that can alter cellular activity, particularly for intracellular CA-expressing tumor cells experiencing rapid pCO_2 fluctuations. The authors also suggested that downregulation of CA_i isoforms may confer a survival advantage of tumor cells over healthy cells, allowing them greater control over pH_i as pCO_2 fluctuates. At the same time, they proposed that cancers cells with high CA_i activity near aberrant blood vessels experiencing sharp pCO_2 fluctuations would experience mTOR-dependent changes in metabolism and perfusion, elicited by changes in intracellular $[Ca^{2+}]$. These results suggest that a technique that can measure temporal pH_i fluctuations could identify tumors or tumor regions that are activating particular oncogenic pathways, thereby facilitating tumor characterization. It also proposes a mechanism by which pH-sensing proteins could become activated or deactivated by temporal pH changes.

3.3. Tumor pH_e Decreases Over Time During Tumorigenesis and Disease Progression

While rapid fluctuations in tumor $pH_{i,e}$ may regulate cancer cell function and metabolism, $pH_{i,e}$ changes over a slower time scale (e.g., weeks to months) may play an important role in cancer progression. For example, it has been demonstrated that changes in pancreatic pH_e result from chronic inflammatory pancreatitis and after secretin administration, and it has been hypothesized that this could drive pancreatic cancer development [58]. This hypothesis is further supported by evidence that low pH_e is associated with local invasion [39] and metastatic disease [59]. Moreover, alterations in metabolic phenotype, including increased production of lactic acid, are upregulated in disease progression, thereby inducing a higher degree of acidosis (Figure 1). These indirect lines of evidence suggest a temporal link between changes in tumor pH and an invasive, metastatic phenotype.

The hypothesis that tumor pH_e decreases during disease progression could be directly tested in spontaneous genetically engineered models (GEM), which allow monitoring of tumors from early precursors to high-grade, metastatic, lethal tumors [60]. Recently, we have evaluated the pH_e of the Transgenic Adenocarcinoma of the Mouse Prostate (TRAMP) model in both early- and late-stage tumors. This is a spontaneous GEM which proceeds from hyperplasia to low-grade tumors, ultimately progressing to high-grade disease, metastasis, and death [61]. We hypothesized that pH_e would decrease based on prior data indicating increased production of lactic acid in high-grade tumors [62], as well as the observation that treatment with sodium bicarbonate blocked tumorigenesis in this model [63]. Supporting the hypothesis, we found that there was a significant decrease in pH_e in mice bearing high-grade tumors compared against low-grade counterparts [64]. Therefore, there is an accumulating body of both indirect and direct evidence supporting the hypothesis that a temporal decrease in pH_e could represent a biomarker of tumor disease progression.

4. Techniques to Measure pH Spatiotemporal Heterogeneity

The interstitial acidification that accompanies cancer was first discovered using pH microelectrodes [3]. Today, many methodologies exist for studying pH changes in time and space, covering a wide range of modalities, including nuclear methods such as positron emission tomography (PET) and single-photon emission computerized tomography (SPECT), fluorescence, and magnetic resonance. The principles underlying chemical agents that detect pH changes are summarized in Figure 2. These techniques rely on a variety of mechanisms to generate image contrast, and they operate over a wide range of spatial resolution scales. To the best of our knowledge, the only techniques that have reported tumor pH_e in patients are microelectrodes (5.85–7.68 over many tumor types) [3], ^{11}C-DMO PET (6.88–7.26 in brain tumors/metastases) [65], and acido-chemical exchange saturation transfer (acidoCEST) MRI (6.58 in metastatic ovarian cancer) [66]. In this section, we will briefly summarize the range of techniques available for studying pH heterogeneity; these have also been discussed in a recent review [67].

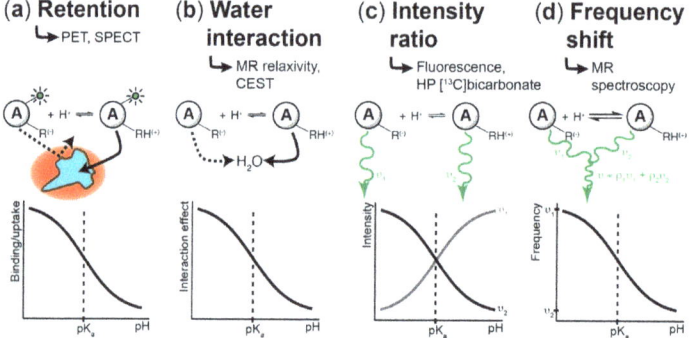

Figure 2. Mechanisms of pH measurement in cells and tissues. As a general rule, a pH-sensing agent must contain at least one functional group with a pK_a within the physiological range of detection to generate image contrast. (**a**) Agents may demonstrate pH-dependent cell binding or uptake. In this case, a pH decrease can trigger a change in cell permeability, membrane binding, or release of a prodrug agent which can bind to cells. Importantly, absolute pH quantification is not possible. This approach is used primarily for pH imaging with positron emission tomography (PET) or single-photon emission computerized tomography (SPECT). (**b**) MR-based agents may interact with water protons in a pH-dependent manner, in which pH induces changes in relaxivity or in exchange (as in acido-chemical exchange saturation transfer, acidoCEST). (**c**) The protonated and deprotonated states of an agent may emit different electromagnetic frequency waves. In this case, the ratio of emission between the two wavelengths can be used to determine the pH. This approach is relevant to fluorescent-based pH probes as well as hyperpolarized (HP) [^{13}C]bicarbonate. (**d**) If the kinetic rate of protonation–deprotonation is much faster than the absolute frequency difference between emission wavelengths, the agent will exhibit a frequency shift rather than two distinct emission wavelengths. The observed frequency depends on the relative populations (ρ) of protonated and deprotonated states, thereby giving the pH. This approach describes pH imaging with MR spectroscopic techniques (^{1}H, ^{31}P, HP ^{13}C).

4.1. Fluorescence-Based Measurements

Various fluorescent dyes and proteins exhibit a wavelength shift upon protonation, enabling ratiometric $pH_{i,e}$ calculation by measuring fluorescent output at each wavelength. In general, fluorescence methods including microscopy have very high spatial resolution (<1 μm), allowing subcellular measurements of pH gradients, although applications to whole animal and clinical imaging are limited by low penetration of light through tissue. An exemplary review covering pH-sensitive fluorescent dyes is Han et al. [68]. Generally, pH imaging studies with fluorescent dyes are constrained to 60 minutes in length. One notable approach to pH measurement in various intracellular compartments involves transfecting cells with a genetic construct encoding a pH-sensitive fluorescent protein (e.g., pHluorin) modified with a targeting domain that will localize the protein to the desired organelle [69,70]. This approach also extends the imaging timescale beyond that achievable with fluorescent dyes. The low depth of tissue penetration for fluorescence in the visible spectrum can be overcome through the use of agents emitting in the near-infrared range, which have a deeper tissue penetration compared with visible light [71,72], allowing imaging in murine models. A different way to overcome the tissue penetration limitations of fluorescence dyes in preclinical in vivo studies is by constructing a dorsal window chamber. Some studies have demonstrated the use of SNARF-1 fluorescent dye with a dorsal window chamber in order to study proton gradients and flow in tumor tissue [36] and to observe tumor cell migration along pH_e gradients [39]. In theory, a similar approach could be utilized for intraoperative fluorescence imaging of pH in patients, which has been reported using other fluorescence molecular imaging probes [73], although this has not been reported to date.

4.2. PET/SPECT-Based Imaging Methods

Several radiolabeled tracers have been developed in order to study pH_e in vivo, including ^{11}C-dimethyloxazolidinedione (DMO) [65], ^{11}CO$_2$ [74], and ^{123}I-labeled derivatives of malonic acid [75]. One elegant example of probe design is ^{64}Cu-conjugated pH-low insertion peptide (pHLIP), which anchors the radioisotope into cell membranes in regions where pH_e is below 7.0. We have reported the synthesis of various caged derivatives of ^{18}F-fluorodeoxyglucose (FDG) that demonstrate pH_e-sensitive localization in vivo by caging group release in acidic pH_e followed by uptake via glucose transporters. By using different amine-containing caging groups varying in pK_a, we could tune the pH sensitivity of FDG uptake [76]. PET/SPECT-based approaches can be readily implemented for in vivo imaging with good spatial resolution (1–2 mm); however, their primary limitation is that they cannot measure absolute pH_e, but only indicate regions below a certain threshold pH_e. Although arterial blood sampling along with imaging can be fit to a model to estimate pH values [65,74], these pH values have not been correlated with microelectrode measurements. Nevertheless, these techniques may prove to be useful in a clinical setting if threshold pH values can be demonstrated to sensitively and selectively identify or characterize lesions.

4.3. MR-Based Techniques

Magnetic resonance offers spectral sensitivity that enables absolute pH quantification with high tissue penetration depth, making it a well-studied technique for $pH_{i,e}$ measurement. Major techniques under investigation include spectroscopic methods and chemical exchange saturation transfer (CEST) based methodologies.

4.3.1. Chemical Exchange Saturation Transfer (CEST)

CEST approaches represent a rapidly-developing field of study for pH_e measurement which has the advantage of high spatial resolution (0.1–2 mm) but potentially low sensitivity; a comprehensive review has been written by Chen et al. [77]. Generally, CEST techniques are able to measure pH_e by determining relative rates of protonation and deprotonation, typically for amide functional groups on either endogenous molecules or administered contrast agents. A recent study demonstrated more robust and accurate measurement of pH_e using the acidoCEST method, which relies upon exogenous contrast agent administration [78]. In an elegant study, Longo et al. combined CEST pH_e measurements with FDG PET imaging, demonstrating an inverse correlation between tumor pH_e and glucose uptake [79]. It is noteworthy that acidoCEST with the FDA-approved CT contrast agent iopamidol to measure pH_e has been demonstrated in patients with high-grade invasive ductal carcinoma and with metastatic ovarian cancer [66].

4.3.2. MR Relaxometry

In this method, paramagnetic contrast agents with a predictable, pH-dependent change in spin-lattice (T_1) relaxation time are administered and used to measure tissue pH. A major strength of this method is high signal-to-noise ratio and spatial resolution (0.2–2 mm); however, a second, pH-insensitive contrast agent must also be administered to accurately measure pH. For example, Gillies et al. used a pH-dependant chelate, GdDOTA-4AmP^{5-}, paired with a pH-independent analog, GdDOTP^{5-}, to generate high spatial resolution maps of tissue pH$_e$ in a rat glioma model [80]. A variety of other agents have been reported [81,82] for this purpose.

4.3.3. MR Spectroscopic Approaches

Magnetic resonance spectroscopy can be used to measure tumor pH$_{i,e}$ by measuring the chemical shift of a nucleus in a molecule with a pK_a close to the physiological range and determining the pH from a previously-constructed MR titration curve. This has been described for a variety of chemical compounds and nuclei, including ^{31}P, ^{1}H, and ^{19}F. ^{31}P MR spectroscopy can be used to measure pH$_i$ based on the chemical shift of the inorganic phosphate peak. Administration of 3-aminopropylphosphonate (3-APP) followed by ^{31}P MR spectroscopy can be used to measure pH$_e$ [83–85]. Similarly, ^{1}H MR spectroscopic imaging of imidazole-containing compounds, notably (±)2-(imidazol-1-yl)3-ethoxycarbonylpropionic acid (IEPA) [86] and (±)2-(imidazol-1-yl)succinic acid (ISUCA) [31,87,88], can generate in vivo pH$_e$ maps and therefore be used to study pH$_e$ heterogeneity. Similar approaches have been reported with ^{19}F-containing agents [89]. With the exception of ^{31}P, MR imaging approaches can capture pH$_e$ heterogeneity with acceptable spatial resolution (1–2 mm) and in a reasonable timeframe (10–30 min), however it cannot measure pH$_i$ or capture kinetic pH changes. Both these limitations are linked with low signal-to-noise or contrast-to-noise ratios.

4.3.4. Hyperpolarized (HP) ^{13}C MR Imaging

The dramatic gain in MR signal attainable through dissolution dynamic nuclear polarization (d-DNP) [90] provides unique opportunities to capture spatial as well as temporal changes in pH$_e$. Importantly, the ability to polarize, inject, and image multiple agents simultaneously [91] or in the same imaging session holds great promise for simultaneously measuring pH and related metabolic or physiological processes, such as glycolysis and perfusion. pH$_e$ mapping with HP [^{13}C]bicarbonate represents the majority of HP pH imaging and has been demonstrated in tumors [91–93], perfused lungs [94,95], and other tissues [96,97]. pH$_i$ can also be quantified from HP ^{13}CO$_2$ produced from [1-^{13}C]pyruvate in organs with high pyruvate dehydrogenase flux, most notably the heart [98,99]. Although the short T_1 of [^{13}C]bicarbonate/^{13}CO$_2$ (~10 s in vivo [91–93,97,100]) poses a significant challenge for obtaining sufficient spatial resolution, recent advances in hyperpolarization approaches, including HP precursor decarboxylation [93,94,101], as well as advanced HP imaging sequences [96,102,103], can provide significant gains in available HP signal and its effective utilization. Nevertheless, HP image resolution (2–10 mm) is currently coarser than other modalities and MR approaches. Figure 3 demonstrates hyperpolarized pH$_e$ imaging using an optimized [^{13}C]bicarbonate method along with HP measures of glycolysis and perfusion in the TRAMP mouse model of prostate cancer. Other ^{13}C-labeled compounds have also demonstrated pH sensitivity that are potentially amenable to in vivo pH$_e$ imaging, including N-(2-acetamido)-2-aminoethanesulfonic acid (ACES) [104], diethylmalonic acid (DEMA) [105], zymonic acid [106,107], and amino acid derivatives [108]. Notably, zymonic acid was applied to pH imaging in kidneys and in a mammary tumor model [106]. Taken together, these data demonstrate robust tumor pH$_e$ measurements using a variety of HP ^{13}C MRI methods.

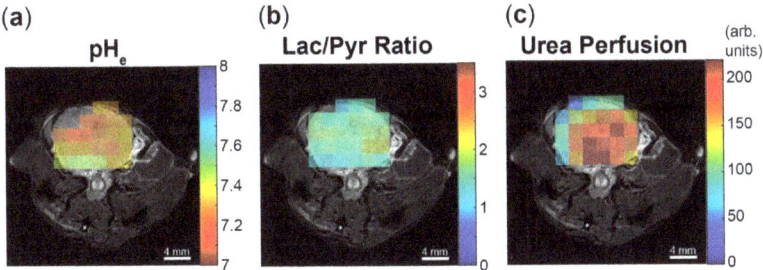

Figure 3. Hyperpolarized Imaging of pH_e, lactate conversion, and perfusion can be performed in a single imaging study. Data are shown for a transgenic adenocarcinoma of the mouse prostate (TRAMP) animal model displaying a consolidated, high-grade tumor confirmed with histology. HP images of (**a**) extracellular pH, (**b**) lactate-to-pyruvate (Lac/Pyr) ratio, and (**c**) urea signal intensity are shown overlaid on ^{1}H anatomical images, enabling voxel-to-voxel correlations in order to study the interplay between metabolism and acidification.

Importantly, high HP signal gains can also be used to measure kinetic phenomena, such as CA-catalyzed [^{13}C]bicarbonate-$^{13}CO_2$ exchange, on a sufficiently short timescale (0.1–1 s resolution). Gallagher et al. studied differences in both pH_e and bicarbonate-CO_2 exchange within HCT116 xenografts that either overexpressed CAIX or did not [56]. The bicarbonate-to-CO_2 forward reaction rate was quantified by selective saturation of the HP $^{13}CO_2$ resonance. They found that CAIX-overexpressing tumors demonstrated a pH_e that was 0.15 units lower, similar to results in cell spheroids [30], but a paradoxically slower exchange rate, which they attributed to a pH-dependent reduction in CAIX activity. It may be possible to measure both pH_e and exchange rate in vivo through MR spectroscopic techniques similar to the ones employed in this study, although the injected HP [^{13}C]bicarbonate must be given sufficient time to equilibrate if pH_e is to be accurately measured.

HP approaches may also enable in vivo kinetic measurements of pH_i, which represents a tantalizing subject of investigation. One elegant example of this was demonstrated in perfused rat hearts, where hyperpolarized [1-^{13}C]pyruvate was decarboxylated to form $^{13}CO_2$, enabling intracellular measurement of pH by comparison with the bicarbonate resonance. The HP bicarbonate/CO_2 data clearly show differences in measured pH_i dynamics with and without CA inhibition, suggesting the ability to quantify CA-catalyzed intracellular bicarbonate-CO_2 interconversion [98]. Similarly, HP ^{13}C-labeled organic phosphates formed from [U-^{13}C,U-^{2}H]glucose, including glyceronephosphate and 3-phosphoglycerate, have been shown to enable pH_i quantification in yeast cells [109]. A similar approach in which a HP ^{13}C-labeled compound is taken up in mammalian cells and subsequently phosphorylated to generate a pH-sensing moiety that may be feasible. Additionally, an existing HP pH agent such as a dicarboxylic acid could be derivatized to form an ethyl ester, as has been demonstrated with [1-^{13}C]pyruvate to enhance blood–brain barrier crossing [110]. The ester groups could then be cleaved inside the cell to generate the carboxylic acid moieties and regain pH-sensing ability. Both these approaches may introduce significant toxicity concerns; nevertheless, these or other HP approaches could open the way to measuring pH_i spatiotemporal fluctuations in vivo.

5. Conclusions

Measuring average pH in tumors provides useful information but fails to describe the complex dynamics of the tumor microenvironment. The spatial heterogeneity surrounding, among and within cells plays a major role in driving the aggressive tumor phenotype. Rather than serving as merely a byproduct of altered metabolism, pH variation throughout a tumor generates the necessary conditions to alter protein functionality throughout cells, preserve cellular differentiation capacity, reduce therapeutic uptake, shut down antitumor immune activity, and promote cellular migration and metastasis. In addition, the kinetic processes that influence pH may hold a great deal of information regarding tumor initiation, metabolism, and cellular maintenance. Many imaging and measurement techniques have been developed in order to study both pH_i and pH_e. Hyperpolarized ^{13}C in particular holds great promise for capturing both spatial and temporal heterogeneity within tumors based on its ability to estimate kinetic rate constants in an imaging setting. Further development of these and other in vivo pH measurement techniques will help to reveal the complex role that proton transport plays in tumor development and therapy.

Funding: R.R.F. acknowledges support from the National Institutes of Health (R21-EB026012), the Department of Defense (Physician Research Training Grant PC150932), University of California Cancer Research Committee Award (CRN-19-581541), a UCSF Research Allocation Program Pilot Award, and the Prostate Cancer Foundation David Blitzer Young Investigator Award.

Conflicts of Interest: The authors declare no conflict of interest.

References

1. Hanahan, D.; Weinberg, R.A. Hallmarks of Cancer: The Next Generation. *Cell* **2011**, *144*, 646–674. [CrossRef] [PubMed]
2. Lawson, D.A.; Kessenbrock, K.; Davis, R.T.; Pervolarakis, N.; Werb, Z. Tumour heterogeneity and metastasis at single-cell resolution. *Nat. Cell Biol.* **2018**, 1–12. [CrossRef]
3. Wike-Hooley, J.L.; Haveman, J.; Reinhold, H.S. The relevance of tumour pH to the treatment of malignant disease. *Radiother. Oncol.* **1984**, *2*, 343–366. [CrossRef]
4. Webb, B.A.; Chimenti, M.; Jacobson, M.P.; Barber, D.L. Dysregulated pH: A perfect storm for cancer progression. *Nat. Rev. Cancer* **2011**, *11*, 671–677. [CrossRef] [PubMed]
5. Damaghi, M.; Wojtkowiak, J.W.; Gillies, R.J. pH sensing and regulation in cancer. *Front. Physiol.* **2013**, *4*. [CrossRef] [PubMed]
6. Corbet, C.; Feron, O. Tumour acidosis: From the passenger to the driver's seat. *Nat. Rev. Cancer* **2017**, *17*, 577–593. [CrossRef] [PubMed]
7. Persi, E.; Duran-Frigola, M.; Damaghi, M.; Roush, W.R.; Aloy, P.; Cleveland, J.L.; Gillies, R.J.; Ruppin, E. Systems analysis of intracellular pH vulnerabilities for cancer therapy. *Nat. Comms.* **2018**, *9*, 2997. [CrossRef]
8. Casey, J.R.; Grinstein, S.; Orlowski, J. Sensors and regulators of intracellular pH. *Nat. Rev. Mol. Cell Biol.* **2010**, *11*, 50–61. [CrossRef] [PubMed]
9. Schönichen, A.; Webb, B.A.; Jacobson, M.P.; Barber, D.L. Considering Protonation as a Posttranslational Modification Regulating Protein Structure and Function. *Annu. Rev. Biophys.* **2013**, *42*, 289–314. [CrossRef] [PubMed]
10. Huang, S.; Cheung, W.Y. H^+ is involved in the activation of calcineurin by calmodulin. *J. Biol. Chem.* **1994**, *269*, 22067–22074.
11. Webb, B.A.; White, K.A.; Grillo-Hill, B.K.; Schönichen, A.; Choi, C.; Barber, D.L. A Histidine Cluster in the Cytoplasmic Domain of the Na-H Exchanger NHE1 Confers pH-sensitive Phospholipid Binding and Regulates Transporter Activity. *J. Biol. Chem.* **2016**, *291*, 24096–24104. [CrossRef] [PubMed]
12. Frantz, C.; Barreiro, G.; Dominguez, L.; Chen, X.; Eddy, R.; Condeelis, J.; Kelly, M.J.S.; Jacobson, M.P.; Barber, D.L. Cofilin is a pH sensor for actin free barbed end formation: Role of phosphoinositide binding. *J. Cell Biol.* **2008**, *183*, 865–879. [CrossRef] [PubMed]
13. Srivastava, J.; Barreiro, G.; Groscurth, S.; Gingras, A.R.; Goult, B.T.; Critchley, D.R.; Kelly, M.J.S.; Jacobson, M.P.; Barber, D.L. Structural model and functional significance of pH-dependent talin-actin binding for focal adhesion remodeling. *Proc. Natl. Acad. Sci. USA* **2008**, *105*, 14436–14441. [CrossRef] [PubMed]
14. White, K.A.; Ruiz, D.G.; Szpiech, Z.A.; Strauli, N.B.; Hernandez, R.D.; Jacobson, M.P.; Barber, D.L. Cancer-associated arginine-to-histidine mutations confer a gain in pH sensing to mutant proteins. *Sci. Signal.* **2017**, *10*, eaam9931. [CrossRef] [PubMed]
15. Stock, C.; Schwab, A. Protons make tumor cells move like clockwork. *Pflugers Arch.—Eur. J. Physiol.* **2009**, *458*, 981–992. [CrossRef] [PubMed]
16. Szpiech, Z.A.; Strauli, N.B.; White, K.A.; Ruiz, D.G.; Jacobson, M.P.; Barber, D.L.; Hernandez, R.D. Prominent features of the amino acid mutation landscape in cancer. *PLoS ONE* **2017**, *12*, e0183273-12. [CrossRef] [PubMed]

17. Kallunki, T.; Olsen, O.D.; Jäättelä, M. Cancer-associated lysosomal changes: Friends or foes? *Oncogene* **2013**, *32*, 1995–2004. [CrossRef] [PubMed]
18. Stransky, L.; Cotter, K.; Forgac, M. The Function of V-ATPases in Cancer. *Physiol. Rev.* **2016**, *96*, 1071–1091. [CrossRef] [PubMed]
19. Grillo-Hill, B.K.; Choi, C.; Jimenez-Vidal, M.; Barber, D.L. Increased H^+ efflux is sufficient to induce dysplasia and necessary for viability with oncogene expression. *eLife* **2015**, *2015*, 1–31. [CrossRef]
20. Humez, S.; Monet, M.; van Coppenolle, F.; Delcourt, P.; Prevarskaya, N. The role of intracellular pH in cell growth arrest induced by ATP. *Am. J. Physiol., Cell Physiol.* **2004**, *287*, C1733–C1746. [CrossRef]
21. Neri, D.; Supuran, C.T. Interfering with pH regulation in tumours as a therapeutic strategy. *Nat. Rev. Drug Discov.* **2011**, *10*, 768–777. [CrossRef]
22. Schornack, P.A.; Gillies, R.J. Contributions of cell metabolism and H+ diffusion to the acidic pH of tumors. *Neoplasia* **2003**, *5*, 135–145. [CrossRef]
23. Latour, L.L.; Svoboda, K.; Mitra, P.P.; Sotak, C.H. Time-dependent diffusion of water in a biological model system. *Proc. Natl. Acad. Sci. USA* **1994**, *91*, 1229–1233. [CrossRef]
24. Gatenby, R.A.; Gillies, R.J. Why do cancers have high aerobic glycolysis? *Nat. Rev. Cancer* **2004**, *4*, 891–899. [CrossRef]
25. Montcourrier, P.; Silver, I.; Farnoud, R.; Bird, I.; Rochefort, H. Breast cancer cells have a high capacity to acidify extracellular milieu by a dual mechanism. *Clin. Exp. Metastasis* **1997**, *15*, 382–392. [CrossRef]
26. Newell, K.; Franchi, A.; Pouyssegur, J.; Tannock, I. Studies with glycolysis-deficient cells suggest that production of lactic acid is not the only cause of tumor acidity. *Proc. Natl. Acad. Sci. USA* **1993**, *90*, 1127–1131. [CrossRef]
27. Yamagata, M.; Hasuda, K.; Stamato, T.; Tannock, I.F. The contribution of lactic acid to acidification of tumours: Studies of variant cells lacking lactate dehydrogenase. *Br. J. Cancer* **1998**, *77*, 1726–1731. [CrossRef]
28. Hulikova, A.; Black, N.; Hsia, L.-T.; Wilding, J.; Bodmer, W.F.; Swietach, P. Stromal uptake and transmission of acid is a pathway for venting cancer cell-generated acid. *Proc. Natl. Acad. Sci. USA* **2016**, *113*, E5344–E5353. [CrossRef]
29. Swietach, P.; Wigfield, S.; Cobden, P.; Supuran, C.T.; Harris, A.L.; Vaughan-Jones, R.D. Tumor-associated carbonic anhydrase 9 spatially coordinates intracellular pH in three-dimensional multicellular growths. *J. Biol. Chem.* **2008**, *283*, 20473–20483. [CrossRef]
30. Swietach, P.; Patiar, S.; Supuran, C.T.; Harris, A.L.; Vaughan-Jones, R.D. The role of carbonic anhydrase 9 in regulating extracellular and intracellular ph in three-dimensional tumor cell growths. *J. Biol. Chem.* **2009**, *284*, 20299–20310. [CrossRef]
31. Lee, S.-H.; McIntyre, D.; Honess, D.; Hulikova, A.; Pacheco-Torres, J.; Cerdán, S.; Swietach, P.; Harris, A.L.; Griffiths, J.R. Carbonic anhydrase IX is a pH-stat that sets an acidic tumour extracellular pH in vivo. *Br. J. Cancer* **2018**, *119*, 622–630. [CrossRef]
32. McIntyre, A.; Hulikova, A.; Ledaki, I.; Snell, C.; Singleton, D.; Steers, G.; Seden, P.; Jones, D.; Bridges, E.; Wigfield, S.; et al. Disrupting Hypoxia-Induced Bicarbonate Transport Acidifies Tumor Cells and Suppresses Tumor Growth. *Cancer Res.* **2016**, *76*, 3744–3755. [CrossRef]
33. Swietach, P.; Hulikova, A.; Vaughan-Jones, R.D.; Harris, A.L. New insights into the physiological role of carbonic anhydrase IX in tumour pH regulation. *Oncogene* **2010**, *29*, 6509–6521. [CrossRef]
34. Ippolito, J.E.; Piwnica-Worms, D. A Fluorescence-Coupled Assay for Gamma Aminobutyric Acid (GABA) Reveals Metabolic Stress-Induced Modulation of GABA Content in Neuroendocrine Cancer. *PLoS ONE* **2014**, *9*, e88667-15. [CrossRef]
35. Ippolito, J.E.; Brandenburg, M.W.; Ge, X.; Crowley, J.R.; Kirmess, K.M.; Som, A.; D'Avignon, D.A.; Arbeit, J.M.; Achilefu, S.; Yarasheski, K.E.; et al. Extracellular pH Modulates Neuroendocrine Prostate Cancer Cell Metabolism and Susceptibility to the Mitochondrial Inhibitor Niclosamide. *PLoS ONE* **2016**, *11*, e0159675. [CrossRef]
36. Gatenby, R.A.; Gawlinski, E.T.; Gmitro, A.F.; Kaylor, B.; Gillies, R.J. Acid-mediated tumor invasion: A multidisciplinary study. *Cancer Res.* **2006**, *66*, 5216–5223. [CrossRef]
37. Park, H.J.; Lyons, J.C.; Ohtsubo, T.; Song, C.W. Acidic environment causes apoptosis by increasing caspase activity. *Br. J. Cancer* **1999**, *80*, 1892–1897. [CrossRef]

38. Williams, A.C.; Collard, T.J.; Paraskeva, C. An acidic environment leads to p53 dependent induction of apoptosis in human adenoma and carcinoma cell lines: Implications for clonal selection during colorectal carcinogenesis. *Oncogene* **1999**, *18*, 3199–3204. [CrossRef]
39. Estrella, V.; Chen, T.; Lloyd, M.; Wojtkowiak, J.; Cornnell, H.H.; Ibrahim-Hashim, A.; Bailey, K.; Balagurunathan, Y.; Rothberg, J.M.; Sloane, B.F.; et al. Acidity Generated by the Tumor Microenvironment Drives Local Invasion. *Cancer Res.* **2013**, *73*, 1524–1535. [CrossRef]
40. Raghunand, N.; He, X.; Van Sluis, R.; Mahoney, B.; Baggett, B.; Taylor, C.W.; Paine-Murrieta, G.; Roe, D.; Bhujwalla, Z.M.; Gillies, R.J. Enhancement of chemotherapy by manipulation of tumour pH. *Br. J. Cancer* **1999**, *80*, 1005–1011. [CrossRef]
41. Fischer, K.; Hoffmann, P.; Voelkl, S.; Meidenbauer, N.; Ammer, J.; Edinger, M.; Gottfried, E.; Schwarz, S.; Rothe, G.; Hoves, S.; et al. Inhibitory effect of tumor cell-derived lactic acid on human T cells. *Blood* **2007**, *109*, 3812–3819. [CrossRef]
42. Calcinotto, A.; Filipazzi, P.; Grioni, M.; Iero, M.; De Milito, A.; Ricupito, A.; Cova, A.; Canese, R.; Jachetti, E.; Rossetti, M.; et al. Modulation of Microenvironment Acidity Reverses Anergy in Human and Murine Tumor-Infiltrating T Lymphocytes. *Cancer Res.* **2012**, *72*, 2746–2756. [CrossRef]
43. Vermeulen, M.; Giordano, M.; Trevani, A.S.; Sedlik, C.; Gamberale, R.; Fernandez-Calotti, P.; Salamone, G.; Raiden, S.; Sanjurjo, J.; Geffner, J.R. Acidosis Improves Uptake of Antigens and MHC Class I-Restricted Presentation by Dendritic Cells. *J. Immunol.* **2004**, *172*, 3196–3204. [CrossRef]
44. Gottfried, E. Tumor-derived lactic acid modulates dendritic cell activation and antigen expression. *Blood* **2006**, *107*, 2013–2021. [CrossRef]
45. Yuan, Y.H.; Zhou, C.F.; Yuan, J.; Liu, L.; Guo, X.R.; Wang, X.L.; Ding, Y.; Wang, X.N.; Li, D.S.; Tu, H.J. NaHCO3 enhances the antitumor activities of cytokine-induced killer cells against hepatocellular carcinoma HepG2 cells. *Oncol. Lett.* **2016**, *12*, 3167–3174. [CrossRef]
46. Hjelmeland, A.B.; Wu, Q.; Heddleston, J.M.; Choudhary, G.S.; MacSwords, J.; Lathia, J.D.; McLendon, R.; Lindner, D.; Sloan, A.; Rich, J.N. Acidic stress promotes a glioma stem cell phenotype. *Cell Death Differ.* **2011**, *18*, 829–840. [CrossRef]
47. Suzuki, A.; Maeda, T.; Baba, Y.; Shimamura, K.; Kato, Y. Acidic extracellular pH promotes epithelial mesenchymal transition in Lewis lung carcinoma model. *Cancer Cell Int.* **2014**, *14*, 129. [CrossRef]
48. Singh, S.; Lomelino, C.L.; Mboge, M.Y.; Frost, S.C.; McKenna, R. Cancer Drug Development of Carbonic Anhydrase Inhibitors beyond the Active Site. *Molecules* **2018**, *23*. [CrossRef]
49. Parks, S.K.; Chiche, J.; Pouyssegur, J. Disrupting proton dynamics and energy metabolism for cancer therapy. *Nat. Rev. Cancer* **2013**, *13*, 611–623. [CrossRef]
50. Tang, H.; Zhao, W.; Yu, J.; Li, Y.; Zhao, C. Recent Development of pH-Responsive Polymers for Cancer Nanomedicine. *Molecules* **2018**, *24*. [CrossRef]
51. Taresco, V.; Alexander, C.; Singh, N.; Pearce, A.K. Stimuli-Responsive Prodrug Chemistries for Drug Delivery. *Adv. Ther.* **2018**, *1*. [CrossRef]
52. Sedlakova, O.; Svastova, E.; Takacova, M.; Kopacek, J.; Pastorek, J.; Pastorekova, S. Carbonic anhydrase IX, a hypoxia-induced catalytic component of the pH regulating machinery in tumors. *Front. Physiol.* **2014**, *4*, 400. [CrossRef]
53. Geers, C.; Gros, G. Carbon dioxide transport and carbonic anhydrase in blood and muscle. *Physiol. Rev.* **2000**, *80*, 681–715. [CrossRef]
54. Hallerdei, J.; Scheibe, R.J.; Parkkila, S.; Waheed, A.; Sly, W.S.; Gros, G.; Wetzel, P.; Endeward, V. T Tubules and Surface Membranes Provide Equally Effective Pathways of Carbonic Anhydrase-Facilitated Lactic Acid Transport in Skeletal Muscle. *PLoS ONE* **2010**, *5*, e15137-11. [CrossRef]
55. Svastova, E.; Hulíková, A.; Rafajová, M.; Zat'ovičová, M.; Gibadulinová, A.; Casini, A.; Cecchi, A.; Scozzafava, A.; Supuran, C.T.; Pastorek, J.; et al. Hypoxia activates the capacity of tumor-associated carbonic anhydrase IX to acidify extracellular pH. *FEBS Lett.* **2004**, *577*, 439–445. [CrossRef]
56. Gallagher, F.A.; Sladen, H.; Kettunen, M.I.; Serrao, E.M.; Rodrigues, T.B.; Wright, A.; Gill, A.B.; McGuire, S.; Booth, T.C.; Boren, J.; et al. Carbonic Anhydrase Activity Monitored In Vivo by Hyperpolarized ^{13}C-Magnetic Resonance Spectroscopy Demonstrates Its Importance for pH Regulation in Tumors. *Cancer Res.* **2015**, *75*, 4109–4118. [CrossRef]

57. Hulikova, A.; Aveyard, N.; Harris, A.L.; Vaughan-Jones, R.D.; Swietach, P. Intracellular carbonic anhydrase activity sensitizes cancer cell pH signaling to dynamic changes in CO2 partial pressure. *J. Biol. Chem.* **2014**, *289*, 25418–25430. [CrossRef]
58. Pedersen, S.F.; Novak, I.; Alves, F.; Schwab, A.; Pardo, L.A. Alternating pH landscapes shape epithelial cancer initiation and progression: Focus on pancreatic cancer. *BioEssays* **2017**, *39*, 1600253-10. [CrossRef]
59. Cardone, R.A.; Casavola, V.; Reshkin, S.J. The role of disturbed pH dynamics and the Na+/H+ exchanger in metastasis. *Nat. Rev. Cancer* **2005**, *5*, 786–795. [CrossRef]
60. Day, C.-P.; Merlino, G.; Van Dyke, T. Preclinical mouse cancer models: A maze of opportunities and challenges. *Cell* **2015**, *163*, 39–53. [CrossRef]
61. Greenberg, N.M.; Demayo, F.; Finegold, M.J.; Medina, D.; Tilley, W.D.; Aspinall, J.O.; Cunha, G.R.; Donjacour, A.A.; Matusik, R.J.; Rosen, J.M. Prostate Cancer in a Transgenic Mouse. *Proc. Natl. Acad. Sci. USA* **1995**, *92*, 3439–3443. [CrossRef]
62. Albers, M.J.; Bok, R.; Chen, A.P.; Cunningham, C.H.; Zierhut, M.L.; Zhang, V.Y.; Kohler, S.J.; Tropp, J.; Hurd, R.E.; Yen, Y.F.; et al. Hyperpolarized ^{13}C Lactate, Pyruvate, and Alanine: Noninvasive Biomarkers for Prostate Cancer Detection and Grading. *Cancer Res.* **2008**, *68*, 8607–8615. [CrossRef]
63. Ibrahim-Hashim, A.; Cornnell, H.H.; Abrahams, D.; Lloyd, M.; Bui, M.; Gillies, R.J.; Gatenby, R.A. Systemic Buffers Inhibit Carcinogenesis in TRAMP Mice. *JURO* **2012**, *188*, 624–631. [CrossRef]
64. Korenchan, D.E.; Bok, R.; Sriram, R.; Delos Santos, R.; Qin, H.; Vigneron, D.B.; Wilson, D.M.; Kurhanewicz, J.; Flavell, R.R. Hyperpolarized in vivo pH imaging reveals grade-dependent interstitial acidification. In Proceedings of the International Society for Magnetic Resonance in Medicine, Paris, France, 16–21 June 2018; Abstract #3711.
65. Rottenberg, D.A.; Ginos, J.Z.; Kearfott, K.G. In vivo measurement of brain tumor pH using [11C] DMO and positron emission tomography. *Ann. Neurol.* **1985**, *17*, 70–79. [CrossRef]
66. Jones, K.M.; Randtke, E.A.; Yoshimaru, E.S.; Howison, C.M.; Chalasani, P.; Klein, R.R.; Chambers, S.K.; Kuo, P.H.; Pagel, M.D. Clinical Translation of Tumor Acidosis Measurements with AcidoCEST MRI. *Mol. Imaging Biol.* **2017**, 1–9. [CrossRef]
67. Anemone, A.; Consolino, L.; Arena, F.; Capozza, M.; Longo, D.L. Imaging tumor acidosis: A survey of the available techniques for mapping in vivo tumor pH. *Cancer Metastasis Rev.* **2019**, *8*, 705–725. [CrossRef]
68. Han, J.; Burgess, K. Fluorescent Indicators for Intracellular pH. *Chem. Rev.* **2010**, *110*, 2709–2728. [CrossRef]
69. Koivusalo, M.; Welch, C.; Hayashi, H.; Scott, C.C.; Kim, M.; Alexander, T.; Touret, N.; Hahn, K.M.; Grinstein, S. Amiloride inhibits macropinocytosis by lowering submembranous pH and preventing Rac1 and Cdc42 signaling. *J. Cell Biol.* **2010**, *188*, 547–563. [CrossRef]
70. Grillo-Hill, B.K.; Webb, B.A.; Barber, D.L. Ratiometric Imaging of pH Probes. In *Quantitative Imaging in Cell Biology*, 1st ed.; Waters, J.C., Wittman, T., Eds.; Elsevier: San Diego, CA, USA, 2014; Volume 123, pp. 429–448.
71. Ni, Y.; Wu, J. Far-red and near infrared BODIPY dyes: Synthesis and applications for fluorescent pH probes and bio-imaging. *Org. Biomol. Chem.* **2014**, *12*, 3774–3791. [CrossRef]
72. Luo, S.; Zhang, E.; Su, Y.; Cheng, T.; Shi, C. A review of NIR dyes in cancer targeting and imaging. *Biomaterials* **2011**, *32*, 7127–7138. [CrossRef]
73. van Dam, G.M.; Themelis, G.; Crane, L.M.A.; Harlaar, N.J.; Pleijhuis, R.G.; Kelder, W.; Sarantopoulos, A.; de Jong, J.S.; Arts, H.J.G.; van der Zee, A.G.J.; et al. Intraoperative tumor-specific fluorescence imaging in ovarian cancer by folate receptor-α targeting: First in-human results. *Nat. Med.* **2011**, *17*, 1315–1319. [CrossRef]
74. Buxton, R.B.; Alpert, N.M.; Babikian, V.; Weise, S. Evaluation of the 11C02 Positron Emission Tomographic Method for Measuring Brain pH. I. pH Changes Measured in States of Altered Pco2. *J. Cereb. Blood Flow Metab.* **1987**, *7*, 709–719. [CrossRef]
75. Bauwens, M.; De Saint-Hubert, M.; Cleynhens, J.; Brams, L.; Devos, E.; Mottaghy, F.M.; Verbruggen, A. Radioiodinated Phenylalkyl Malonic Acid Derivatives as pH-Sensitive SPECT Tracers. *PLoS ONE* **2012**, *7*, e38428. [CrossRef]
76. Flavell, R.R.; Truillet, C.; Regan, M.K.; Ganguly, T.; Blecha, J.E.; Kurhanewicz, J.; VanBrocklin, H.F.; Keshari, K.R.; Chang, C.J.; Evans, M.J.; et al. Caged [^{18}F]FDG Glycosylamines for Imaging Acidic Tumor Microenvironments Using Positron Emission Tomography. *Bioconjug. Chem.* **2016**, *27*, 170–178. [CrossRef]
77. Chen, L.Q.; Pagel, M.D. Evaluating pH in the Extracellular Tumor Microenvironment Using CEST MRI and Other Imaging Methods. *Adv. Radiol.* **2015**, *2015*, 1–25. [CrossRef]

78. Lindeman, L.R.; Randtke, E.A.; High, R.A.; Jones, K.M.; Howison, C.M.; Pagel, M.D. A comparison of exogenous and endogenous CEST MRI methods for evaluating in vivo pH. *Magn. Reson. Med.* **2018**, *79*, 2766–2772. [CrossRef]
79. Longo, D.L.; Bartoli, A.; Consolino, L.; Bardini, P.; Arena, F.; Schwaiger, M.; Aime, S. In Vivo Imaging of Tumor Metabolism and Acidosis by Combining PET and MRI-CEST pH Imaging. *Cancer Res.* **2016**, *76*, 6463–6470. [CrossRef]
80. Martin, M.G.; Martinez, G.V. High resolution pHe imaging of rat glioma using pH-dependent relaxivity. *Magn. Reson. Med.* **2006**, 309–315. [CrossRef]
81. Kálmán, F.K.; Woods, M.; Caravan, P.; Jurek, P.; Spiller, M.; Tircsó, G.; Király, R.; Brücher, E.; Sherry, A.D. Potentiometric and relaxometric properties of a gadolinium-based MRI contrast agent for sensing tissue pH. *Inorg. Chem.* **2007**, *46*, 5260–5270. [CrossRef]
82. Raghunand, N.; Howison, C.; Sherry, A.D.; Zhang, S.; Gillies, R.J. Renal and systemic pH imaging by contrast-enhanced MRI. *Magn. Reson. Med.* **2003**, *49*, 249–257. [CrossRef]
83. Gillies, R.J.; Liu, Z.; Bhujwalla, Z. ^{31}P-MRS measurements of extracellular pH of tumors using 3-aminopropylphosphonate. *Am. J. Physiol., Cell Physiol.* **1994**, *267*, C195–C203. [CrossRef]
84. McCoy, C.L.; Parkins, C.S.; Chaplin, D.J.; Griffiths, J.R.; Rodrigues, L.M.; Stubbs, M. The Effect of Blood-Flow Modification on Intra- and Extracellular Ph Measured by P-31 Magnetic-Resonance Spectroscopy in Murine Tumors. *Br. J. Cancer* **1995**, *72*, 905–911. [CrossRef]
85. Bhujwalla, Z.M.; McCoy, C.L.; Glickson, J.D.; Gillies, R.J.; Stubbs, M. Estimations of intra- and extracellular volume and pH by P-31 magnetic resonance spectroscopy: Effect of therapy on RIF-1 tumours. *Br. J. Cancer* **1998**, *78*, 606–611. [CrossRef]
86. Garcia-Martin, M.L.; Herigault, G.; Remy, C.; Farion, R.; Ballesteros, P.; Coles, J.A.; Cerdan, S.; Ziegler, A. Mapping extracellular pH in rat brain gliomas in vivo by H-1 magnetic resonance spectroscopic imaging: Comparison with maps of metabolites. *Cancer Res.* **2001**, *61*, 6524–6531.
87. Provent, P.; Benito, M.; Hiba, B.; Farion, R.; Lopez-Larrubia, P.; Ballesteros, P.; Remy, C.; Segebarth, C.; Cerdan, S.; Coles, J.A.; et al. Serial In vivo Spectroscopic Nuclear Magnetic Resonance Imaging of Lactate and Extracellular pH in Rat Gliomas Shows Redistribution of Protons Away from Sites of Glycolysis. *Cancer Res.* **2007**, *67*, 7638–7645. [CrossRef]
88. Pacheco-Torres, J.; Mukherjee, N.; Walko, M.; López-Larrubia, P.; Ballesteros, P.; Cerdán, S.; Kocer, A. Image guided drug release from pH-sensitive Ion channel-functionalized stealth liposomes into an in vivo glioblastoma model. *Nanomedicine* **2015**, *11*, 1345–1354. [CrossRef]
89. Ojugo, A.S.E.; McSheehy, P.M.J.; McIntyre, D.J.O.; McCoy, C.; Stubbs, M.; Leach, M.O.; Judson, I.R.; Griffiths, J.R. Measurement of the extracellular pH of solid tumours in mice by magnetic resonance spectroscopy: A comparison of exogenous19F and31P probes. *NMR Biomed.* **1999**, *12*, 495–504. [CrossRef]
90. Ardenkjaer-Larsen, J.H.; Fridlund, B.; Gram, A.; Hansson, G.; Hansson, L.; Lerche, M.H.; Servin, R.; Thaning, M.; Golman, K. Increase in signal-to-noise ratio of > 10,000 times in liquid-state NMR. *Proc. Natl. Acad. Sci. USA* **2003**, *100*, 10158–10163. [CrossRef]
91. Wilson, D.M.; Keshari, K.R.; Larson, P.E.Z.; Chen, A.P.; Hu, S.; Criekinge, M.V.; Bok, R.; Nelson, S.J.; Macdonald, J.M.; Vigneron, D.B.; et al. Multi-compound polarization by DNP allows simultaneous assessment of multiple enzymatic activities in vivo. *J. Magn. Reson.* **2010**, *205*, 141–147. [CrossRef]
92. Gallagher, F.A.; Kettunen, M.I.; Day, S.E.; Hu, D.-E.; Ardenkjaer-Larsen, J.H.; Zandt, R.I.T.; Jensen, P.R.; Karlsson, M.; Golman, K.; Lerche, M.H.; et al. Magnetic resonance imaging of pH in vivo using hyperpolarized ^{13}C-labelled bicarbonate. *Nature* **2008**, *453*, 940–943. [CrossRef]
93. Korenchan, D.E.; Flavell, R.R.; Baligand, C.; Sriram, R.; Neumann, K.; Sukumar, S.; VanBrocklin, H.; Vigneron, D.B.; Wilson, D.M.; Kurhanewicz, J. Dynamic nuclear polarization of biocompatible ^{13}C-enriched carbonates for in vivo pH imaging. *Chem. Commun.* **2016**, *52*, 3030–3033. [CrossRef]
94. Ghosh, R.K.; Kadlecek, S.J.; Pourfathi, M.; Rizi, R.R. Efficient production of hyperpolarized bicarbonate by chemical reaction on a DNP precursor to measure pH. *Magn. Reson. Med.* **2014**, *74*, 1406–1413. [CrossRef]
95. Drachman, N.; Kadlecek, S.; Pourfathi, M.; Xin, Y.; Profka, H.; Rizi, R. In vivo pH mapping of injured lungs using hyperpolarized [1-^{13}C]pyruvate. *Magn. Reson. Med.* **2016**, *78*, 1121–1130. [CrossRef]
96. Scholz, D.J.; Janich, M.A.; Köllisch, U.; Schulte, R.F.; Ardenkjaer-Larsen, J.H.; Frank, A.; Haase, A.; Schwaiger, M.; Menzel, M.I. Quantified pH imaging with hyperpolarized ^{13}C-bicarbonate. *Magn. Reson. Med.* **2014**, *73*, 2274–2282. [CrossRef]

97. Scholz, D.J.; Otto, A.M.; Hintermair, J.; Schilling, F.; Frank, A.; Köllisch, U.; Janich, M.A.; Schulte, R.F.; Schwaiger, M.; Haase, A.; et al. Parameterization of hyperpolarized ^{13}C-bicarbonate-dissolution dynamic nuclear polarization. *Magn. Reson. Mater. Phys.* **2015**, *28*, 591–598. [CrossRef]
98. Schroeder, M.A.; Swietach, P.; Atherton, H.J.; Gallagher, F.A.; Lee, P.; Radda, G.K.; Clarke, K.; Tyler, D.J. Measuring intracellular pH in the heart using hyperpolarized carbon dioxide and bicarbonate: A ^{13}C and 31P magnetic resonance spectroscopy study. *Cardiovasc. Res.* **2010**, *86*, 82–91. [CrossRef]
99. Lau, A.Z.; Miller, J.J.; Tyler, D.J. Mapping of intracellular pH in the in vivo rodent heart using hyperpolarized [1-^{13}C]pyruvate. *Magn. Reson. Med.* **2017**, *77*, 1810–1817. [CrossRef]
100. Martínez-Santiesteban, F.M.; Dang, T.P.; Lim, H.; Chen, A.P.; Scholl, T.J. T1nuclear magnetic relaxation dispersion of hyperpolarized sodium and cesium hydrogencarbonate-^{13}C. *NMR Biomed.* **2017**, *30*, e3749-8. [CrossRef]
101. Maptue, N.; Jiang, W.; Harrison, C.; Funk, A.M.; Sharma, G.; Malloy, C.R.; Sherry, D.; Khemtong, C. Esterase-Catalyzed Production of Hyperpolarized ^{13}C-Enriched Carbon Dioxide in Tissues for Measuring pH. *ACS Sensors* **2018**, *3*, 2232–2236. [CrossRef]
102. Lau, A.Z.; Chen, A.P.; Cunningham, C.H. Integrated Bloch-Siegert B$_1$ mapping and multislice imaging of hyperpolarized ^{13}C pyruvate and bicarbonate in the heart. *Magn. Reson. Med.* **2012**, *67*, 62–71. [CrossRef]
103. Korenchan, D.E.; Gordon, J.W.; Subramaniam, S.; Sriram, R.; Baligand, C.; VanCriekinge, M.; Bok, R.; Vigneron, D.B.; Wilson, D.M.; Larson, P.E.Z.; et al. Using bidirectional chemical exchange for improved hyperpolarized [13 C]bicarbonate pH imaging. *Magn. Reson. Med.* **2019**, *82*, 959–972. [CrossRef]
104. Flavell, R.R.; von Morze, C.; Blecha, J.E.; Korenchan, D.E.; Van Criekinge, M.; Sriram, R.; Gordon, J.W.; Chen, H.-Y.; Subramaniam, S.; Bok, R.; et al. Application of Good's buffers to pH imaging using hyperpolarized ^{13}C MRI. *Chem. Commun.* **2015**, *51*, 14119–14122. [CrossRef]
105. Korenchan, D.E.; Taglang, C.; von Morze, C.; Blecha, J.E.; Gordon, J.W.; Sriram, R.; Larson, P.E.Z.; Vigneron, D.B.; VanBrocklin, H.F.; Kurhanewicz, J.; et al. Dicarboxylic acids as pH sensors for hyperpolarized (13)C magnetic resonance spectroscopic imaging. *Analyst* **2017**, *142*, 1429–1433. [CrossRef]
106. Düwel, S.; Hundshammer, C.; Gersch, M.; Feuerecker, B.; Steiger, K.; Buck, A.; Walch, A.; Haase, A.; Glaser, S.J.; Schwaiger, M.; et al. Imaging of pH in vivo using hyperpolarized. *Nature* **2017**, *8*, 1–9.
107. Hundshammer, C.; Düwel, S.; Köcher, S.S.; Maltee, G.; Feuerecker, B.; Scheurer, C.; Haase, A.; Glaser, S.J.; Schwaiger, M.; Schilling, F. Deuteration of Hyperpolarized ^{13}C-Labeled Zymonic Acid Enables Sensitivity-Enhanced Dynamic MRI of pH. *ChemPhysChem* **2017**, *18*, 2422–2425. [CrossRef]
108. Hundshammer, C.; Düwel, S.; Ruseckas, D.; Topping, G.; Dzien, P.; Müller, C.; Feuerecker, B.; Hövener, J.B.; Haase, A.; Schwaiger, M.; et al. Hyperpolarized Amino Acid Derivatives as Multivalent Magnetic Resonance pH Sensor Molecules. *Sensors* **2018**, *18*, 600. [CrossRef]
109. Jensen, P.R.; Meier, S. Hyperpolarised organic phosphates as NMR reporters of compartmental pH. *Chem. Commun.* **2016**, *52*, 2288–2291. [CrossRef]
110. Hurd, R.E.; Yen, Y.-F.; Mayer, D.; Chen, A.; Wilson, D.; Kohler, S.; Bok, R.; Vigneron, D.; Kurhanewicz, J.; Tropp, J.; et al. Metabolic imaging in the anesthetized rat brain using hyperpolarized [1-^{13}C] pyruvate and [1-^{13}C] ethyl pyruvate. *Magn. Reson. Med.* **2010**, *63*, 1137–1143. [CrossRef]

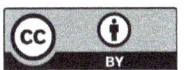

© 2019 by the authors. Licensee MDPI, Basel, Switzerland. This article is an open access article distributed under the terms and conditions of the Creative Commons Attribution (CC BY) license (http://creativecommons.org/licenses/by/4.0/).

MDPI
St. Alban-Anlage 66
4052 Basel
Switzerland
Tel. +41 61 683 77 34
Fax +41 61 302 89 18
www.mdpi.com

Cancers Editorial Office
E-mail: cancers@mdpi.com
www.mdpi.com/journal/cancers

www.ingramcontent.com/pod-product-compliance
Lightning Source LLC
LaVergne TN
LVHW070203100526
838202LV00015B/1991